Surgical Endocrinopathies

Janice L. Pasieka • James A. Lee
Editors

Surgical Endocrinopathies

Clinical Management and the Founding
Figures

Editors
Janice L. Pasieka
Divisions of General Surgery and
Surgical Oncology
Faculty of Medicine, University of Calgary
Calgary
Alberta
Canada

James A. Lee
Department of Surgery
Columbia University Medical Center
New York
New York
USA

ISBN 978-3-319-13661-5   ISBN 978-3-319-13662-2 (eBook)
DOI 10.1007/978-3-319-13662-2

Library of Congress Control Number: 2015935936

Springer Cham Heidelberg New York Dordrecht London
© Springer International Publishing Switzerland 2015

Printed on acid-free paper

Springer is part of Springer Science+Business Media (www.springer.com)

To my father ARP, a 'founding figure' in my life. I miss you dad.

JP

Dedicated to Gretchen, Elizabeth, and Matthew—My unending source of joy and inspiration.

JL

Foreword

Endocrine surgery is both an exciting and satisfying area to work in, with outcomes meeting patient and surgeon expectations to a high level.

Fifty years ago, the volume of endocrine surgical work in most hospitals was not sufficient to allow full endocrine specialization for all but a few select surgeons, with the majority of clinical surgical activity being centered around the thyroid gland. Endocrine surgery had become much safer, but there were still surgeons who performed the occasional thyroidectomy and who did not maintain acquaintance with the advancing clinical science or technical surgical improvement. The outcomes in such cases were not necessarily ideal. This situation needed to be addressed.

Change has occurred; sound governance is now maintained through international and national organizations of endocrine surgeons. These organizations have been the drivers of progress and the catalyst for clinical cooperation and friendships. There is now provision of regular scientific meetings, support for research, clinical and research exchange, and clinical and research fellowships. In each of these areas there are good levels of success. This is readily seen from the free flow of clinical and research papers at scientific meetings with these research papers providing evidence of the overall work patterns and outcomes, the volume of cases and the quality of endocrine surgical units around the world.

The increasing volume of activity has presaged the need for collation of publications for ready access and review and for reference purposes.

Most trainees and their mentors are familiar with the range of publications in each endocrine system, together with newer methods of surgical access, pathology, genetic, biochemical, and imaging requirements and also with the advances in multiple endocrine neoplasia and its ancillary demands. This is an overall satisfactory situation.

There are however some reservations about the knowledge of some younger surgeons who are mentors and faculty members and their trainees about the Founding Figures of Endocrine Surgery. Some seem to have forgotten, overlooked, or plainly never learned about those observant doctors of yesteryear and overlooked, on occasions, those who have more recently brought their contemporary observations to all of us interested in improving the understanding of endocrine diseases and endocrine surgery. All of these founding figures and current leaders have provided clear information on their areas of interest, have taken classical histories of patients, recorded and reported fully on their observational and clinical findings and given strong outlines of their self-propelled clinical research. Even if recorded over a hundred years ago, such information can today mobilize a clinician's focus and guide confirmation of a sound working diagnosis. This was particularly true of the work of Graves and von Basedow, where research continues to unlock the underlying cause of the diseases that for many years have carried their names.

It is to be expected that the efforts made by Dr. Janice Pasieka and her co-editor Dr. James Lee and their illustrious cast of authors and biographers in compiling their textbook "Surgical

Endocrinopathies: Clinical Management and the Founding Figures" clinical and research material that can rekindle interest in the Founding Figures of endocrine surgery and perhaps open new windows that light the way for new research and further advancement of endocrine surgery.

A space awaits for this publication on my bedside table, where my favored books are available to be read to provide me with knowledge, enjoyment, and comfort.

Tom Reeve
Emeritus Professor of Surgery
The University Sydney

Foreword

As an endocrinologist with a long interest in endocrine surgery (and endocrine surgeons), it is with great pleasure that I write this foreword for a truly unique and outstanding endocrine surgery text. While I fully expected the in-depth and outstanding coverage of the wide range of medical and surgical issues associated with endocrine disease, I was completely surprised and delighted with the historical details provided in the chapters on the founding figures that have defined and shaped our current management approaches. While we often provide one or two brief sentences about these famous clinicians/scientists in our reviews, none of our standard textbooks provide this level of detail with regard to the historical background, their families, their colleagues and their patients that so significantly impacted their observations and discoveries. It is amazing to see how often their major discoveries (for which they are so well remembered today) went against the prevailing management paradigms of the time. These historical accounts also vividly remind us that success seldom came easily or quickly to these founding figures. More commonly, their discoveries and observations were the product of prolonged periods of work, often in the face of significant opposition by peers who were reluctant to embrace new findings. This should serve as a note of great encouragement to those of us trying to change one or more of the long-held endocrine beliefs!

So, it is with great pleasure that I can highly recommend "Surgical Endocrinopathies: Clinical Management and the Founding Figures" as required reading for all clinicians (surgeons and endocrinologist alike) who care for patients with endocrine diseases. All critical aspects of diagnosis and management are carefully described in the scientific chapters. But even more importantly, the in-depth historical reviews remind us of where we have been and how difficult it was to get where we are. Furthermore, the insights provided by biographies should stimulate us to continue to question our current treatment approaches, develop novel research questions, and live up to the wonderful endocrine legacy that has been provided to us by this amazing cast of characters. It is only through continued learning, research, and hard work that we can hope to provide the best possible care to our patients with endocrine disorders.

Dr. Janice Pasieka and Dr. James Lee are to be congratulated on assembling a remarkable cohort of authors and organizing one of the most unique textbooks on endocrine disease that I have ever seen. I have no doubt that many of the facts about these founding giants will find their way into my future lectures and papers.

While most of my textbooks remain on the shelf in my office, this one will likely stay on my coffee table at home: where I can read the historical vignettes for pleasure at my leisure and reflect on the clinicians and scientists that have laid the groundwork for our current understanding of endocrine diseases.

R. Michael Tuttle, MDEndocrinology Service
Memorial Sloan Kettering Cancer Center
New York, NY

Preface

The concept for this book started at the scrub sink…

Surgeon: How does one make the diagnosis of an insulinoma?

Junior resident: Well, one starts with a good history and physical exam followed by demonstrating Whipple's Triad during a prolonged fast.

Surgeon: Excellent. Who was Whipple?

Junior resident: Pardon me?

Surgeon: Tell me about Allen Whipple and when did he describe Whipple's Triad?

(*Silence*)

Senior resident: I guess he was a surgeon, you know, the one who invented the Whipple procedure.

Surgeon: Yes, he was a surgeon. When do you think he developed the triad?

(*More silence and vigorous scrubbing*)

Senior resident: Uh, I would be guessing but was it in the early 1800s?

Surgeon: Hmm, wouldn't you agree that it is unlikely he described the triad before the discovery of insulin?

Residents: Yes, that makes sense.

Surgeon: So, when was insulin discovered?

(*More vigorous scrubbing and rinsing*)

Medical student: I know. It was a long time ago, in the early 1960s.

Surgeon: The 1960s, long time ago?? *(gulp)* You mean when the Beatles became famous?

Medical student: The Who?

Surgeon: *(Sigh)* Yes, them too…

And so it goes. With each new generation, the knowledge of our founding figures, those astute clinicians that unearthed the bedrock of clinical endocrinology, gradually erodes. Their names have morphed into eponyms without any sense of the history behind their discoveries. Who were the people behind the names? What spark of intuition led them to their revelations? This textbook is meant to bring to light the giants on whose shoulders we stand. Following each clinical chapter several figures who played a prominent role in the diseases discussed are highlighted. Of course, the limitations of time and space preclude including all of the founding figures whose contributions guide us to this day. For that we apologize, but do not let them become mere eponyms and make a point of sharing their stories next time you stand at the scrub sink or on the ward rounding with the team.

We hope you will relish reading about our shared history as much as we have enjoyed compiling it.

Janice L. Pasieka
James A. Lee

Contents

Contributors

Peter Angelos Endocrine Surgery Research Program, Department of Surgery, University of Chicago Pritzker School of Medicine, Chicago, IL, USA

Yasmine Assadipour Surgical Oncology, National Cancer Institute, National Institutes of Health, Bethesda, MD, USA

Courtney J. Balentine Chief of Endocrine Surgery, University of Wisconsin, Madison, WI, USA

Elpidio Manuel Barajas-Fregoso Endocrine Surgery, Department of Surgery, Instituto Nacional de Ciencias Medicas y Nutricion "Salvador Zubiran", Mexico D.F., Mexico

Jean M. Butte Hepato-Pancreato-Biliary, Foothills Medical Centre, University of Calgary, Calgary, AB, Canada

Angela L. Carrelli Department of Medicine, Columbia University College of Physicians & Surgeons, New York, NY, USA

Sally E. Carty Division of Endocrine Surgery, University of Pittsburgh, Pittbsurgh, PA, USA

Anthony J. Chambers Department of Surgical Oncology, St. Vincent's Hospital and University of New South Wales, Darlinghurst, NSW, Australia

Herbert Chen Division of General Surgery, K3-705 Clinical Science Center, University of Wisconsin, Madison, WI, USA

Orlo Clark Department of Surgery, University of California San Francisco Medical Center, San Francisco, CA, USA

Leigh W. Delbridge Surgery, University of Sydney, Sydney, NSW, Australia

Michael J. Demeure Integrated Cancer Genomics, Translational Genomics Research Institute, Phoenix, AZ, USA

Elijah Dixon Division of General Surgery, Faculty of Medicine, University of Calgary, EG - 26, Foothills Medical Centre, Calgary, AB, Canada

Kimlynn B. Do Brigham and Women's Hospital, Westminster, CA, USA

Gerard M. Doherty Department of Surgery, Boston University, Boston, MA, USA

Nancy Dugal Perrier Surgical Oncology, MD Anderson Cancer Center, The University of Texas, Houston, TX, USA

Quan-Yang Duh Department of Surgery, Section of Endocrine Surgery, University of California, San Francisco, CA, USA

Surgical Service, VA Medical Center, San Francisco, CA, USA

William S. Duke Department of Otolaryngology-Head and Neck Surgery, GRU Thyroid and Parathyroid Center, Georgia Regents University, Augusta, GA, USA

Benzon M. Dy Endocrine Surgery, Mayo Clinic, Rochester, MN, USA

Konstantinos P. Economopoulos Department of Surgery, Massachusetts General Hospital, Boston, MA, USA

Dawn M. Elfenbein Department of Surgery, University of Wisconsin, Madison, WI, USA

Thomas J. Fahey Division of Endocrine Surgery, General Surgery, New York Presbyterian/ Weill Cornell Medical Center, New York, NY, USA

Josefina C. Farra Department of Surgery, University of Miami Miller School of Medicine, Miami, FL, USA

Jessica Furst Endocrinology, Department of Medicine, Columbia University Medical Center, New York, NY, USA

Paul G. Gauger Surgery, University of Michigan, Ann Arbor, MI, USA

Jason A. Glenn Department of Surgery, Division of Surgical Oncology, Medical College of Wisconsin, Milwaukee, WI,, USA

Clive S. Grant Department of Surgery, Mayo Clinic, Rochester, MN, USA

Raymon H. Grogan Department of Surgery, The University of Chicago Pritzker School of Medicine, Chicago, IL, USA

Philip I. Haigh Department of Surgery, Kaiser Permanente Los Angeles Medical Center, Los Angeles, CA, USA

David A. Hanley Medicine, Oncology and Community Health Sciences, Division of Endocrinology and Metabolism, University of Calgary, Calgary, AB, Canada

Adrian Harvey Department of Surgery, Surgery and Oncology, Foothills Medical Center, University of Calgary, Calgary, AB, Canada

Ian D. Hay Endocrine Research, Division of Endocrinology, Metabolism, Nutrition and Internal Medicine, Mayo Clinic College of Medicine, Rochester, MN, USA

Jon A. van Heerden General Surgery, Medical University of South Carolina, Charleston, SC, USA

Per Hellman Department of Surgery, University Hospital, Uppsala, Sweden

Miguel F. Herrera Endocrine Surgery, Department of Surgery, Instituto Nacional de Ciencias Medicas y Nutricion "Salvador Zubiran", Mexico D.F., Mexico

Marybeth S. Hughes Director of the Surgical Oncology Research Fellowship, Thoracic and Gastrointestinal Oncology Branch, Center for Cancer Research, National Cancer Institute, National Institutes of Health, Bethesda, MD, USA

William B. Inabnet III Department of Surgery, Division of Metabolic, Endocrine and MIS, Surgical Sciences, Metabolism Institute, Mount Sinai Medical Center, New York, NY, USA

Benjamin C. James Chairman, Department of Surgery, The University of Chicago Pritzker School of Medicine, Chicago, IL, USA

Michael G. Johnston General Surgery, Uniformed Services University of the Health Sciences, Portsmouth, VA, USA

Edwin L. Kaplan Endocrine Surgery, Section of General Surgery, The University of Chicago Pritzker School of Medicine, Chicago, IL, USA

Electron Kebebew Endocrine Oncology Branch, National Institutes of Health-National Cancer Institute, Bethesda, MD, USA

Gregory A. Kline Department of Medicine, Endocrinology, University of Calgary, Calgary, AB, Canada

Jennifer H. Kuo Surgery Department, New York Presbyterian Hospital, Columbia University Medical Center, New York, NY, USA

Salila Kurra Department of Medicine, Columbia University Medical Center, New York, NY, USA

Grace S. Lee Department of Surgery, Mayo Clinic, Rochester, MN, USA

James A. Lee Associate Professor, Department of Surgery, Columbia University Medical Center, New York, NY, USA

Jane S. Lee Surgery, Mount Sinai Hospital, New York, NY, USA

Thomas W. J. Lennard Surgery, Clinical Academic Office, Newcastle University, Newcastle, Tyne and Wear, UK

Steven K. Libutti Surgery and Genetics, Albert Einstein College of Medicine, Broonx, USA

Department of Surgery, Montefiore Einstein Center for Cancer Care, Montefiore Medical Center, Broonx, NY, USA

Carrie C. Lubitz Department of Surgery, Harvard Medical School, Massachusetts General Hospital, Boston, MA, USA

Peter J. Mazzaglia Rhode Island Hospital, Warren Alpert School of Medicine, Brown University, Providence, RI, USA

Kelly L. McCoy Division of Endocrine Surgery, University of Pittsburgh, Pittbsurgh, PA, USA

Christopher R. McHenry Department of Surgery, MetroHealth Medical Center, Cleveland, OH, USA

Catherine McManus Department of Surgery, New York Presbyterian Hospital Columbia Campus, New York, NY, USA

Jacob Moalem Endocrine Surgery and Endocrinology, Surgery Department, University of Rochester, Rochester, NY, USA

Maureen Daly Moore General Surgery, New York Hospital Weill-Cornell Medical Center, New York, NY, USA

Sapna Nagar Department of Surgery, University of Chicago, Pritzker School of Medicine, Chicago, IL, USA

Vladimir Neychev Endocrine Oncology Branch, National Institutes of Health-National Cancer Institute, Bethesda, MD, USA

Naris Nilubol Endocrine Oncology Branch, National Cancer Institute, The National Institutes of Health, Bethesda, MD, USA

Sareh Parangi Department of Surgery, Harvard Medical School, Massachusetts General Hospital, Boston, MA, USA

Janice L. Pasieka Divisions of General Surgery and Surgical Oncology, Faculty of Medicine, University of Calgary, Calgary, AB, Canada

Latha V. Pasupuleti Surgery Department, New York Presbyterian Hospital, Columbia University Medical Center, New York, NY, USA

Kepal N. Patel Division of Endocrine Surgery, Surgery, Otoloaryngology and Biochemistry, NYU Langone Medical Center, New York, NY, USA

Adriana G. Ramirez Department of Surgery, University of Virginia, Charlottesville, VA, USA

Melanie L. Richards Department of Surgery, Mayo Clinic, Rochester, MN, USA

Kevin Ro Section of Endocrine Surgery, UCLA David Geffen School of Medicine, Los Angeles, CA, USA

Steven E. Rodgers Department of Surgery, University of Miami Miller School of Medicine, Miami, FL, USA

Minerva Angélica Romero Arenas Surgery, Sinai Hospital of Baltimore, Baltimore, MD, USA

Daniel T. Ruan General and GI Surgery, Endocrine Surgery, Brigham and Women's Hospital, Harvard Medical School, Boston, MA, USA

Endocrine Surgery, Harvard Medical School, Boston, MA, USA

Jonathan W. Serpell Monash University Endocrine Surgery Unit, Alfred Hospital, Melbourne, Vic, Australia

Wen T. Shen Department of Surgery, UCSF/ Mt. Zion Medical Center, University of California, San Francisco, CA, USA

Shonni J. Silverberg Department of Medicine, Columbia University College of Physicians & Surgeons, New York, NY, USA

Rebecca S. Sippel Chief of Endocrine Surgery, University of Wisconsin, Madison, WI, USA

Robert C. Smallridge Division of Endocrinology & Metabolism, Mayo Clinic, Jacksonville, FL, USA

Philip W. Smith Department of Surgery, University of Virginia, Charlottesville, VA, USA

Meredith J. Sorensen General Surgery, Dartmouth Hitchcock Medical Center, Lebanon, NH, USA

Julie Ann Sosa Department of Surgery, Section of Endocrine Surgery, Surgery and Medicine (Oncology), Endocrine Neoplasia Diseases Group, Duke Cancer Institute, Durham, NC, USA

Cord Sturgeon Endocrine Surgery, Northwestern University, Chicago, IL, USA

Sonia L. Sugg Department of Surgery, Division of Surgical Oncology and Endocrine Surgery, University of Iowa Carver College of Medicine, Iowa City, IA, USA

Mark Sywak Endocrine Surgical Unit, University of Sydney, St. Leonards, NSW, Australia

David J. Terris Otolaryngology-Head and Neck Surgery, Georgia Regents University, Augusta, GA, USA

Geoffrey B. Thompson Surgery, College of Medicine, Mayo Clinic, Rochester, MN, USA

Scott M. Thompson Medical Scientist Training Program, College of Medicine, Mayo Clinic, Rochester, MN, USA

Robert Udelsman Surgery & Oncology, Yale-New Haven Hospital, Yale University School of Medicine, New Haven, CT, USA

Jon A. van Heerden General Surgery, Medical University of South Carolina, Charleston, SC, USA

Kuan-Chi Wang Endocrine Surgical Unit, University of Sydney, St. Leonards, NSW, Australia

Tracy S. Wang Division of Surgical Oncology, Section of Endocrine Surgery, Medical College of Wisconsin, Milwaukee, WI, USA

Scott M. Wilhelm Surgery Department, Case Medical Center, University Hospitals, Cleveland, OH, USA

Stuart D. Wilson Division of Surgical Oncology, Department of Surgery, Froedtert Hospital/Medical College of Milwaukee, Milwaukee, WI, USA

Mathias Worni General Surgery, Division of Surgical Oncology, Duke University Medical Center, Durham, NC, USA

James X. Wu Section of Endocrine Surgery, UCLA David Geffen School of Medicine, Los Angeles, CA, USA

Michael W. Yeh Section of Endocrine Surgery, UCLA David Geffen School of Medicine, Los Angeles, CA, USA

Tina W.F. Yen Department of Surgery, Medical College of Wisconsin, Milwaukee, WI, USA

Linwah Yip Division of Endocrine Surgery and Surgical Oncology, Department of Surgery, University of Pittsburgh, Pittsburgh, PA, USA

William F. Young Division of Endocrinology, Diabetes, Metabolism, and Nutrition, Mayo Clinic College of Medicine, Rochester, MN, USA

Hannah Y. Zhou Department of Surgery, University Hospitals Case Medical Center, Cleveland, OH, USA

Part I
The Thyroid Gland

Thyroid Physiology

Meredith J. Sorensen and Paul G. Gauger

Produced by the thyroid gland and precisely regulated both centrally and peripherally, thyroid hormone (TH) is essential for normal development and metabolism in all vertebrates. Appearing around embryonic day 22 in humans, the thyroid gland is the first endocrine organ to develop, and circulating endogenous fetal TH is detectable by 11–13 weeks of gestation [2]. TH equilibrium in the fetus, which is maintained by a combination of endogenously produced hormone and maternal TH, is necessary for normal growth and development and is especially crucial for neural differentiation [1–3]. Although some of the most profound effects of TH are observed during development, it regulates metabolism and influences the function of nearly every organ system throughout all stages of life [1, 4, 5].

Thyroid Gland Anatomy and Histology

A basic knowledge of the cellular and microscopic structure of the thyroid gland is necessary to understand the physiology of TH synthesis. Two types of cells comprise the mature thyroid gland: follicular cells (which originate from the embryonic endoderm) and parafollicular cells, also called C cells (which originate from embryonic ectoderm and migrate into the thyroid gland during its development) [2, 4]. Follicular cells, arranged in a single layer, form the walls of spherical thyroid follicles. These follicles are filled with colloid, a proteinaceous substance primarily composed of thyroglobulin, which is a glycoprotein dimer essential for both the synthesis and storage of TH [4] (Fig. 1). The C cells produce calcitonin, which works together with parathyroid

hormone (PTH) and vitamin D to maintain serum calcium homeostasis, although calcitonin's direct impact on calcium levels is minimal in higher mammals [4].

Thyroid Hormone Synthesis

The thyroid gland produces two main types of TH: thyroxine (T4) and triiodothyronine (T3). They share a nearly identical molecular structure—phenolic rings joined by an ether link and iodinated at either three (T3) or four (T4) positions (Fig. 2). Since only T3 is biologically active, T4 is considered a prohormone and requires conversion to T3 in the peripheral tissues [2]. Both types of TH are synthesized in the follicular cells, a process that involves concentration of iodine, organification and coupling, and, finally, secretion or storage [2, 4] (Fig. 3).

Iodine Metabolism

Only 7 years after the discovery of iodine in 1812, Coindet published a description of the element being used for the treatment of goiter [6, 7]. Throughout the nineteenth century, observational evidence mounted connecting iodine deficiency to goiter, cretinism, and myxedema, but the presence of iodine in the thyroid gland was not formally demonstrated until 1896, and TH was not isolated until 1919—exactly 100 years after Coindet's publication [7].

Iodine's role as a key ingredient for TH synthesis (it accounts for 65% of the molecular weight of T4 and 59% of T3) is now well understood [8]. Iodine is an essential micronutrient that can be acquired only via dietary sources [6, 8, 9]. It circulates in the bloodstream in its ionized form, iodide (I−). Since up to 90% of ingested iodine is excreted in the urine, the thyroid evolved a very efficient mechanism to "trap" and concentrate iodide [6, 10, 11]. In order to provide the adult thyroid with the 60 µg of I− per day required to synthesize normal amounts of TH, the recommended daily in-

M. J. Sorensen (✉)
General Surgery, Dartmouth Hitchcock Medical Center, Lebanon, NH 03756, USA
e-mail: Meredith.J.Sorensen@hitchcock.org

P. G. Gauger
Surgery, University of Michigan, Ann Arbor, MI 48109, USA

J. L. Pasieka, J. A. Lee (eds.), *Surgical Endocrinopathies,* DOI 10.1007/978-3-319-13662-2_1,
© Springer International Publishing Switzerland 2015

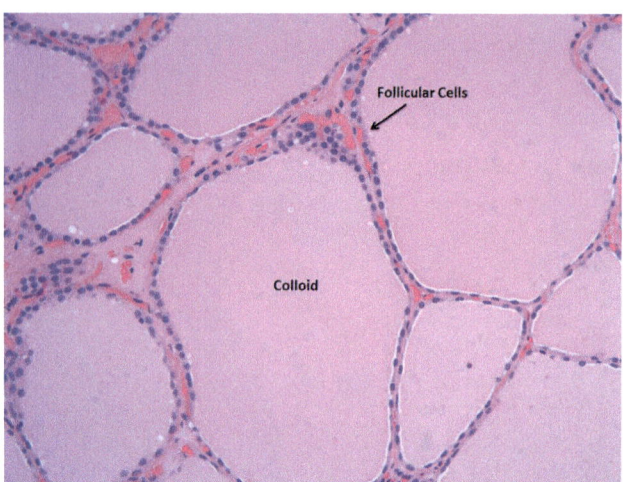

Fig. 1 Histological section of normal thyroid, magnified 20×. Each colloid-filled follicle is surrounded by a single layer of thyroid follicular cells

take of iodine is 150 μg [6, 9, 12]. Under normal physiologic conditions, the thyroid contains more than 90 % of the total body iodide, with an I− concentration 20–40 times higher than that of serum [13].

The mechanism for the gland's ability to accumulate I− against its concentration gradient was a subject of considerable research and debate until the cloning of the Na^+/I− symporter (NIS) in 1996 [6, 14]. Located at the basolateral plasma membrane of the follicular cells, the NIS has 13 transmembrane segments [6, 15]. It uses the inwardly directed Na^+ gradient generated by the Na^+/K^+ ATPase to couple movement of Na^+ and I− from the blood to the follicular cell cytoplasm. Two Na^+ ions enter for every I−, and this 2:1 stoichiometry generates a positively charged inward current [6, 15]. Activity of the NIS and uptake of iodide are regulated by thyroid-stimulating hormone (TSH) and by iodide itself [15].

Once I− is inside the follicular cell, the electrochemical gradient drives it to the apical surface of the cell. The mechanism of the efflux of I− from the cell cytoplasm into the follicular lumen is less well defined [13, 16]. Another transmembrane protein, pendrin, is thought to play a role in apical iodide transport. This anion exchanger is mutated in Pendred's syndrome, leading to a partial defect in organification of iodide. The syndrome is characterized by hereditary sensorineural deafness and occasionally euthyroid goiter [6, 13, 15, 16]. However, the fact that Pendred's syndrome patients living in iodine-replete regions do not tend to develop goiter, combined with the findings that pendrin knockout mice have normal thyroid size and function, suggests that other routes for I− efflux exist as well [6, 13, 16]. Several anion transporters and channels known to transport chloride, including the Cl^-/H^+ antiporter (CLC-5), the sodium-monocarboxylic acid transporter (SMCT1), and the cystic fibrosis transmembrane conductance regulator (CFTR), have been proposed as alternate candidates to mediate the translocation of I− to the follicular lumen [6, 16].

Before it can be incorporated into the tyrosine residues on thyroglobulin, I− must be oxidized [2, 13]. This process is catalyzed by the enzyme thyroperoxidase (TPO) and requires the presence of hydrogen peroxide (H_2O_2) [8, 13]. A multispanning membrane protein called dual oxidase 2 (Duox2), a calcium-dependent nicotinamide adenine dinucleotide phosphate (NADPH) oxidase, plays a key role in generating the necessary H_2O_2 on the luminal surface of the apical follicular cell membrane [6, 13]. Although the substrates and catalyst for this reaction are well understood, the exact nature of the oxidized iodinating species is still not known [17, 18]. Several models have been proposed, including hypoiodite (OI−), hypoiodous acid (HOI), or iodonium (I^+) [13, 18].

Thyroglobulin

Synthesized in the follicular cells, thyroglobulin is the most highly expressed protein in the thyroid gland [19]. With a dimeric molecular mass of 660 kDa, it is one of the largest proteins in the human body, and it consists of a signal peptide sequence and approximately 2750 amino acid residues [19, 20]. The protein has a homogeneous structure in all verte-

Fig. 2 The molecular structures of thyroxine (*T4*) and triiodothyronine (*T3*)

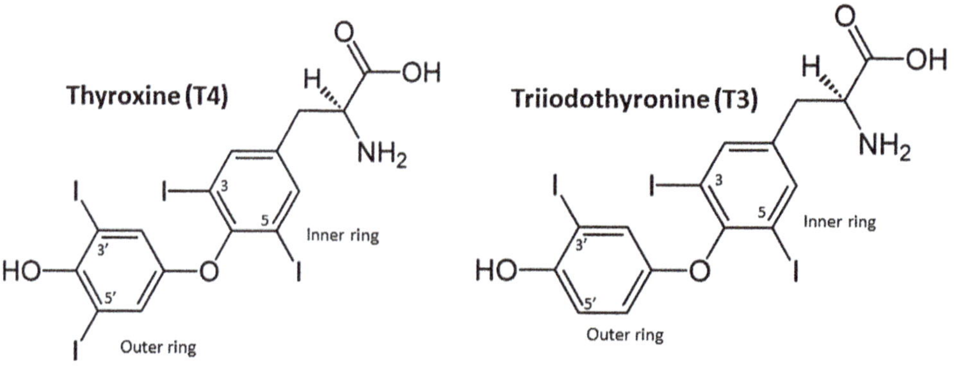

Thyroxine (T4)

Triiodothyronine (T3)

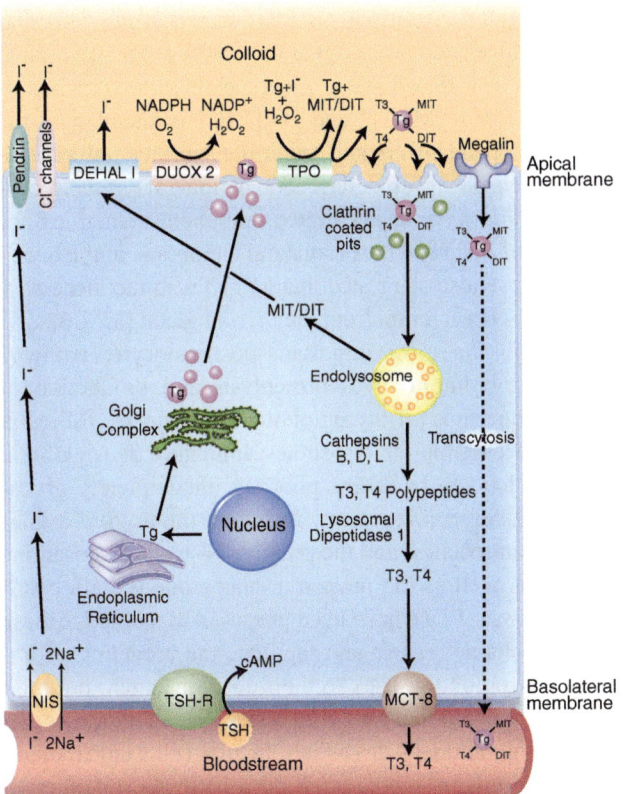

Fig. 3 The synthesis and secretion of thyroid hormone by the thyroid follicular cell. Thyroid hormone synthesis is stimulated by binding of TSH to the TSHR, which increases intracellular cAMP. Iodide enters the thyroid gland via the Na$^+$/I$^-$ symporter (*NIS*). The intracellular electrochemical gradient then drives I$-$ to the apical surface of the cell, where it exits into the follicular lumen either through pendrin or chloride channels or both. The I$-$ is then oxidized by the enzyme thyroperoxidase (*TPO*) in the presence of hydrogen peroxide (H$_2$O$_2$), which is generated by dual oxidase 2 (Duox2), an NADPH oxidase. Oxidized iodide attaches to tyrosyl residues of thyroglobulin to form monoiodotyrosine (*MIT*) or diiodotyrosine (*DIT*) residues, a process also catalyzed by TPO. MIT and DIT then combine to form T3 and T4, all still incorporated within the thyroglobulin molecule. Iodinated thyroglobulin is then taken up by clathrin-coated pits on the apical surface of the follicular cell, which invaginate to form intracellular vesicles. These fuse with the endolysosomal system. MIT, DIT, T4, and T3 residues are selectively removed from the molecule. MIT and DIT residues are deiodinated by DEHAL1 and the iodide is recycled. The T3- and T4-containing polypeptides are further processed to become free T3 and T4, which are then released into the circulation via a hormone transporter, MCT8. A small proportion of iodinated thyroglobulin binds to a protein called megalin before being internalized by the thyrocyte and is transported through the cell before being released intact into the bloodstream. This process is called transcytosis. *TSH* thyroid-stimulating hormone, *TSHR* thyroid-stimulating hormone receptor, *NADPH* nicotinamide adenine dinucleotide phosphate, *MCT* monocarboxylate transporter

brates, consisting of four distinct regions: three cysteine-rich repetitive domains (Tg1, Tg2, and Tg3) and the cholinesterase-like (ChEL) domain (C-terminus of the molecule), which is highly homologous to acetylcholine [19, 21, 22]. Production of thyroglobulin is regulated by TSH and several transcription factors, including thyroid transcription factor 1 (TTF-1), TTF-2, and paired box gene 8 (Pax-8) [19]. As the nascent thyroglobulin polypeptide chains emerge from the polyribosomes, they enter the cytosolic side of the endoplasmic reticulum, where each region undergoes an independent oxidative folding process [19, 22, 23]. All the cysteine residues ultimately become incorporated into disulfide bonds, although the number of intra/interchain bonds creates significant potential for errant folding [22, 23]. Thyroglobulin molecules also undergo glycosylation and dimerization [19, 21]. Several molecular chaperones, including BiP, GRP94, GRP170, ERp29, ERp72, and calnexin, are involved in the maturation of thyroglobulin and act as intracellular quality control to ensure that only properly folded and glycosylated thyroglobulin molecules are ultimately released [8, 19, 20]. The process is relatively lengthy, with a half-time of 90–120 min for newly synthesized thyroglobulin to arrive at the Golgi complex [22]. There it is incorporated into exocytic vesicles that migrate to the apical membrane of the follicular cell, where the organification and coupling process takes place [8, 19].

Organification and Coupling

Although organification and coupling are often discussed as discrete steps, both reactions are catalyzed by TPO and in fact occur simultaneously [13]. The process by which oxidized iodide attaches to tyrosyl residues of thyroglobulin is referred to as organification. The reaction leads to the formation of monoiodotyrosine (MIT) or diiodotyrosine (DIT) residues, still located within the thyroglobulin molecule [8, 13]. Of the 132–140 tyrosyl residues in each molecule of dimerized human thyroglobulin (the reported number varies because of refinements in complementary DNA (cDNA) sequencing), only a small subset are actually susceptible to iodination [8, 13, 21, 24]. While each molecule of mature thyroglobulin contains 5–50 iodine atoms, only certain iodinated sites are ultimately involved in hormonogenesis because of their spatial orientation [8, 13].

Once MIT and DIT form, the coupling reaction occurs: two DIT residues combine to form T4 or one MIT combines with one DIT to create T3 [8, 13]. In this reaction, also catalyzed by TPO and mediated by H$_2$O$_2$, the iodinated phenyl group of a tyrosyl residue is donated to become the outer ring of the iodothyronine acceptor site [13]. Tyrosines 5, 2554, and 2747 are the most important acceptor sites, while tyrosines 130, 847, and 1448 are the dominant donors [13, 24]. About one-third of T4 is created by the acceptor–donor pair of tyrosine 5 and tyrosine 130 [8]. After the coupling reaction, the newly formed T3 and T4 are still incorporated within the thyroglobulin molecule [8]. Under normal conditions (normal iodine supply and normal thyroid function), the average thyroglobulin molecule contains 2.5 residues of T4 residues, 0.7 of T3, 4.5 of DIT, and 5 of MIT [8].

Secretion and Storage

Once organification and coupling are complete, the mature, iodinated thyroglobulin is released into the follicular lumen, where it comprises more than 95 % of the colloid [8, 25]. About two-thirds of thyroglobulin in the colloid is in the soluble 660 kDa dimerized form, but free monomers and tetramers are also found in minimal amounts [8, 25]. The other 34 % of thyroglobulin exists in a dense, highly concentrated insoluble form (i-Tg), with high iodine content but nearly undetectable TH residues [8, 11, 25].

When follicular cells are stimulated by TSH, thyroglobulin is mobilized from the colloid and reenters the thyrocyte via a process called micropinocytosis. Because of their physical proximity to the apical membrane and solubility, newly secreted thyroglobulin molecules are taken up first (the "last-come-first-served" principle first described by Schneider et al. in 1964) [11, 25, 26]. Clathrin-coated pits form on the luminal side of the apical membrane of thyrocytes and internalize thyroglobulin. These pits then invaginate to form intracellular vesicles, which shed their clathrin coats and quickly fuse with early endosomes [8, 25, 27]. This process is thought to occur via a combination of nonspecific fluid-phase uptake (which likely is the main route of thyroglobulin uptake leading to degradation and TH release) and receptor-mediated uptake (which appears to lead to other post-endocytic pathways) [8, 25, 28].

The intracellular thyroglobulin molecules then follow one of at least three different pathways: proteolytic destruction into its component parts, recycling back to the follicular lumen, or transcytosis [8, 25, 28]. In the first pathway, thyroglobulin travels through the endosomal system to lysosomes, where MIT, DIT, T4, and T3 residues are selectively removed from the molecule [8, 29]. Free MIT and DIT residues released from lysosomes cannot combine to synthesize hormone; rather, they are deiodinated to produce I− and tyrosine, both of which are then reused for novel thyroglobulin synthesis and organification. The enzyme primarily responsible for this iodide recycling process is iodotyrosine dehalogenase 1 (DEHAL 1), an NADPH-dependent transmembrane protein located at the apical membrane of follicular cells [30, 31]. Finally, cathepsins D, B, and L, which are lysosomal proteases, act at specific cleavage sites on thyroglobulin to produce hormone-enriched polypeptides. These are then further hydrolyzed by exopeptidases (most importantly lysosomal dipeptidase I) to release free TH into the cytoplasm [32–34].

Conventionally, the secretion of TH into the bloodstream has been attributed to passive diffusion, but more recent evidence supports a transport system located at the follicular cell basolateral membrane. Over the past few decades, transmembrane TH transporters, most notably monocarboxylate transporter 8 (MCT8) and OATP1C1 (a member of the sodium-independent organic anion-transporting polypeptide family), have been well described in peripheral tissue. Recent animal studies have demonstrated immunohistochemical localization of MCT8 to the basolateral membrane of the thyrocyte and have also suggested that MCT8 is in fact necessary for normal TH secretion from the thyroid gland [35, 36].

Although the most important post-endocytic pathway for thyroglobulin involves proteolysis and production of free hormone, not all thyroglobulin taken up by follicular cells is processed in the lysosomes. Immature thyroglobulin molecules tend to be iodine poor and incompletely glycosylated [8]. Several receptors, including the thyroid asialoglycoprotein receptor and the putative N-acetylglucosamine receptor, as well as the molecular chaperone protein disulfide isomerase (PDI), have been proposed to recognize these immature characteristics and facilitate the recycling of immature thyroglobulin back to the follicular lumen, but their exact roles remain unclear [8, 25]. Megalin, another receptor found on the luminal side of the follicular cell's apical membrane, is known to mediate the third pathway for internalized thyroglobulin called transcytosis. Thyroglobulin that binds to megalin before being internalized by the thyrocyte escapes the lysosomal pathway and instead is transported intact to the basolateral membrane with subsequent release into the bloodstream [37, 38]. With normal TSH stimulation, the expression of megalin is relatively low and very little thyroglobulin is transcytosed. When TSH is elevated, however, megalin expression increases, leading to significantly greater amounts of transcytosis. By diverting thyroglobulin from lysosomal proteolysis, this may serve to reduce free hormone release under conditions of massive TSH stimulation [25, 38].

Peripheral Actions of Thyroid Hormone

Under normal circumstances, 90 % of the hormone secreted by the thyroid gland is in the form of T4 and the other 10 % is T3 [2]. Only a very small fraction of the released TH (about 0.03 % of total T4 and 0.3 % of total T3) circulates as free hormone [39]. The rest of the released TH binds to carrier proteins, with 95 % bound to either thyroid-binding globulin (TBG), transthyretin (TTR), or albumin. The remaining 4–5 % is bound to other minor TH carriers, including lipoproteins, immunoglobulins, and lipocalins [39, 40]. These carrier proteins serve both as a stable reservoir of extrathyroidal TH and as protection for the extremely hydrophobic free hormone from its aqueous environment [2, 39, 40]. Because of this method of distribution and buffering, T4 has the longest half-life of any hormone (6–7 days), and its serum concentration of 0.1 μM is second only to cortisol [40].

Circulating free TH can be taken up by peripheral cells at any time, and both T4 and T3 can rapidly dissociate from their carrier proteins to increase the availability of free hormone when necessary [2, 40]. The entry of free T4 or T3 into target cells is mediated by a variety of plasma membrane transporters, including the aforementioned monocarboxylate transporters (including MCT8 and MCT10) and OATP1C1, as well as the Na$^+$-taurocholate cotransporting polypeptide, the L-type amino acid transporters (LAT1 and LAT2), and fatty acid translocase [35, 36, 41]. To date, the roles of the MCT and OATP families are best understood. While the MCT transporters are widely expressed in most tissues, OATP1C1 is much more specific, expressed predominantly in the brain and testes [36, 42]. The transporters also vary in their ligand specificity, with MCT10 demonstrating increased affinity for T3 and OATP1C1 demonstrating strong preference for T4 [36, 42]. The exact mechanisms by which these transporters facilitate TH uptake are still under investigation [35, 41, 42]. The clinical importance of TH transporters is manifested in the Allan–Herndon–Dudley syndrome. First described in 2004, this X-linked syndrome of severe psychomotor retardation and elevated T3 levels, results from mutations in the MCT8 gene [41, 42].

Once inside the cytosol of the target cells, T4 (and sometimes T3) is deiodinated by the iodothyronine deiodinase family of selenoproteins. Outer (5′)-ring deiodination of the prohormone T4 produces the active form of T3, while inner (5)-ring deiodination produces the inactive metabolite (reverse T3; rT3) [43, 44]. Although they share an overall 50% sequence homology and similar catalytic properties, the three deiodinases differ with regard to function and tissue specificity [2, 43, 45].

Type 1 deiodinase (D1), anchored on the cytosolic side of the plasma membrane, is the only enzyme of the three that is capable of deiodinating either the inner or the outer ring [43, 44]. Although it is believed to be an important source of T3 to the circulation, D1 is much less efficient than D2 in catalyzing the T4 to T3 conversion [44]. D1 also displays a strong preference for rT3 as its outer ring deiodination substrate. Consequently, it has been proposed that the more important role of D1 is as a scavenger enzyme, clearing inactive iodothyronines from the circulation and recycling the iodine [43, 44]. It is primarily expressed in the thyroid, liver, and kidney [43]. Increased thyroidal activity of D1 is thought to play a major role in the disproportionate overproduction of T3 observed in Graves' disease and multinodular toxic goiter, while reduced hepatic and renal D1 activity may account for the decreased levels of T3 associated with nonthyroidal illness syndrome (NTIS) [44].

Type 2 deiodinase (D2), located in the endoplasmic reticulum, is considered the major prohormone activator, as it exclusively catalyzes the conversion of T4 to T3 by 5′ deiodination [43, 45]. In order to maintain a relatively constant level of free T3 even when levels of T4 fluctuate, expression of D2 is tightly regulated at both the transcriptional and posttranslational levels [45]. One essential mechanism of protein homeostasis is the ubiquitin/proteasome system. Lysine residues within unneeded proteins are tagged with ubiquitin molecules, which induce a structural change that facilitates uptake by proteasomes and subsequent degradation. The D2 protein, with its 15 lysine residues, appears to be particularly susceptible to ubiquitination, a process that is even further accelerated in the presence of its natural substrate, T4 [45]. Distributed primarily in the brain, pituitary gland, thyroid gland, skeletal muscle, and brown adipose tissue, D2 is particularly important for the development of sensory organs (including the cochlea and retina), the regulation of the hypothalamus–pituitary–thyroid (HPT) axis, the cell maturation of bone and muscle, and thermogenesis [45].

Type 3 deiodinase (D3) is considered the major TH-inactivating enzyme. Located in the plasma membrane, it catalyzes inner ring deiodination of T4 and T3 to produce rT3 and 3,3′-diiodothyronine (T2), both inactive [43, 46]. D3 is very highly expressed in the placenta and in most fetal tissues, where it acts to limit fetal exposure to TH [43, 46]. With the exception of the brain, skin, and pregnant uterus, D3 is not active in normal adult tissues. However, it is often referred to as an oncofetal protein because it is reactivated in several human tumors, including astrocytomas, oligodendrogliomas, glioblastoma multiforme, basal cell carcinoma, infantile hemangioma, and adult hemangioendothelioma [46]. While the exact tumorigenic mechanism of D3 overexpression is not fully understood, it has been hypothesized that underproduction of T3 may be a way for tumor cells to escape normal differentiation [46]. D3 activity also increases significantly in inflammatory states, during tissue regeneration (such as after hepatectomy), and after ischemic events, including stroke and myocardial infarction [46].

At a cellular level, T3 can act within the nucleus, at the plasma membrane, in the cytoplasm, and at the mitochondrion [47]. The action of TH in the nuclei, called genomic action, involves the binding of T3 to TH nuclear receptors (TR), which then function as T3-inducible transcription factors that upregulate the expression of TH-responsive genes [1, 2, 47]. There are two major subtypes of TRs, each of which has several isoforms. Located on chromosome 17, the TRα gene encodes TRα1, which binds T3, as well as two other non-T3-binding products: TRα2 and TRα3 [1, 47]. TRα1 is constitutively expressed during embryonic development, while in postnatal life, it is predominantly expressed in brain, heart, bone, and skeletal muscle [1, 47]. There are three T3-binding TRβ isoforms encoded by the TRβ gene on chromosome 3: TRβ1 is expressed widely, TRβ2 primarily in brain, retina, and inner ear, and TRβ3 in kidney, liver, and lung [1, 47]. The phenotypic consequences of this tissue-specific TR expression are still under investigation.

The actions of T3 at the plasma membrane, cytoplasm, and mitochondria are referred to as nongenomic actions and are being increasingly recognized [1]. TH binding to sites on the plasma membranes of various types of cells has been shown to activate certain signal transduction pathways, as well as modulate the activity of the calcium pump, the sodium pump, and the sodium–proton exchanger. Some of the action of TH within the cytoplasm may be attributable to the presence of extranuclear TRs, but several other cytoplasmic proteins, including pyruvate kinase, are also known to bind T3 [47]. While it is well established that TH increases the number of mitochondria within a cell, the mechanism by which it does so is poorly understood, as are its effects on mitochondrial energetics and heat generation [47].

Regulation of Thyroid Hormone

Although TH homeostasis involves many complex local and systemic pathways, the most classic understanding of TH regulation is based on the negative feedback system of the HPT axis [2, 48–51] (Fig. 4). In this model, thyrotropin-releasing hormone (TRH) neurons located in the paraventricular nucleus of the hypothalamus (PVH) sense the circulating levels of TH. While other regions of the hypothalamus, including the lateral and ventromedial nuclei, also express TRH, only the PVH is tightly regulated by TH [48]. TH binds to the TRβ2 isoform in the PVH and influences TRH gene expression via a negative feedback fashion: When

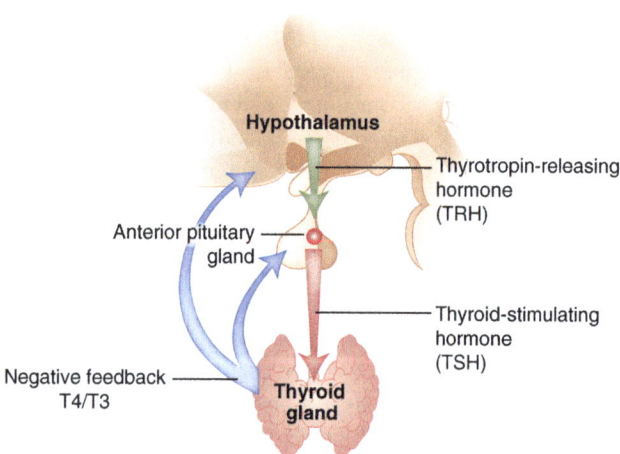

Fig. 4 The negative feedback system of the hypothalamic–pituitary–thyroid (*HPT*). Thyrotropin-releasing hormone (*TRH*) produced in the hypothalamus stimulates the anterior pituitary gland to synthesize and secrete thyroid-stimulating hormone (*TSH*). TSH binds to TSH receptors on thyroid follicular cells to stimulate synthesis of thyroid hormone (T3 and T4). Circulating T3 and T4 then exert a negative feedback effect on both the hypothalamus and the pituitary glands to decrease subsequent production of TRH and TSH

TH levels are high, TRH expression is low and vice versa [48, 50]. The pituitary portal vasculature then delivers TRH to the anterior pituitary gland, where TSH (also called thyrotropin) is synthesized and secreted. TH exerts a negative feedback effect on this step as well. After it is released from the pituitary gland, TSH binds to TSH receptors (TSHR) on the basal membrane of follicular cells, which triggers an intracellular cascade, including the activation of adenylate cyclase [11, 49, 50]. The resultant increase in cyclic adenosine monophosphate (cAMP) stimulates nearly every step in TH synthesis, including iodine uptake, synthesis of thyroglobulin, organification and coupling, and follicular cell uptake of thyroglobulin from the colloid [50].

Another key component of TH regulation is the availability of iodine. As previously discussed, iodine is essential for TH synthesis. In patients with iodine deficiency, TSH secretion is increased, which stimulates follicular growth and goiter formation [52]. The behavior of the thyroid gland under conditions of iodine excess is more complex. Large quantities of iodine are found in some medications, topical antiseptics, radiology contrast agents, and food preservatives [9, 52]. The tolerable upper limits of daily iodine ingestion have been reported from 600 to 1100 μg per day, but exposure above this limit is generally very well tolerated [12].

Under normal conditions, iodine essentially produces an intrathyroidal negative feedback system: Excess iodine inhibits its own organification, which prevents overproduction of TH [12, 49, 52]. This phenomenon was described in vitro by Morton and colleagues in 1944 and then in vivo in 1948 by **Wolff** and **Chaikoff**, after whom it was named [52]. Although it has been nearly 60 years since these original publications, the mechanism of the Wolff–Chaikoff effect remains elusive. It is hypothesized to be due to inhibition of TPO by intrathyroidal organic iodocompounds, but reduced intrathyroidal deiodinase activity also seems to play a role [12, 52]. In normal subjects, the inhibition of TH synthesis is transient (lasting 24–48 h), even with continued administration of excess iodine [9, 12, 49]. Within 24 h after an acute iodine load, there is a decreased expression of the NIS, resulting in reduced thyroidal uptake of iodine and resumption of normal TH synthesis [12, 49, 52]. This so-called escape from the Wolff–Chaikoff effect prevents development of iodine-induced hypothyroidism.

Iodine-induced hypothyroidism is observed in patients with underlying thyroid disease, neonates, the elderly, patients taking medications such as lithium and amiodarone (which can also cause thyrotoxicosis), and patients with certain nonthyroidal illnesses, such as cystic fibrosis and chronic renal insufficiency [52]. In these patients, the escape from the Wolff–Chaikoff effect fails. Likely because the NIS is not downregulated, they continue to have high concentrations of intrathyroidal inorganic iodine. The increased supply of iodine inhibits the synthesis of new TH, so the intrathyroidal and serum supplies of T3 and T4 are rapidly depleted, leading to increased serum TSH. However, TSH cannot overcome the inhibitory effects of iodine on TPO—instead, it stimulates expression of the NIS, which serves to further increase the intrathyroidal iodine concentration [12, 52]. With few exceptions, previously euthyroid patients who develop iodine-induced hypothyroidism return to normal within 2–8 weeks after iodine withdrawal. (Amiodarone-induced hypothyroidism takes longer to resolve because of the drug's long half-life.) However, many of these patients will eventually develop permanent hypothyroidism because of their underlying thyroid disease [52].

In another group of patients, excess iodine triggers hyperthyroidism. Iodine-induced thyrotoxicosis is termed the Jöd-Basedow phenomenon, after the German word for iodine (Jöd) and the German physician **Karl von Basedow** [12]. Although it has been described in patients with clinically normal thyroids, it is usually seen in people with a history of diffuse or nodular goiters, often in the setting of underlying iodine deficiency [9, 53]. The biologic basis of this phenomenon is believed to be thyroid autonomy, which becomes unmasked when iodine repletion (in endemic iodine-deficient areas) or iodine excess (in iodine-sufficient areas) provides the substrate for additional TH synthesis [9, 53]. As in iodine-induced hypothyroidism, normal thyroid function is usually restored after removing the excess iodine source [12].

Nonthyroidal Illness Syndrome (Euthyroid Sick Syndrome)

Acute or chronic nonthyroidal illness commonly induces predictable abnormalities in serum TH parameters (decreased T3, normal or decreased T4, and normal or decreased TSH) [54–57]. Once called "euthyroid sick syndrome," the term NTIS is now more commonly used to describe this constellation of thyroid function test derangements, which has been reported in up to 70 % of hospitalized patients [56, 57]. Most patients appear to be clinically euthyroid, and whether NTIS represents an appropriate physiologic adaptation to illness or a pathologic phenomenon that warrants correction remains a matter of debate [54, 55].

The etiology of NTIS is multifactorial. For years, altered deiodinase activity (particularly the inhibition of hepatic and renal D1) was thought to be responsible for the decreased levels of serum T3 during illness [55, 57]. However, recent mouse studies have shown that the decrease in serum T3 precedes the decreased D1 gene expression and also that, in the setting of experimental illness, serum T3 decreases even in D1 knockout mice [55, 56]. Changes to the hypothalamic–pituitary axis probably have a more significant contribution to the pathophysiology of NTIS. Diminished calorie intake and inflammatory cytokines (including IL-6, TNF-α, NFκB,

IL-1, and IFN-α) have been implicated in decreased production of TRH by the PVN [54, 56, 57]. This leads to either low TSH or the failure of TSH to rise appropriately in the presence of low circulating levels of serum THs. Additionally, the major binding proteins (TTR and TBG) are acute phase reactants and therefore decrease markedly during acute illness [57]. Reduced availability of binding proteins can significantly reduce the serum levels of total T3 and T4. Impaired transport of T4 into the peripheral tissues during acute illness has also been postulated, although no studies have demonstrated downregulation of TH transporters [55, 57].

An association between NTIS and worse outcomes, including mortality, has been described in patients with surgical sepsis, trauma, respiratory failure, acute stroke, myocardial infarction, and other critical illnesses [54, 56, 58, 59]. In a prospective study of 480 intensive care unit (ICU) patients, Wang and colleagues demonstrated that free T3 level was an independent predictor of ICU mortality, and therefore proposed that it be added to the Acute Physiology and Chronic Health Evaluation II (APACHE II) scoring system [60]. Despite the negative prognostic significance of low T3, however, no evidence currently exists to support TH replacement therapy in patients with NTIS [54–57]. Further study is needed to determine whether treatment would improve the clinical outcomes in these patients, and, if so, whether T3 or T4 would be the more appropriate preparation.

Key Summary Points

- TH is essential for normal development and metabolism in all vertebrates.
- Both types of TH, T4, and T3 are synthesized in the follicular cells via a process that involves concentration of iodine, organification and coupling, and secretion or storage.
- Through the NIS, iodine enters thyroid follicular cells against its concentration gradient.
- Thyroglobulin, a protein synthesized in the thyroid follicular cells, is an essential building block of TH.
- TH synthesis primarily occurs on the apical membrane of the follicular cell.
- TPO catalyzes the oxidation and organification of iodine, which leads to formation of MIT or DIT residues.
- In the coupling reaction, two DIT residues combine to form T4 or one MIT combines with one DIT to create T3.
- TSH stimulates iodinated thyroglobulin to mobilize from the colloid and reenter the thyrocyte. It is then processed by the endolysosomal system to form T4 and T3, which are secreted into the bloodstream via a transporter, MCT8.
- Under normal circumstances, 90 % of the hormone secreted by the thyroid gland is in the form of T4 and the other 10 % is T3.

- Peripherally, T4 is converted to T3 by tissue-specific deiodinases.
- TH synthesis is regulated by the negative feedback of HPT axis.
- The Wolff–Chaikoff effect describes the phenomenon whereby excess iodine inhibits its own organification, which prevents overproduction of TH.
- The Jöd-Basedow phenomenon, often seen in the setting of underlying iodine deficiency, refers to iodine-induced thyrotoxicosis.
- NTIS or euthyroid sick syndrome occurs when acute or chronic nonthyroidal illness induces predictable abnormalities in serum TH parameters (decreased T3, normal or decreased T4, and normal or decreased TSH).

References

1. Brent GA. Mechanisms of thyroid hormone action. J Clin Invest. 2012;122(9):3035–43.
2. Stathatos N. Thyroid physiology. Med Clin North Am. 2012;96(2):165–73.
3. Schmaltz C. Thyroid hormones in the neonate: an overview of physiology and clinical correlation. Adv Neonatal Care. 2012;12(4):217–22.
4. Chiasera JM. Back to the basics: thyroid gland structure, function and pathology. Clin Lab Sci. 2013;26(2):112–7.
5. Warner A, Mittag J. Thyroid hormone and the central control of homeostasis. J Mol Endocrinol. 2012;49(1):R29–35.
6. Portulano CM, Paroder-Belenitsky M, Carrasco N. The Na+/I− symporter (NIS): mechanism and medical impact. Endocr Rev. 2014;35(1):106–49.
7. Towery BT. The physiology of iodine. Bull World Health Organ. 1953;9(2):175–82.
8. Dunn JT, Dunn AD. Update on intrathyroidal iodine metabolism. Thyroid. 2001;11(5):407–14.
9. Roti E, Uberti ED. Iodine excess and hyperthyroidism. Thyroid. 2001;11(5):493–500.
10. Dobson JE. The iodine factor in health and evolution. Geogr Rev. 1998;88(1):1–28.
11. Colin IM, et al. Recent insights into the cell biology of thyroid angiofollicular units. Endocr Rev. 2013;34(2):209–38.
12. Leung AM, Braverman LE. Iodine-induced thyroid dysfunction. Curr Opin Endocrinol Diabetes Obes. 2012;19(5):414–9.
13. Kopp P. Thyroid hormone synthesis. In: Braverman LE, Utiger R, editors. Werner & Ingbar's the thyroid: a fundamental and clinical text. Philadelphia: Lippincott Williams & Wilkins; 2005. p. 52–76.
14. Dai G, Levy O, Carrasco N. Cloning and characterization of the thyroid iodide transporter. Nature. 1996;379(6564):458–60.
15. Carrasco N. Thyroid iodine transport. In: Braverman LE, Utiger R, editors. Werner & Ingbar's the thyroid: a fundamental and clinical text. Philadelphia: Lippincott Williams & Wilkins; 2005. p. 37–52.
16. Fong P. Thyroid iodide efflux: a team effort? J Physiol. 2011;589(Pt 24):5929–39.
17. Ohtaki S, et al. Thyroid peroxidase: experimental and clinical integration. Endocr J. 1996;43(1):1–14.
18. Ruf J, Carayon P. Structural and functional aspects of thyroid peroxidase. Arch Biochem Biophys. 2006;445(2):269–77.
19. Arvan P, Di Jeso B. Thyroglobulin structure, function, and biosynthesis. In: Braverman LE, Utiger R, editors. Werner & Ingbar's the thyroid: a fundamental and clinical text. Philadelphia: Lippincott Williams & Wilkins; 2005. p. 77–95.
20. Yoshihara A, et al. Regulation of dual oxidase expression and H$_2$O$_2$ production by thyroglobulin. Thyroid. 2012;22(10):1054–62.
21. Belkadi A, et al. Phylogenetic analysis of the human thyroglobulin regions. Thyroid Res. 2012;5(1):3.
22. Di Jeso B, et al. Transient covalent interactions of newly synthesized thyroglobulin with oxidoreductases of the endoplasmic reticulum. J Biol Chem. 2014;289(16):11488–96.
23. Kim PS, Arvan P. Folding and assembly of newly synthesized thyroglobulin occurs in a pre-golgi compartment. J Biol Chem. 1991;266(19):12412–8.
24. Xiao S, et al. Selectivity in tyrosyl iodination sites in human thyroglobulin. Arch Biochem Biophys. 1996;334(2):284–94.
25. Marino M, McCluskey RT. Role of thyroglobulin endocytic pathways in the control of thyroid hormone release. Am J Physiol Cell Physiol. 2000;279(5):C1295–306.
26. Schneider PB. Thyroidal iodine heterogeneity: "last come, first served" system of iodine turnover. Endocrinology. 1964;74:973–80.
27. Bernier-Valentin F, et al. Coated vesicles from thyroid cells carry iodinated thyroglobulin molecules. First indication for an internalization of the thyroid prohormone via a mechanism of receptor-mediated endocytosis. J Biol Chem. 1990;265(28):17373–80.
28. Botta R, et al. Binding, uptake, and degradation of internalized thyroglobulin in cultured thyroid and non-thyroid cells. J Endocrinol Invest. 2011;34(7):515–20.
29. Rousset B, et al. Thyroid hormone residues are released from thyroglobulin with only limited alteration of the thyroglobulin structure. J Biol Chem. 1989;264(21):12620–6.
30. Gnidehou S, et al. Iodotyrosine dehalogenase 1 (DEHAL1) is a transmembrane protein involved in the recycling of iodide close to the thyroglobulin iodination site. FASEB J. 2004;18(13):1574–6.
31. Gnidehou S, et al. Cloning and characterization of a novel isoform of iodotyrosine dehalogenase 1 (DEHAL1) DEHAL1C from human thyroid: comparisons with DEHAL1 and DEHAL1B. Thyroid. 2006;16(8):715–24.
32. Dunn AD, Crutchfield HE, Dunn JT. Thyroglobulin processing by thyroidal proteases. Major sites of cleavage by cathepsins B, D, and L. J Biol Chem. 1991;266(30):20198–204.
33. Dunn AD, Crutchfield HE, Dunn JT. Proteolytic processing of thyroglobulin by extracts of thyroid lysosomes. Endocrinology. 1991;128(6):3073–80.
34. Dunn AD, Myers HE, Dunn JT. The combined action of two thyroidal proteases releases T4 from the dominant hormone-forming site of thyroglobulin. Endocrinology. 1996;137(8):3279–85.
35. Di Cosmo C, et al. Mice deficient in MCT8 reveal a mechanism regulating thyroid hormone secretion. J Clin Invest. 2010;120(9):3377–88.
36. Friesema EC, et al. Thyroid hormone transport by the human monocarboxylate transporter 8 and its rate-limiting role in intracellular metabolism. Mol Endocrinol. 2006;20(11):2761–72.
37. Marino M, et al. Targeting of thyroglobulin to transcytosis following megalin-mediated endocytosis: evidence for a preferential pH-independent pathway. J Endocrinol Invest. 2003;26(3):222–9.
38. Marino M, et al. Megalin in thyroid physiology and pathology. Thyroid. 2001;11(1):47–56.
39. Benvenga S. Thyroid hormone transport proteins and the physiology of hormone binding. In: Braverman LE, Utiger R, editors. Werner & Ingbar's the thyroid: a fundamental and clinical text. Philadelphia: Lippincott Williams & Wilkins; 2005. p. 97–108.
40. Schussler GC. The thyroxine-binding proteins. Thyroid. 2000;10(2):141–9.
41. van der Deure WM, Peeters RP, Visser TJ. Molecular aspects of thyroid hormone transporters, including MCT8, MCT10, and OATPs, and the effects of genetic variation in these transporters. J Mol Endocrinol. 2010;44(1):1–11.

42. Fu J, Dumitrescu AM. Inherited defects in thyroid hormone cell-membrane transport and metabolism. Best Pract Res Clin Endocrinol Metab. 2014;28(2):189–201.

43. Dentice M, et al. The deiodinases and the control of intracellular thyroid hormone signaling during cellular differentiation. Biochim Biophys Acta. 2013;1830(7):3937–45.

44. Maia AL, et al. Deiodinases: the balance of thyroid hormone: type 1 iodothyronine deiodinase in human physiology and disease. J Endocrinol. 2011;209(3):283–97.

45. Arrojo e Drigo R, Bianco AC. Type 2 deiodinase at the crossroads of thyroid hormone action. Int J Biochem Cell Biol. 2011;43(10):1432–41.

46. Dentice M, Salvatore D. Deiodinases: the balance of thyroid hormone: local impact of thyroid hormone inactivation. J Endocrinol. 2011;209(3):273–82.

47. Cheng SY, Leonard JL, Davis PJ. Molecular aspects of thyroid hormone actions. Endocr Rev. 2010;31(2):139–70.

48. Hollenberg AN. The role of the thyrotropin-releasing hormone (TRH) neuron as a metabolic sensor. Thyroid. 2008;18(2):131–9.

49. Sellitti DF, Suzuki K. Intrinsic regulation of thyroid function by thyroglobulin. Thyroid. 2014;24(4):625–38.

50. Zoeller RT, Tan SW, Tyl RW. General background on the hypothalamic-pituitary-thyroid (HPT) axis. Crit Rev Toxicol. 2007;37(1–2):11–53.

51. Dietrich JW, Landgrafe G, Fotiadou EH. TSH and thyrotropic agonists: key actors in thyroid homeostasis. J Thyroid Res. 2012;2012:351864.

52. Markou K, et al. Iodine-induced hypothyroidism. Thyroid. 2001;11(5):501–10.

53. Stanbury JB, et al. Iodine-induced hyperthyroidism: occurrence and epidemiology. Thyroid. 1998;8(1):83–100.

54. Bello G, et al. The role of thyroid dysfunction in the critically ill: a review of the literature. Minerva Anestesiol. 2010;76(11):919–28.

55. Farwell AP. Nonthyroidal illness syndrome. Curr Opin Endocrinol Diabetes Obes. 2013;20(5):478–84.

56. Pappa TA, Vagenakis AG, Alevizaki M. The nonthyroidal illness syndrome in the non-critically ill patient. Eur J Clin Invest. 2011;41(2):212–20.

57. Warner MH, Beckett GJ. Mechanisms behind the non-thyroidal illness syndrome: an update. J Endocrinol. 2010;205(1):1–13.

58. Bello G, et al. Nonthyroidal illness syndrome and prolonged mechanical ventilation in patients admitted to the ICU. Chest. 2009;135(6):1448–54.

59. Todd SR, et al. The identification of thyroid dysfunction in surgical sepsis. J Trauma Acute Care Surg. 2012;73(6):1457–60.

60. Wang F, et al. Relationship between thyroid function and ICU mortality: a prospective observation study. Crit Care. 2012;16(1):R11.

Emil Theodor Kocher

1841–1917

Mathias Worni and Julie Ann Sosa

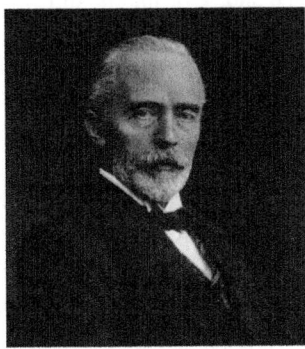

Emil Theodor Kocher (From National Institutes of Health, unknown photographer)

Emil Theodor Kocher was an outstanding personality, self-critical, systematic, modest, laborious and driven by a tremendous thrive for innovation. His capacity to link a clinical observation to its hitherto mostly unknown physiological basis was his fundament to revolutionize the surgical field and influence innumerable young surgeons across the world. Albeit described as a reserved personality, he entertained long lasting friendship with most great surgeons at his time including William Halsted, **Harvey Cushing**, and **Theodor Billroth**. Those and many more connections together with his scientific and surgical achievements helped to leverage the Inselspital—founded in 1354 and later transformed to the University Clinic of Bern—to worldwide fame at the end of the 19th century. It goes without saying that the receipt of the Nobel Prize was the culmination of his success awarding his greatest accomplishment, mastering thyroid surgery and more importantly understanding its physiology. When he died the entire Swiss government attended his funeral and all children of the city of Bern, the capital of Switzerland, had a day off school. It is impressive to observe how lasting Kocher's heritage is in "his" Inselspital and in our collective memories. Prof. D. Candinas

J. A. Sosa (✉)
Department of Surgery, Section of Endocrine Surgery, Duke University Medical Center, DUMC #2945, Durham, NC 27710, USA
e-mail: julie.sosa@duke.edu

M. Worni
Division of Advanced Oncology and General Surgery, Duke University Medical Center, Durham, NC 27710, USA

Emil Theodor Kocher was born on August 25, 1841, in the capital of Switzerland, Bern. As the son of the chief engineer of the canton of Bern, Jakob Alexander Kocher, the young Kocher grew up in a peaceful, culturally sophisticated, and religious atmosphere. He was characterized as a quiet, unassuming, but sometimes mischievous boy. After finishing secondary school, he trained without interruption at the University of Bern, from which he graduated and obtained his doctorate in 1865 [1]. He started his surgical career after medical school in Bern, but his talent and purposefulness took him to advanced studies at academic centers such as Zurich, Berlin, London, Paris, and Vienna. There, he learned under famous teachers, including Hermann Askan Demme (1802–1867), Georg Albert Lücke (1829–1894), Theodor Billroth (1829–1894), and Bernhard von Langenbeck (1810–1887). As associate professor, he returned to Bern, where he worked as a surgical assistant under Professor Georg Lücke. It was no surprise that in 1872 he was promoted to full professor of surgery; at this time, he also became director of the University Surgical Clinic in Bern as the position became vacant. He was only 31 years old when he was appointed to this job. He held the position until his death on July 27, 1917, 45 years later; this was an unprecedented feat. Even for those early years, selection as chair of a surgical department at age 31 was an outstanding honor. Whenever Kocher was invited to consider other lofty academic surgery positions around Europe, including Prague, Vienna, and Berlin, he deferred [2]. Throughout his career, he remained committed to his beloved hometown of Bern, where he found ideal conditions for his work. He was a humble man and reserved by nature; however, by report, he was very warm with patients, who uniformly loved him [3].

It was still very early in his medical and surgical career when Kocher described a new method for reducing shoulder dislocations and first received the attention of Theodor Billroth, who would become one of his critical mentors. Kocher intensively studied the pathologic anatomy of the shoulder and was then able to demonstrate his newly developed reduction technique on a patient with an old subcoracoid dis-

J. L. Pasieka, J. A. Lee (eds.), *Surgical Endocrinopathies,* DOI 10.1007/978-3-319-13662-2_2,
© Springer International Publishing Switzerland 2015

location. During a conference, all attempts to reduce the patient's shoulder by multiple physicians, including Billroth, failed. Kocher then volunteered to give his newly developed technique a try in front of multiple visiting physicians—and it worked on the first attempt! He called his technique for reducing shoulder dislocations the "Kocher method" [4]. His method was soon widely accepted, as it was shown to be simple, safe, and applicable for chronic and acute dislocations.

Kocher started his surgical career shortly after the appreciation of antiseptic treatment of wounds. He was heavily influenced by Sir Joseph Lister (1827–1912), a pioneer of antiseptic surgery. Kocher steadily supported the transition to using sterile technique, as he understood its immense importance and benefit for most patients. He was also one of the first surgeons who worked in a completely aseptic fashion. He benefited from close collaboration with Ernst Tavel (1858–1912) from the University of Bern, who was famous for his bacteriological studies [1]. They summarized their findings in the second edition of "Vorlesungen über chirurgische Infektionskrankheiten" (lectures on surgical infectious diseases), which was published in 1895 [5]. The University Clinic in Bern, Inselspital, remained for many years an international centerpiece among physicians who favored the antiseptic approach.

Aside from extensive work on antiseptic treatment, Kocher started to publish widely on a diverse set of topics in general surgery. One early publication included experiments about hemostasis (by torsion of the arteries); this pleased **Billroth**, especially, and it was published in Langenbecks Archive, Vol II [1]. Kocher also performed studies on gunshot wounds, as he had to give courses to military doctors. He worked on acute osteomyelitis (1878) and the theory of strangulated hernias (1877). He developed a new theory of hernia strangulation that was called the "dilation theory"; this received attention in the field of ileus research. He published regarding a new technique for gastric resection, describing pylorectomy with subsequent gastroduodenostomy. In addition, Kocher advanced the surgical procedure initiated by Kraske, where part of the coccyx was removed during rectal surgery to facilitate additional removal of a portion of the sacrum (1874), and he described gallstone excision from the lowest portion of the bile duct. One of the most important procedures he described in detail was the mobilization of the duodenum and pancreatic head from its posterior attachments and neighboring organs, including the inferior vena cava. This helped to advance many surgical procedures, including surgery on the duodenum, extrahepatic bile duct, pancreas, and stomach. This crucial step of early mobilization is employed as part of many larger upper gastrointestinal (GI) operations, and it is named the Kocher maneuver, or Kocher mobilization.

The list of his contributions seems to be endless, as he also published on simplified cholecystectomy procedures, ileus treatment, vertebral column fractures, traumatic epilepsy, brain damage, and trepanation. Most surgical specialties have benefited from the findings, inventions, and descriptions of Kocher. He also was respected by his peers because he reported his own patient outcomes regularly. His transparency regarding his own outcomes was novel. Importantly, Kocher for the first time demonstrated an association between increased (surgeon) volume and improved (patient) outcomes. Indeed, Kocher's outcomes following thyroidectomy improved dramatically over the course of his prolific career. Until his death at age 76 years, he was able to keep up with the same pace and rigor that he did when he started his surgical and scientific career.

While any of these achievements might have led to a durable legacy, Theodor Kocher is still best known and remembered for his advancements with regard to the physiology, pathology, and surgery of the thyroid gland. Thomas Wharton, an English anatomist, first named the thyroid in 1656; unfortunately, he believed that its purpose was "to fill the neck and make it shapely." Kocher's research on the thyroid gland significantly moved our understanding forward, and for this he was awarded the Nobel Prize in Physiology or Medicine in 1909. He was the first surgeon to receive the Nobel Prize in the field of science. His pioneering work

> "…gave a comprehensive exposition, which has been of fundamental importance to the latter development of thyroid surgery as well as to other important areas of our knowledge of this gland. Through Kocher's exposition, it became quite clear that complete extirpation of the thyroid is reprehensible. A portion of the gland which is capable of functioning must be left behind at the operation."

While debate today continues about the relative merits of total thyroidectomy versus thyroid lobectomy, Kocher established the importance of not performing total thyroidectomy in an era prior to the evolution of exogenous thyroid hormone supplementation or replacement. But it was not just Kocher's exposition about surgical approach that advanced the field of thyroidology forward, but also his studies

> "…into the causes of endemic occurrence of goiter in certain regions and into the cretinism connected with disturbances in thyroid function."

The money he received for this prize (200,000 Swiss francs) was fully donated by him to his University (of Bern) to build a Research Institute for Biology. The Theodor Kocher Institute of the Medical Faculty of the University of Bern is active today, addressing molecular mechanisms involved in inflammation, with a special focus on studying immune cell migration during immune surveillance and inflammation [6].

In the 1850s, thyroid surgery was only performed for vital indications, as operative mortality rates were often higher than 40%. The principal reasons for fatal outcomes were uncontrollable bleeding and/or infectious complications. Indeed, in the early days, thyroid surgery was considered such a dangerous operation that it was prohibited in France. It is worth noting, for example, that Lücke, the predecessor of Kocher, operated on ten goiters from 1866 to 1872, and nine of his patients succumbed to complications from their surgeries. Many voices were raised against thyroidectomy, and thyroid surgery had a reputation for being a thankless, dangerous, and reckless pursuit [7]. Samuel Gross, a surgical contemporary of Kocher's who worked in the USA, wrote in 1866:

> If a surgeon should be so adventurous, or foolhardy, as to undertake thyroidectomy, I shall not envy him… Every step he takes will be environed with difficulty, every stroke of his knife will be followed by a torrent of blood, and lucky will it be for him if his victim lives long enough to enable him to finish his horrid butchery… No honest and sensible surgeon, it seems to me, would ever engage in it. [8]

Using advanced surgical techniques described by Kocher and Billroth, in particular, the mortality rate was significantly reduced over the coming years. Kocher's first paper on thyroid gland pathology and surgery in 1874 reported his series of 13 patients, and only 2 of these patients died. He described a technique where he first ligated the major arteries and veins to the thyroid gland; in turn, he identified the recurrent laryngeal nerve. After achieving this control, the external capsule of the gland was split, and the isthmus was removed. This helped to avoid profuse bleeding and spared the recurrent laryngeal nerves [3]. Most of the surgeries were performed under ether anesthesia and using local infiltration of cocaine. Kocher reported his surgical mortality rate in 1883 at the German Congress of Surgery; by that time, he had performed 101 goiter operations with an associated mortality rate of only 13%, which was groundbreaking for his time. In this surgical series, 18 patients developed the typical presentation of myxedema and altered mental status; all of this subset had undergone total thyroidectomy. Kocher closely followed his patients in the postoperative setting, and he found that those who underwent total thyroidectomy died within 7 years after surgery. Patients who underwent intended total thyroidectomy but who did not die were seen to develop a new, but smaller goiter. In autopsy studies, no thyroid tissue was found in the patients who died. This led Kocher to describe the cretinoid pattern, which he named "cachexia strumipriva"; this was first thought to be related to chronic asphyxia due to damage to the trachea and only later related to profound hypothyroidism [1]. In 1893, Kocher reported that ingestion of raw thyroid tissue could im-

prove the severe symptoms of "cachexia strumipriva," and others subsequently confirmed this finding. In turn, Kocher changed his earlier view that the thyroid gland's main purpose was just to regulate blood flow to the brain [9].

In 1889, Kocher published a series of 250 goiter resections and described precisely the surgical procedure he called "enucleation resection," including the typical transverse collar incision of the skin; today, this is still referred to as a Kocher incision. He also described why it is necessary to leave a minimum amount of healthy thyroid tissue behind to allow for continued thyroid function, and why it is essential to preserve the function of the recurrent laryngeal nerves as well as the parathyroid glands. However, in Kocher's time, the function of the parathyroid glands was still unknown. For many years, the Kocher operation (advocating for less than total thyroidectomy) was standard of care; only recently has there been a shift toward total thyroidectomy for the purpose of reduced risk of recurrence. Only with the later development of exogenous thyroid hormone supplementation and replacement has total thyroidectomy been rendered safe.

Tetany and hypoparathyroidism were not yet understood in Kocher's time, but his (relatively) bloodless technique permitted him to have fewer complications postoperatively compared to his contemporaries [1]. Kocher was renowned for his purposeful and precise style of performing thyroidectomy. With fastidious technique and integration of advanced antiseptic surgical methods, Kocher was able to reduce his perioperative mortality rate to 0.5% by 1912 [10]. By that time, he had performed more than 5000 thyroid operations, making him perhaps the earliest "high-volume" endocrine surgeon, and the first surgeon who demonstrated that with increasing experience, patient outcomes are optimized.

Kocher also was interested in the etiology of the development of goiters, and he performed a large study examining thousands of schoolchildren living in the canton of Bern; in this study, he described a total goiter prevalence rate that ranged from 20 to 100% [11]. He realized that there were significant geological differences regarding the prevalence of goiter and cretinism, and further studies focused on its etiology with the aim being to provide prophylaxis for the Swiss population. Shortly before his death, Kocher recommended that iodine supplementation be provided at a population level in order to prevent goiters. However, he was convinced at that time that iodine deficiency was not the cause of the development of goiters but rather an entity that could antagonize the real, unknown goitrogen. It was not until 1914 that thyroxine was identified by Kendall, and later, in 1926, first synthesized by Harrington in London.

Over the course of his career, Kocher published 249 scientific articles and books, operated on thousands of patients, and trained new generations of surgeons. His way of teach-

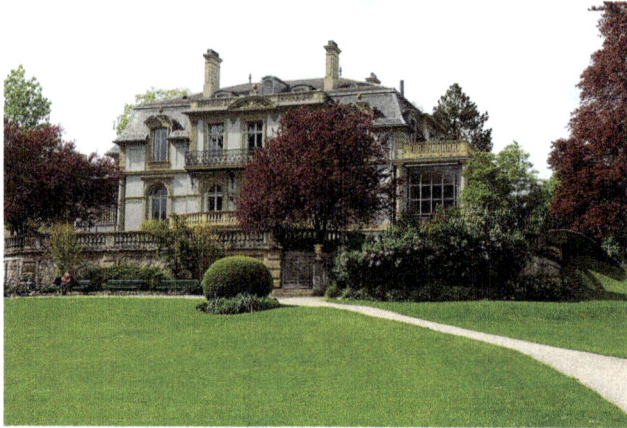

Fig. 1 Kocher Park with House of University, Bern. (Photograph courtesy of Bruno Worni)

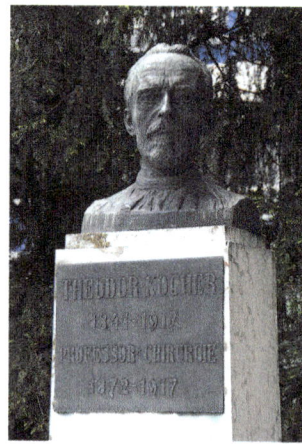

Fig. 3 Bust of Kocher in front of the Inselspital, Bern. (Photograph courtesy of Bruno Worni)

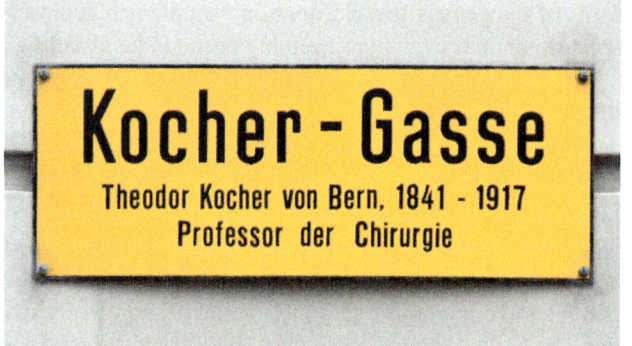

Fig. 2 Street sign of the Kochergasse. (Photograph courtesy of Bruno Worni)

ing is still contemporary and has applications for the purpose of ensuring the highest quality surgical care. Fausto Chiesa summarized his strategy in an editorial around four points: (1) the importance of meticulous and repeated observations; (2) the knowledge of anatomy, pathology, and surgical techniques; (3) the accuracy, care, and patience that are necessary during surgical procedures (It is more important to be safe than fast!); and (4) the critical audit of results [12].

His fame and reputation as the first premier high-volume thyroid surgeon is robust today; rarely does a day go by when surgical trainees do not learn about the importance of the Kocher maneuver during pancreaticoduodenectomy, or perform a Kocher incision during thyroidectomy, or utilize or pass a Kocher clamp. His name and spirit continue to live

in the city of Bern in the Theodor Kocher Institute, the Kocher Park (Fig. 1), Kochergasse (Fig. 2), as well as in two Kocher busts, one placed in front of his so loved Inselspital, the University Clinic of Bern (Fig. 3).

Acknowledgments Daniel Candinas, MD FRCS, Chair of the Department of Surgery, University Clinic of Bern, Inselspital, Switzerland.

References

1. "Theodor Kocher—Biographical". Nobelprize.org. Nobel Media AB 2013. 2013. <http://www.nobelprize.org/nobel_prizes/medicine/laureates/1909/kocher-bio.html>. Accessed 13 April 2014.
2. Tröhler U. The subtle knife: a revolution in surgery. Karger Gazette; No 71 Swiss Pioneers in Science and Medicine 2010:12–4.
3. Tan SY, Shigaki D. Emil Theodor Kocher (1841–1917): thyroid surgeon and nobel laureate. Singap Med J. 2008;49(9):662–3.
4. Kocher T. Eine neue Reductionsmethode für Schulterverrenkung. (Berliner Wochenschrift) Berl Wkly Clin. 1870;7(9):101–05.
5. Kocher T, Tavel E. Vorlesungen über chirurgische Infectionskrankheiten. Basel: Verlag von Carl Sallmann; 1895.
6. Theodor Kocher Institute. http://www.tki.unibe.ch/.
7. Diffenbach J. Die operative Chirurgie II. Leipzig: FA Brockhaus; 1848. p. 331.
8. Grant CS. Presidential address: boiling water to iodine—a story of unparalleled collaboration. Surgery. 2002;132(6):909–15.
9. Sawin C. Werner and Inbar's the thyroid: a fundamental and clinical test. 7th ed. Philadelphia: Lippincott-Raven; 1991.
10. Choong C, Kaye AH. Emil theodor kocher (1841–1917). J Clin Neurosci. 2009;16(12):1552–4.
11. Kocher T. Vorkommen und Vertheilung des Kropfes im Kanton Bern. Berne: KJ Wyss; 1889.
12. Chiesa F. The 100 years anniversary of the nobel prize award winner Emil Theodor Kocher, a brilliant far-sighted surgeon. Acta Otorhinolaryngol Ital. 2009;29(6):289.

Karl von Basedow

1799–1854

Tina W.F. Yen

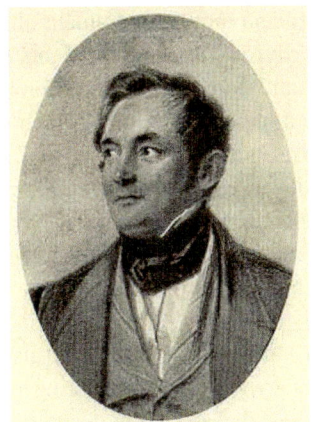

Karl Adolph von Basedow.

Karl Adolph von Basedow was born on March 28, 1799, in Dessau, Germany, a town located between Berlin and Leipzig (Fig. 1). He was the son of an aristocratic family. His grandfather, Johann Bernhard Basedow, was a German educational reformer, teacher, and writer. In 1774, he founded the "Philanthropinum" in Dessau, a short-lived but influential progressive school inspired by the French philosopher J. J. Rousseau. Von Basedow's father held a prominent position as president of the council of the principality of Anhalt [1].

Little is known about von Basedow's youth. He had two sisters and one brother [1]. Basedow went to school in Dessau and then studied medicine at the University of Halle (south of Dessau), where he received his doctorate of medicine and surgery in January 1821 at the age of 22. His thesis, which was written in Latin, addressed a new method of lower leg amputation. After spending 2 years on the surgical services at two famous hospitals in Paris, Hòtel de Dieu and Charité, von Basedow obtained his license certifying him as a general practitioner, surgeon, and obstetrician in June 1822. In the summer of 1822, at the age of 23, Basedow settled in Merseburg (Fig. 1), a district town of about 8000 inhabitants, and began practicing as a general physician.

On April 23, 1823, von Basedow married Louise Friederike Scheuffelhuth, the daughter of a district notary. They had three daughters and one son; their youngest daughter died at 6 months of age from tuberculosis [1]. Von Basedow was described as an affectionate father, taking time to play music with his daughters. He loved not only listening to music and concerts but also hiking, was an avid hunter and fisherman, and enjoyed socializing [2]. The evening soirées at the von Basedow's were quite popular in the community.

In 1841, von Basedow was appointed Royal Medical Counselor, and in 1848, he was selected from among eight other candidates as state physician/chief medical officer ("Kreisphysikus") for the district of Merseburg, a position he held until his untimely death. After pricking his finger while performing an autopsy on a patient who died of typhus or spotted fever, von Basedow developed a fever and died 3 days later of sepsis on April 11, 1854, at the age of 55 [2, 3]. Von Basedow was buried in the Sixtus Cemetery in Merseburg on Good Friday, April 14, 1854.

As a physician, von Basedow had a reputation as a kind, talented, and skilled family doctor with extensive knowledge of all aspects of medical practice who also possessed a social conscience [2]. He was the "round-the-clock" physician for "the town and country," caring for not only aristocrats but also the poorest, sometimes without seeking payment. In 1831, he voluntarily helped to fight the cholera epidemic in Magdeburg; an invaluable experience that he would later draw from when cholera afflicted Merseburg. He performed the autopsies of many of his patients, including his youngest child. The comprehensive care provided by von Basedow as a general practitioner during these times is truly remarkable.

Von Basedow was not only an astute and dedicated physician but he was also extremely dedicated to public health issues. He sought to end the "unchristian breast-feeding by paid wet nurses," introduced testing of drinking water, and,

T. W. Yen (✉)
Department of Surgery, Medical College of Wisconsin, 9200 W. Wisconsin Avenue, Milwaukee, WI 53226, USA
e-mail: tyen@mcw.edu

J. L. Pasieka, J. A. Lee (eds.), *Surgical Endocrinopathies*, DOI 10.1007/978-3-319-13662-2_3,
© Springer International Publishing Switzerland 2015

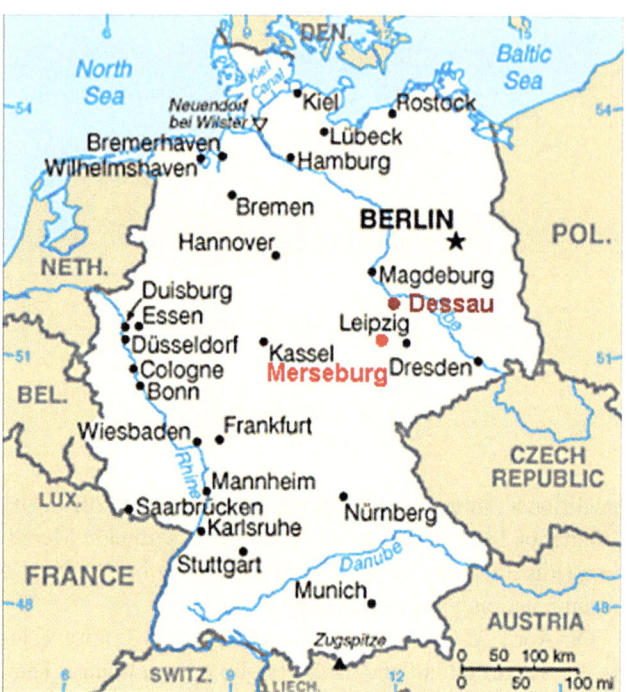

Fig. 1 Map of Germany, indicating Dessau, von Basedow's hometown, and Merseburg, the town where he practiced as a family physician and was laid to rest

after observing the detrimental effects of arsenic-containing paints ("Schweinfurter Grün," "poison green"), vehemently fought to ban paints containing arsenic [1, 2].

From a scientific standpoint, von Basedow became a member of the Medical Society of Leipzig in 1838 and was recognized as a very accomplished scholar with excellent insight and foresight. Similar to his clinical practice, he had extensive, broad, and diverse scientific interests, which were documented in approximately 60 publications. The majority of his contributions addressed topics related to surgery, internal medicine, and obstetrics and gynecology. However, articles also focused on diseases of the eye, ear, nose, and throat, dermatology, neurology, and pediatrics, reflecting von Basedow's extensive and different scientific interests [4].

Von Basedow's most significant contribution to medicine was the first description of "Basedow disease" in the German language on March 28, 1840, entitled "Exophthalmos due to hypertrophy of the cellular tissue in the orbit" [5]. In this seminal article, von Basedow describes "…there appeared an eminent protrusion of the eyeballs, which by the way were absolutely healthy and had a completely full sight. In spite of this, the sick woman was sleeping with open eyes and had a frightening appearance." This initial publication was followed by several others and the phrase "glotzaugencachexie" or "google eyes cachexia" was coined [6, 7]. These publications represent von Basedow's observations of four patients over periods ranging from 2 to 11 years. In his 1840 publication, von Basedow masterfully described

the relationship between three characteristic symptoms: exophthalmos, palpitations, and goiter [5]. In 1851, these three cardinal symptoms characterizing the disease became known as "Merseburg triad."

Von Basedow had impressive observation skills and depicted this illness meticulously, vividly, and accurately, describing a frequent pulse that was irregular and sometimes accelerated, a swollen thyroid gland, and eyeballs that could not be pushed back with movements that were hindered such that the patients slept with their eyes open [2]. He also remarkably described the symptoms of heat intolerance (during cold weather, women would wear open or light clothing), profound sweating, diarrhea, and weight loss in the presence of increased appetite, as well as weakness, tremor, pretibial myxedema, and temperament change [2]. His two most severely thyrotoxic female patients displayed an "unnatural gaiety and carelessness," and one, Madame F, was even placed in a lunatic asylum, although she never had any ill intentions or "abnormal expressions of will."

Although the long-standing and extreme alterations of untreated disease are scarcely seen today, von Basedow clearly describes these processes such as observed in Herr M who lost his eyesight after his "prominent like a crayfish's eyes" were gradually destroyed by infections, leaving residual craters [1]. In his female patients, he also reported on the amelioration of hyperthyroidism during pregnancy, as well as deterioration of disease in the postpartum period [2]. Regarding treatment, von Basedow reported that mineral waters that contained iodine and bromide and digitalis would improve the symptoms of hyperthyroidism [1].

There has been a long dispute over who first described these diagnostic features as these symptoms had been previously reported by Irish physician **Robert James Graves** in 1835 [8], Italians Antonio Giuseppe Testa in 1810 [9] and Giuseppe Flajani in 1802 [10], and British Caleb Hilier Parry in 1825 [11]. However, none of these other descriptions were as extensive and complete as von Basedow's, and von Basedow was the first to associate the large and complex symptomatology to a single underlying disease process. Since 1858, this disease has been most commonly referred to as "Morbus Basedow" or Basedow's disease in Europe and Graves' disease in English-speaking countries [3].

Von Basedow not only described the relationship between these symptoms but also attempted to explain the pathophysiology of this unusual combination of symptoms and involved organs. He recognized that the exophthalmos was not due to any change in the eyeball but rather to hypertrophy of the surrounding tissues of the eye [5]. In addition, von Basedow was correct in postulating that the etiology of this disease was mediated via the circulation when he hypothesized that "dyscrasia" (inadequate mixture) of the blood was responsible for the orbital swelling and goiter [12]. He proposed that the disease was due to a wrong mixing of the blood resulting in cell tissue congestion and glandular vegetation in the affected organs [2].

During the next 100 years, over 50 publications proposed various etiologies for this disease process, but it was not until the late 1950s, when Adams and Purves discovered the antibody-mediated origin of this disease [13, 14]. It is now well accepted that Basedow's disease is an organ-specific autoimmune process that differs from all other autoimmune diseases since it is associated with target organ hyperfunction and not organ destruction [15]. If we accept that "dyscrasia" describes circulating antibodies and immune imbalance and "cell tissue congestion and glandular vegetations" depict the cellular infiltration seen with autoimmune orbitopathy and thyroiditis, we can contemplate whether much progress has been made since von Basedow's astute observations [2]. In March 1990, von Basedow's outstanding contributions to this disease process were the focus of an international convention, "150 Years of Morbus Basedow," which was held in Halle and Merseburg, Germany.

Today, 160 years after the death of its describer, the exact etiology for autoantibody production resulting in the triad of symptoms known as Basedow's disease and Graves' disease remains to be determined. However, to this day, we are indebted to Dr. Karl von Basedow for his remarkable clinical observations and description of this disease process, as well as its potential pathophysiology, management, and treatment. In this modern era of technology and science, we should not forget the power of observation, the gift of astute reasoning, and the genius of Karl von Basedow.

References

1. Wenzel KW. European Thyroid Association. Milestones in European Thyroidology (MET): Carl Adolph von Basedow (1799–1854) 2013. http://www.eurothyroid.com/about/met/basedow.html. Accessed 17 May 2014.

2. Meng W. Carl Adolph von Basedow–150th anniversary of his death. Z fur arztl Fortbild Qualitatssicherung. 2004 May;98(Suppl 5):7–12. PubMed PMID: 15255307. Carl Adolph von Basedow–Zu seinem 150. Todestag.

3. Duntas LH. A tribute to Carl Adolph von Basedow: to commemorate 150 years since his death. Hormones. 2004 Jul-Sep;3(3):208–9. PubMed PMID: 16982595.

4. Goring HD. Carl Adolph von Basedow on the on the occasion of the 150th anniversary of the day he died. J Deutsch Dermatol Ges (J Ger Soc Dermatol: JDDG). 2004 Nov;2(11):963–7. PubMed PMID: 16281617. Carl Adolph von Basedow aus Anlass seines 150. Todestages.

5. Basedow CA. Exophthalmos durch Hypertrophie des Zellgewebes in der Augenhöhle. Wochenschr Gesammte Heilkd. 1840;13:197–204, 20–8.

6. Basedow CA. Die Glotzaugen. Wochenschr Gesammte Heilkd. 1848;49:769–77.

7. Basedow CA. Ueber Exophthalmos, ebenda. Wochenschr Gesammte Heilkd. 1848;26:414–6.

8. Graves RJ. New observed affection of the thyroid gland in females. Lond Med Surg J. 1835;7:516–7.

9. Testa AG. Delle malattie del cuore, loro cagioni, specie, segni e cura. 2nd ed. Bologna: Presso Giuseppe Lucchesini; 1810.

10. Flajani G. Sopra un tumor freddo nell'anterior parte del collo broncocele (Osservazione LXVII). Collezione d'osservazioni e reflessioni di chirurgia. A Ripa Presso Lino Contedini. 1802;3:270–3.

11. Parry CH. Enlargement of the thyroid gland in connection with enlargement or palpitations of the heart. In: Parry CH, editor. Collections from the unpublished medical writings of H. Parry. London: Underwoods; 1825. p. 111–129.

12. Hennemann G. Historical aspects about the development of our knowledge of morbus Basedow. J Endocrinol Invest. 1991 Jul-Aug;14(7):617–24. PubMed PMID: 1940068.

13. Adams DD, Purves HD. The role of thyrotrophin in hyperthyroidism and exophthalmos. Metab: Clin Exp. 1957 Jan;6(1):26–35. PubMed PMID: 13386966.

14. Adams DD. The presence of an abnormal thyroid-stimulating hormone in the serum of some thyrotoxic patients. J Clin Endocrinol Metab. 1958 Jul;18(7):699–712. PubMed PMID: 13549548.

15. Chen CR, Pichurin P, Nagayama Y, Latrofa F, Rapoport B, McLachlan SM. The thyrotropin receptor autoantigen in Graves disease is the culprit as well as the victim. J Clin Invest. 2003 Jun;111(12):1897–904. PubMed PMID: 12813025. Pubmed Central PMCID: 161420.

Jan Wolff and Israel L. Chaikoff

1925–; 1902–1966

James X. Wu, Kevin Ro and Michael W. Yeh

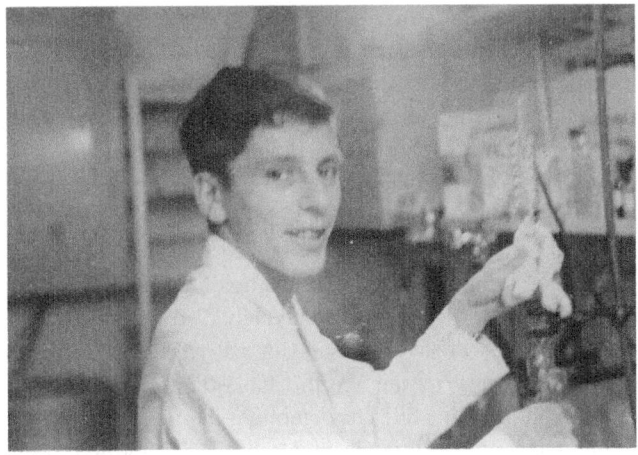

Dr. Jan Wolff (April 25, 1925). Photo of young Dr. Wolff in laboratory

Born in Germany, Dr. Wolff was displaced to Holland at a young age as Hitler came into power. His father was a Jewish pediatrician, and his mother was Dutch. At age 12, he would be relocated again, this time to San Francisco, where his father would repeat his pediatric residency.

Dr. Wolff's high school chemistry teacher kindled his initial interest in chemistry and science research. This interest would later inspire him to major in chemistry and biochemistry at University of California (UC) at Berkeley, the university where he would stay for his undergraduate, master's, and doctorate degrees in physiology. He was drawn to Dr. Chaikoff's laboratory because he offered a salary—a rare thing at the time—of US$ 100 a month. This was no small amount since tuition fees were US$ 25 per semester. Joining as an undergraduate student, Dr. Wolff spent a total of 4 years in Dr. Chaikoff's laboratory.

Wolff's accomplishments in the Chaikoff laboratory were made at a time when scientific research was grueling in comparison to modern standards. Dr. Wolff assembled his own Geiger tubes. To measure thyroxine, he digested thyroid glands from animals, performed an extraction with *n*-butanol, then distilled the liquid with a Chaney still. At first, the laboratory bombarded tellurium on a copper target with deuterons to create radioactive iodine.

Wolff's relationship with Chaikoff was often challenging. Chaikoff was very demanding, but at the same time, he empowered his trainees to shoo him away if they were concentrating on an experiment—something a busy Dr. Wolff would often do. In addition to laboratory work, writing papers together was equally arduous. Always maintaining a high standard, Dr. Chaikoff insisted that all papers went through the English department. Ultimately, the results were routinely superb and the added effort would prove worthwhile. Chaikoff's passion and drive were infectious, and propelled Wolff into excellence early in his career.

Following his time at UC Berkeley, Wolff went to medical school at Harvard, followed by a medical internship at Massachusetts General Hospital. During his internship, he realized that patient care always left him unsatisfied and perpetually curious about underlying mechanisms. Thus, he was drawn back to basic science research, and joined the National Institute of Health (NIH). At the NIH, after continuing thyroid studies, his later research focus shifted to the study of tubulin and microtubule assembly.

To this day, Dr. Wolff is frequently contacted to discuss the use of iodine in the event of nuclear accidents. His expertise was sought following hydrogen bomb testing at the Marshall Islands during the 1950s and after the Chernobyl accident in 1986. He was an early recruit to the clinical endocrinology branch of the National Institute of Diabetes and Digestive and Kidney Diseases (NIDDK), and later became the chief of the Endocrine Biochemistry Section of the Laboratory of Biochemistry and Genetics at NIDDK. Now retired from research, he continues to be academically active and teaches at the NIH.

M. W. Yeh (✉) · J. X. Wu · K. Ro
Section of Endocrine Surgery, UCLA David Geffen School of Medicine, 10833 Le Conte Ave, 72-228 CHS, 956904, Los Angeles, CA 90095, USA
e-mail: myeh@mednet.ucla.edu

J. L. Pasieka, J. A. Lee (eds.), *Surgical Endocrinopathies*, DOI 10.1007/978-3-319-13662-2_4,
© Springer International Publishing Switzerland 2015

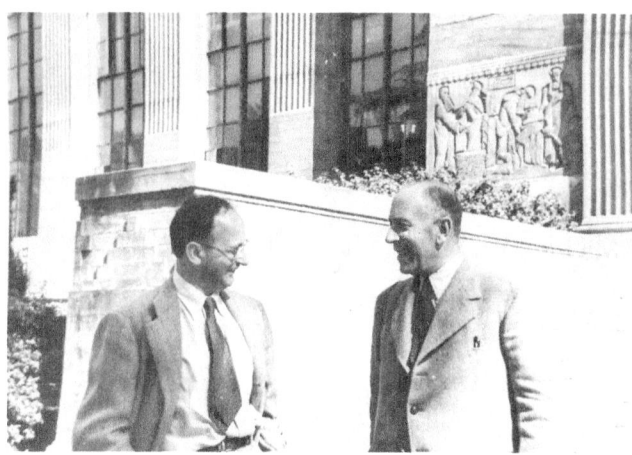

Dr. Israel Lyon Chaikoff (July 2, 1902–January 25, 1966; Born in London, England). Photo of Dr. Chaikoff (*left*) with colleague Dr. Walter Griesbach

Dr. Israel Chaikoff joined the UC Berkeley in 1930, after obtaining his PhD and MD degrees from the University of Toronto. During his time at the University of Toronto, on the same campus, **Dr. Frederick Banting** performed his series of experiments that led to the discovery of insulin in the 1920s. That discovery sparked Chaikoff's interest in endocrine research, which focused on fat and carbohydrate metabolism. Chaikoff gained early recognition as an outstanding lecturer in endocrinology.

When Chaikoff arrived at Berkeley, the Department of Physiology was in its infancy. The faculty comprised one full professor and four assistant professors, all of whom been present for less than 3 years. Focused and determined, Chaikoff often worked on experiments well into the night. Until he married, he lived mostly in the Faculty Club.

His doggedness would prove very fruitful. By the end of his career, Dr. Chaikoff would contribute more than 400 publications. He also pioneered the use of radioactive isotopes in research, including I^{131} in thyroid metabolism and disease, P^{32} in phospholipid membrane turnover, and C^{14} in the study of hepatic steatosis. In addition to describing the Wolff–Chaikoff effect and other aspects of thyroid physiology, he made significant contributions to the study of adrenal hormones, fatty acid metabolism, and cholesterol synthesis. Chaikoff later become co-chairman of his department and received numerous accolades, including the Endocrine Society medal in 1958. Today, the Chaikoff Memorial Award is given each year to an undergraduate student at UC Berkeley who distinguishes him or herself in the area of molecular and cell biology.

Chaikoff was afflicted with severe asthma. Despite his condition, he continued to lecture, mentor his graduate students, and conduct world-class research. The condition also did not prevent him from enjoying one of his most beloved meals once a month, spaghetti al pesto, despite the mild re-

action that would inevitably follow. Sadly, Chaikoff's career was cut short in 1966, when he passed away from status asthmaticus. Chaikoff's legacy lies not only in his discoveries, the significance of which echoes into modern day, but also in his teachings, which shaped many great scientists, including Dr. Wolff, Dr. Isadore Perlman, Dr. Gordon Tomkins, and many others.

Discovery of the Wolff–Chaikoff Effect

In the 1940s, iodine was available to the public and had been used to treat thyroid disease and other ailments for some time before Wolff and Chaikoff made their discovery. Lugol's solution, a solution of elemental iodine and potassium iodide, was first made in 1829. It was used to treat hyperthyroidism, though its mechanism of action was poorly understood. Surgeons of that era also used it to reduce thyroid vascularity prior to thyroid operations. Iodine deficiency as a cause of goiter formation and cretinism gained wide recognition in the late eighteenth and early nineteenth centuries. This led to the development of iodized salt in Switzerland. Subsequently, iodized salt was championed in the USA by the University of Michigan, and widely distributed throughout the USA by the Morton Salt Company in 1924.

The discovery of the Wolff–Chaikoff effect was based upon a simple objective: to determine the degree to which iodine supplementation can increase thyroid hormone production. Wolff and Chaikoff hypothesized that plasma iodide would exert a sigmoidal effect on endogenous thyroxine production in rats; in other words, that increasing doses of iodine would increase thyroxine production until the thyroid gland became saturated, at which point hormone production would plateau. To their surprise, higher doses of iodine paradoxically resulted in less thyroidal iodine organification compared to smaller doses. After repeated trials and other researchers confirmed the effect, they concluded that plasma iodine levels above a certain threshold inhibit thyroid hormone production by the thyroid: a phenomenon now known as the Wolff–Chaikoff effect [1]. The Wolff–Chaikoff effect is now seen as an autoregulatory, homeostatic mechanism that protects against the wide fluctuations in thyroxine levels that would otherwise result if thyroxine production were purely a function of dietary iodine intake.

The mechanisms underlying the Wolff–Chaikoff effect are still being studied, but are now hypothesized to involve the formation of inhibitory iodolipids. Currently, it is known that high serum and thyroidal iodide levels trigger cell signaling cascades that lead to downregulation of the sodium/iodide symporter on the thyrocyte cell surface, resulting in decreased availability of intracellular iodide for organification [2]. Excess serum iodide also has a number of effects on intracellular signaling molecules and interactions with cell membrane phospholipids. Though the clinical significance of many of these individual interactions remains unknown, the net effect is downregulation of many thyroidal as well as systemic metabolic functions. Further research has also revealed an "escape phenomenon," by which the normal thyroid regains normal thyroid hormone production after 2–6 days of exposure to persistently high serum iodide levels. A related effect, the Jod-Basedow phenomenon, also deserves mention. The Jod-Basedow phenomenon describes altered thyroid physiology in patients with endemic goiter due to chronic iodine deficiency. In direct contrast to the inhibitory effect described by Wolff and Chaikoff, a small percentage of chronically iodine-deficient patients can develop hyperthyroidism upon receiving iodine supplementation, an effect not seen in individuals with normal thyroid glands; this represents a failure of the Wolff–Chaikoff effect in these individuals.

Clinical Applications

The Wolff–Chaikoff effect underpins the use of iodine as a treatment for autoimmune hyperthyroidism (Graves' disease). Patients with autoimmune thyroid disease display abnormal autoregulation and "fail to escape" from the Wolff–Chaikoff effect. Hence, strong iodine preparations such as supersaturated potassium iodide (SSKI) and potassium iodide–iodine solution (Lugol's) can be used to medically manage Graves' disease for weeks. Today, a short course (5–10 days) of iodine is commonly administered to lower thyroxine concentrations and decrease gland vascularity to prepare for thyroidectomy in Graves' disease.

Iodine is also given prior to diagnostic scanning with I^{131}-labeled metaiodobenzylguanidine (mIBG, used to image pheochromocytomas and paragangliomas) to protect the thyroid gland from damage from the radioisotope. Iodinated intravenous contrast is frequently administered to enhance imaging with computed tomography. In patients with differentiated thyroid cancer, at least 1 month must be allowed to pass following the administration of contrast for iodine to "wash out" through urinary excretion prior to eligibility for therapeutic radioactive iodine [3]. Different contrast media preparations release iodine at different rates, requiring tailoring of new recommendations to individual contrast agents. These clinical applications are both mediated by the Wolff–Chaikoff effect.

Radiation Safety Applications

The Wolff–Chaikoff effect carries a number of societal implications that extend beyond the realm of patient care. At present, more than 400 nuclear power plants are functioning worldwide, providing approximately 15 % of the world's energy [4]. Radioactive iodine isotopes, including I^{129} and I^{131}, are volatile products of nuclear fission that have the potential to disperse rapidly into the environment unless properly contained. I^{129} has a half-life of 15.7 million years, and thus is not a safety concern, but it can be used for long-term monitoring of artificial products of nuclear fission. In contrast, I^{131} is a beta-emitting isotope with a relatively short half-life of 8 days; ionizing radiation from I^{131} exposure can lead to thyroid injury, thyroiditis, and increased risk of thyroid cancer. As evidenced by the rise in thyroid cancer incidence in Belarus and Ukraine following the 1986 Chernobyl nuclear disaster, the accidental release of radioactive I^{131} from nuclear power plants can have serious deleterious health effects [5]. Despite progress in nuclear safety over time, the recent Fukushima Daiichi nuclear accident (which released approximately 10 % of the amount of radioactive iodine that was released during the Chernobyl accident) highlights the continued importance of population preparedness for nuclear fallout [6].

In the event of a nuclear power plant accident, the prophylactic administration of iodine will prevent thyroidal uptake and concentration of radioactive iodine isotopes via the Wolff–Chaikoff effect. Ideally, the prophylactic dose should be distributed in advance, within a large radius around any nuclear reactors. Following the Chernobyl accident, potassium iodide was widely distributed by the Polish government to children and the elderly. In the USA, the Public Health Security and Bioterrorism Preparedness and Response Act of 2002 states that the federal government will provide potassium iodide for distribution in a 10-mile radius around all domestic nuclear reactors [7]. However, the governing bodies of many reactors have waived this provision, arguing that evacuation and sheltering are more effective means of preventing radiation poisoning.

Though prophylactic iodide supplementation is often discussed in the setting of possible terrorist attacks involving a "dirty bomb" device, it would likely be of little practical use. A dirty bomb is a theoretical weapon that would use conventional explosives to disperse radioactive material. The wide dispersal area of radioactive particles would make dirty bombs a tool for generating injury, panic, and fear, though the doses of radiation exposure would likely be nonlethal. If such a device were to contain radioactive iodine, then prophylactic iodine would help reduce thyroidal uptake of the radioactive material. However, dirty bombs are very unlikely to contain I^{131} in large amounts, and iodine supplementation would not protect against other radioactive materials. If a dirty bomb were to be employed, it would more likely utilize radioactive materials with a longer half-life, such as strontium-90 (half-life 29 years). The radioactivity of other fissile, biologically hazardous materials would have rapidly decayed before such a device could be detonated. In the event of a nonradioactive iodine-based bomb, only evacuation and sheltering would be effective in preventing or minimizing radiation exposure.

Acknowledgments A special thanks to Dr. Jan Wolff for sharing his experiences and expertise.

Editors' Note: We want to thank the authors and Dr. Wolff for taking the time to get together with the authors to provide such exquisite detail for this chapter.

References

1. Wolff J, Chaikoff IL. Plasma inorganic iodide as a homeostatic regulator of thyroid function. J Biol Chem. 1948;174(2):555–64.
2. Eng PH, Cardona GR, Fang SL, et al. Escape from the acute Wolff–Chaikoff effect is associated with a decrease in thyroid sodium/iodide symporter messenger ribonucleic acid and protein. Endocrinology. 1999;140(8):3404–10.
3. Padovani RP, Kasamatsu TS, Nakabashi CC, et al. One month is sufficient for urinary iodine to return to its baseline value after the use of water-soluble iodinated contrast agents in post-thyroidectomy patients requiring radioiodine therapy. Thyroid. 2012 Sep;22(9):926–30.
4. Britannica E. Nuclear power. Encyclopædia Britannica Online 2014. 2014. http://www.britannica.com/EBchecked/topic/421749/nuclear-power. Accessed 28 May 2014.
5. Robbins J, Schneider AB. Radioiodine-induced thyroid cancer: studies in the aftermath of the accident at Chernobyl. Trends Endocrinol Metab: TEM. 1998 Apr;9(3):87–94.
6. Schneider AB, Smith JM. Potassium iodide prophylaxis: what have we learned and questions raised by the accident at the Fukushima Daiichi Nuclear Power Plant. Thyroid. 2012 Apr;22(4):344–6.
7. Congress US. Public health security and bioterrorism preparedness and response act of 2002. Public Law. 2002;107(188):188.

Hyperthyroidism and Thyroiditis

Kepal N. Patel

Hyperthyroidism

Hyperthyroidism is the overproduction of thyroid hormones resulting in thyrotoxicosis. Symptoms of hyperthyroidism can vary depending on the severity of thyrotoxicosis and the age of the patient. Common symptoms include nervousness, increased sweating and heat intolerance, palpitations, fatigue, weight loss, dyspnea, and weakness. These symptoms are often well tolerated in younger patients. Older patients can present with cardiovascular symptoms, depression, lethargy, and weakness (termed "apathetic hyperthyroidism") [1]. The diagnosis is made on the basis of elevated free T4 or T3 level and suppressed thyroid-stimulating hormone (TSH) level. In subclinical hyperthyroidism, the mildest form of hyperthyroidism, only the TSH is abnormal.

The most common cause of hyperthyroidism is Graves' disease, an autoimmune disease resulting in production of TSH-receptor-stimulating antibodies. Other causes include toxic adenoma, toxic multinodular goiter (TMG), postpartum thyroiditis, and subacute and rarely suppurative thyroiditis. Symptoms are similar but can vary depending on the degree of thyroiditis and patients with **Graves'** disease may have symptoms related to the nonthyroidal manifestations (exophthalmos, dermopathy, acropachy). The diagnosis is often made on clinical presentation and examination; however, studies such as iodine-123 scans (I-123), ultrasonography (US), and laboratory values are required for an accurate diagnosis. Treatment strategies are tailored to the etiology and the individual patient and can range from medical management to surgical intervention.

Graves' Disease

Graves' disease is the most common type of thyrotoxicosis affecting approximately 2 % of women and 0.2 % of men [2, 3]. The peak incidence is in the third to fourth decades of life. In the USA, it accounts for 75 % of thyrotoxic patients [4]. In Graves' disease, the thyrotropin receptor on the follicular cells is the target for thyroid autoantibodies that bind to these receptors, stimulating them just as TSH triggers the receptor. This results in constant autonomous thyroid function, hyperthyroidism, and diffuse enlargement of the thyroid gland without focal nodules, referred to as diffuse toxic goiter. Pathologically, there is diffuse hyperplasia of the follicular epithelial cells and depletion of colloid, with increased vascularity. In addition to the autoimmune basis for Graves' disease, other factors likely play an important role. Graves' disease is likely the result of a complex interaction between autoimmune, genetic, and environmental factors.

The autoimmune basis for Graves' disease involves a group of immunoglobulin G (IgG) autoantibodies that are produced by B lymphocytes which bind and activate the thyrotropin or TSH receptor (TSHR). These IgG antibodies are variably termed thyroid-stimulating antibody (TSAb), thyroid-stimulating immunoglobulin (TSI), or thyrotropin receptor antibody (TRAb), and stimulate the thyrocyte in a similar fashion to TSH, causing secretion of T3 and T4, resulting in hyperthyroidism [5]. Serologic tests (i.e., TSI level) can help confirm the diagnosis of Graves' disease in patients with hyperthyroidism. The initiating cause for the production of the autoantibodies is still unknown. Environmental and genetic factors may play a role.

Studies of monozygotic twins have shown that Graves' disease may have a genetic component with a familial predisposition. Concordance rates of disease occurrence as high as 60 % have been reported in monozygotic twins. This is in contrast to 3–9 % in dizygotic twins and 0.2 % of the general population [6].

An environmental influence, or some sort of triggering event, has long been sought as a contributing factor to the

K. N. Patel (✉)
Division of Endocrine Surgery, Surgery, Otoloaryngology
and Biochemistry, NYU Langone Medical Center, 530 First Ave.,
Suite 6H, New York, NY 10016, USA
e-mail: Kepal.Patel@nyumc.org

J. L. Pasieka, J. A. Lee (eds.), *Surgical Endocrinopathies*, DOI 10.1007/978-3-319-13662-2_5,
© Springer International Publishing Switzerland 2015

Table 1 Symptoms and signs of Graves' disease

Symptoms
Nervousness
Heat intolerance
Insomnia
Anxiety
Hyperhidrosis
Weight loss
Fatigue
Muscle weakness
Decreased menstrual flow
Palpitations
Signs
Tachycardia
Ophthalmopathy
Dermopathy (pretibial myxedema)
Proximal muscle weakness
Diffuse goiter (+/− bruit)
Fine tremor
Spooning of nails

Table 2 Radionuclide scanning and hyperthyroidism

Scan findings
Graves' disease intense diffuse uptake
Toxic adenoma focal uptake with suppressed adjacent tissue
Toxic multinodular goiter areas of patchy uptake

development of Graves' disease. Although bacteria, viruses, tobacco, and stress have been implicated in the pathogenesis of Graves' disease, there is no clear evidence of cause and effect.

The clinical features of Graves' disease are listed in Table 1. The hyperthyroid features of Graves' disease are nonspecific and occur with all types of thyrotoxicosis, regardless of etiology including tachycardia, widened pulse pressure, warm skin, proximal muscle weakness, and fine tremor. Unique features of Graves' disease include ophthalmopathy (proptosis) and dermopathy (pretibial myxedema).

Graves' disease is characterized by suppressed TSH level and an elevated serum-free T4. The suppressed TSH level helps exclude other conditions in which the serum T4 may be elevated, such as estrogen therapy, nonthyroidal illness, TSH-secreting pituitary adenoma, or central thyroid hormone resistance [7].

Once the diagnosis of thyrotoxicosis is established, radionuclide scintigraphy may be useful in differentiating Graves' disease from other causes of hyperthyroidism. In Graves' disease, the thyroid gland is diffusely enlarged with intense, diffuse radiotracer uptake often as high as 80 % in 24 h. The uptake is homogeneous whereas in TMG there are areas of both increased and decreased uptake. The overall uptake in TMG is not as avid as in Graves' disease. In toxic adenoma, there is focal uptake in a single nodule, often with suppression of the remaining normal glandular tissue (Table 2).

On ultrasound, patients with Graves' disease have a diffusely enlarged thyroid gland, with a smooth but lobular surface contour. The thyroid gland may range from being isoechoic to diffusely hypoechoic, and is typically homogeneous and with increased vascularity often referred to as "the thyroid inferno" [8].

The treatment of Graves' disease is directed at decreasing the B-adrenergic symptoms by administering a B-blocking drug and inhibiting the synthesis and release of thyroid hormone thus reversing the catabolic effects. B-blocking agents such as propranolol and atenolol can quickly reduce symptoms of palpitations, nervousness, sweating, and tremor. Inhibition of thyroid hormone synthesis and release can be achieved by thionamide drugs, radioiodine (RAI) therapy, and surgery (Table 3).

The two most common thionamide drugs are methimazole (Tapazole, MMI) and propylthiouracil (PTU). Both agents are equally effective. MMI has a greater potency and longer biological half-life, whereas PTU has the theoretical advantage of a more rapid fall in serum T3 levels because of its property of inhibiting peripheral conversion of T4 to T3 [9]. Biochemical euthyroidism is usually established within 6–8 weeks and doses are adjusted accordingly. The drugs are well tolerated with minimal side effects. Approximately 20 % of patients are allergic to both agents, necessitating the use of RAI or surgery. The most serious side effect of the drugs is agranulocytosis, which is rare and can occur in 0.2–0.5 % of patients, and can be fatal. However, elevations in liver enzymes may also necessitate cessation of thionamides [10, 11].

Complete remission rates with thionamides vary considerably; however, studies have shown up to 75 % remission rate with high-dose therapy. Most relapses following cessation of thionamide therapy occur shortly after the drugs are discontinued. In some cases, relapses can occur even several years later; therefore, these patients need to be followed closely for extended periods of time. Patients who fail thionamide therapy will require definitive therapy, either RAI or total thyroidectomy.

In the USA, RAI therapy is the most common choice of therapy for Graves' disease [12]. Its benefits include general effectiveness, relatively low expense, and minimal side effects. However, RAI therapy may take months to have an effect. The most common side effect is dry mouth which may be temporary and in rare cases permanent. The most considerable side effect is hypothyroidism which is actually the intended goal of therapy. The risk of secondary malignancies from RAI therapy for Graves' disease is very small and usually not considered significant for adult patients [13, 14]. The risk of developing deleterious genetic, carcinogenic, teratogenic, and reproductive effects from RAI therapy for Graves' disease is negligible [15–17]. Contraindications for

Table 3 Hyperthyroidism and treatment options

	Thionamides	RAI	Surgery
Graves' disease	a	a	a
Toxic adenoma	–	c	a
Toxic multinodular goiter	–	b	a

a Recommended
b Sometimes recommended
c Rarely recommended
(–) Not recommended
RAI radioiodine

RAI therapy include pediatric age, pregnancy, and nursing mothers. Patients treated with RAI therapy should avoid becoming pregnant for at least 6 months [15].

Surgical management of Graves' disease is becoming more common in the USA [18]. Advantages to surgery include its high success rate, rapid onset of effect, and relative safety. Both thionamide and RAI therapy can take weeks to months to achieve euthyroidism. Thyroidectomy offers immediate therapeutic response. The risk of surgery, including hypoparathyroidism and vocal cord paralysis, is very low in high-volume surgeons [18, 19]. Unlike the high relapse rate after discontinuation of thionamides, surgery reliably provides a cure with only a small chance of recurrent hyperthyroidism.

Patients who would certainly benefit from surgery are those with large goiters likely to be resistant to RAI, patients with compressive symptoms, and those with coincidental thyroid nodules concerning for malignancy. Approximately 13 % of patients with Graves' disease have thyroid nodules suspicious for carcinoma [20]. Studies have shown that the incidence of malignancy for a solid, cold nodule is the same as for a patient without the disease, 15–20 %. Some studies suggest that thyroid carcinoma in patients with Graves' disease is more likely to be aggressive, with increased lymph node metastasis and local invasion [21, 22]. Multiple other studies report no difference in the prognosis of carcinoma for patients with or without Graves' disease.

Other indications for surgical management of Graves' disease include medically noncompliant patients, thyroid storm unresponsive to medical therapy, amiodarone-induced thyrotoxicosis, and thyroid-associated ophthalmopathy (TAO). TAO can be seen in up to 50 % of patients with Graves' disease [23]. Some studies have shown that total thyroid ablation by surgery or RAI decreases initiation and halts progression of TAO [24–26]. Studies have also reported that RAI may worsen TAO. Of the two ablative therapies, surgery appears to be more effective than RAI.

Preoperative preparation is recommended to avoid intraoperative or postoperative thyroid storm. Many different regimens have been utilized. Most regimens consist of a combination of thionamide therapy, iodine (SSKI, Lugol's solution), and/or B-blocking agent. The choice of operation also varies based on surgeon preference and should be individualized for each patient. The three main operations are total thyroidectomy, bilateral subtotal thyroidectomy, and total lobectomy with contralateral subtotal lobectomy. The goal is to avoid hypoparathyroidism and injury to the recurrent laryngeal nerves, and at the same time minimize the chance of recurrent hyperthyroidism. Most authors recommend total thyroidectomy when possible. The other options leave remnant tissue and are associated with an increased rate of recurrent hyperthyroidism. After surgery, most patients are rendered hypothyroid and life-long thyroid hormone replacement therapy should be anticipated.

Toxic Nodular Goiter

The term toxic nodular goiter refers to two entities: toxic adenoma, implying a single lesion, and toxic multinodular goiter (TMG), in which more than one hyperfunctioning nodule exists. Toxic nodular goiter was first described as a type of thyrotoxicosis clinically distinct from Graves' disease by **Henry Plummer** in 1913. Often the term Plummer's disease is used to describe thyrotoxicosis resulting from either a single nodule or multiple autonomous nodules.

Toxic Adenoma

Toxic adenomas are discrete, solitary nodules that may occur at any age. They are most common in the third to fourth decade of life and they are rare in children [27, 28]. Toxic adenoma synthesizes and secretes thyroid hormone independent of TSH control. This results in TSH suppression, with increased T3 and T4 levels. Usually the nodule is the only functioning tissue with the extranodular tissue becoming dormant. This is highlighted in the hotspots seen with radionuclide scanning (Table 2). Toxic adenomas seem to be more prevalent in regions of iodine deficiency and recently it has been shown that a mutation of the gene for the TSHR may be associated with their development. This mutation results in the constitutive activation of the cyclic adenosine monophosphate (cAMP) cascade, causing hypersecretion of thyroid hormone and tissue growth [29–32].

Most toxic adenomas are follicular adenomas with carcinoma being very rare. Hyperthyroidism usually does not occur until the nodule is 2.5–3.0 cm in diameter. The symptoms and signs of hyperthyroidism are milder than in Graves' disease and do not include ophthalmopathy and dermopathy. The diagnosis is usually established by a suppressed TSH and elevated free T3 or free T4 levels. In subclinical thyrotoxicosis, serum levels of T3 and T4 may be normal. Confirmation of the diagnosis may require radionuclide scanning, showing concentration of RAI in the nodule with inhibition of RAI uptake in surrounding thyroid tissue. Fine-needle aspiration biopsy of toxic adenomas is not recommended. They are rarely malignant and more importantly, cytologic features of toxic adenomas can be misleading. These lesions often exhibit cellular atypia suggestive of a follicular neoplasm or well differentiated thyroid cancer [33].

The treatment for toxic adenomas is either ablation or surgery (Table 3). Unlike Graves' disease, there is no role for thionamides in the management of toxic adenomas. Long-lasting remission rarely occurs with thionamide therapy and after therapy is stopped, the chance of recurrent hyperthyroidism is high. Radioiodine therapy can be effective but the doses required are usually higher than those used in Graves' disease. Also, complete nodule regression with RAI therapy is not common and continued surveillance is necessary. This makes RAI therapy less desirable than surgery. Sclerosing agents such as ethanol have been shown to be effective in several small series [34, 35]. However, multiple injections are often needed (3–13) and exacerbation of hyperthyroidism and temporary vocal cord paralysis have been reported with ethanol injection [36, 37].

Surgery is commonly employed in the treatment of toxic adenomas and is usually the treatment of choice. Unilateral thyroid lobectomy is the preferred procedure by most authors. It is very effective with low risk of hypothyroidism since the contralateral lobe is not removed. Surgery also provides tissue for pathologic diagnosis in the rare cases of suspected carcinoma.

Toxic Multinodular Goiter

The prevalence of TMG is significantly higher in areas of endemic goiter and iodine deficiency. In areas where iodine repletion has occurred, the prevalence of TMG has decreased [38]. A genetic predisposition and female gender also seem to play a role in the development of TMG.

TMG seems to evolve over many years from sporadic, diffuse goiter to the development of functional autonomy and eventual clinical thyrotoxicosis. The pathogenesis of TMG likely involves iodine deficiency which leads to a decreased production of thyroid hormone, resulting in an increase in TSH secretion, promoting goiter formation [39, 40]. Multiple nodules develop which in time become autonomous. Autonomous areas eventually grow large enough to secrete increased amounts of thyroid hormone and suppress TSH. Hyperthyroidism can be precipitated in nontoxic multinodu-

lar goiter both with autonomy and without autonomy and in TMG by iodides (i.e., intravenous (IV) contrast media) [41]. This is referred to as the **Jod-Basedow** phenomenon.

Due to the many years it takes to develop, TMG generally occurs in older persons. The hyperthyroidism tends to be insidious in onset, may be mild to severe, and is unaccompanied by the infiltrative ophthalmopathy and dermopathy of Graves' disease. In older patients, the hyperthyroidism may be masked and the patient may present with cardiac findings such as atrial fibrillation, tachycardia, congestive heart failure, angina, weight loss, anxiety, insomnia, or muscle wasting. Patients with TMG often have no thyromegaly on clinical examination.

The diagnosis of TMG is a clinical one, based on physical examination and laboratory confirmation. Serum levels of free T3 and free T4 are elevated with a suppressed TSH. Radionuclide scanning reveals a multinodular gland with areas of increased patchy uptake (Table 2).

The principal treatment options for TMG include RAI therapy or surgery (Table 3). Since remission does not occur with TMG, the long-term use of thionamides is not indicated unless there are contraindications to the use of RAI therapy or surgery. Patients with TMG often require multiple doses of RAI to control hyperthyroidism because of the larger gland size and lower uptake of RAI, when compared to patients with Graves' disease. Although RAI treats the hyperthyroidism, studies show that it does not significantly reduce goiter size, compressive symptoms, or substernal extension, because TMG contains areas of fibrosis, calcifications, and nonfunctioning nodules [42, 43].

Surgery is usually recommended in younger, healthier patients with large goiters and/or compressive symptoms. Either bilateral subtotal thyroidectomy or total thyroidectomy is the preferred operation. Bilateral subtotal thyroidectomy has the potential advantage of decreased hypoparathyroidism, decreased vocal cord paralysis, and decreased hypothyroidism. However, the incidence of recurrent hyperthyroidism is greater than in total thyroidectomy patients. Total thyroidectomy results in near-zero recurrence but nearly all patients are rendered hypothyroid, requiring thyroid hormone supplementation. Total thyroidectomy for patients with TMG is a safe operation in experienced hands with low rates of hypoparathyroidism and vocal cord paralysis [44].

Thyroiditis

Thyroiditis, infiltration of the thyroid gland with inflammatory cells, may be seen in a diverse group of autoimmune, inflammatory, and infectious processes. It comprises a diverse group of disorders that are among the most common endocrine abnormalities encountered. The diagnosis of thyroiditis is based on the clinical presentation and laboratory

Table 4 Different types of thyroiditis

Hashimoto's thyroiditis (chronic lymphocytic thyroiditis)
Subacute (painless) lymphocytic thyroiditis
Sporadic silent thyroiditis
Postpartum thyroiditis
Subacute (painful) granulomatous thyroiditis (de Quervain's thyroiditis, giant cell thyroiditis)
Acute suppurative thyroiditis
Riedel struma (Riedel's thyroiditis, invasive fibrous thyroiditis)

analysis of thyroid function. Thyroiditis can be classified as (1) chronic, which includes Hashimoto's thyroiditis and Riedel struma, (2) subacute, which includes lymphocytic and granulomatous, and (3) acute suppurative, which is rare (Table 4).

Hashimoto's Thyroiditis

Hashimoto's thyroiditis, also called chronic lymphocytic thyroiditis, is the prototypical autoimmune thyroiditis. Hashimoto's is the most common cause of goiter and hypothyroidism in the USA and affects approximately 2% of the general population [45]. **Hakaru Hashimoto** first described this disorder in 1912 and termed it "struma lymphomatosa."

Pathologically, the thyroid gland is initially enlarged and has lymphocytic and plasma-cell infiltration, follicular cell atrophy, and interlobular fibrosis, eventually leading to a shrunken fibrotic gland [46]. The normal follicular cells are altered and often replaced with pink oxyphilic or Hurthle cells. Classically, Hashimoto's thyroiditis occurs as a painless diffuse goiter in young to middle-aged women in their third and fourth decades and is frequently associated with asymptomatic hypothyroidism [47]. Hashimoto's thyroiditis has also been reported to occur with increased frequency in patients with other autoimmune disorders such as lupus, Graves' disease, and pernicious anemia [48].

The hallmarks of this disorder are high circulating titers of antibodies to thyroid peroxidase (90% of patients) and thyroglobulin (20–50% of patients). Antibodies to the TSHR have also been identified. The inciting event that triggers the development of antithyroid antibodies remains unclear. There does appear to be a genetic predisposition, with reported associations with human leukocyte antigen (HLA)-DR3, HLA-DR5, and HLA-B8 [49–51]. Viral etiologies and smoking have also been implicated. Although the exact pathogenesis is not known, it is clear that thyroid autoimmunity drives the lymphocytic collection and is responsible for thyroid epithelial cell damage. Progressive, immune-mediated thyroid cell damage leads to goiter formation and thyroid gland failure.

The clinical presentation varies, depending on the stage at the time of presentation. The patient may be completely asymptomatic or present with hypothyroid symptoms. Physical examination typically reveals a firm, bumpy, nontender goiter, often symmetric, with a palpable pyramidal lobe. Usually there are no discrete nodules. Single or dominant nodules should be evaluated and if indicated a fine-needle aspiration biopsy should be performed to exclude malignancy. Thyroid hormone levels may also vary based on time of presentation. They may be normal with a normal TSH (euthyroid), low with an elevated TSH (hypothyroid), or normal with an elevated TSH (subclinically hypothyroid). Euthyroid individuals with Hashimoto's thyroiditis develop hypothyroidism at a rate of approximately 5% per year [52]. Mild thyrotoxicosis ("Hashitoxicosis") has been reported to be the initial presentation in up to 5% of patients with Hashimoto's thyroiditis [53]. The clinical course for Hashimoto's thyroiditis is variable. Up to 50% of patients can become subclinically hypothyroid and 5–40% can become clinically hypothyroid, emphasizing the importance of following thyroid function tests in these patients [54].

Imaging studies for Hashimoto's thyroiditis are not particularly useful. Radionuclide scanning usually reveals patchy nonspecific uptake with minimal clinical significance. Ultrasound reveals marked hypoechogenicity with coarse echogenic bands. If a dominant nodule is found, then follow-up with repeat sonography and/or fine-needle biopsy may be warranted. Patients with Hashimoto's thyroiditis can be at increased risk of developing B-cell lymphoma, and as such, rapid growth in the setting of Hashimoto's thyroiditis should raise concern about the possibility of thyroid lymphoma [55, 56].

The treatment of Hashimoto's thyroiditis consists of thyroid hormone replacement for hypothyroidism. Levothyroxine is the hormone of choice for replacement therapy because of its consistent potency and prolonged duration of action. In patients who remain symptomatic on levothyroxine alone, combination therapy with liothyronine may be beneficial. Surgery is indicated only for large symptomatic goiters or persistent painful Hashimoto's thyroiditis.

Subacute (Painless) Lymphocytic Thyroiditis

There are two forms of painless thyroiditis, sporadic silent and postpartum, both sharing very similar features. It is characterized by destruction of the thyroid gland by lymphocytes (destruction-induced thyroiditis), absence of pain, and temporary thyroid dysfunction. Sporadic silent thyroiditis and postpartum thyroiditis are probably variants of the same disorder, distinguished only by their relationship to pregnancy.

The etiology is unclear, but the immune system is likely involved because it has been found in patients with a wide variety of autoimmune diseases. HLA-DR3 is present in increased frequency in both sporadic and postpartum thyroiditis [57]. HLA-DR5 is also increased in frequency in postpartum thyroiditis [57]. Histopathology shows extensive lymphocytic infiltration, collapsed follicles, and degeneration of follicular cells [58, 59]. The changes can be either focal or diffuse, with lymphoid follicles being present in about half of the patients [59]. Unlike Hashimoto's thyroiditis, there is usually no stromal fibrosis, oxyphilic changes, or germinal centers.

Clinically, the patient typically passes through four phases: thyrotoxic, euthyroid, hypothyroid, and euthyroid, although not all phases are seen in all patients. The initial thyrotoxicosis is caused by a release of preformed hormone and not because of sustained overproduction of the hormone and therefore is not true hyperthyroidism [60]. The thyrotoxicosis typically lasts from 3 to 6 months but can persist up to a year. Postpartum thyroiditis typically occurs 4–6 weeks following delivery. It occurs in up to 5% of postpartum women and may recur with subsequent pregnancy [61]. The process usually resolves after transient hypothyroidism; however, some patients (20%) progress to chronic lymphocytic thyroiditis.

Symptoms are generally mild; however, in certain cases they can be severe. The initial thyrotoxic phase in postpartum thyroiditis is usually milder than in sporadic silent thyroiditis. The thyroid is symmetrical, slightly enlarged, and painless. The erythrocyte sedimentation rate (ESR) is usually normal. Because the hyperthyroid phase is usually transient and mild, most patients do not require treatment.

Subacute (Painful) Granulomatous Thyroiditis

Subacute granulomatous thyroiditis is also referred to as de Quervain's thyroiditis, giant cell thyroiditis, pseudogranulomatous thyroiditis, and subacute painful thyroiditis. The pathology of this disorder was first described by **Fritz de Quervain** in 1904 [62]. He showed giant cells and granulomatous changes in the thyroid gland of affected patients.

Like sporadic silent and postpartum thyroiditis, subacute granulomatous thyroiditis is a spontaneous, remitting, inflammatory disorder that may last for weeks to months. As with other thyroid disorders, subacute granulomatous thyroiditis is more common in women, with a peak incidence in the fourth and fifth decades of life and is rarely seen in children or the elderly [62].

The pathogenesis of subacute granulomatous thyroiditis is unclear. It does not seem to be an autoimmune disease. A viral etiology has been implicated; however, the evidence is largely indirect [63–65]. Subacute thyroiditis has been associated with adenovirus, Coxsackie, Epstein–Barr, and influenza viruses [66, 67]. Subacute granulomatous thyroiditis often follows an upper respiratory tract infection and occasionally includes a prodromal phase of muscular aches, pains, fever, and malaise. The primary events in the pathology of subacute granulomatous thyroiditis are destruction of the follicular epithelium and loss of follicular integrity; however, the histopathological changes are distinct from those found in Hashimoto's thyroiditis. The characteristic follicular lesion is a central core of colloid surrounded by multinucleate giant cells. These lesions progress to form granulomas [68, 69].

The most prominent physical finding is an enlarged thyroid gland that is exquisitely tender to palpation. The pain is usually constant, gradual to sudden in onset, and often severe, involving the entire thyroid gland. Pain is often aggravated by turning the head or swallowing and may radiate to the jaw, ear, or occiput on the ipsilateral side. Frequently, patients present with tachycardia and hyperpyrexia, with temperatures elevated up to 102 °F. Unlike subacute (painless) lymphocytic thyroiditis, the ESR is consistently high and the white blood cell count may be elevated. Thyroid function tests may be normal, elevated, or low depending on the stage of the disease at the time of presentation. The clinical course of subacute granulomatous thyroiditis is self-limited and is similar to painless thyroiditis. Similar to painless thyroiditis, patients go through the initial phases of thyrotoxicosis for a few months. The thyrotoxicosis is a result of the release of stored thyroid hormones from acute destruction of the thyroid parenchyma. Subsequent to that, they become euthyroid. In rare, severe cases, patients can then develop hypothyroidism which is usually transient with 90% of the patients returning to a euthyroid state.

Salicylates and nonsteroidal anti-inflammatory drugs are often adequate to decrease pain in mild to moderate cases. In more severe cases, oral glucocorticoids may provide dramatic relief of pain and swelling.

Acute Suppurative Thyroiditis

This rare entity usually occurs from a bacterial infection and rarely from nonbacterial infections of the thyroid [70]. This disease tends to affect younger patients and typically occurs in the 30s to 40s. The pathogenesis primarily involves decreased resistance of the thyroid gland to infection. Infection may reach the gland via blood, lymphatics, or directly through a persistent thyroglossal duct or a nearby internal fistula such as a piriform sinus fistula [71]. Bacterial thyroiditis is often preceded by an upper respiratory infection.

Treatment of acute bacterial thyroiditis requires admission to the hospital, drainage of any abscess and parenteral antimicrobial therapy aimed at the causative agent. Since a piriform sinus fistula is a very common route of infection in bacterial thyroiditis, a barium swallow, computed tomography (CT), or magnetic resonance imaging (MRI), and possibly hypopharynx endoscopy should be performed to look for communicating fistulas in most patients with their first episode and in all patients with recurrent episodes. Such fistulas must be surgically excised for definitive cure and prevention of recurrent infection [72, 73]. In the adult, *Staphylococcus aureus* and *Streptococcus pyogenes* are the offending pathogens in approximately 80% of patients [70]. Mortality has markedly improved for acute bacterial thyroiditis, from 25% down to 8.6% in recent years [70]. However, the mortality is close to 100% if the diagnosis is delayed and antimicrobial therapy not initiated [70].

Nonbacterial infection of the thyroid gland is very rare. Known causes are *Aspergillus, Coccidioides immitis, and Candida*. The treatment consists of appropriate antimicrobial therapy and analgesics.

Riedel Struma

Also known as invasive fibrous thyroiditis or Riedel's thyroiditis, it is a very rare disorder of unknown etiology which is characterized by intense infiltration of the thyroid parenchyma by inflammatory cells and subsequent replacement by dense fibrosis and collagen [74]. This disorder results in an extremely fibrotic thyroid gland. Riedel's thyroiditis is not a primary disorder of the thyroid but involves the thyroid and represents a systemic disease. This disease may involve other sites such as the mediastinum, orbit, retroperitoneum, and biliary tract. It is named after Bernhard Riedel, who initially described this entity in 1893. Riedel struma affects mainly women in their fourth to fifth decade of life.

The clinical presentation is a painless goiter which is firm, fixed, and "woody" in texture [74]. The extensive, progressive fibrosis may eventually cause compression of the trachea and esophagus. Most patients are euthyroid, but may progress to hypothyroidism when the gland is sufficiently replaced by the fibroid tissue. The clinical presentation may be confused with an aggressive thyroid malignancy such as anaplastic carcinoma. Imaging studies and fine-needle aspiration or open biopsy can help differentiate the two. Unlike the CT findings of locally advanced thyroid malignancies, in Riedel struma the infiltrative mass is isodense with the neck muscles, hypodense with the normal thyroid tissue, and does not enhance with contrast [75, 76].

This condition is benign and usually self-limiting. Nonetheless, surgery may be warranted to alleviate compression symptoms. Extensive resection is often impossible, but wedge resections, especially over the isthmus, to relieve tracheal compression, can be very effective [77]. Recurrent obstruction after resection is rare. Medical therapy, especially if started early, may be successful in preventing compressive symptoms. Effective agents include corticosteroids, tamoxifen, and methotrexate [78–81].

Key Summary Points

- The most common cause of hyperthyroidism is Graves' disease.
- Graves' disease is an autoimmune disease.
- Graves' disease may have nonthyroidal symptoms such as exophthalmos and dermopathy.
- Surgery can be performed safely with excellent results for patients with Graves' disease and toxic nodular goiter.
- Thyroiditis comprises a diverse group of disorders ranging from chronic, subacute, and acute.
- Hashimoto's thyroiditis is the most common cause of goiter and hypothyroidism in the USA.
- Treatment for thyroiditis is focused on relieving the symptoms and correcting thyroid hormone levels.

References

1. Campbell AJ. Thyroid disorders in the elderly. Difficulties in diagnosis and treatment. Drugs. 1986;31(5):455–61.
2. Vanderpump MP, et al. The incidence of thyroid disorders in the community: a twenty-year follow-up of the Whickham Survey. Clin Endocrinol (Oxf). 1995;43(1):55–68.
3. Tunbridge WM, et al. The spectrum of thyroid disease in a community: the Whickham survey. Clin Endocrinol (Oxf). 1977;7(6):481–93.
4. Pearce EN, Braverman LE. Hyperthyroidism: advantages and disadvantages of medical therapy. Surg Clin North Am. 2004;84(3):833–47.
5. Baker JR Jr. Immunologic aspects of endocrine diseases. JAMA. 1992;268(20):2899–903.
6. Stenszky V, et al. The genetics of Graves' disease: HLA and disease susceptibility. J Clin Endocrinol Metab. 1985;61(4):735–40.
7. McDermott MT, Ridgway EC. Central hyperthyroidism. Endocrinol Metab Clin North Am. 1998;27(1):187–203.
8. Ralls PW, et al. Color-flow Doppler sonography in Graves disease: "thyroid inferno". AJR Am J Roentgenol. 1988;150(4):781–4.
9. Chopra IJ. A study of extrathyroidal conversion of thyroxine (T4) to 3,3',5-triiodothyronine (T3) in vitro. Endocrinology. 1977;101(2):453–63.
10. Cooper DS. Antithyroid drugs. N Engl J Med. 1984;311(21):1353–62.
11. Cooper DS, et al. Agranulocytosis associated with antithyroid drugs. Effects of patient age and drug dose. Ann Intern Med. 1983;98(1):26–9.
12. Graham GD, Burman KD. Radioiodine treatment of Graves' disease. An assessment of its potential risks. Ann Intern Med. 1986;105(6):900–5.
13. Saenger EL, Thoma GE, Tompkins EA., Incidence of leukemia following treatment of hyperthyroidism. Preliminary report of the cooperative thyrotoxicosis therapy follow-up study. JAMA. 1968;205(12):855–62.

14. Ron E, et al. Cancer mortality following treatment for adult hyperthyroidism. Cooperative thyrotoxicosis therapy follow-up study group. JAMA. 1998;280(4):347–55.

15. Dobyns BM, et al. Malignant and benign neoplasms of the thyroid in patients treated for hyperthyroidism: a report of the cooperative thyrotoxicosis therapy follow-up study. J Clin Endocrinol Metab. 1974;38(6):976–98.

16. Safa AM, Schumacher OP, Rodriguez-Antunez A. Long-term follow-up results in children and adolescents treated with radioactive iodine (131I) for hyperthyroidism. N Engl J Med. 1975;292(4):167–71.

17. Fujii H. A long-term follow-up study of late-onset hypothyroidism and prognosis of hyperthyroid patients treated with radioiodine. Kaku Igaku. 1991;28(9):1067–73.

18. Liu J, et al. Total thyroidectomy: a safe and effective treatment for Graves' disease. J Surg Res. 2011;168(1):1–4.

19. Prasai A, et al. Total thyroidectomy for safe and definitive management of Graves' disease. J Laryngol Otol. 2013;127(7):681–4.

20. Carnell NE, Valente WA. Thyroid nodules in Graves' disease: classification, characterization, and response to treatment. Thyroid. 1998;8(7):571–6.

21. Ozaki O, et al. Thyroid carcinoma in Graves' disease. World J Surg. 1990;14(3):437–40, discussion 440–1.

22. Behar R, et al. Graves' disease and thyroid cancer. Surgery. 1986;100(6):1121–7.

23. Falk SA, Birken EA, Ronquillo AH. Graves' disease associated with histologic Hashimoto's thyroiditis. Otolaryngol Head Neck Surg. 1985;93(1):86–91.

24. Gwinup G, Elias AN, Ascher MS. Effect on exophthalmos of various methods of treatment of Graves' disease. JAMA. 1982;247(15):2135–8.

25. Marushak D, Faurschou S, Blichert-Toft M. Regression of ophthalmopathy in Graves' disease following thyroidectomy. A systematic study of changes of ocular signs. Acta Ophthalmol (Copenh). 1984;62(5):767–79.

26. Vana S, et al. Surgical treatment of endocrine orbital disease. Indications, methods, results. Vnitr Lek. 1992;38(9):897–902.

27. Hamburger JI. Evolution of toxicity in solitary nontoxic autonomously functioning thyroid nodules. J Clin Endocrinol Metab. 1980;50(6):1089–93.

28. Hamburger JI. Solitary autonomously functioning thyroid lesions. Diagnosis, clinical features and pathogenetic considerations. Am J Med. 1975;58(6):740–8.

29. Russo D, et al. Thyrotropin receptor gene alterations in thyroid hyperfunctioning adenomas. J Clin Endocrinol Metab. 1996;81(4):1548–51.

30. Russo D, et al. Genetic alterations in thyroid hyperfunctioning adenomas. J Clin Endocrinol Metab. 1995;80(4):1347–51.

31. Derwahl M, et al. Constitutive activation of the Gs alpha protein-adenylate cyclase pathway may not be sufficient to generate toxic thyroid adenomas. J Clin Endocrinol Metab. 1996;81(5):1898–904.

32. Arturi F, et al. Thyrotropin receptor mutations and thyroid hyperfunctioning adenomas ten years after their first discovery: unresolved questions. Thyroid. 2003;13(4):341–3.

33. Walfish PG, Strawbridge HT, Rosen IB. Management implications from routine needle biopsy of hyperfunctioning thyroid nodules. Surgery. 1985;98(6):1179–88.

34. Monzani F, et al. Five-year follow-up of percutaneous ethanol injection for the treatment of hyperfunctioning thyroid nodules: a study of 117 patients. Clin Endocrinol (Oxf). 1997;46(1):9–15.

35. Papini E, et al. Percutaneous ultrasound-guided ethanol injection: a new treatment of toxic autonomously functioning thyroid nodules? J Clin Endocrinol Metab. 1993;76(2):411–6.

36. Papini E, et al. Long-term results of echographically guided percutaneous ethanol injection in the treatment of the autonomous thyroid nodule. Minerva Endocrinol. 1993;18(4):173–9.

37. Livraghi T, et al. Treatment of autonomous thyroid nodules with percutaneous ethanol injection: 4-year experience. Radiology. 1994;190(2):529–33.

38. Baltisberger BL, Minder CE, Burgi H. Decrease of incidence of toxic nodular goitre in a region of Switzerland after full correction of mild iodine deficiency. Eur J Endocrinol. 1995;132(5):546–9.

39. Vassart G, Dumont JE. The thyrotropin receptor and the regulation of thyrocyte function and growth. Endocr Rev 1992;13(3):596–611.

40. Dumont JE, et al. Physiological and pathological regulation of thyroid cell proliferation and differentiation by thyrotropin and other factors. Physiol Rev. 1992;72(3):667–97.

41. Blum M, et al. Thyroid storm after cardiac angiography with iodinated contrast medium. Occurrence in a patient with a previously euthyroid autonomous nodule of the thyroid. JAMA. 1976;235(21):2324–5.

42. Heimann P. Should hyperthyroidism be treated by surgery? World J Surg. 1978;2(3):281–7.

43. Huysmans D, et al. Radioiodine for nontoxic multinodular goiter. Thyroid. 1997;7(2):235–9.

44. Smith JJ, et al. Toxic nodular goiter and cancer: a compelling case for thyroidectomy. Ann Surg Oncol. 2013;20(4):1336–40.

45. Hay ID. Thyroiditis: a clinical update. Mayo Clin Proc. 1985;60(12):836–43.

46. Volpe R. The pathology of thyroiditis. Hum Pathol. 1978;9(4):429–38.

47. Intenzo CM, et al. Clinical, laboratory, and scintigraphic manifestations of subacute and chronic thyroiditis. Clin Nucl Med. 1993;18(4):302–6.

48. Weetman AP, Walport MJ. The association of autoimmune thyroiditis with systemic lupus erythematosus. Br J Rheumatol. 1987;26(5):359–61.

49. Weetman A. A hundred years of Hashimoto's thyroiditis. Thyroid. 2013;23(2):135–6.

50. Weetman AP. The immunopathogenesis of chronic autoimmune thyroiditis one century after hashimoto. Eur Thyroid J. 2013;1(4):243–50.

51. Weetman AP. Autoimmune thyroiditis: predisposition and pathogenesis. Clin Endocrinol (Oxf). 1992;36(4):307–23.

52. Tunbridge WM, et al. Natural history of autoimmune thyroiditis. Br Med J (Clin Res Ed). 1981;282(6260):258–62.

53. Fatourechi V, McConahey WM, Woolner LB. Hyperthyroidism associated with histologic Hashimoto's thyroiditis. Mayo Clin Proc. 1971;46(10):682–9.

54. Hayashi Y, et al. A long term clinical, immunological, and histological follow-up study of patients with goitrous chronic lymphocytic thyroiditis. J Clin Endocrinol Metab. 1985;61(6):1172–8.

55. Holm LE, Blomgren H, Lowhagen T. Cancer risks in patients with chronic lymphocytic thyroiditis. N Engl J Med. 1985;312(10):601–4.

56. Kato I, et al. Chronic thyroiditis as a risk factor of B-cell lymphoma in the thyroid gland. Jpn J Cancer Res. 1985;76(11):1085–90.

57. Farid NR, Hawe BS, Walfish PG. Increased frequency of HLA-DR3 and 5 in the syndromes of painless thyroiditis with transient thyrotoxicosis: evidence for an autoimmune aetiology. Clin Endocrinol (Oxf). 1983;19(6):699–704.

58. Inada M, et al. Reversible changes of the histological abnormalities of the thyroid in patients with painless thyroiditis. J Clin Endocrinol Metab. 1981;52(3):431–5.

59. Mizukami Y, et al. Silent thyroiditis: a histologic and immunohistochemical study. Hum Pathol. 1988;19(4):423–31.

60. Woolf PD, Thyroiditis. Med Clin North Am. 1985;69(5):1035–48.

61. Hamburger JI. The various presentations of thyroiditis. Diagnostic considerations. Ann Intern Med. 1986;104(2):219–24.

62. Singer PA. Thyroiditis. Acute, subacute, and chronic. Med Clin North Am. 1991;75(1):61–77.

63. Volpe R. Subacute (de Quervain's) thyroiditis. Clin Endocrinol Metab. 1979;8(1):81–95.
64. Volpe R. Subacute thyroiditis. Prog Clin Biol Res. 1981;74:115–34.
65. Volpe R. The management of subacute (DeQuervain's) thyroiditis. Thyroid. 1993;3(3):253–5.
66. Volpe R, Row VV, Ezrin C. Circulating viral and thyroid antibodies in subacute thyroiditis. J Clin Endocrinol Metab. 1967;27(9):1275–84.
67. Stancek D, et al. Isolation and some serological and epidemiological data on the viruses recovered from patients with subacute thyroiditis de Quervain. Med Microbiol Immunol. 1975;161(2):133–44.
68. Mizukami Y, et al. Immunohistochemical and ultrastructural study of subacute thyroiditis, with special reference to multinucleated giant cells. Hum Pathol. 1987;18(9):929–35.
69. Mizukami Y, et al. Chronic thyroiditis: thyroid function and histologic correlations in 601 cases. Hum Pathol. 1992;23(9):980–8.
70. Berger SA, et al. Infectious diseases of the thyroid gland. Rev Infect Dis. 1983;5(1):108–22.
71. Takai SI, et al. Internal fistula as a route of infection in acute suppurative thyroiditis. Lancet. 1979;1(8119):751–2.
72. Miyauchi A. Thyroid gland: a new management algorithm for acute suppurative thyroiditis? Nat Rev Endocrinol. 2010;6(8):424–6.
73. Miyauchi A, et al. Piriform sinus fistula: an underlying abnormality common in patients with acute suppurative thyroiditis. World J Surg. 1990;14(3):400–5.
74. Schwaegerle SM, Bauer TW, Esselstyn CB Jr. Riedel's thyroiditis. Am J Clin Pathol. 1988;90(6):715–22.
75. Ozgen A, Cila A. Riedel's thyroiditis in multifocal fibrosclerosis: CT and MR imaging findings. AJNR Am J Neuroradiol. 2000;21(2):320–1.
76. Perez Fontan FJ, et al. Riedel thyroiditis: US, CT, and MR evaluation. J Comput Assist Tomogr. 1993;17(2):324–5.
77. Lorenz K, et al. Riedel's thyroiditis: impact and strategy of a challenging surgery. Langenbecks Arch Surg. 2007;392(4):405–12.
78. Soh SB, et al. Novel use of rituximab in a case of Riedel's thyroiditis refractory to glucocorticoids and tamoxifen. J Clin Endocrinol Metab. 2013;98(9):3543–9.
79. Pritchyk K, et al. Tamoxifen therapy for Riedel's thyroiditis. Laryngoscope. 2004;114(10):1758–60.
80. Few J, et al. Riedel's thyroiditis: treatment with tamoxifen. Surgery. 1996;120(6):993–8, discussion 998–9.
81. Lo JC, et al. Riedel's thyroiditis presenting with hypothyroidism and hypoparathyroidism: dramatic response to glucocorticoid and thyroxine therapy. Clin Endocrinol (Oxf). 1998;48(6):815–8.

Robert James Graves

1795–1853

Melanie L. Richards

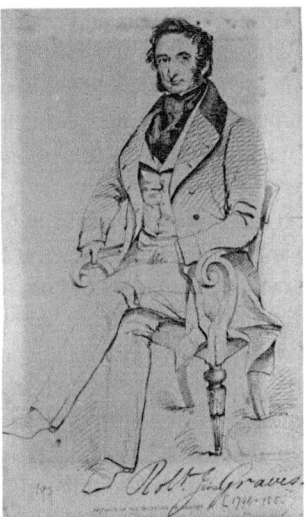

Robert James Graves. (Etching by Sherman & Smith. Image from the History of Medicine (NLM))

As a lecturer Professor Graves was endowed with peculiar capabilities. To a remarkable person he added great powers of arresting attention in the very outset of his discourse, which by an almost startling impressiveness he maintained throughout; his ideas were conveyed in a bold, fluent and classic style; in his language he was always forcible and elegant, and though frequently eloquent he never sacrificed his subject for flowers of rhetoric, or lost sight of his text in the froth of metaphor; for whether discussing the investigations of others, or detailing the results of his own enquiries, he ever manifested the same critical acumen, the same powers of the same piercing analysis. (William Wilde, father of Oscar Wilde, editor of the Dublin University Magazine [1])

This portrait of Robert James Graves by his friend and former student William Wilde was published in 1839, when Graves was 44 years old. His words reflect the unique abili-

ties of Graves as an educator. Graves was a masterful teacher and lecturer, which were his greatest contributions to medicine. Ironically, the syndrome that bears his name was but a fragment of his medical career.

Graves' Disease

It was in 1835 that Robert Graves shared his clinical observations of three patients with toxic goiter during a lecture at Meath Hospital. The article, "Newly observed affection of the thyroid gland in females" was transcribed from his lecture and published in the *London Medical and Surgical Journal* in May 1835 [2]. His classical description was, "I have lately seen three cases of violent and long continued palpitations in females, in each of which the same peculiarity presented itself, viz. enlargement of the thyroid gland; the size of this gland, at all times considerably greater than natural, was subject to remarkable variations in every one of these patients. When the palpitations were violent the gland used notably to swell and become distended, having all the appearance of being increased in size in consequence of an interstitial and sudden effusion of fluid into its substance. The swelling immediately began to subside as the violence of the paroxysm of palpitation decreased, and during the intervals the size of the gland remained stationary. Its increase of size and the variation to which it was liable had attracted forcibly the attention both of the patients and of their friends. There was not the slightest evidence of anything like the inflammation of the gland." One patient was described as having audible heartbeats as far as 4 ft. away from her chest. The sudden enlargement of the thyroid was reported to be associated with a feeling of suffocation. Graves described these attacks as a "hysteric paroxysm or hysterical fit," as palpitations of the heart were common in hysterical and nervous females. Eye manifestations were described in a 20-year-old woman. "The eyes assumed a singular appearance, for the eyeballs were apparently enlarged, so that when she slept or tried to shut her eyes, the lids were incapable

M. L. Richards (✉)
Department of Surgery, Mayo Clinic, 200 First Street SW, Rochester, MN 55905, USA
e-mail: richards.melanie@mayo.edu

J. L. Pasieka, J. A. Lee (eds.), *Surgical Endocrinopathies,* DOI 10.1007/978-3-319-13662-2_6,
© Springer International Publishing Switzerland 2015

of closing. When the eyes were open, the white sclerotic could be seen, to a breadth of several lines, all round the cornea."

Robert Graves' description was not the first of exophthalmic goiter, Caleb Hillier Parry from Bath, England, described the syndrome in 1786, but it was not documented on until a posthumous and unpublished collection of his writings were completed in 1825, 10 years earlier than Graves' publication [3]. Guiseppe Flajani, an Italian surgeon and anatomist, reported on a patient with exophthalmos and goiter in 1802 [4]. In Germany, von Basedow reported on exophthalmic goiter in 1840 [5]. In most of Europe, this syndrome is referred to as von Basedow's disease. The USA, Britain, and other English-speaking areas will refer to it as Graves' disease. This has been attributed to **Armand Trousseau** (Trousseaus' sign in hypocalcemia), who published in London a textbook, *Clinique Medicale de L'Hotel Dieu de Paris*, that had a chapter, "Du Goitre Exophthalmique, ou Maladie de Graves'." It is a mystery why Caleb Parry was not given full credit despite it being given to him in Sir William *Osler's Textbook of Medicine,* the gold standard text in English-speaking countries for many years.

Personal and Professional Life

Robert James Graves (1796–1853) was born in Dublin, Ireland. He was the seventh of ten children. His father, Richard, and maternal grandfather were both educated at Trinity College in Dublin. Richard studied theology and published several books of his sermons. He was both a preacher and a teacher, reaching the rank of professor of divinity at Trinity. Robert's mother, Eliza Draught, was the daughter of a professor. Robert Graves also pursued his undergraduate studies at Trinity College. He stayed on at Trinity to complete his medical degree. His interest in the basic sciences prompted him to spend a lot of time in the anatomy laboratory, which had been traditionally reserved only for those destined to be surgeons. Following graduation, at the top of his class, in 1818, he spent 3 years traveling throughout Europe visiting leading medical schools. This was a testament to his quest for knowledge, as there was no requirement for additional postgraduate or residency training at the time. A medical school graduate could begin their medical practice as soon as they graduated. He spent the majority of his time in England, Germany, Denmark, and Italy. The German approach to medical education involved the integration of the sciences with bedside clinical teaching. This was of greatest impact to Graves.

Robert Graves had a colorful and slightly histrionic personality. He was very outgoing with confident and boundless energy. His physical presence was also commanding with his dark complexion and tall height. These characteristics, which would later contribute to his success as a lecturer, placed him into some interesting life experiences. During his travels, he developed skills as an artist when he became a traveling partner with Joseph William Mallord Turner, a famous painter at the time. Interestingly, he was not aware of Turner's identity until after they had traveled together for months. Graves was also a natural at learning other languages. So much so, that he was actually accused of being a German spy in Austria because he spoke the language so well. He had forgotten his passport and ended up in prison and it took 10 days to prove his identity before his release. One interesting part of his travels was when he was aboard a ship from Genoa to Sicily. According to his friend William Stokes, they encountered a storm, and the boat began to fill with water as the pumps failed. This led the crew to attempt to abandon the ship, with a plan to leave Graves and one other passenger behind. Graves boldly stated, "it is a pity to part good company," as he took an axe to the lifeboat to dissuade them from leaving. He then proceeded to fix the pump, using the leather from his shoes, saving all and thus transitioning to the next chapter in his career.

Graves' medical career began in 1821 at Meath Hospital, Dublin, where he applied the knowledge he acquired on his travels. Graves appreciated the roles of both teacher and student. He helped found the Park Street School of Medicine and introduced bedside teaching at his hospital. His contributions to medical education were pioneering, and many believe that they are his greatest contributions to medicine. He engaged students on the wards. Traditional rounds were done with the attending physician leading the crowd of students, lecturing to the group with no expectation of questions and no direct examination of the patient. Rounds with Graves were actually teaching rounds where the students were treated like junior colleagues and encouraged to ask questions. He gave them direct responsibility in the care of the patients and expected them to have a reason for their clinical decision making. Graves treated his patients in a similar way, with respect and kindness. He was a physician who would sit on the edge of the bed, always giving them his full attention and time for listening.

Graves was a lifelong student who practiced scientific thinking, searching knowledge about specific diseased and treatments that were supported by scientific evidence. This differed from his colleagues who were quite content to conduct teaching rounds without scientific support for their teachings. To put things in perspective, there were few treatments for specific diseases or symptoms available. Most were plant concoctions available at the apothecary. The few that remain useful today include opiates and digitalis. He was well ahead of his time with his commitment to the basic sciences as the foundation for knowledge of the clinical sciences.

Graves' ability to skillfully deliver stimulating lectures created a large following of students and physicians.

At 4:00 p.m. sharp, he would lecture at Sir Patrick Dun's Hospital on a daily basis. He was always on time, and the crowd was never less than 140. He spoke on a variety of topics ranging from the esoteric, such as "the infinity of life" to the doctrine of modern metaphysics, to the physiology of the senses. Many of his lectures were published and 20 were even incorporated into a book as a memorial to Graves by his brother and William Stokes, a former student. He was also a prolific author, making contributions in nearly every aspect of medicine, many of which were purely observations or case reports and also writing on current events. One of his greatest contributions was his book, *A System of Clinical Medicine,* which was published in 1843 and sold out in months. The second edition was a worldwide best seller and was translated into three languages.

Graves had a very successful professional career despite hardship in his personal life. He married Matilda Jane Eustace the year he began his medical practice in 1821. Soon after, they had a daughter, Eliza Drewe. In 1825, at the age of 29 years, he suffered the loss of both his wife, Matilda Jane, and his daughter Eliza Drewe. The next year he married Sarah Jane Brinkley, only to have her and their daughter, Sara-Jane, both die the following year in 1827. His third marriage was to Anna Grogan in 1830 and they remained together, having six children. She was an active socialite and focused much of her energy outside the home. They are reported to have lived very separate lives, which likely would have been necessary, as Graves would have definitely fallen under the category of workaholics by today's standards. Robert Graves died of liver cancer at the age of 56 in 1853.

References

1. Eponymists in Medicine. Robert Graves the golden years of Irish medicine. Selwyn Taylor. Editor-in-Chief Hugh L'Etang. Copyright 1989 Royal Society of Medicine Services Limited.
2. Graves RJ. New observed affection of the thyroid gland in females. (Clinical lectures). Lond Med Surg J (Renshaw). 1835;7:516–7. (Reprinted in Medical Classics, 1940;5:33–6).
3. Parry CH. Enlargement of the thyroid gland in connection with enlargement or palpitations of the heart. Posthumous. In: Collections from the unpublished medical writings of C.H. Parry. London: Underwood's Fleet-Street; 1825, pp. 111–129.
4. Flanjani G. Collezione d'osservanioni e reflessioni di chirurgia. Vol. 3. Rome: Michele A Ripa Presso Lino Contedini; 1802. pp 270–3.
5. von Basedow KA. Exophthalmus durch hypertrophie des zellgewebes in der augenh Öhle. (Caspers'). Worchenschr für die gesammte Heilkund. 1840;6:197–204. (Berlin).

Henry Stanley Plummer

1874–1936

Robert C. Smallridge and Ian D. Hay

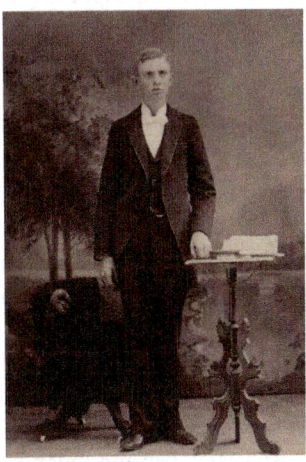

Henry Plummer, photographed at age 26, soon after graduating with his medical degree from Northwestern University and just before being recruited by the Mayo doctors. (By Permission of the Mayo Historical Unit, Mayo Clinic, Rochester, Minnesota)

Henry S. Plummer has been described by a colleague with an intimate knowledge of his life as being both an "eccentric" and a "genius" [1, 2]. Helen Clapesattle, a former director of the University of Minnesota Press, was commissioned to write the history of the Mayo family from the 1850s to 1939, and through her interviews with **Drs. Charles** and **William Mayo**, as well as friends and colleagues at the Mayo Clinic, she was able to compile examples of both the brilliance and the mannerisms of Dr. Plummer [2]. Subsequently, Dr. F. A. Willius, a cardiologist at Mayo Clinic and longtime friend and colleague, wrote a detailed and insightful description of Dr. Plummer from his childhood until his final days and

described therein not only his remarkable and diverse professional accomplishments but also several anecdotes about his personal characteristics and his private life [1].

Born on March 3, 1874, to Isabelle Steer Plummer, a schoolteacher, and Dr. Albert Plummer, a country doctor in southern Minnesota, Henry Plummer was drawn to medicine at an early age. It is said that as a toddler he loved looking at the illustrations in his father's copy of Gray's Anatomy and as a child accompanied his father on house calls, traveling by horse and buggy [1]. He attended his local high school, then the University of Minnesota for 2 years, and subsequently received his M.D. diploma from the Medical School of Northwestern University of Chicago in 1898 [1]. Henry joined his father as a general practitioner for 3 years, and in 1900 a chance occurrence changed the futures of both Dr. Plummer and the Mayo Clinic. On that day, **Dr. William Mayo** traveled to Racine, Minnesota, to accompany Dr. Albert Plummer on a house call. Not feeling well, the senior Dr. Plummer sent his son, Henry, with Dr. Mayo. Henry had a long-standing interest in engineering and had developed an interest in laboratory procedures. He brought with him a microscope, discussed its usefulness with Dr. Mayo, and demonstrated its value in examining a blood sample during their visit with the patient who had leukemia [1]. Upon his return to Rochester, Dr. Will Mayo said to his brother, "that son of Dr. Plummer's is an extraordinary young man. I believe we ought to get him up here to take charge of our laboratories; he would do us a lot of good" [2].

Henry thus moved to Rochester as one of the early members of the Mayo brothers' practice. His younger brother, William Albert, also later became a Mayo Clinic physician. On October 4, 1904, Henry married Daisy Berkman, a niece of the Mayo brothers. Henry and Daisy adopted two children, Robert and Gertrude (Fig. 1). His career can be divided into three areas of interest. The most far-reaching was his vision for the practice of medicine. He saw the value of an integrated practice and the need for specialization. With this in mind, he was entrusted by the Mayo brothers to oversee the design and construction of not one, but two clinic buildings (the latter, completed in 1928, is now named the Plummer building). He designed exam rooms, lighting, and com-

R. C. Smallridge (✉)
Division of Endocrinology
& Metabolism, Mayo Clinic, 4500 San Pablo Road, Jacksonville, FL 32224, USA
e-mail: smallridge.robert@mayo.edu

I. D. Hay
Endocrine Research, Division of Endocrinology, Metabolism, Nutrition and Internal Medicine, Mayo Clinic College of Medicine, 200 First St., SW, Rochester MN 55905, USA

J. L. Pasieka, J. A. Lee (eds.), *Surgical Endocrinopathies,* DOI 10.1007/978-3-319-13662-2_7,
© Springer International Publishing Switzerland 2015

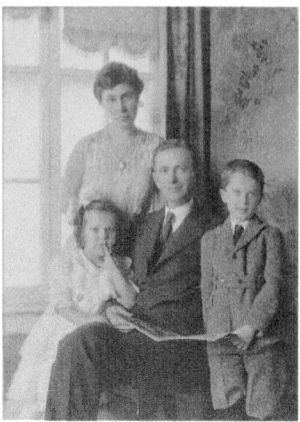

Fig. 1 Henry Plummer, photographed with his wife and two adopted children. (By Permission of the Mayo Historical Unit, Mayo Clinic, Rochester, Minnesota)

munication systems that streamlined the flow of patients. He recognized that the system of patient records, where entries were placed in ledgers and kept in individual physician's offices, was inefficient. He, therefore, developed a single medical record that contained all of a patient's records, each catalogued by type—history, laboratory, operative note, etc. The records were then maintained centrally but transported as needed via a pneumatic tube system. The records were designed to facilitate review for research on, and future publication of, patient outcomes. In essence, he created an early version of today's electronic medical record. Dr. Plummer was also placed in charge of modernizing the laboratories, introducing x-ray machines to the clinic, as well as electrocardiograms (ECGs) and measurements of O_2 requirements [1].

A second area of Dr. Plummer's professional interests pertained to esophageal diseases, including foreign bodies, strictures, and cardiospasm [3]. During the period of his clinical practice, accidental lye ingestion was a common occurrence with devastating consequences. Henry became adept in bronchoscopy and esophagoscopy, and with his background interest in mechanics and engineering he created equipment such as dilators in his home workshop to assist in esophageal instrumentation. He established and published on his specialty referral practice in esophageal disorders; he is remembered for describing the "Plummer–Vinson" syndrome [3].

Clinically, however, Henry Plummer is best known for his many contributions to the field of thyroidology. His interest in the thyroid began as a teenager when he observed one of his father's patients with a goiter that progressively enlarged, causing respiratory symptoms and eventually being resected by Dr. William Mayo. He apparently continued his interest in patients with goiter as a medical student, and it was therefore not unexpected that he should pursue thyroid disease as an area of clinical focus when he joined the Mayo

brothers [1]. Goiters were very common at the beginning of the twentieth century. Iodine deficiency was common, particularly in the Midwest, and these goiters when they became greatly enlarged required surgical resection. Surgery, however, was associated with a significant mortality rate, and so patients traveled to centers with expertise in thyroidectomy. Dr. Charles Mayo had such an interest and became known as "the American father of thyroid surgery," performing and reporting results on thousands of such operations.

Some of the larger goiters seen by the Mayo doctors presented with thyrotoxicosis and, not surprisingly, Dr. Plummer found himself leading a multispecialty team with expertise in the diagnosis and management of hyperthyroidism. Their chosen pathologist, Dr. Louis B. Wilson, reviewed **Dr. Charles Mayo's** surgical cases of hyperthyroidism due to exophthalmic goiter (Graves' disease) from 1898 to 1908 and divided them into pathological groups [4]. He then had Dr. Plummer review his clinical notes and separate patients into four groups: (a) acute hyperthyroidism (mild, moderate, severe, very severe); (b) prior severe, but examined when in remission; (c) prior severe, but current symptoms related to end-organ (e.g., cardiac) symptoms; and (d) mild, chronic hyperthyroidism. The results showed "an almost complete parallel was found to exist between the pathological conjectures and the clinical facts in about 80% of the cases" [4]. The same Dr. Wilson later became much better known for his development of the frozen section technique to assist surgeons.

In his first paper on the subject, Dr. Plummer reported 2917 new cases undergoing surgery in 1909–1912. He described patients as having either a hyperplastic or nonhyperplastic goiter and constitutionally being either toxic or atoxic as follows:

–	Toxic (%)	Atoxic (%)
Hyperplastic (42.8%)	99.2	0.8
Nonhyperplastic (57.2%)	23.3	76.7

The temporal onset of thyrotoxicity differed also: hyperplastic goiters were detected on average at age 32, with toxicity noted shortly thereafter, at 32.9 years. In contrast, nonhyperplastic goiters were discovered at age 22, but toxicity was not apparent until age 36.5 years [5].

In 1914, Dr. Wilson received a letter from Dr. Edward C. Kendall, a research chemist in New York City, inquiring about a job at Mayo Clinic. Kendall was working on isolating the active product from thyroid glands, an effort of interest to both Dr. Charles Mayo and Dr. Plummer. Plummer had concluded that patients with exophthalmic goiter had both a normal and an abnormal product in their thyroid glands. Kendall might be able to answer this question, and so he was hired. On Christmas day, 1914, Kendall isolated a crystalline structure that contained 60% iodine and proved to be the elusive substance which he called thyroxin [2]. Later in his career, while working for the Mayo Clinic in Rochester, Minnesota, Dr. Kendall received the Nobel Prize for his isolation and characterization of cortisone.

As part of his responsibilities in overseeing the laboratories, Plummer also recruited Dr. Walter M. Boothby from Boston in 1916 [1]. In March 1917, a metabolic laboratory opened under the direction of Dr. Boothby and Irene Sandiford, Ph.D., with Dr. Plummer serving as the clinical director. Boothby and Sandiford published a manual of their technique for measuring basal metabolic rate (BMR), and in 1920 the results of an elevated BMR in 1917 cases of exophthalmic goiter were reported [6]. Also noted was that within 2 weeks of thyroidectomy, the BMR decreased from +31 to +5%, and the pulse rate from 104 to 84 beats/min [6].

Plummer was keenly interested in the role of iodine in various types of hyperthyroidism. He confirmed earlier observations by Kocher that some patients with adenomatous goiter without hyperthyroidism when given iodine may become hyperthyroid [7, 8], and the condition may persist for months or years [7]. Plummer postulated that "the cause of exophthalmic goiter is unknown" and "that intensive stimulation of unknown source, acting on the entire gland, drives it to the point of producing an active agent abnormal in quality as well as quantity (or an excessive amount of the normal active agent), which in the tissues of the body causes all the phenomena of the disease" [7]. This unknown source we now know today to be the thyroid-stimulating immunoglobulin or thyroid-stimulating hormone (TSH) receptor antibody. He also subsequently suggested "the possibility of an incompletely iodized thyroxin molecule being driven from the thyroid by intensive stimulation" [9], thereby foreseeing the discovery decades later of triiodothyronine, T3.

From his extensive studies of goitrous patients, Plummer concluded that in contrast to patients with adenomatous goiter, who were often clinically worsened by iodine, in patients with exophthalmic goiters administration of iodine could actually prove to be beneficial. Therefore, at the Mayo Clinic, "the first extensive study of the effect of iodine in exophthalmic goiter was initiated by Plummer in March 1922" [8]. Two years later, in 1924, Plummer and Boothby reported that the optimal dose of Lugol's solution is ten drops and that if "not tolerated by mouth, it is given in similar doses by rectum" [8]. They demonstrated that patients had a prompt decrease in pulse rate and BMR, an increase in body weight, and cessation of nausea and vomiting in those with severe disease. They also recommended "postponing operative procedures until it is evident that no further improvement is to be obtained from Lugol's solution. Maximal improvement usually occurs after…eight or ten days" [8]. A year later, in 1925, Plummer wrote that "large doses (of iodine) might tend partially to reverse the absorption and discharge

mechanism of the gland. This led me to the trial of much larger doses of iodine than theory seemed to indicate and of Lugol's solution" [9].

As would be expected with clinical improvement, "the use of iodine in the clinic decreased the surgical mortality from approximately 3.5% to approximately 1% in cases in which operation was performed in Rochester" [9]. Furthermore, staged operations, which included ligation of thyroid arteries followed later by thyroidectomy was no longer necessary. Mayo and Plummer provided more detailed mortality figures the following year [10]:

	1921	1922	1923	1924 (8 mos.)
No. cases	561	491	564	600
Mortality (%) surgical	3.38	2.24	1.41	0.66

In Rochester, Dr. Plummer was highly respected among his Mayo Clinic colleagues for his diagnostic skills (Fig. 2), and he was acknowledged for his ability to integrate physiologic principles into his teaching. He presided over a weekly "goiter lunch" at the Kahler Hotel (which still stands in 2014, immediately adjacent to the clinic buildings). In Plummer's time, the Kahler Hotel actually had medical wards within it, designed principally to deal with the challenges of thyrotoxic patients, considered to be at risk of "thyroid storm". The "goiter lunch," under Plummer's leadership, proved to be a popular meeting, which was regularly attended by not only internists and surgeons but also pathologists and chemists, who gathered to discuss thyroid topics and the clinicopathological details of unusual cases of particular interest [2].

Dr. Plummer, in addition to his numerous contributions to the advancement of medicine, had many interests in his personal and family life. He loved the outdoors and enjoyed camping and boating. He and his wife purchased a cruiser

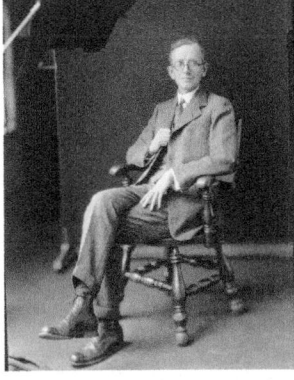

Fig. 2 Henry Plummer, around 1935, in Rochester, Minnesota, posing in the plummer building photographic studio for his Mayo Clinic staff portrait. In 2014, a copy of this photo still hangs above the fireplace in the Plummer Hall of the Mayo Clinic Library. (By Permission of the Mayo Historical Unit, Mayo Clinic, Rochester, Minnesota)

and navigated it inland from New York City to Minnesota less than a year before his death. He was an accomplished gardener and horticulturist, and he had a home workshop where he created medical instruments and designed furniture. He had remarkable skills in engineering and interior design; his architectural abilities, working in association with the C.F. Ellerbe firm from the Twin Cities, resulted in two elegant, but practical, Mayo Clinic buildings and a remarkable Tudor home for his family, which was subsequently gifted to the city. He strongly believed that physicians should read beyond the medical literature, and he created the Browsing Room Library and donated many classics from his personal library.

Henry Plummer died on December 31, 1936. The day before, while driving home, he became ill and needed assistance into his home. Ever the clinician, he gathered his family and told them he would soon become unconscious. He went into a coma and passed away the following evening. Dr. F. A. Willius, who trained under and worked with Dr. Plummer for years, described him as "a pioneer in many phases of medicine" [1].

Acknowledgments I wish to thank Renee Ziemer of the Mayo Historical Unit for assistance in obtaining archived documents and Kathleen Norton for typing the manuscript.

References

1. Willius FA. Henry Stanley Plummer—a diversified genius. Springfield: Charles C. Thomas; 1960.
2. Clapesattle H. The doctors Mayo. Rochester: Mayo Foundation for Medical Education & Research; 1969.
3. Plummer HS, Vinson PP. Cardiospasm: a report of 301 cases. Med Clinic N Am. 1921;5(Sept):355–69.
4. Wilson LB. The pathological changes in the thyroid gland, as related to the varying symptoms in Graves' disease. Am J Med Sci. 1908;cxxxvi:851–61.
5. Plummer HS. The clinical and pathologic relationships of hyperplastic and non-hyperplastic goiter. JAMA. 1913;LXI:650–1.
6. Sandiford I. The basal metabolic rate in exophthalmic goitre (1917 cases) with a brief description of the technic used at the Mayo Clinic. Endocrinology. 1920;iv:71–87.
7. Plummer HS, Wilson LB, Boothby WM. Diseases of the thyroid gland. In: Christian HA, Mackenzie J, editors. Oxford medicine . Vol. 3, Chapter XV-A. New York: Oxford University Press; 1922. pp. 838–963.
8. Plummer HS, Boothby WM. The value of iodin in exophthalmic goiter. J Iowa State Med Soc. 1924;xiv:66–73.
9. Plummer HS. The function of the thyroid gland. Coll Pap Mayo Clin. 1925;17:473–99.
10. Mayo CH, Plummer HS. The results of iodine administration in exophthalmic goiter. Tr Am S A. 1926;42:541–56.

Hakaru Hashimoto

1881–1934

Sapna Nagar and Peter Angelos

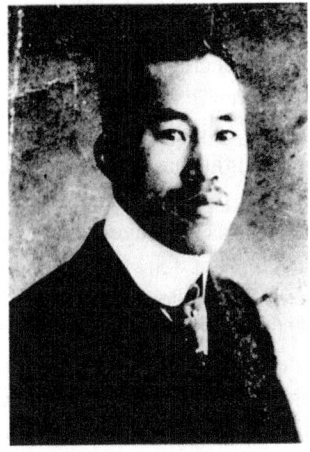

Hakaru Hashimoto is pictured here at 31 years old. It was at this age that he wrote his most famous work. (Picture is courtesy of The Japan Endocrine Society)

Early Life

Hakaru Hashimoto was born on May 5, 1881, in the village of Midai, Nishitsuge. He was the third son born to a family that had practiced medicine for generations within this small town [1]. Today, this historical village would be considered a part of the larger town of Iga Ueno. This castle town surrounded by mountains in the Kinki district was the birthplace of Iga Ninja and is where the Iga Ninja School was established in the fifteenth century. It was also the hometown of the famous Haiku poet, Basho Matsuo.

Hashimoto spent his childhood in the village of his birth and then left to enter the First Mie Prefectural Junior High School at Tsu [1]. This is around the time when he consid-

S. Nagar (✉)
Department of Surgery, University of Chicago, Pritzker School of Medicine, Chicago, IL, USA
e-mail: snagar29@gmail.com

P. Angelos
Endocrine Surgery Research Program, Department of Surgery, University of Chicago Pritzker School of Medicine, Chicago, IL, USA

ered an education in medicine. He was in an environment that seemed to foster these early career aspirations given that many of his friends eventually went on to also become involved in medicine. More specifically, the influence of his grandfather, Gen'i Hashimoto, sealed Hashimoto's fate as a physician. Gen'i was a well-known physician within the region who had studied Dutch medicine at the end of the Edo era [1].

Hashimoto went on to attend the National High School at Kyoto, and in 1903, he entered the Department of Medicine at Kyusyu Imperial University in Fukuoka. Hashimoto was in the first graduating class in 1907. Following graduation from medical school, he entered the First Department of Surgery and studied under Professor Hayari Miyake for 4 years. It was here, while he was completing his studies in surgery, that Hashimoto encountered the thyroid glands of four women who had a completely distinct histopathology never before described [1–4].

Life Overseas

After the publication of his original paper at the young age of 31 years, Hashimoto went to Germany for further study. He had a particular interest in pathology and worked under Professor Kaufman at Goettingen University, but his time in Germany was shorter than planned. After 2 years of living in Germany, he was forced to return to Japan in 1914 as a result of the outbreak of World War I in Europe [5] (Fig. 1).

His Return to Japan

Hashimoto returned to Japan and joined his alma mater for a short time. However, due to financial pressures, he soon decided to move back to his hometown to take over the family practice [1]. He began his surgical practice in the spring of 1916 at the age of 35 years. His practice could best be described as that of a private practice surgeon. He became

J. L. Pasieka, J. A. Lee (eds.), *Surgical Endocrinopathies,* DOI 10.1007/978-3-319-13662-2_8,
© Springer International Publishing Switzerland 2015

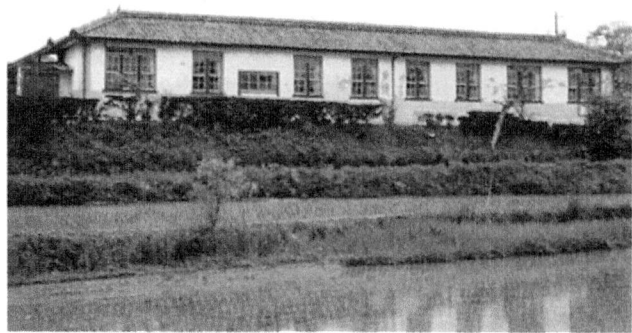

Fig. 1 Seen here is the hospital in Dr. Hashimoto's hometown. This is his place of practice for most of his career and is where he performed his surgical procedures. (Picture is courtesy of The Japan Endocrine Society)

widely known within the area that he served for his impeccable training and generosity [1]. His dedication to his patients was evidenced by the fact that he reportedly would travel great distances using a rickshaw within the countryside to see his patients. He treated all patients irrespective of class or income [1].

After 4 years in practice, he married at the age of 39. He and his wife eventually had four children: three sons and a daughter. During the prime of his life, Hashimoto contracted typhoid fever very suddenly from one of his patients. He ultimately succumbed to his illness and died at the age of 52 years on January 9, 1934 [1, 3]. His contribution to medicine had gone unnoticed during his lifetime, and he died without the recognition he deserved for his discovery (Fig. 2).

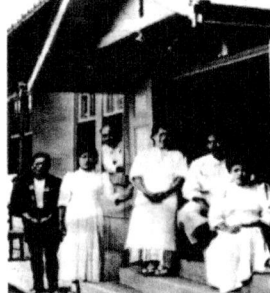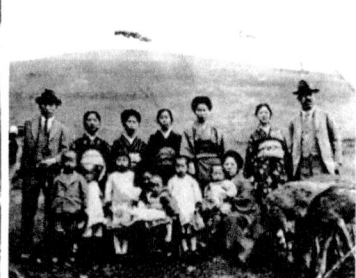

Fig. 2 The picture on the left shows Dr. Hashimoto with other hospital employees posing at the entrance of the town hospital. He is standing third from the *left* looking out from the window. The picture on the *right* shows Dr. Hashimoto standing with his family at a picnic. He is the first man on the *right*. (Pictures is courtesy of The Japan Endocrine Society)

Hakaru Hashimoto's Discovery

The Initial Description

At the time of his discovery, Hashimoto was finishing his surgical training at the Kyusyu Imperial University. During this time, the primary treatment modality for a thyroid goiter was surgery and thyroidectomies were commonplace. As a result, Hashimoto had the opportunity to study the histology of many resected thyroid specimens. Over the span of 7 years, he came across the thyroid glands of four women who underwent partial thyroidectomy for the indication of goiter. The description of the histology of these glands constituted his most famous piece of work entitled "Zur Kenntniss der lymphomatosen Veranderung der Schilddruse (struma lymphomatosa)" [6]. He decided to publish this article in the German journal *Archiv für Klinishe Chirurgie* because German was the primary scientific language of the time. Ironically enough, he thought that the information in his article would disseminate most quickly this way.

The article itself was 30 pages long with five sections consisting of the introduction, clinical case presentations, histological description, review of previous reports, and discussion [1, 6]. The bulk of the article involved a very thorough histologic description of the thyroid goiters in the four patients. He explained the extensive lymphocytic infiltration and lymphoid follicles that had not been reported prior. Additionally, he described eosinophilic changes to follicular cells and interstitial fibrosis along with round cell infiltration [1, 6, 7].

The remainder of the article reviewed the reports available at the time differentiating this entity from other known etiologies of thyroid goiter. In meticulous detail, he explained the histological differences of struma lymphomatosa from Riedel's thyroiditis and the clinical differences of struma lymphomatosa from Graves' disease [6, 7]. He was confident that this was a new histologic finding within thyroid goiters [6]. Additionally, he made efforts to point out the histological similarities of struma lymphomatosa and Mikulicz's disease, thought to be Sjögren's syndrome today. He recognized that histologically this was similar to a modern-day autoimmune disease. He understood that a still unrecognized stimulus was responsible for the histologic changes to these thyroid glands stating, "we can assume that...the lymphocytic elements are stimulated by a certain factor" but that "at present we cannot say anything definite about the cause" [2, 6].

A Lost Discovery

After publication in 1912, Hashimoto's work received some recognition in Germany. The next year, in 1913, a German pathologist by the name of Simmonds mentioned Hashimoto's work, but was unsure whether it was a distinct pathologic entity of the thyroid [8]. Then, in 1914, a German surgeon thought it was a form of chronic thyroiditis [9]. However, during this time, major texts in the British and American literature failed to make mention of Hashimoto or his work when discussing inflammatory disorders of the thyroid gland [2]. Today, many believe the reasons for this relative obscurity were because it was a rare disease compared to endemic goiter; it was harder to access given the need for translation from German, and also because after World War I broke out, the perception of German scientific work on the world stage had changed [2].

In the 1920s, there continued to be more citations of his discovery limited to German journals. They were also limited to pathology journals [2]. North American and European clinicians continued to fail to recognize his contribution. In 1925, a British pathologist independently described what he thought was a new disease terming it "lymphadenoid goiter." In his literature review, he failed to identify that it had been described previously [10]. The Western world continued to neglect Hashimoto's contribution.

Final Recognition

It was not until the 1930s when Allen Graham, a surgeon from the Cleveland Clinic, pointed out that lymphomatous goiter was a distinct histologic type. He confirmed that it was different from other inflammatory conditions of the thyroid, namely Riedel's thyroiditis [11]. He made a clear connection between Hashimoto's description and what he had encountered, giving proper credit to him [11, 12]. After these articles were published, surgeons in the USA who had once failed to mention him a decade earlier now included Hashimoto's work in their textbooks [13]. Hashimoto's name became attached with the disease process. The British also followed suit, and a surgeon by the name of Cecil Joll admitted his error of not recognizing Hashimoto's description. He later wrote a paper explicitly describing Hashimoto's disease and crediting him with its discovery [14].

By the end of the 1930s, Hashimoto's thyroiditis had now become a distinct disease within the spectrum of chronic thyroiditis. In fact, the Third International Thyroid Conference in 1938 held in Washington, DC, had an entire session devoted to Hashimoto's disease. Despite all of these new advancements, Hashimoto's disease was still considered to be a rare thyroid disorder. Also, the connection between the disease and hypothyroidism still had not been made. Surgical intervention was still the treatment of choice during this time [2].

The Discovery of an Antibody

Though the scientific community had embraced Hashimoto's disease as a distinct histopathology of the thyroid gland, physicians still had not recognized its association with hypothyroidism or its etiology. There was speculation that the insulting agent might be a mysterious chemical, but no investigation into why there was lymphocytic infiltration into the thyroid gland had been conducted primarily due to World War II [2]. During the 1940s and early 1950s, this disease remained a strange histology encountered rarely among patients with thyroid goiter [2].

The first inclination that Hashimoto's disease was an immunologic abnormality was when Fromm and associates detected an elevation of plasma gamma globulin fraction in patients with chronic thyroiditis [15]. This was followed by identification of abnormalities in serum flocculation tests in these patients [16]. Taken together, these preliminary experiments indicated that the disease might be related to a complex autoimmune reaction [17].

In 1956, the work of two independent groups changed the way physicians understood Hashimoto's disease. Noel Rose and Ernst Witebsky were immunologists in Buffalo, New York, who showed that when rabbits were immunized with thyroid cells, they would form antibodies to thyroglobulin. When they analyzed the thyroid glands of these animals under the microscope, they found the same lymphocytic infiltration observed by Hashimoto 40 years earlier [18]. They were also able to demonstrate the presence of these autoantibodies in the serum of patients with chronic thyroiditis and published this in a landmark paper [19]. Also in 1956, Ivan Roitt, Deborah Doniach, and colleagues from England were able to demonstrate the presence of antibodies to thyroglobulin in the serum of patients with Hashimoto's disease [20].

Up until this time, the idea of autoimmunity had existed but was never taken seriously. Now, with these new findings, this concept was a valid theory. This work allowed for a connection to be established between the histology of the thyroid glands that Hashimoto observed and the physiologic underpinnings [2, 3]. Even more impressively, the identification of close to 80 autoimmune diseases affectin g almost every organ of the body began from this work (Fig. 3).

Hashimoto's Thyroiditis Today

Epidemiology

Early epidemiologic studies investigating the prevalence of this disease in large populations elucidated that Hashimoto's disease was more common than initially thought with close

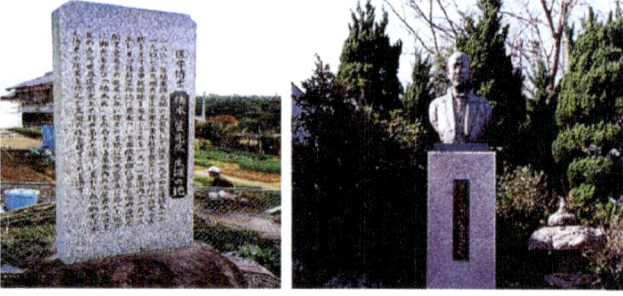

Fig. 3 Dr. Hashimoto is beloved by the people of his hometown and country of Japan for his contributions. There are numerous symbolic monuments and roads built in his honor. The picture on the right is a monument located in his birthplace of Midai, Nishitsuge, commemorating his life. The picture on the right is a statue of Dr. Hashimoto located in the public hall in the city of Iga. (Pictures is courtesy of The Japan Endocrine Society)

to 2 % of subjects having overt hypothyroidism, 10–26 % of subjects with evidence of anti-thyroid peroxidase (TPO) antibodies present in their serum, and 7.5–30 % of subjects with elevated serum thyroid-stimulating hormone (TSH) [21–24]. Today, Hashimoto's disease is considered the most common autoimmune disease, most common endocrine disorder, and the most common cause of hypothyroidism [25]. It exists in populations at a much higher rate than what is diagnosed clinically [17]. The current estimated incidence is approximately 1 case per 1000 persons, and the prevalence is 8 cases per 1000 persons. The prevalence is 46 cases per 1000 when subjects have biochemical evidence of hypothyroidism and thyroid autoantibodies [25].

We also know that the incidence and prevalence of Hashimoto's disease are increasing. A review article by McLeod and Cooper analyzed epidemiological studies performed worldwide. They found increases in the incidence and prevalence of Hashimoto's disease in different geographic areas, with advancing age, in female gender, and in iodine-sufficient populations [26]. A recent review of pathologic records from 1889 to 2012 at the Johns Hopkins Hospital revealed that 6 % of all thyroidectomies reported Hashimoto's thyroiditis. Interestingly, the first time Hashimoto's name appeared in a pathology report was in 1942 [27].

Clinical Features

Hashimoto's disease was originally described as a chronic inflammatory change of the thyroid gland resulting in a goiter. However, the histological changes can also be seen in atrophic glands. In patients who develop goiterous change, the clinical–pathological spectrum of Hashimoto's disease includes one of the following forms: classic, fibrosing variant, immunoglobulin G4 (IgG4)-related variant, juvenile

form, Hashitoxicosis variant, and painless (sporadic, postpartum) [25].

In considering symptomatic disease, there are local and systemic symptoms. Local symptoms include vague discomfort of the neck and compression of cervical structures resulting in dysphonia, dyspnea, and dysphagia. Systemic manifestations are a result of a loss of normal thyroid function (hypothyroidism) causing disturbances in the gastrointestinal, cardiovascular, reproductive, and pulmonary systems of the body [17, 25]. Patients may also suffer from psychiatric disturbances [28].

Up to 20 % of patients with Hashimoto's disease will have mild symptoms of hypothyroidism [17]. In patients who progress from euthyroidism to hypothyroidism, it is usually considered irreversible. However, there is evidence that up to 25 % of these patients may spontaneously recover [17, 29]. In fact, in children who are initially euthyroid with Hashimoto's disease, only 50 % will go on to develop hypothyroidism at 5 years [30].

Association with Other Disease Processes

Autoimmune Diseases

Hashimoto's disease and Graves' disease are on opposite ends of the spectrum of autoimmune thyroid disease. Both conditions have complex autoimmune pathways to alter the function of follicular cells as the end organ [31–38]. The details of these elegant studies are beyond the scope of this review. Suffice to say, pathogenesis involves activation of $CD4^+$ and $CD8^+$ T cells leading to cytokine-mediated apoptosis of follicular cells [32–36, 38]. In addition to Hashimoto's disease being related to Graves' disease, it is also associated with Sjögren's syndrome, polyglandular autoimmune disease, and IgG4-related pancreatitis (autoimmune pancreatitis), among other autoimmune diseases [7, 39–42].

Papillary Thyroid Cancer
The association between papillary thyroid cancer and Hashimoto's disease has been studied extensively. Hashimoto's thyroiditis was first thought to be associated with thyroid cancer in 1955 [43]. A recent meta-analysis of 38 studies concluded that papillary thyroid carcinoma was significantly associated with pathologically confirmed Hashimoto's disease [44]. The common pathway between the two may involve the PI3k/Akt pathway [45]. Papillary thyroid cancer associated with Hashimoto's disease has more favorable clinicopathologic features when compared to sporadic papillary thyroid cancer [44, 46, 47]. There may be a protective effect of the lymphocytic infiltration and inflammatory response in these patients.

Thyroid Lymphoma

Hashimoto's disease has also been associated with thyroid lymphomas. Thyroid lymphomas are rare [48]. However, there have been reports of B cell lymphomas and Hashimoto's disease [49]. There are close histologic, immunohistologic, and clinical similarities between non-Hodgkin's lymphomas and the lymphocytic infiltration seen in Hashimoto's disease. Also, a report of T cell lymphoma arising in the background of Hashimoto's disease has been reported [50] (Fig. 3).

Summary

The year 2013 marked the centennial anniversary of Hashimoto's initial description of struma lymphomatosa. His discovery was lost to the scientific community for the greater part of the last century; however, he was ultimately properly credited decades later. His discovery allowed those who followed to elucidate the true epidemiology, pathophysiology, and immunology of Hashimoto's disease. As a result of the tireless work of the scientists who followed, our understanding of Hashimoto's disease has come a long way. We now know that Hashimoto's disease is the most common endocrine disease, autoimmune disease, and cause of hypothyroidism.

Hashimoto's life as a physician was one of service and commitment. He was known in his community as a conscientious surgeon who worked tirelessly to ensure that his patients were well looked after. Coming from generations of physicians, he carried on the tradition of his honored family. He was considered a hero by the people he touched directly in Japan. And though it took some time for him to be recognized, he later became a hero to people around the world that he touched indirectly with his discovery.

References

1. Amino Nobuyuki, Tada Hisato, Hidaka Yoh, Hahimoto K. Hashimoto's disease and Hakaru Hashimoto. Endocr J. 2002;49(4):393–7.
2. Savin CT. The heritage of Dr. Hakaru Hashimoto (1881–1934). Endocr J. 2002;49(4):399–403.
3. Weetman A. A hundred years of Hashimoto's thyroiditis. Thyroid. 2013;23(2):135–6.
4. Duntas LH, Hiromatsu Y, Amino N. Centennial of the description of Hashimoto's thyroiditis: two thought-provoking events. Thyroid. 2013;23(6):643–5.
5. Hiromatsu Y, Satoh H, Amino N. Hashimoto's thyroiditis: history and future outlook. Hormones (Athens). 2013;12:12–8.
6. Hashimoto H. Zur Kenntniss der lymphomatosen Veränderung der Schilddrüse (Struma lymphomatosa). Arch Klin Chir. 1912;97(219):219–248.
7. Ahmed R, Al-Shaikh S, Akhtar M. Hashimoto thyroiditis: a century later. Adv Anat Pathol. 2012;19(3):181–6.
8. Simmonds M. Uber lymphatische herde in der schilddrüse. Virch Arch Patholog Anat Physiol. 1913;211:73–9.
9. Heinke. Die chronische thyreoiditis. Frankf Zeit F Pathol. 1914;28:141–50.
10. Williamson GS, Pearse IH. The pathological classification of goitre. J Pathol Bacteriol. 1925;28:361–7.
11. Graham A. Riedel's struma in contrast to struma lymphomatosa (Hashimoto). West J Surg. 1931;39:681–9.
12. McCullagh EP, Graham A. Atrophy and fibrosis associated with lymphoid tissue in the thyroid. Struma lymphomatosa (Hashimoto). Arch Surg. 1932;22:584–7.
13. Hertzler AE. Surgical pathology of the thyroid gland. Philadelphia: J.B. Lippincott; 1935.
14. Joll C. The pathology, diagnosis, and treatment of Hashimoto's disease (struma lymphomatosa). Br J Surg. 1939;27:351–9.
15. Fromm GA, Lascano EF, Bur GE, Escalante D. Tiroiditis cronica inespecifica. Rev Assoc Med Arg. 1953;67:162.
16. Cooke RT, Luxton RW. Hashimoto's struma lymphomatosa: diagnostic value and significance of serum-flocculation reactions. Lancet 1956;271(6934):105–109.
17. Akamizu T, Amino N, De Groot LJ. Hashimoto's thyroiditis. De Groot L J. Thyroid Disease Manager 2012. www.thyroidmanager.org.
18. Rose NR, Witebsky E. Studies on organ specificity. V. Changes in the thyroid glands of rabbits following active immunization with rabbit thyroid extracts. J Immunol. 1956;76(6):417–27.
19. Witebsky E, Rose NR, Terplan K, Paine JR, Egan RW. Chronic thyroiditis and autoimmunization. J Am Med Assoc. 1957;164(13):1439–47.
20. Campbell PN, Doniach D, Hudson RV, Roitt IM. Auto-antibodies in Hashimoto's disease (lymphadenoid goitre). Lancet. 1956;271(6947):820–1.
21. Gordin A, Maatela J, Miettinen A, Helenius T, Lamberg BA. Serum thyrotrophin and circulating thyroglobulin and thyroid microsomal antibodies in a Finnish population. Acta Endocrinol (Copenh). 1979;90(1):33–42.
22. Buchanan WW, Harden RM. Primary hypothryoidism and Hashimoto's thyroiditis. A continuous spectrum. Arch Intern Med. 1965;115:411–7.
23. Tunbridge WMG, Evered DC, Hall R, Appleton D, Brewis M, Clark F, et al. The spectrum of thyroid disease in a community: the Whickham survey. Clin Endocrinol (Oxf). 1977;7(6):481–3.
24. McConahey WM, Keating JR FR, Beahrs OH, Wooner LB. On the increasing occurrence of Hashimoto's thyroiditis. JCEM. 1962;22(5):542–4.
25. Caturegli P, De Remigis A, Rose NR. Hashimoto thyroiditis: clinical and diagnostic criteria. Autoimmun Rev. 2014;13(4–5):391–7.
26. McLeod DS, Cooper DS. The incidence and prevalence of thyroid autoimmunity. Endocrine. 2012;42(2):252–5.
27. Caturegli P, De Remigis A, Chuang K, Dembele M, Iwama A, Iwama S. Hashimoto's thyroiditis: celebrating the centennial through the lens of the Johns Hopkins hospital surgical pathology records. Thyroid. 2013;23(2):142–50.
28. Hall RC, Popkin MK, Devaul R, Hall AK, Gardner ER, Beresford TP. Psychiatric manifestations of Hashimoto's thyroiditis. Psychosomatics. 1982;23(4):337–42.
29. Takasu N, Yamada T, Takasu M, Komiya I, Nagasawa Y, Asawa T, et al. Disappearance of thyrotropin-blocking antibodies and spontaneous recovery from hypothyroidism in autoimmune thyroiditis. N Engl J Med. 1992;326(8):513–8.
30. Radetti G, Gottardi E, Bona G, Corrias A, Salardi S, Loche S. Study Group for Thyroid Diseases of the Italian Society for Pediatric Endocrinology and Diabetes (SIEDP/ISPED). The natural history of euthyroid Hashimowto's thyroiditis in children. J Pediatr. 2006;149(6):827–32.
31. Tomer Y. Mechanisms of autoimmune thyroid diseases: from genetics to epigenetics. Annu Rev Pathol. 2014;9:147–56.

32. Kawakami Y, Fisfalen ME, DeGroot LJ. Proliferative responses of peripheral blood mononuclear cells from patients with autoimmune thyroid diseases to synthetic peptide epitopes of human thyroid peroxidase. Autoimmunity. 1992;13(1):17–26.

33. Kotani T, Aratake Y, Hirai K, Fukazawa Y, Sato H, Ohtaki S. Apoptosis in thyroid tissue from patients with Hashimoto's thyroiditis. Autoimmunity. 1995;20(4):231–6.

34. Li D, Cai W, Gu R, Zhang Y, Zhang H, Tang K, et al. Th17 cell plays a role in the pathogenesis of Hashimoto's thyroiditis in patients. Clin Immunol. 2013;149(3):411–20.

35. Ng HP, Kung AW. Induction of autoimmune thyroiditis and hypothyroidism by immunization of immunoactive T cell epitope of thyroid peroxidase. Endocrinology. 2006;147(6):3085–92.

36. Figueroa-Vega N, Alfonso-Pérez M, Benedicto I, Sánchez-Madrid F, González-Amaro R, Marazuela M. Increased circulating pro-inflammatory cytokines and Th17 lymphocytes in Hashimoto's thyroiditis. J Clin Endocrinol Metab. 2010;95(2):953–62.

37. Chistiakov DA. Immunogenetics of Hashimoto's thyroiditis. J Autoimmune Dis. 2005;2(1):1.

38. Dong Z, Takakuwa T, Takayama H, Luo W-J, Takano T, Amino N, et al. Fas and Fas ligand gene mutations in Hashimoto's thyroiditis. Lab Invest. 2002;82(12):1611–6.

39. Eisenbarth GS, Wilson PW, Ward F, Buckley C, Lebovita H. The polyglandular failure syndrome: disease inheritance, HLA type, and immune function. Ann Intern Med. 1979;91(4):528–33.

40. Komatsu K, Hamano H, Ochi Y, Takayama M, Muraki T, Yoshizawa K, et al. High prevalence of hypothyroidism in patients with autoimmune pancreatitis. Dig Dis Sci. 2005;50(6):1052–7.

41. Effraimidis G, Wiersinga WM. Mechanisms of endocrinology: autoimmune thyroid disease: old and new players. Eur J Endocrinol. 2014;170(6):R241–252.

42. Loviselli A, Mathieu A, Pala R, Mariotti S, Cau S, Marongiu C, et al. Development of thyroid disease in patients with primary and secondary Sjögren's syndrome. J Endocrinol Invest. 1988;11(9):653–6.

43. Dailey ME, Lindsay S, Skahen R. Relation of thyroid neoplasms to Hashimoto disease of the thyroid gland. AMA Arch Surg. 1955;70(2):291–7.

44. Lee JH, Kim Y, Choi JW, Kim YS. The association between papillary thyroid carcinoma and histologically proven Hashimoto's thyroiditis: a meta-analysis. Eur J Endocrinol. 2013;168(3):343–9.

45. Larson SD, Jackson LN, Riall TS, Uchida T, Thomas RP, Qiu S, Evers BM. Increased incidence of well-differentiated thyroid cancer associated with Hashimoto thyroiditis and the role of the PI3k/Akt pathway. J Am Coll Surg. 2007;204(5):764–73; discussion 773–5.

46. Marotta V, Guerra A, Zatelli MC, Uberti ED, Di Stasi V, Faggiano A, et al. BRAF mutation positive papillary thyroid carcinoma is less advanced when Hashimoto's thyroiditis lymphocytic infiltration is present. Clin Endocrinol (Oxf). 2013;79(5):733–8.

47. Dvorkin S, Robenshtok E, Hirsch D, Strenov Y, Shimon I, Benbassat CA. Differentiated thyroid cancer is associated with less aggressive disease and better outcome in patients with coexisting Hashimotos thyroiditis. J Clin Endocrinol Metab. 2013;98(6):2409–14.

48. Freeman C, Berg JW, Cutler SJ. Occurrence and prognosis of extranodal lymphomas. Cancer. 1972;29(1):252–60.

49. Hyjek Elisabeth IPG. Primary B-cell lymphoma of the thyroid and its relationship to Hashimoto's thyroiditis. Hum Pathol. 1988;19(11):1315–26.

50. Abdul-Rahman ZH, Gogas HJ, Tooze JA, Anderson B, Mansi J, Sacks NP, Finlayson CJ. T-cell lymphoma in Hashimoto's thyroiditis. Histopathology. 1996;29(5):455–9.

Fritz de Quervain

1868–1940

Jonathan W. Serpell

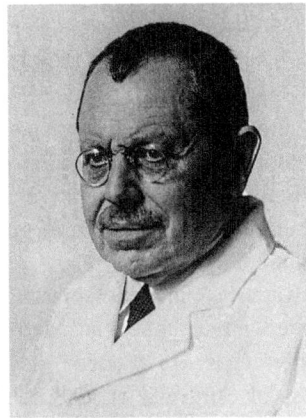

Fritz de Quervain, MD

Fritz de Quervain is regarded as one of the last surgical giants, and his obituary appeared in *Nature* after his death on January 24, 1940 [1].

De Quervain's most prolific contributions were in thyroid surgery, but he was a true generalist and published widely in diverse areas of surgery.

He was born in Sion, the capital of the Swiss Canton of Valais on May 4, 1868. His family were of Huguenot stock, and de Quervain was one of the ten siblings, most of whom made their own names with substantial achievements in their own right. His recorded birth name was Johann Friedrich de Quervain, but later he called himself Fritz.

De Quervain attended the Lerber School in Bern and, in 1887, began his medical education at the University of Bern. He matriculated at the University of Bern in 1888, and completed medical school in 1892.

During his medical course, de Quervain had the great fortune to be influenced by four eminent individuals—Kocher, Kronecker, Langhans, and Sahli, who helped make the Bern

Medical School famous at that time. De Quervain was first an assistant to Hugo Kronecker, a physiologist at the University of Bern, between 1889 and 1891. He was then an assistant to Theodor Langhans, a pathologist in 1891 and 1892. Langhans—who was influenced by Virchow and von Recklinghausen—described the giant cells of the tubercle granuloma. Later in his career, Langhans was particularly interested in the pathology of goitres and cretinism. Another teacher was Hermann Sahli, a notable physician and professor of internal medicine, with particular interests in haematology and haemodynamics.

After graduating in 1892, de Quervain became an assistant in **Emil Theodor Kocher's** surgical clinic in Bern at the *Inselspital*. Within 18 months, he had become the first assistant within that clinic, and eventually succeeded Kocher. Kocher won the Nobel Prize in Physiology or Medicine in 1909 for his work on the physiology, pathology, and surgery of the thyroid gland. While these four giants in physiology, pathology, medicine, and surgery at the Bern Medical School profoundly influenced de Quervain, his professors noted that de Quervain, as a student, demonstrated a clear intellect, a tremendous capacity for work, and an extraordinary memory.

In 1894, de Quervain moved to La Chaux-de-Fonds, a watch-making district in the Neuchâtel Mountains. De Quervain was to remain in La Chaux-de-Fonds for 15 years, and became director of the Surgical Clinic there in 1897. It was during this time that he published prolifically in many areas in surgical journals and textbooks. In La Chaux-de-Fonds, he described the stenosing tendovaginitis affecting the tendons at the wrist, which was subsequently named after him.

Of enterprising nature, de Quervain worked not only in the local hospital at La Chaux-de-Fonds but he also developed his own private clinic and, subsequently, a more modern hospital. In 1898, de Quervain acquired the necessary parts and constructed an X-ray machine in his clinic, only 3 years after X-rays were discovered by Röntgen in 1895.

With this extensive general surgical practice, he had a large pool of patients and became a pioneer in what would now be regarded as clinical research.

J. W. Serpell (✉)
Monash University Endocrine Surgery Unit, Alfred Hospital, Commercial Road, Prahran, Melbourne, Vic 3181, Australia
e-mail: jonathan.serpell@alfred.org.au

J. L. Pasieka, J. A. Lee (eds.), *Surgical Endocrinopathies,* DOI 10.1007/978-3-319-13662-2_9,
© Springer International Publishing Switzerland 2015

De Quervain's syndrome of repetitive stress injury affecting the thumb, in particular the tendons of abductor pollicis longus and extensor pollicis brevis at the level of the wrist over the radial styloid process, was described in 1895. It is of interest that his mentor, Theodor Kocher, was consulted on this new syndrome of stenosing tendovaginitis. They exchanged details on a number of cases, but it was de Quervain who published his findings, describing five cases in an article in 1895 entitled "On a Form of Chronic Tendovaginitis" [2]. The description and the surgical treatment of this condition have changed little over the past 120 years. De Quervain's syndrome of stenosing tendovaginitis has had various interesting synonyms attached to it, including mother's wrist, washerwoman's sprain, and, in more modern-day parlance, gamer's thumb, "BlackBerry" thumb, or texting thumb.

During his time in La Chaux-de-Fonds, de Quervain's intellect was apparent in other areas. He developed a new and advanced autoclave, which enabled sterilisation of all instruments, drapes, and dressings. The key feature of the new autoclave was that it could create a pressure of 2 atm, compared to the then standard of 0.5 atm.

He also developed an innovative operating table, which could have its height adjusted and which supported the patient's head. These advances were popular and led to the table's worldwide adoption.

At La Chaux-de-Fonds, de Quervain wrote extensively. He co-edited *The Encyclopedia of Entire Surgery* with Kocher, which was published in 1901 [3]. Putting together his extensive clinical experience and research, he produced *Clinical Surgical Diagnosis for Students and Practitioners* in 1907 [4]. This ultimately went to six editions and was translated into a number of languages, becoming a major reference for surgeons at the time and ensuring de Quervain became widely known around the world. In 1908, he also wrote a chapter on surgery of the head and neck for Wullstein and Wilm's *Textbook of Surgery* [5].

De Quervain retained his interest in clinical research and thyroid disease, undoubtedly stimulated by his mentor, Kocher. His doctoral thesis in 1893 was titled "On the Change of the Central Nervous System by Experimental Hypothyroid Cachexia". In 1902, he presented his work on non-bacterial thyroid inflammation, entitled "Subacute Non-suppurative Thyroiditis" [6] which was subsequently published in 1904 [7]. This condition would later be known as de Quervain's thyroiditis, and otherwise as subacute or granulomatous thyroiditis.

A less well-known syndrome described by de Quervain in 1923, is complete testicular feminisation, which is the most common form of male pseudohermaphroditism [8].

Overall, it is believed that de Quervain published over 300 papers, many of which were devoted to thyroid disease, ranging from technical aspects of thyroidectomy to the epidemiology of thyroid disease. Perhaps his greatest contribution to thyroid disease was based on his epidemiological work and the introduction of iodised salt for the prevention of goitre.

In recognition of his substantial achievements in academic surgery, and with the aid of his mentor, Theodor Kocher, de Quervain was appointed to the position of Titular Professor at Bern in 1907. In 1910, he was appointed Professor of Surgery at the University of Basel and remained there until 1918. He expected to finish his surgical career at Basel, finding it an agreeable position, gaining wide respect, and remaining very productive. However, in July 1917, Theodor Kocher died suddenly and unexpectedly. Unusually for the time, rather than advertise the position, the faculty at Bern voted to offer the position of Professor of Surgery at Bern to de Quervain. It would seem appropriate that de Quervain succeeded his mentor to the chair of surgery in Bern. De Quervain became the head of the University Clinic of Surgery at Bern in 1918, and remained there for two decades until he retired in 1938.

De Quervain remained a strong proponent of his general approach to the patient, and is attributed as one of the earliest clinicians to realise that "postoperative pneumonia" was often in fact a pulmonary infarct due to pulmonary embolism, rather than an infection.

De Quervain was active in the international medical community and visited many colleagues and attended many international conferences. He attended the inaugural International Congress of Surgeons in 1905, and also the first meeting of the Swiss Society for Surgery, of which he was president from 1919 to 1920. He was Dean of the Faculty from 1923 to 1924, and Rector of the University between 1935 and 1936.

De Quervain retired from the University of Bern in 1938, but remained active and continued to perform surgery and research. However, he died suddenly of complications due to acute pancreatitis, on January 24, 1940, at the age of 70.

While he is remembered principally for de Quervain's syndrome, the stenosing tendovaginitis of the wrist, de Quervain's subacute or granulomatous thyroiditis, and for introducing iodised table salt to prevent endemic goitre, de Quervain had major influence in many areas of clinical observation, epidemiology, operative surgery, technologies such as radiology, sterilisation, and operating tables, and is remembered as a father of modern clinical research [9].

References

1. Obituary Prof Fritz de Quervain. Nature 1940;145:291. doi:10.1038/145291b0.
2. de Quervain F. Ueber eine Form von chronischer Tendovaginitis. Korrespondenzblatt für Schweiz Arzte 1895;25:389–94.
3. de Quervain F. Spezielle chirurgische Diagnostik für Studierende und Arzte. Leipzig: Vogel; 1907.
4. Kocher T, de Quervain F. Die Encyklopädie der gesamten Chirurgie. Leipzig: Vogel; 1903.

5. Wullstein L, Wilms M. Lehrbuch der Chirurgie. Jena: Fischer; 1908. p. 360–449.

6. de Quervain F. Ueber acute, nicht eiterige Thyreoiditis. Arch Klinis-chechir. 1902;67:706–14.

7. de Quervain F. Die acute, nicht eitrige Thyreoiditis und die Beteiligung der Schilddrüse an akuten Intoxikationen und Infektionen überhaupt. Jena: Fischer; 1904. p. 1–23.

8. de Quervain F. Ein Fall von Pseudohermaphrodismus masculinus. Schweizerische Medizinische Wochenschr. 1923;53:563.

9. Ahuja NK, Chung KC. Fritz de Quervain, MD (1868–1940): stenosing tendovaginitis at the radial styloid process. J Hand Surg. 2004;29(6):1164–70.

George W. Crile

1864–1943

Edwin L. Kaplan, Benjamin C. James and Raymon H. Grogan

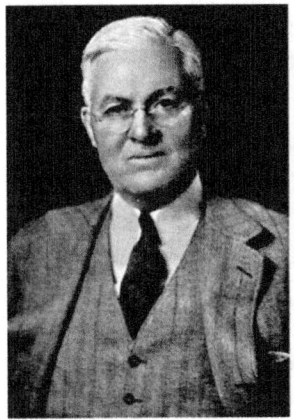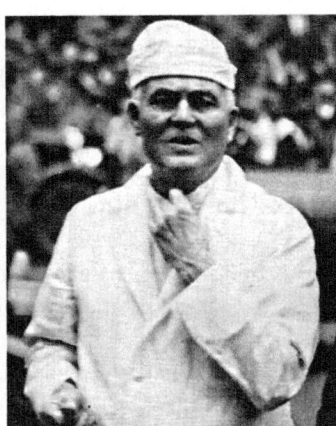

Dr. George W. Crile. (From [5]. Reprinted with permission, Cleveland Clinic Center for Medical Art & Photography © 2014. All Rights Reserved)

Introduction

Born in 1864 in Chili, Ohio, Dr. George Washington Crile became one of the most distinguished surgeons of the early twentieth century worldwide [1]. He was a founder and the second president of the American College of Surgeons, and cofounder of the Cleveland Clinic. He served in the Spanish American War and in World War I, where he became very interested in shock. He was the head of experimental clinical research for the American Expeditionary Force, and ultimately rose to the rank of general. He is credited with giving the first human blood transfusion. He designed a hemostat which bears his name. He developed the use of narcotics and

E. L. Kaplan (✉)
Endocrine Surgery, Section of General Surgery, The University of Chicago Pritzker School of Medicine, 5841 S. Maryland Avenue, MC 4052, Chicago, IL 60637, USA
e-mail: ekaplan@surgery.bsd.uchicago.edu

B. C. James · R. H. Grogan
Department of Surgery, The University of Chicago Pritzker School of Medicine, Chicago, IL, USA

regional anesthesia with general anesthesia, now called "balanced anesthesia." For his work on "shockless surgery," he received a gold medal from the National Institute of Social Sciences. In World War II, the *SS George Crile* was named after him. A lunar crater "Crile" also bears his name. These latter two honors certainly attest to the high esteem in which he was held.

All of his accomplishments are beyond the scope of this chapter. We focus on his greatness as a surgeon, especially on the early development of an effective operation for thyrotoxicosis at a time when this disease was associated with a very high mortality rate. Furthermore, we discuss how he translated his experimental work on shock into clinical practice to benefit the most difficult patients with recurrent hyperthyroidism from Graves' disease. The brain, he felt, was central as a cause of *Graves'* disease; fear and other harmful emotions were to be avoided. "Stealing the thyroid" and using adrenal denervation to produce a state of anociassociation and shockless surgery were used in the treatment of the most serious cases of recurrent thyrotoxicosis. These terms and the procedures that he used are described in detail.

Shock and Anociassociation

For much of his life, Dr. Crile was interested in the mechanism of shock. He wrote that low blood pressure, failing respiration, changes in chemistry of the blood, mental and muscular weakness, and the exudation of serum through the walls of the blood vessels were not the cause of shock, but rather the result of shock [2]. He found that these manifestations of shock could be almost completely prevented by the use of morphine, nitrous oxide, and spinal anesthesia. Thus, he felt that the causes of shock were psychic or neural impulses reaching the brain. By preventing the brain from receiving these stimuli, called a state of *anociassociation*, one could prevent the manifestations of shock.

The adrenal gland and adrenaline were very important in changes in blood pressure and shock during operations in man [3]. Crile realized that strong emotions, such as fear before an operation, might produce shock and severe complications of the operation. He attempted to allay fear by "psychic suggestion," and when an operation was necessary, by anesthetizing the operative area by use of local anesthesia before giving general anesthesia. Thus, by blocking nerve communication between the affected part and the brain by use of local or regional anesthesia, he could achieve a shockless operation. He used these principles in the treatment of severe cases of thyrotoxicosis.

Thyroid Surgery and Graves' Disease

The 1920s were a period of great excitement for thyroid surgeons. In 1922, Dr. **Henry Plummer** showed that when patients with Graves' disease were given iodine, their hyperthyroidism could be partially controlled, and thyroidectomy was made relatively safe [4]. Prior to that time, thyroid storm and bleeding made this operation extremely dangerous. Only the most courageous surgeon would operate on a patient with **Graves'** disease. Now for the first time, many patients who were being followed were considered operative candidates. Furthermore, the Cleveland area and the Midwest were considered a "goiter belt" and huge nontoxic goiters were common. Iodine supplementation to prevent and treat goiters was not yet common in medical practice.

Dr. Crile was perhaps one of the most prolific surgeons of his time [5]. He and his group were ready for an ever-increasing number of thyroid operations. In 1927, these reached a peak when 2700 thyroid operations were performed in a single year. The largest number of operations performed by Crile in 1 day was 35. Throughout his career, Crile performed more than 25,000 thyroid operations. It has been written that "the original (Cleveland) Clinic and Hospital buildings were paid for mainly by the receipts from thyroidectomies." His operative techniques and procedures are briefly discussed in the following sections.

Fear, Thyroid Storm, and "Stealing the Thyroid"

The greatest danger when operating on a thyrotoxic patient in the 1920s was thyroid storm or crisis. The pulse soared, the heart often fibrillated, the temperature rose to 105 or 106 °F, and the patient "literally consumed himself in the fire of metabolism" [5]. Ice bags and oxygen were applied. There were no medications to slow the pulse. There were no corticosteroids for possible adrenal insufficiency. The peak of a thyroid crisis occurred on the second night after operation, and then subsided if the patient were to survive. These events followed general anesthesia, an operation, an infection, or a frightening episode.

Crile believed that emotion, especially fear, was the cause of thyroid storm [3, 5]. He developed a system to prevent the patient's fear which became known as "stealing the thyroid." The thyrotoxic patient consented to operation but was never told when the operation would take place. Each morning, breakfast was held and the anesthetist would come into the room and administer nitrous oxide–oxygen analgesia by mask—enough to make the patient giddy and confused. On the morning when the operation was to be done, the routine was the same, but deeper analgesia was obtained. The thyroid operation was performed most often in the patient's bed. The patient never had a chance to become afraid. A modification of this system was sometimes used by other surgeons. Each day saline was injected intravenously into a patient's arm vein. On the day when the operation was to be performed, morphine, other sedatives, or an anesthetic agent was injected, and the patient was operated upon.

Operative Technique

The patient, in a sedated and euphoric state from the nitrous oxide, was positioned while still in bed and sterilely prepped and draped. Commonly, Dr. Crile would operate in stages [5]. Particularly if the patient was considered a bad risk, one or both superior thyroid arteries were ligated as a definitive operation or as a first step. In other patients, a subtotal lobectomy was performed; often, the same procedure was performed on the other side several days later. Dr. Crile would run from room to room, changing his gown, gloves, and instruments, usually with a group of visiting surgeons following him. He often lectured to them on his theories of the relation of the adrenal glands to hyperthyroidism while he performed surgery. It has been written that he operated rapidly and never clamped any bleeders. That was the job of the assistants. A team was ready to transfuse the patient or to perform a tracheostomy, if necessary. Crile recommended leaving the posterior capsule of the thyroid when performing a thyroid resection (Fig. 1) [6]. He called the area near the recurrent laryngeal nerve and parathyroids "no man's land." "It is not to be palpated; it is subject to the least possible traction and no division of tissue is made" within this area. By these precautions, he wrote that "temporary and permanent injury of the recurrent laryngeal nerve may be completely eliminated."

Crile wrote that "compared to peripheral nerves, the recurrent laryngeal nerves are exceedingly soft…and the slightest direct or even indirect pressure on the recurrent nerve interferes with nerve conduction" [6]. If the nerve trunk is exposed during operation, it will be covered by scar formation, and scar produces a "physiologic severance of the nerve." Thus, the nerve should never be seen during thyroid resection. In this way, the parathyroids would be preserved

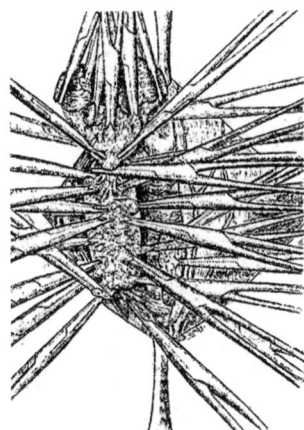

Fig. 1 Dr. Crile's technique for thyroid lobectomy. The posterior part of the thyroid lobe was always left in place in order to avoid "no man's land." The recurrent laryngeal nerve was purposely never seen. As he cut across the lobe, assistants clamped the bleeding points with numerous hemostats placed transversely. Tissue was then suture-ligated with fine catgut. (From [6], Chap. XXXII. Reprinted with permission from Elsevier)

CLEVELAND CLINIC HOSPITAL
Schedule of Operations
Date – June 7, 1928

1.	8:00	Dr. Crile	Lobectomy or Closure, R.
2.	8:15		Lobectomy or Closure, R.
3.	8:30		Thyroidectomy, R.
4.	8:45		Lobectomy or Closure, R.
5.	9:00		Thyroidectomy, R.
6.	9:15		Lobectomy or Closure, R.
7.	9:30		Thyroidectomy, R.
8.	9:45		Thyroidectomy, R.
9.	10:00		Lobectomy, R.
10.	10:15		Lobectomy or Closure, R.
11.	10:30		Ligation, R.
12.	10:40		Lobectomy, R.
13.	10:55		Thyroidectomy, R.
14.	11:10		Ligation, R.
15.	11:20		Ligation, R.
16.	11:30		Ligation, R.
17.	11:40		Lobectomy or Closure, R.
18.	11:55		Ligation, R.
19.	12:05		Thyroidectomy, R.
20.	12:20		Thyroidectomy, R.
21.	12:35		Lobectomy, R.
22.	12:50		Lobectomy or Closure, R.
23.	1:05		Final lobectomy, R.
24.	1:20		Thyroidectomy, R.
25.	1:35		Thyroidectomy, R.
26.	1:50		Thyroidectomy, R.
27.	2:05		Ligation, R.
28.	2:15		Thyroidectomy, R.
29.	2:30		Thyroidectomy, R.
30.	3:00		Ligation, R.
31.	3:10		Left adrenalectomy

Fig. 2 Typical operating day for Dr. Crile. He moved from patient bed to patie nt bed, operating rapidly. Ligation of a superior thyroid artery was scheduled for 10 min and thyroid lobectomy for 15 min. Surgical assistants then finished the operation after he left the room. (From [5]. Reprinted with permission, Cleveland Clinic Center for Medical Art & Photography © 2014. All Rights Reserved.)

as well. Today, using this technique of thyroidectomy is considered a very dangerous practice.

The average thyroid operation took Crile approximately 10–15 min to perform (Fig. 2) [5]. Then, it took the assistant about 30 min to stop the bleeding and close the wound. Thus, operating in the patient's room, instead of in the four operating rooms, proved to be very efficient and allowed him to perform many more operations.

In 1932, Crile wrote that he and his associates had performed 22,441 operations on the thyroid—5533 had been ligations and 16,908 had been thyroidectomies of which 12,747 had been for hyperthyroidism [7]. The last 5000 thyroidectomies were performed with a mortality rate of 0.84%—a remarkable feat at that time! Vocal cord paralyses, mostly unilateral, occurred in 1.08%. Temporary or persistent hypoparathyroidism occurred in 0.97% of the entire series. Postoperative hypothyroidism was treated with thyroid extract and checked by measurement of the basal metabolic rate. Crile stated that it was also important to treat these patients with dilute hydrochloric acid to correct low gastric acid and gastrointestinal (GI) hypomotility.

Recurrent hyperthyroidism was found to occur only in 3.03% of his patients; half of these occurred within 2 years [7]. When this occurred, he recommended reoperation on the thyroid in most patients unless he was certain that the surgeon had removed enough thyroid gland at the first operation. If enough had been removed, he wrote that "it is evident that the recurrence is caused by local infection somewhere in the body or that the patient is being subjected to social maladjustments, worry, overwork, or some other strain not disclosed by the clinical investigations." *In such cases of re-current hyperthyroidism, it was necessary to cure them by operating on their adrenal glands.*

Adrenalectomy or Adrenal Denervation for Recurrent Hyperthyroidism

Crile became very interested in the brain–thyroid–adrenal sympathetic system which he called the *kinetic system.* When this system became hyperkinetic, he postulated that it led to a number of diseases in man—hyperthyroidism, neurocirculatory asthenia, peptic ulcer, and probably diabetes [3]. Neurocirculatory asthenia was defined as a rapid heartbeat, nervousness, and fatigue. This caused incapacitation in soldiers at the front (called soldier's heart) and similar problems in civilians. It was due to severe stress, he postulated. The control of these diseases was therefore "rationalization" (or what we call psychiatric help) and if this was insufficient, by the performance of one or more of the following operations either singly or in combination: removal of the thyroid, excision of certain sympathetic ganglia, or the division of the nerves leading from the adrenal glands. The adrenal glands, he postulated, played a very important role in the pathogenesis of these diseases [8].

Fig. 3 a Diagram of the efferent nerves from the adrenal gland. **b** These adrenal nerves were divided sharply first and any remaining nerves were divided manually thereafter. Adrenal denervation was used to cure the most difficult cases of recurrent thyrotoxicosis. (From [3]. Permission requested)

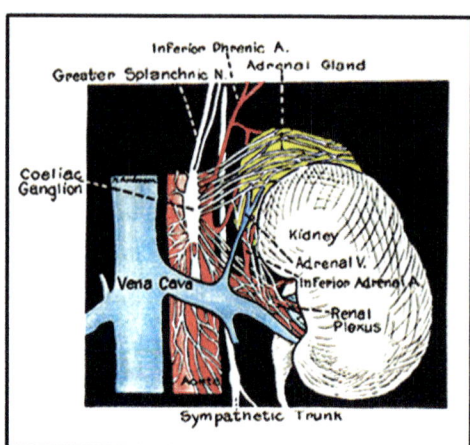
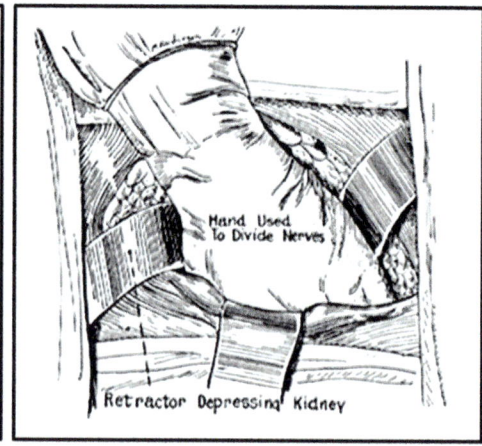

Latarjet and Bertrand had shown that there are 30–40 efferent nerves from the adrenal glands which go to the celiac plexuses or the celiac ganglia (Fig. 3a) [9]. By dividing these nerves, Crile stated that activity of the kinetic system could be reduced and the patient cured of a number of diseases. A standard kidney incision was made. Novocaine was infused around the adrenal gland to prevent the hypertension that might occur by dissecting tissue and nerves around this gland and to prevent these efferent nerves from signaling the brain. The adrenal gland was elevated by a special instrument, and the nerves, but not the blood vessels, were attempted to be divided. Then the surgeon's hand was inserted and any remaining nerves were manually divided (Fig. 3b) [8].

Crile performed an adrenalectomy, but more commonly, a unilateral or bilateral denervation of the adrenal as primary treatment for some primary cases of hyperthyroidism, but used this technique especially for very difficult cases of recurrent thyrotoxicosis due to Graves' disease. Following denervation in 68 thyrotoxic patients, he reported a cure rate of 93.7 % [10]. Similar cure rates or clinical improvement followed adrenal denervation in patients with neurocirculatory asthenia or with peptic ulcers. He felt that this operation would also benefit patients with diabetes.

This was a different time. There were no antithyroid medications other than iodine, no beta-blockers for thyrotoxicosis, no oral diuretics, and no antibiotics until sulfa drugs were introduced in the late 1930s. Crile's results, as reported, especially in treating patients with severe thyrotoxicosis of Graves' disease, were remarkable, although he stated that effective follow-up of the patients was quite difficult to achieve.

Of greatest importance to the authors is the fact that Dr. Crile's legacy and his dedication and love for endocrine surgery have not been lost. His DNA was transmitted to his son, Dr. George (Barney) Crile, Jr., a very accomplished thy

roid and breast surgeon. Finally, two of his granddaughters married very prominent leaders in endocrine surgery—Dr. Caldwell Esselstyn and Dr. Roger Foster.

Dr. Crile died in 1943 at the age of 78. He was a great man. He will be long remembered for being a founder of the Cleveland Clinic and, along with Dr. **Charles Mayo**, for being one of the foremost thyroid surgeons of the early twentieth century.

Acknowledgment The authors wish to thank Ms. Patricia Schaddelee for the preparation of this manuscript.

References

1. Crile GW. Wikipedia, http://en.wikipedia.org. Accessed 8 Feb 2015.
2. Crile G. An autobiography, vol. 2. In: Crile G, editor. Philadelphia: JB Lippincott; 1947. p. 585.
3. Crile G. Diseases peculiar to civilized man. Clinical management and surgical treatment. New York: MacMillan; 1934. pp. 89–94.
4. McConahey W, Pady DS. Henry Stanley Plummer. Endocrinology 1991;129:2271–3.
5. Bunts AT, Crile G Jr. To act as a unit. The story of the Cleveland Clinic. Ohio: The Cleveland Clinic Foundation; 1971. pp. 83–103.
6. Crile George and Associates. Diagnosis and treatment of diseases of the thyroid gland. Philadelphia: WB Saunders; 1932. pp. 377–418.
7. Crile George and Associates. Diagnosis and treatment of diseases of the thyroid gland. Philadelphia: WB Saunders; 1932. pp. 483–91.
8. Crile G. Diseases peculiar to civilized man. Clinical management and surgical treatment. New York: MacMillan; 1934. pp. 109–17.
9. Latarjet A, Bertrand P. Innervation of the suprarenals, kidneys, and upper ureters. Lyon Chir. 1923;20:452–62.
10. Crile G. Diseases peculiar to civilized man. Clinical management and surgical treatment. New York: MacMillan; 1934. p. 151.

Multinodular Goiter

Scott M. Wilhelm

Introduction

Perhaps one of the most common thyroid disorders is the thyroid nodule. Solitary palpable nodules can be found in up to 4–7 % of the adult population [1–3]. However, autopsy studies have shown this number to be higher at up to 50 % [4]. Radiographic studies utilizing ultrasound agree with this finding that thyroid nodules are seen in approximately 40–70 % of patients [5]. In addition, ultrasound performed in patients with a known thyroid nodule will reveal the finding of additional nodules in as many as 48 % of patients [6]. While the general etiologies and surgical management for the solitary nodule and multinodular goiter (MNG) are similar, there are some unique elements to the management of MNG which this chapter tries to elucidate.

Etiology

MNG is a term that has been traditionally used to describe an enlarged thyroid gland containing multiple areas of nodular hyperplasia. MNG has been found to be one of the most common endocrine disorders in the world affecting between 500 and 600 million individuals [7]. The most common cause for this disorder is generally related to dietary issues such as iodine deficiency or the consumption of goitrogens, which reduce the body's ability to uptake and process iodine for the production of thyroid hormone. The most potent goitrogens include those from the cruciferous family of vegetables, including things, such as broccoli, cauliflower, and cabbage. The African fruit cassava is another common goitrogen [8]. Much of the research for iodine deficiency leading to goiters was initiated by Dr. David Marine in Cleveland, OH, at Case Western Reserve University. He was one of the first researchers to develop the concept that the enlargement of the thyroid gland is due to an increased production of thyroid-stimulating hormone (TSH) from the anterior pituitary gland [9]. He demonstrated that iodine deficiency leads to decreased thyroid hormone production, which in turn leads to the typical feedback mechanism of increased TSH production. Selwyn Taylor, surgeon and first president of the International Association of Endocrine Surgeons (IAES), then expanded upon this theory and created a hypothesis that the follicular cells of the thyroid will undergo diffuse hyperplasia in the setting of TSH stimulation [10]. Some of the individual cells may have clonal abnormalities that allow them to grow into true nodules. This theory has been substantiated by Studer et al. [11], who demonstrated the existence of both monoclonal and polyclonal nodules within a multinodular thyroid gland.

Once nodules have begun to form, they may then become encapsulated by compression from surrounding thyroid tissue. As these nodules grow, they begin a process of colloid storage which leads to nodular growth. Nodules may ultimately outlive their blood supply, at which time they undergo necrosis and internal hemorrhage. That cycle is then followed by a typical inflammatory and fibrotic reaction allowing for a cyclical pattern of ongoing nodular growth [12].

In countries such as the USA where iodine deficiency is rare, other causes of MNG have been found that are genetic in nature. A gene on chromosome 14q, which has been named MNG-1, has been associated with a familial form of nontoxic MNG [13]. In addition, a research team at the Mayo Clinic [14] has identified an abnormality in codon 727 of the human TSH receptor, which has been linked to the development of toxic MNGs. Regardless of the mechanism, once MNGs have formed, they may go on to medical or surgical evaluation based on symptoms or a concern for malignancy.

S. M. Wilhelm (✉)
Surgery Department, Case Medical Center, University Hospitals, 11100 Euclid Avenue, Cleveland, OH 44106, USA
e-mail: Scott.Wilhelm@UHhospitals.org

J. L. Pasieka, J. A. Lee (eds.), *Surgical Endocrinopathies,* DOI 10.1007/978-3-319-13662-2_11,
© Springer International Publishing Switzerland 2015

Clinical Evaluation and Treatment Indications

Patients are generally referred for surgical evaluation of an MNG based on a variety of symptoms or complaints. In most cases, these can be broken down into three categories including that of (1) functional nodules, (2) compressive symptoms, or (3) concern for thyroid malignancy.

Functional Nodules in MNG

Toxic MNG or Plummer's syndrome named after **Dr H Plummer** relates to nodules that have taken on autonomous production of thyroid hormone leading to classic symptoms of hyperthyroidism such as tachycardia, hypertension, weight loss, insomnia, heat intolerance, etc. This topic and other functional thyroid nodules are covered in another chapter and will not be addressed in detail here. Routine laboratory testing including TSH, free T3 and free T4 levels can usually determine if an MNG is the cause of functional symptoms. An assessment of thyroid function should take place for all patients undergoing thyroid surgery.

Compressive Symptoms with MNG

Compressive MNG symptoms most often include dysphagia, dyspnea, and rarely vocal complaints. MNGs are typically slow-growing processes. As such, if they occur in the cervical area, the overlying skin, soft tissues, and musculature can gradually adapt and patients can have fairly large goiters that remain asymptomatic despite being visible on simple neck inspection (Fig. 1). (*Note:* This type of goiter would be classified by the World Health Organization as a grade 3 lesion (see below).)

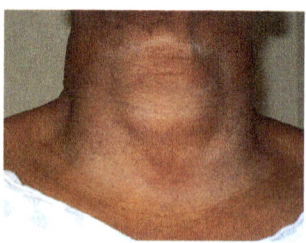

Fig. 1 Pt with visible but asymptomatic cervical multinodular goiter. Grade 3 by World Health Organization goiter classification system

However, goiters which become substernal in their growth pattern have a higher likelihood to become symptomatic. As the goiter grows below the sternal notch and into the thoracic inlet, the trachea and esophagus can become compressed between the sternum and thyroid anteriorly and the cervical and upper thoracic spine posteriorly (see Fig. 2).

This compression can lead to true dysphagia characterized by difficulty in swallowing solid foods or odynophagia with pain upon swallowing. This should be distinguished from a complaint of a "globus pharyngeus" which implies a sensation of lump in the back of the throat where no lump is actually felt on exam or visualized on inspection or radiographic imaging. The most common causes of globus are gastroesophageal reflux (GERD), sinus drainage, or dis-coordination of the muscles involved in the swallowing mechanism. While patients who have true compressive symptoms or even sleep apnea related to their MNG may benefit clinically from surgery [15, 16], patients with globus sensations should be cautioned that thyroidectomy may or may not improve their symptoms and other evaluations such as laryngoscopy, video endoscopy (esophagogastroduodenoscopy (EGD)), barium swallow, and treatment of other causes as listed above should be considered before undertaking surgery.

World Health Organization (WHO) Grading of Thyroid Goiter

Grade 0: No goiter found, thyroid impalpable/invisible

Grade 1a: Thyroid palpable but invisible even with full neck extension

Grade 1b: Thyroid palpable in neutral position/visible with neck extension

Grade 2: Goiter visible, no palpation required to make diagnosis

Grade 3: Goiter clearly visible at a distance

Of note: Substernal goiters may not meet typicalclassificationdependingontheamountofthe goiter present in the neck.

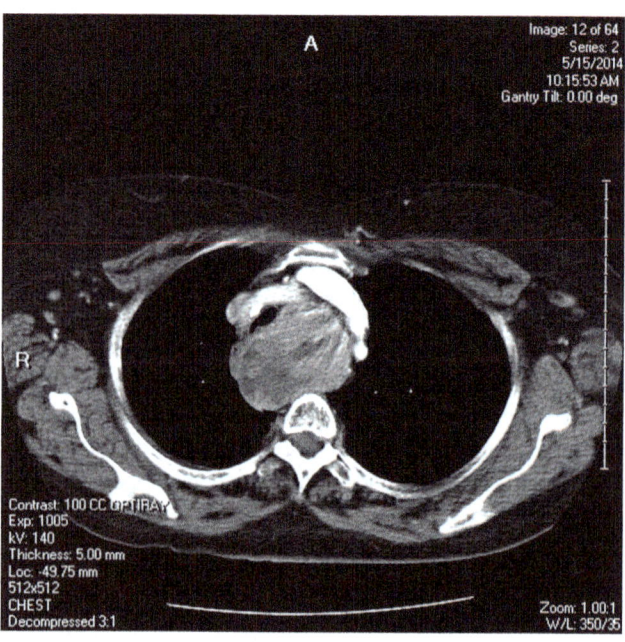

Fig. 2 Substernal goiter leading to significant tracheal deviation and compression with symptomatic dyspnea on exertion

Another form of compression results from tracheal compression, which again usually occurs in the setting of a multinodular substernal goiter (SG). Patients may complain of dyspnea on exertion or positional dyspnea (PD)—worsening shortness of breath when reclined or lying flat. Stang et al. from the University of Pittsburgh provided an evaluation of almost 200 patients with PD in the setting of SG. They demonstrated that SG led to some degree of tracheal compression in 97% of their patients when evaluated by computed tomography (CT) scan. Improvement in PD after surgical resection was predicted by a gland weight of >100 g (normal thyroid is approximately 15–20 g) or tracheal compression of >35% of tracheal diameter [17]. In the office, the surgeon should ask detailed questions regarding respiratory status both at rest and during exertion. The patient should be questioned about orthopnea and sleeping habits. On physical examination, if the lower extent of the thyroid cannot be palpated during swallowing, an SG should be suspected. Pemberton's sign [18] can also be a useful physical exam finding to point to a goiter as the cause of compressive symptoms. Named for **Dr. Hugh Pemberton** who in 1946 described the maneuver, Pemberton's sign can be used to detect compression at the thoracic inlet from goiter or other anterior mediastinal masses. The patient is asked to extend their arms over their head next to their face which raises the clavicles, posteriorly displaces the upper ribs and narrows the thoracic inlet. If an anterior mediastinal mass is present, the additional compression will result in facial congestion, cyanosis, or respiratory distress in <1 min.

Patients with subjective complaints of compressive symptoms accompanied by a physical exam suggestive of an SG or positive Pemberton's sign should undergo a CT scan of the neck and chest to determine the extent of the SG and degree of tracheal compression to aid in surgical and anesthetic planning [19].

In regard to vocal changes associated with MNG, persistent hoarseness of the voice should prompt preoperative vocal cord assessment. Vocal cord paresis strongly suggests the presence of invasive thyroid malignancy. Persistent vocal changes in the setting of benign MNG are uncommon.

Risk of Malignancy in MNG

The final consideration of surgical intervention in the setting of MNG is the risk of malignancy. A common misconception is that an MNG implies a benign etiology or has a substantially lower risk of malignancy when compared to a solitary nodule. Several independent studies have shown the risk of malignancy in MNG to be 10–31% [20–22]. A recent large meta-analysis (23,000 patients) review by Brito et al. evaluated the risk of malignancy of single nodule versus MNG [23]. While their overall conclusion was that single nodules

had a slightly higher risk of malignancy compared to solitary thyroid nodules, the overall risk of malignancy in surgically resected MNG was 8–15%.

Thus, the evaluation for cancer in MNG should not differ from solitary nodules. Patients with nodules identified on physical exam or by other radiographic tests such as CT scan, positron emission tomography (PET) scan, and carotid duplex should undergo a dedicated thyroid ultrasound to accurately measure nodules and characterize them to see if they meet American Thyroid Association guidelines for biopsy [24]. Nodules >1 cm should undergo biopsy. Nodules less than 1 cm with atypical features or in patients with a family history of thyroid cancer or personal history of radiation exposure should be "considered" for biopsy.

Ultrasound may also be very helpful in determining which nodules to biopsy based on ultrasonographic criteria that have been shown to predict a higher incidence of malignancy (see below). Biopsies performed under ultrasonographic guidance by experienced physicians have excellent sensitivity, specificity, and accuracy (95, 87.7, and 89%, respectively) [25].

Ultrasonographic Features Worrisome for Thyroid Malignancy

1. Irregular borders
2. Microcalcifications
3. Lesions that are taller than they are wide
4. Hypoechoic lesions
5. Hypervascular thyroid nodules (central not peripheral pattern)
6. Abnormal lymph nodes (microcalcifications, loss of fatty hilum)

One question that frequently occurs in the setting of MNG is how many nodules should be biopsied to predict that the remaining nodules are benign. Ultrasonography as mentioned above can guide biopsy of nodules with worrisome features. Thyroid uptake scanning (I-123) has also been used to some extent [26] to find "cold" nodules which have a generally accepted rate of malignancy of 10–20%. However, this test cannot reliably exclude malignancy in a thyroid nodule. Some texts have advocated simply biopsying the "dominant" or "largest" nodule. Returning to Frates et al. [22], we see that when they biopsied either solitary thyroid nodules or MNG, the rate of cancer in both groups was similar at 14.8 and 14.9%, respectively. On subgroup analysis of the MNG patients, if they had only biopsied the largest nodule in patients with at least two nodules >1 cm in size, they would have missed a cancer in the nondominant nodule in 14% of patients. If the MNG contained at least three nodules (>1 cm), biopsy of the dominant lesion would have missed another malignancy in 50% of patients. Thus, they advocate biopsying up to four nodules in the setting of MNG to exclude a risk of cancer in additional nodules.

Treatment Options for MNG

Medical Treatment

Medical treatment options generally employ either TSH suppression with levothyroxine (LT4) administration or radioactive iodine thyroid ablation. In the setting of hypothyroidism, excess TSH production can result in hyperplasia, nodular growth, and a general increase in goiter size. Here, the use of LT4 to induce a euthyroid state has been clearly documented to decrease goiter size [9, 10]. However, in the circumstance of the euthyroid MNG, simple LT4 administration is unlikely to have any meaningful effect. Therefore, some groups have advocated high-dose LT4 administration in suppressive doses to significantly lower TSH. Moalem and Duh [27] provide an evidence-based review of the literature on its effectiveness. They reviewed two large meta-analyses, including over 13 major studies and nine randomized trials. In 2002, Castro et al. [28] found six randomized trials comprising almost 350 patients who had a benign solitary thyroid nodule treated with high-dose suppressive LT4. And 22% of patients treated with LT4 had a 50% decrease in nodule volume compared to only 10% of patients treated with placebo; however, *p* values were not significant. In a follow-up study, Sdano et al. [29] expanded on this work by including nine randomized trials (650 patients and some with MNG). 22% of patients who underwent suppressive LT4 therapy had a 50% decrease in nodular size, whereas patients who received no treatment or placebo therapy only had a 10% rate of significant decrease in nodular volume. These results were statistically significant, but as Moalem et al. indicated, "eight patients (with nodular thyroid disease) would need to be treated in order to have one patient benefit," from suppressive LT4 therapy. While these data do hold some promise, there is a concern with LT4 medical treatment that should be raised. This treatment method may often be employed in patients who are poor surgical candidates (elderly, cardiac disease, pulmonary disease, etc.). These are the very patients who may also experience complications due to high-dose LT4 treatment, including osteoporosis [30], atrial fibrillation, and other cardiac arrhythmias. Based on these complications, the American Thyroid Association issued a concern regarding long-term treatment of nontoxic MNG with LT4 therapy and stated, that it is, "generally not recommended." The medical community has also commented that, "as a result of poor efficacy and potential side effects from the induction of subclinical hyperthyroidism," LT4 treatment of MNG has fallen out of favor [31, 32]. Finally, it

must be noted that if LT4 therapy is chosen for the management of MNG, it must be continued indefinitely as it is has been shown that the goiter and nodules may return to their original size within as little as 3 months after discontinuation of suppressive treatment [33].

Another option for the medical treatment of MNG is the use of radioactive iodine (I-131) in ablative doses. This treatment modality is often used for Graves' disease or for toxic MNG. In addition, it has been successfully used to treat MNG for more than 25 years, where it has been shown to cause a decrease in overall thyroid volume of up to 40% in the first year and 50–60% 2 years after treatment [34, 35]. However, its effects are dependent on the ability of the thyroid and its nodules to both uptake and organify iodine. Many nontoxic MNG contain "cold" nonfunctional nodules which can limit the effectiveness of I-131 treatment. Therefore, several groups have employed an off-label use for recombinant human TSH (RhTSH) to increase the uptake of I-131 (radioactive iodine uptake, RAIU) up to two- to threefold [36]. Several trials have demonstrated this improved RAIU with RhTSH pretreatment. These studies have also shown that with RhTSH pretreatment, you can use a decreased dose of I-131, still leading to improved reduction of compressive goiters [37, 38] and even lessen the degree of tracheal compression from SG [39].

While these results are impressive, the advocates of medical treatment of MNG freely admit that it cannot be used in all circumstances and acknowledge that it has potential side effects and drawbacks. I-131 treatment +/− RhTSH is considered contraindicated for patients with an MNG with suspicion of malignancy, goiter during pregnancy, and in patients with severe tracheal compression and overt symptoms. I-131 can lead to acute swelling of MNG which could worsen tracheal compression or other symptoms. RAI use should also be considered a relative contraindication for young patients with large goiter, in patients requiring rapid decompression of compressive goiter, or if prior I-131 treatment has failed to provide adequate relief of symptoms. Its best use may be for patients with mild to moderate compressive symptoms, elderly patients with comorbid conditions that preclude surgery, or in patients who have undergone prior thyroidectomy in which reoperative surgery is considered too risky. This should only be done once cancer has been excluded by biopsy.

Surgical Management

Surgical Indications

The most clear-cut indication for surgical management of an MNG is for the definitive treatment of thyroid cancer. As mentioned above, the overall risk of malignancy in an MNG ranges from 10 to 31%; the majority of these, approximately

60%, are papillary thyroid carcinomas [20–22, 40] which are often multifocal. Thyroidectomy for lesions "suspicious for malignancy," including Bethesda class 3–5 lesions [41] (BC 3: atypia of undetermined significance, BC 4: follicular/Hurthle neoplasms, and BC 5: suspicious for papillary thyroid carcinoma), can give definitive pathologic diagnosis, eliminate the need for long-term ultrasonographic surveillance, and potentially allow for surgical cure of cancer.

For patients with compressive symptoms, thyroidectomy can improve symptoms of tracheal compression, including dyspnea on exertion, orthopnea, PD, and may even improve obstructive sleep apnea [16, 17, 42]. It can also help patients with dysphagia due to extrinsic compression of the esophagus which would usually only be seen in the setting of a substernal MNG.

Surgery would also be indicated for patients who have failed or are not candidates for medical therapy (LT4 suppression or I-131 ablation), have significant obstructive symptoms and cannot wait for medical therapy to take effect, or have compressive or toxic MNG in the setting of pregnancy. Due to the small potential risk for secondary malignancies from I-131 treatment, younger patients should also be considered for a surgical approach [43].

Risks of Surgery

Surgery for MNG carries the standard risks seen for all thyroid surgery, including bleeding +/– neck hematoma, hypocalcemia due to hypoparathyroidism, and recurrent laryngeal nerve (RLN) injury. In addition, patients undergoing total thyroidectomy (TT) will require thyroid hormone replacement therapy. Some of these risks have been correlated to goiter size, intrathoracic or substernal goiter, disease process (toxic MNG and thyroid cancer with localized invasion), and, in some older studies, the extent of thyroid surgery. Probably the most controversial of these is the extent of thyroidectomy. Proponents of subtotal thyroidectomy (ST) argue that by leaving a thyroid remnant, they can reduce the incidence of RLN injury, avoid devascularization of parathyroid glands, and preserve functional thyroid tissue. The concern with this technique is that up to 10–30% of patients who undergo ST will have a recurrence of their disease [44]. In addition, despite leaving "adequate functional" thyroid tissue, up to 60–80% of patients may still become hypothyroid and ultimately require replacement thyroid hormone [45]. Thus, like the trend being seen in other thyroid diseases (cancer [15] and Graves' disease [46]), many dedicated endocrine surgical groups are moving toward TT for the management of MNG. Delbridge et al. [47] examined almost 3500 patients who underwent either ST ($n=1838$) or TT ($n=1251$) for the management of MNG. They saw no significant difference in the rate of permanent RLN injury, permanent hypoparathyroidism, or neck hematoma between ST or TT. Impressively, they did not have a rate higher than 1.4% for

any of these complications in either study arm. At the same time, they saw their recurrence rate of MNG in the setting of ST drop from 19% to zero with TT. Rios-Zambudio et al. showed similar findings in a prospective study of 300 MNG patients. "Definitive" or permanent complications of RLN injury and hypoparathyroidism occurred in <1% of their patients undergoing TT [48]. One possible issue with both of these studies is that they were carried out by groups with a great deal of expertise in thyroid surgery. Therefore, Moalem et al. [27] looked at 13 studies over the past 20 years comparing surgical approaches to MNG (ST vs. TT). When looking at all types of studies, comparative, prospective, and meta-analyses with varying numbers of patients and group experience, the rate of temporary RLN injury (1–10 vs. 0.9–6%), permanent RLN injury (0–1.4 vs. 0–1.4%), and permanent hypoparathyroidism (0–1.4 vs. 0–4%) for ST versus TT was not statistically different. The only difference that was noted was a slightly higher rate of temporary hypocalcemia following TT (9–35%) versus ST (0–18%). This did however resolve to equivalency in the rates of permanent hypoparathyroidism as seen above. Thus, TT should be the preferred approach to the surgical treatment of MNG.

Surgical resection of the MNG offers complete tissue diagnosis of all nodular disease, definitive resection of thyroid malignancy, and immediate relief of compressive symptoms. It has been shown that in experienced centers, TT can be carried out safely with low morbidity. TT also all but eliminates the risk of recurrent MNG which can occur in up to 10–30% of patients undergoing ST [44]. This is important because reoperative surgery for MNG versus initial TT does carry a significantly increased risk for both permanent hypoparathyroidism (0–22 vs. 0–4%) and RLN injury (0–13 vs. 0–4%) [27].

Summary

MNGs have specific nuances when compared to the solitary thyroid nodule which require a thorough evaluation. Patients should be evaluated for functional status to rule out hypothyroidism as a source of MNG or a toxic MNG. A detailed history and physical examination, including neck ultrasound, will elucidate risk factors for malignancy, clarify compressive symptoms, and help guide the need for thyroid biopsies. If malignant disease or nodules with an increased risk for malignancy are found, the patient should proceed on to formal definitive surgical management. If a benign MNG is discovered, patients should be treated based on the degree of compressive or other functional symptoms with medical or surgical treatment as dictated by extent of symptoms, success/failure of medical therapy, and patient choice. Radioactive iodine ablation and thyroid hormone suppressive therapy may play a role in patients with smaller, less symptomatic goiters or in elderly patients or those with extensive comorbidities that would preclude surgical intervention. Surgical resection is favored for younger patients with larger goiters, compressive symptoms, and substernal MNG. CT scan plays a role in the diagnosis and surgical planning for SGs. In the modern era, TT has been shown to be a safe technique in experienced centers that can provide definitive treatment for compressive or toxic MNG that virtually eliminates the risk of recurrent disease. As such it should become the preferred method of surgical management of the MNG.

Key Summary Points

- The etiology of MNGs is multifactorial but can include iodine deficiency, goitrogens, sporadic nodule development, and genetic abnormalities.
- Surgical indications for the MNG can include functional symptoms (toxic MNG), compressive symptoms, or the risk for malignancy.
- MNGs carry an overall risk of malignancy of 10–31 %.
- Medical management may be favored for patients with smaller, less symptomatic MNG or elderly patients with significant comorbidities precluding surgery.
- TT is rapidly becoming the standard operative choice for the management of MNG.

References

1. Vander JB, Gaston EA, Dawber TR. The significance of nontoxic thyroid nodules: final report of a fifteen year study of the incidence of thyroid malignancy. Ann Intern Med. 1968;69:537–40.
2. Turnbridge WM, Evered DC, Hall R, Appleton D, Brewis M, Clark F, et al. The spectrum of thyroid disease in a community: the Whickham survey. Clin Endocrinol. 1977;7:481–93.
3. Hegedus L. Clinical practice. The thyroid nodule. N Engl J Med. 2004;351(17):1764–71.
4. Mortensen JD, Woolner LB, Bennett WA. Gross and microscopic findings in clinically normal thyroid glands. J Clin Endocrinol Metab. 1955;15:1270–80.
5. Brander A, Viikinkowski P, Nickels J, Kivisaari L. Thyroid gland: US screening in a random adult population. Radiology 1991;181:683–7.
6. Ezzat S, Sarti DA, Cain DR, Braunstein GD. Thyroid incidentalomas. Prevalence by palpation and ultrasonography. Ann Intern Med. 1994;154:1838–40.
7. Matovinovic J. Endemic goiter and treatment of cretinism at the dawn of the third Millennium. Annu Rev Nutr. 1983;3:341–412.
8. http://thyroid.about.com/od/symptomsrisks/a/All-About-Goitrogens-thyroid.htm. Accessed 20 Dec 2014.
9. Marine D. Etiology and prevention of simple goiter. Medicine 1924;3:453.
10. Taylor S. The evolution of nodular goiter. J Clin Endocrin Metab 1953;13:1232.
11. Studer H, Peter HJ, Gerber H. Natural heterogeneity of thyroid cells: the basis for understanding thyroid function and nodular growth. Endocr Rev. 1989;10:125.
12. Day TA, Chu A, Hoang KG. Multinodular goiter. Otolarynol Clin N Am. 2003;36:35–54.
13. Neumann S, Willgerrodt H, Ackerman F, et al. Linkage of familial euthyroid goiter to the multinodular goiter-1 locus and exclusion of the candidate genes thyroglobulin, thyroid peroxidase, and Na+/I-symporter. J Clin Endocrin Metab 1999;84:3750–6.
14. Gabriel EM, Begert ER, Grant CS, et al. Germline polymorphism of codon 727 of human thyroid-stimulating hormone receptor is associated with toxic multinodular goiter. J Clin Endocrin Metab. 1999;84:3328–35.
15. Chen AY, Bernet VJ, Carty SE, et al. American Thyroid Association Statement on optimal surgical management of goiter. Thyroid 2014;24(2):181–9.
16. Reiher AE, Mazeh H, Schaefer S, Chen H, Sippel RS. Thyroidectomy decreases snoring and sleep apnea symptoms. Thyroid 2012;22(11):1160–4.
17. Stang MT, Armstrong MJ, Ogilivie JB, et al. Positional dyspnea and tracheal compression as indications for goiter resection. Arch Surg. 2012;147(7):621–6.
18. Pemberton HS. Sign of submerged goiter. Lancet 1946;251:509.
19. Dempsey GA, Schnell JA, Coathup R, Jones TM. Anaesthesia for massive retrosternal thyroidectomy in a tertiary referral centre. Br J Anaesth. 2013;111(4):594–9.
20. Hanumanthappa MB, Gopinathan S, Suvarna R, et al. The incidence of malignancy in multi-nodular goiter: a prospective study at a tertiary care academic centre. J Clin Diag Res. 2012;6(2):267–70.
21. Luo, J, McMannus C, Chen H, Sippel RS. Are there predictors of malignancy in patients with multinodular goiter. J Surg Res. 2011;174:207–10.
22. Frates MC, Benson CB, Doubilet PM, et al. Prevalence and distribution of carcinoma in patients with solitary and multiple thyroid nodules on sonography. J Clin Endocrinol Metab. 2006;91(9):3411–7.
23. Brito JP, Yarur AJ, Prokop LJ, et al. Prevalence of thyroid cancer in multinodular goiter versus single nodule: review and meta-analysis. Thyroid 2013;23(4):449–55.
24. Cooper DS, Doherty GM, Haugen BR, et al. Revised American Thyroid Association management guidelines for patients with thyroid nodules and differentiated thyroid cancer. Thyroid 2009;19:1167–214.
25. Cochand-Priollet B, Guillausseau PJ, Chagnon S, et al. The diagnostic value of fine-needle aspiration biopsy under ultrasonography in nonfunctional thyroid nodules: a prospective study comparing cytologic and histologic findings. Am J Med. 1994;97:152–7.
26. Wilhelm SM. Utility of I-123 thyroid uptake scan in incidental thyroid nodules: an old test with a new role. Surgery 2008;144(4):511–7.
27. Moalem J, Suh I, Duh QY. Treatment and prevention of recurrence of multinodular goiter: an evidence based review of the literature. World J Surg. 2008;32:1301–12.
28. Castro MR, Caraballo PJ, Morris JC. Effectiveness of thyroid hormone suppressive therapy in benign solitary thyroid nodules: a meta-analysis. J Clin Endocrinol Metab. 2002;87:4154–9.
29. Sdano MT, Falciglia M, Welge JA, et al. Efficacy of thyroid hormone suppression for benign thyroid nodules: a meta-analysis of randomized trials. Otolaryngol Head Neck Surg. 2005;133:391–6.
30. Wesche MF, Tiel VBMM, Lips P, et al. A randomized trial comparing levothyroxine with radioactive iodine in the treatment of sporadic non-toxic goiter. J Clin Endocrinol Metab. 2001;86:998–1005.
31. Surks MI, Ortiz e, Daniels GH, et al. Subclinical thyroid disease: scientific review and guidelines for diagnosis and management. J Am Med Assoc. 2004;291:228–38.
32. Bonnema SJ, Hegedus L. A 30 year perspective on radioiodine therapy of benign nontoxic multinodular goiter. Curr Opin Endocrinol Diabetes Obes. 2009;16:379–84.
33. Berghout A, Wiersinga WM, Drexhage HA, et al. Comparison of placebo with L-thyroxine alone or with carbimazole for treatment of sporadic non-toxic goiter. Lancet 1990;336:193–7.

34. Nygaard B, Hegedus L, Gervil M, et al. Radioiodine treatment of multinodular nontoxic goiter. Br Med J. 1993;307:828–32.

35. Nygaard B, Hegedus L, Ulriksen P, et al. Radioiodine therapy for multinodular toxic goiter. Arch Intern Med. 1999;159:1364–8.

36. Fast S, Nielsen VE, Bonnema SJ, Hegedus L. Time to reconsider non surgical therapy of benign nontoxic multinodular goiter: focus on recombinant human TSH augmented radioiodine therapy. Eur J Endocrinol. 2009;160:517–28.

37. Maurer AH, Charkes ND. Radioiodine treatment for nontoxic multinodular goiter. J Nucl Med. 1999;40:1313–6.

38. Ceccarelli C, Brozzi F, Bianchi F, Santini P. Role of recombinant human TSH in the management of large euthyroid multinodular goiter: a new therapeutic option? Pros and cons. Minerva Endocrinol 2010;35(3):161–71.

39. Bonnema SJ, Nielsen VE, Boel-Jorgensen H, et al. Recombinant human thyrotropin-stimulated radioiodine therapy of large nodular goiters facilitates tracheal decompression and improves inspiration. J Clin Endcrinol Metab. 2008;93:3981–4.

40. Gandolfi PP, Frisina A, Raffa M, et al. The incidence of thyroid carcinoma in multinodular goiter: retrospective analysis. Acto Biomed 2004;75:114–7.

41. Cibas E, Syed Z. The Bethesda system for reporting cytopathology. Thyroid 2009;19(11):1159–65.

42. Schneider A, Bourhala K, Petiau C, et al. Role of thyroid surgery in the obstructive sleep apnea syndrome. World J Surg. 2014;38(8):1990–4.

43. Ron E, Doody MM, Becker DV, et al. Cancer mortality following treatment for adult hyperthyroidism. Lancet 1999;353:2111–5.

44. Reeve TS, Delbridge L, Cohen A, et al. Secondary Thyroidectomy: a twenty-year experience. World J Surg. 1988;12:449–53.

45. Vaiman M, Nagiban A, Hagag P, et al. Hypothyroidism following partial thyroidectomy. Otolaryngol Head Neck Surg. 2008;138:98–100.

46. Wilhelm SM, McHenry CR. Total Thyroidectomy is superior to subtotal thyroidectomy for the management of Graves' disease in the United States. World J Surg. 2010;34:1261–4.

47. Delbridge L, Guinea AI, Reeve TS. Total Thyroidectomy for benign multinodular goiter. Arch Surg. 1999;134:1389–93.

48. Rios-Zambudio A, Rodriguez J, Riquleme J, et al. Prospective study of postoperative complications after total thyroidectomy for multinodular goiters by surgeons with experience in endocrine surgery. Ann Surg. 2004;240:18–25.

Hugh Spear Pemberton

1890–1956

Hannah Y. Zhou and Christopher R. McHenry

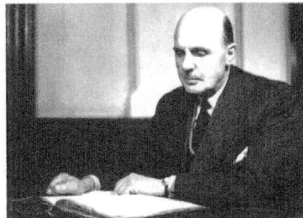

Hugh Spear Pemberton [2]. (By courtesy of the University of Liverpool Library)

Hugh Spear Pemberton was born on June 3, 1890, in Liverpool, England, the youngest son of Thomas Shepherd Pemberton and Elizabeth Marion [1]. He attended the Liverpool Institute and Liverpool University and graduated in 1913 with first class honors with M.B. and Ch.B. degrees. In the fall of 1913 after obtaining his qualifying medical degrees, he became a resident physician and joined the staff at the David Lewis Northern Hospital in Liverpool where he worked for his entire career. Dr. Pemberton married Sarah Ann Hanley in 1914 and his daughter, Lesley Mary, was born in 1916 [2].

His tenure at the David Lewis Northern Hospital was interrupted by World War I, in which he served in the Royal Army Medical Corps in France and Russia. He returned to the David Lewis Northern Hospital in 1918 and was appointed junior physician. He became a member of the Royal College of Physicians in 1921 and achieved the rank of senior consultant at the David Lewis Northern Hospital in 1924.

Dr. Pemberton was a lecturer in clinical medicine at Liverpool University and was recognized for his skills as a teacher. In addition to the Northern Hospital, he also worked at Liverpool Hospital for Women, the Liverpool

C. R. McHenry (✉)
Department of Surgery, MetroHealth Medical Center, 2500 MetroHealth Drive, Cleveland, OH 44109-1998, USA
e-mail: cmchenry@metrohealth.org

H. Y. Zhou
Department of Surgery, University Hospitals Case Medical Center, Cleveland, OH, USA

Radium Institute and the Neston, Hoylake and West Kirby Cottage Hospitals. He became a fellow of the Royal College of Physicians in 1941. He was chairman of the Birkenhead and Wirral Division of the British Medical Association from 1946 to 1950 and vice president of the Section of Medicine in 1950.

Dr. Pemberton had special interests in diabetes mellitus, peripheral vascular disease, thyroid disease, and hospital planning, publishing several papers in the *British Medical Journal* over the course of his career. In 1922, he founded a diabetes clinic, thought to be the first of its kind in England, at the David Lewis Northern Hospital. He also helped found the peripheral vascular disease clinic at the Northern Hospital. He was the principal author of the Northern Hospital's diet book, first published in 1935. He was actively involved with the diagnosis and management of diabetic patients with peripheral vascular disease.

Dr. Pemberton was a dedicated clinician who worked long hours at the hospital and rarely took a day off. He was meticulous, paying close attention to detail and staying late to care for his patients. He was an outstanding teacher who enjoyed discussing medicine with younger colleagues and students. They enjoyed learning from him so much that it became competitive to obtain a position on his team, which was affectionately known as "Pem's firm" [3]. His devotion to the Northern Hospital was especially evident during World War II when he organized and led the evacuation of patients to a local collegiate institution.

Hugh Spear Pemberton was the first to describe an important physical examination finding in patients with substernal goiter that would later become known as Pemberton's sign. In a short letter published in the October 5, 1946, issue of *The Lancet,* Pemberton wrote, "There is a useful sign given by a submerged or intrathoracic goiter which I have employed and taught for many years. It consists in getting the patient to elevate both arms until they touch the sides of the head; after a moment or so, congestion of the face, some cyanosis, and lastly distress become apparent—presumably from narrowing of the thoracic inlet and obstruction of the venous return.

J. L. Pasieka, J. A. Lee (eds.), *Surgical Endocrinopathies,* DOI 10.1007/978-3-319-13662-2_12,
© Springer International Publishing Switzerland 2015

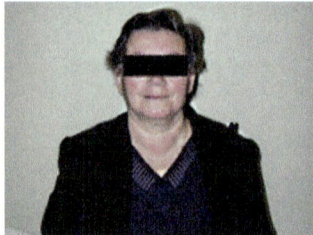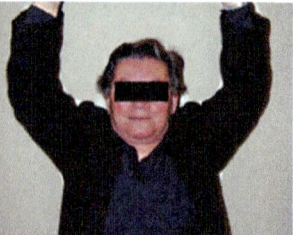

Fig. 1 A patient with a positive Pemberton sign. (Reprinted with permission from Dr. Bill Fleming)

I have not seen it in superior mediastinal block. Doubtless the sign has been described before and even bears a name, but I am unaware of it" [4] (Fig. 1). This finding was subsequently termed Pemberton's sign and has been widely referred to ever since its first description.

Pemberton's wife died in 1950 and he married Dorothy Alice Parker in 1951. He continued to work as a senior physician at the Northern Hospital until his mandatory retirement in June 1955 at the age of 65. He died in his home in Neston, Cheshire less than 6 months after his retirement on January 15, 1956, at the age of 65.

The Superior Thoracic Aperture

Pemberton's sign is a manifestation of impingement on the already limited space in the superior thoracic aperture. The superior thoracic aperture is bounded anteriorly by the sternum, posteriorly by the upper border of the first thoracic vertebra (T1), and laterally by the first ribs [5]. It is approximately 5 cm in anteroposterior diameter (manubrium to T1) and 10 cm in width (rib to rib). The superior aperture can be divided into right lateral, left lateral, and medial compartments. The lateral compartments contain the apices of the lung and pleura, the brachial plexus, and vasculature of the upper extremities. The medial area contains the trachea, esophagus, the sympathetic trunk, the vagus, recurrent laryngeal and phrenic nerves, the vertebral and common carotid arteries, and the internal jugular and inferior thyroid veins.

Substernal Goiters

The term substernal goiter has traditionally been used to describe thyroid enlargement with at least 50 % of the thyroid tissue extending below the superior thoracic aperture [6–9] (Fig. 2). However, patients may experience compressive symptoms related to impingement on vital structures from a retrosternal component that is less than 50 % of the total thyroid mass. As a result, a more liberal definition is often used, consisting of an estimated 3 cm of thyroid tissue below the sternal notch when the patient's neck is extended [10]. The

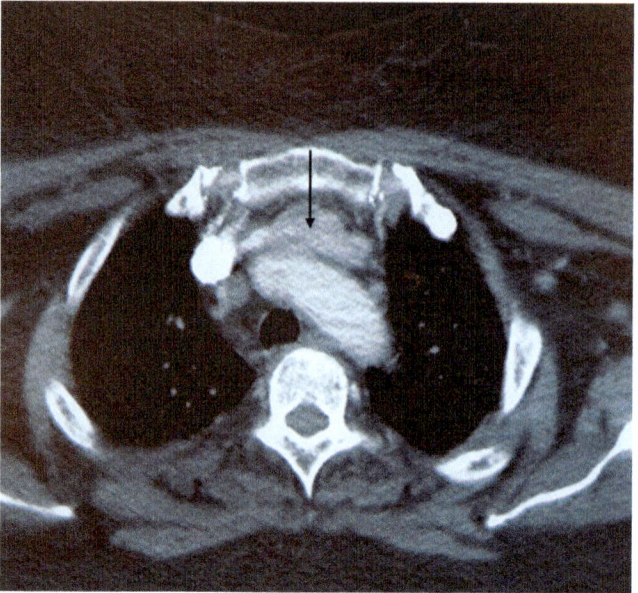

Fig. 2 Computed tomography showing a substernal goiter (*arrow*) extending to the level of the aortic arch

normal swallowing mechanism, the negative intrathoracic pressure, and the force of gravity are factors that are felt to contribute to the development of a substernal goiter [11].

A substernal goiter can be unilateral or bilateral. The reported incidence ranges from 0.05 to 0.5 % of the general population [12, 13] and from 2.6 to 26 % of patients undergoing thyroidectomy [11, 14–17]. The wide variation in incidence is primarily due to the lack of a standardized definition and classification system in the literature. Substernal goiter has become less common with the increase in dietary iodine, especially with iodized salt as well as the effective treatments of hypothyroidism with levothyroxine [18].

Given the limited space within the superior thoracic aperture, a patient with substernal extension of a goiter may experience compressive symptoms [19, 20]. Compression of the trachea can lead to dyspnea, intermittent coughing or choking, and stridor. Compression of the recurrent laryngeal nerve can lead to hoarseness. Esophageal compression may result in dysphagia, more commonly in patients with a posterior mediastinal goiter. Compression of the superior vena cava, pulmonary artery, or carotid artery may lead to superior vena cava syndrome, pulmonary hypertension, and transient ischemic attacks, respectively [21–23]. In addition to Pemberton's sign, physical findings in a patient with a symptomatic substernal goiter include tracheal deviation, distention of neck veins, facial and upper extremity edema, and Horner's syndrome. Horner's syndrome is due to compression or invasion of the cervical sympathetic chain.

The recommended treatment for symptomatic substernal goiters is resection to avoid potential airway compromise and worsening symptoms from compression. For asymptomatic

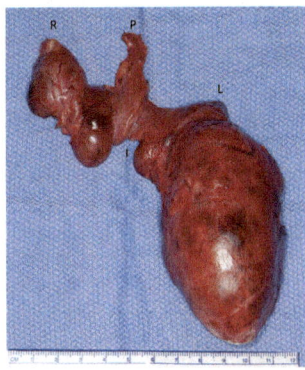

Fig. 3 Intraoperative image of a secondary substernal goiter (*arrow*) that extended inferiorly from the left lobe of the thyroid gland. *R* right thyroid, *L* left thyroid, *I* isthmus, *P* pyramidal lobe

substernal goiters, indications for thyroidectomy include an abnormal fine-needle aspiration biopsy (FNAB), progressive thyroid enlargement, and radiographic evidence of tracheal or esophageal compression. The majority of these goiters are resectable via a cervical incision with careful dissection to avoid vessel or nerve injury. Median sternotomy or thoracotomy is necessary for the treatment of patients with invasive malignancy or primary intrathoracic goiter, defined as a goiter confined to the chest without a cervical component, whose blood supply comes from the internal thoracic artery. Figure 3 shows the specimen following resection of a substernal goiter via a cervical incision.

References

1. Pemberton HS. Munk's roll, vol. V. http://munksroll.rcplondon. ac.uk/Biography/Details/3509. Accessed 20 Oct 2014.
2. Vandyk. Court Photographer (ca. 1940s). Dr Hugh Spear Pemberton: copy of portrait photograph [PDF]. Reference D1017. Special Collections and Archives. University of Liverpool Library, UK; 1940.
3. Obituary: H.S. Pemberton, M.B., F.R.C.P. Brit Med J. 1956 Jan 28;237–8.
4. Pemberton HS. Sign of submerged goitre. Lancet 1946;248:509.
5. Colborn GL, Weidman TA, Mirilas PS, Symbas P, Skandalakis JE. Thoracic wall and pleurae. In: Skandalakis JE, editor. Skalandaladis' surgical anatomy. vol. 1, 14th ed. Athens: Paschalidis Medical Publications.
6. Newman E, Shaha AR. Substernal goiter. J Surg Oncol. 1995;60:207–12.
7. Mack E. Management of patients with substernal goiters. Surg Clin North Am. 1995;75:377–94.
8. Singh B, Lucente FE, Shaha AR. Substernal goiter: a clinical review. Am J Otolaryngol. 1994;15:409–16.
9. Katlic MR, Wang C, Grillo HC. Substernal goiter. Ann Thorac Surg. 1985;39:391–9.
10. Hedayati N, McHenry CR. The clinical presentation and operative management of nodular and diffuse substernal thyroid disease. Am Surg. 2002;68(3):245–52.
11. Lahey F, Swinton N. Intrathoracic goiter. Surg Gynecol Obstet. 1934;59:627–37.
12. Reeves TS, Rubenstein C, Rundle FF. Intrathoracic goitre: its prevalence in Sydney metropolitan mass X-ray survey. Med J Austr. 1957;2:149–51.
13. Rundle FF. Intrathoracic goiter. West J Surg Obstet Gynecol. 1959;67:213–5.
14. Pemberton J. Surgery of substernal and intrathoracic goiters. Arch Surg. 1955;71:347–56.
15. Wax MK, Briant DR. Management of substernal goitre. J Otolaryngol. 1992;21:165–70.
16. Sanders LE, Rossi RL, Shahian DM, Williamson WA. Mediastinal goiter. The need for an aggressive approach. Arch Surg. 1992;127:609–13.
17. Shaha AR, Alfonso AE, Jaffe BM. Operative treatment of substernal goiters. Head Neck 1989;11:325–30.
18. Shambaugh E, Seed R, Korn A. Airway obstruction in substernal goiter: clinical and therapeutic implications. J Chronic Dis. 1973;26:737–43.
19. James R, James J, Vij AS, Dhaliwal AS, Singh A. Case report – Pemberton's sign in retrosternal goitre. Ind J Med Case Rep. 2013;2:36–9.
20. O'Brien KE, Gopal V, Mazzaferri E. Pemberton's sign associated with a large multinodular goiter. Thyroid 2003;13(4):407–8.
21. Vadasz P, Kotsis L. Surgical aspects of 175 mediastinal goiters. Eur J Cardio-Thorac Surg. 1998;14:393–7.
22. Michel LA, Bradpiece HA. Surgical management of substernal goiter. Br J Surg. 1988;94:969–77.
23. Abboud B, Badaoui G, Aoun Z, Tabet G, Jebara VA. Substernal goiter: a rare cause of pulmonary hypertension and heart failure. J Laryngol Otol. 2000;114:719–20.

Medullary Thyroid Carcinoma

Marybeth S. Hughes and Yasmine Assadipour

Introduction

Medullary thyroid cancer (MTC), which develops from para-follicular cells of the thyroid gland, is caused in most cases by an activating mutation in the rearranged during transfection (RET) proto-oncogene, and in some sporadic cases, by a mutation in the rat sarcoma (RAS) proto-oncogene. Patients with a known germ-line risk factor should be screened for serum calcitonin levels. Diagnosis is made by nodules on ultrasound which can be fine-needle aspirated and tested for calcitonin. All patients diagnosed with MTC should be offered genetic screening. Lymph node involvement is very common. Up to one third of patients have distant metastases on diagnosis. Appropriate surgical management includes a total thyroidectomy, central neck lymph node dissection, and lateral neck lymph node dissection if clinically indicated. Calcitonin and carcinoembryonic antigen are useful as tumor markers in surveillance. Local recurrences and isolated distant metastases should be addressed surgically. New modalities developed based on the specific genetic makeup of MTCs are being introduced for patients with metastatic disease, including tyrosine kinase inhibitors.

Anatomy and Physiology of Parafollicular Cells

The parafollicular cells from which MTC originates are embryologically derived from the neural crest [1]. These cells migrate from the third and fourth branchial pouches to the superolateral aspects of each thyroid lobe, and account for approximately 1 % of the cells in the gland [2].

The parafollicular cells are also referred to as C cells for the hormone they secrete, Calcitonin. Calcitonin is a 32-amino-acid protein which interacts with surface receptors on osteoclasts to decrease calcium absorption. However, calcitonin ultimately has a minimal impact on peripheral serum calcium levels, and patients with elevated calcitonin levels very rarely have drastic hypocalcemia. Calcitonin as a tumor marker is integral to the diagnosis of MTC in sporadic and hereditary syndromes, and for the detection of recurrence in the follow-up of patients with MTC. If the basal serum level is elevated but not confirmatory, diagnosis can be confirmed with a stimulated level. Calcitonin secretion can be stimulated by intravenous infusion of pentagastrin, although this is no longer available in many countries. High-dose intravenous calcium stimulation has also been reintroduced into clinical practice to stimulate calcitonin secretion [3]. C cells additionally release carcinoembryonic antigen (CEA), which can also be used as a tumor marker to detect recurrence on follow-up [4].

Risk Factors for Medullary Carcinoma

The most significant risk factor in the carcinogenesis of parafollicular cells is an activating mutation in the RET proto-oncogene. The RET proto-oncogene is located on chromosome 10q11.12, and encodes a tyrosine kinase receptor highly expressed on cells derived from the neural crest, branchial arches, and the urogenital system [5]. Upon ligand binding, the RET receptor dimerizes and several cytoplasmic tyrosine residues are phosphorylated, leading to the induction of downstream signal transduction pathways. RET mutations in MTC cause constitutive activation of the mitogen-activated protein kinase (MAPK) pathway, leading to cell division and proliferation. The (PI3)-K/AKT pathway is also activated, inhibiting apoptosis [6]. This combination of uncontrolled cell division and resistance to apoptotic stimuli leads to

M. S. Hughes (✉)
Director of the Surgical Oncology Research Fellowship, Thoracic and Gastrointestinal Oncology Branch, Center for Cancer Research, National Cancer Institute, National Institutes of Health, 10 Center Drive MSC 1201 Room 4W-3742, Bethesda, MD 20892, USA
e-mail: hughesm@mail.nih.gov

Y. Assadipour
Surgical Oncology, National Cancer Institute, National Institutes of Health, Bethesda, MD, USA

J. L. Pasieka, J. A. Lee (eds.), *Surgical Endocrinopathies,* DOI 10.1007/978-3-319-13662-2_13,
© Springer International Publishing Switzerland 2015

tumor formation. Fifty percent of sporadic MTC cases have a documented somatic RET mutation. Additionally, familial medullary thyroid cancer (FMTC), multiple endocrine neoplasia (MEN) 2A, and MEN2B, which account for 25 % of MTC cases, are all caused by RET mutations [7–9]. Specific mutations in RET leading to the respective phenotypes of FMTC, MEN2A, and MEN2B have been identified [10, 11]. Half of FMTC incidences are related to mutations on exon 10, 13, and 14. Mutations that highly activate RET have an increased risk for developing MTC and an earlier age of presentation. The American Thyroid Association (ATA) has developed a risk stratification system correlating genotype to risk level for aggressive MTC, with level A being the lowest risk and level D being the highest risk for aggressive MTC. FMTC mutations are generally less aggressive, with no level D mutations found in families with FMTC (Table 1).

RAS mutations have also been identified in spontaneous MTC. The RAS proto-oncogenes code for three highly similar GTPases, H-RAS, on chromosome 11p15.5, K-RAS, on chromosome 12p12.1, and N-RAS on chromosome 1p13.2. These GTPases have been shown to play an important role in many human cancers through activation of the MAPK cascade. H-RAS and K-RAS mutations are found in over 50 % of RET-negative MTCs [12]. The fact that RAS and RET mutations in MTC are almost mutually exclusive of one another suggests that both RET and RAS can act as driver mutations in MTC [13].

Table 1 Common RET mutations in sporadic and FMTC and ATA risk stratification

Phenotype	Exon	Codon	ATA risk
Sporadic MTC	13	768	A
–	16	918	D
–	–	–	–
FMTC	11	630	B
–	–	631	B
–	–	634	B or C[a]
–	–	649	A
–	–	666	A
–	13	768	A
–	14	804	A
–	–	819	A
–	–	833	A
–	–	844	A
–	15	866	A
–	–	891	A

MTC medullary thyroid cancer, *FMTC* familial medullary thyroid cancer, *ATA* American Thyroid Association
Category A: Lowest risk of aggressive MTC
Category B: Second lowest risk of aggressive MTC
Category C: Second highest risk of aggressive MTC
Category D: Highest risk of aggressive MTC
[a] 634-bp duplication confers a risk level B; 634-point mutations confer a risk level C

Diagnosis of Medullary Thyroid Cancer

In patients with a known hereditary risk factor, MTC usually presents as an elevated screening calcitonin level or nodule(s) on screening thyroid and neck ultrasounds. These patients tend to have a lower incidence of lymph node involvement and higher cure rates as a result of the routine screening. Patients with sporadic MTC often present with a palpable thyroid nodule or neck mass. The presence of a thyroid nodule in the setting of elevated serum calcitonin is essentially diagnostic of MTC. MTC can also be confirmed with ultrasound-guided fine needle aspiration (FNA) demonstrating C cells on cytology, and more accurately, measuring calcitonin levels in the aspiration needle washout, a test known as FNA calcitonin [14, 15].

There are important gender differences in calcitonin levels, with males having more parafollicular C cells and higher calcitonin levels at baseline than women. Therefore, gender-specific thresholds have been determined, with a basal calcitonin level of 20 pg/mL in women and 100 pg/mL in men, and stimulated calcitonin level of 250 pg/mL in women and 500 pg/mL in men having a positive predictive value of 100 % in detecting an occult MTC [16].

Clinical Features of Medullary Thyroid Cancer

MTCs account for 5 % of all thyroid cancers. The most common age range of presentation is 35–45 years of age. The incidence in men and women is more evenly matched than other thyroid cancer histologies, with only slightly more than half of the patients with MTC being women.

Sporadic MTCs are usually solitary lesions, while hereditary MTC presents with multicentric and bilateral disease in over 80 % of cases. Involvement of both central and lateral cervical lymph nodes is common in both sporadic and hereditary MTC. Early lymph node involvement is very common, with lymph node metastases occurring even with small primary tumors less than 1 cm in size (Fig. 1). The incidence of lymph node metastases increases with the size of the primary tumor [17]. In both sporadic and hereditary MTC, microscopic lymph node involvement in the central compartment level VI nodes was observed in 50–80 % of patients. High rates of micrometastases to the lateral neck level III and IV nodes were also appreciated, including the contralateral lateral neck nodes in patients with unilateral disease [17, 18]. Distant metastases are most frequently to the liver, lung, and bones. Rarely, brain and skin can also be sites of metastases.

Patients with MTC may experience anterior neck pain, which was found to be more common in MTC as compared to other differentiated thyroid cancers. In one series, the presence of neck pain translated to a more advanced stage

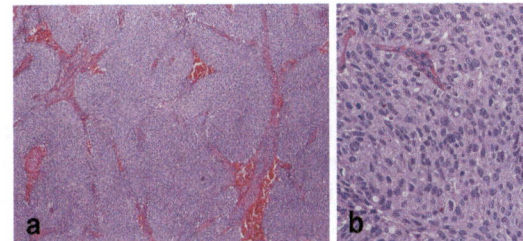

Fig. 1 Thyroid gland and right lateral lymph node compartments from a patient with bilateral synchronous lesions, lymph node metastases, and liver metastases: **a** *left* thyroid gland with primary tumor measuring 4 mm in greatest diameter, **b** *right* thyroid gland with primary tumor measuring 6 mm in greatest diameter, **c** *right* lateral neck compart-ments III, IV, and V had significant tumor burden involving the phrenic nerve, which was spared. Note that despite the primary tumors being small, lymph node involvement was extensive and the patient also had liver metastases. (Courtesy of Martha Quezado, M.D., Department of Pathology, National Institutes of Health)

of disease, with 82% of patients with anterior neck pain being stage III or IV, and only 36% of patients without pain being stage III or IV [19]. In addition to calcitonin and CEA, MTCs can also secrete vasoactive intestinal peptide (VIP), and infrequently, adrenocorticotropic hormone (ACTH) [20]. Therefore, in rare circumstances patients may have **Cushing's** syndrome as part of their presentation. Patients presenting with systemic symptoms related to calcitonin or VIP burden, including bone pain, diarrhea, or flushing, al-most universally have distant metastases [21].

Meeting the criteria for FMTC necessitates two genera-tions with MTC and no evidence of hyperparathyroidism or pheochromocytoma as first described by **Dr John Farndon** [22]. Other proposed definitions include MTC in four family members with no evidence of other MEN2 manifestations [23]. Overall, FMTC has a later age of presentation and is less aggressive biologically than MTCs in the sporadic or MEN2 setting [22]. Whether FMTC is a distinct entity or a specific phenotypic presentation of MEN2A is not con-cretely defined at this time, and some consider FMTC to be a variant of MEN2A.

Pathologic Features

MTCs are usually found in the upper third of the thyroid gland, due to the normal anatomic location of parafollicu-lar cells. Grossly, the tumors appear well circumscribed, and nonencapsulated. Histologically, hyperchromatic spindle and polygonal tumor cells can be appreciated in sheets or nests separated by fibrovascular septa. The vast majority of MTCs have extracellular deposits of amyloid protein visible on microscopic examination. On immunohistochemistry, they stain positively for calcitonin and CEA (Fig. 2). In addi-tion to the tumor, there are often areas of C cell hyperplasia (CCH) in patients with hereditary MTC. The diagnosis of CCH is made when three low power fields (area 1.93 mm^2) contain over 50 calcitonin-positive cells which do not dem-onstrate any nuclear abnormalities, defects in the follicular basal lamina, or infiltration of the thyroid interstitium, as such qualities would be indicative of microscopic MTC [24].

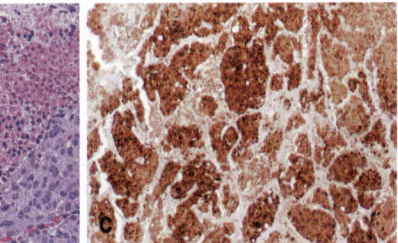

Fig. 2 Histopathology of medullary thyroid cancer: **a** hematoxylin and eosin stained MTC at 4× magnification view, demonstrating sheets and nests of tumor cells separated by fibrovascular septa, **b** at 20× magni-fication view, spindle and polygonal tumor cells with hyperchromatic nuclei can be appreciated, **c** MTCs are highly positive for calcitonin on immunohistochemistry, which stains brown. (Courtesy of Martha Quezado, M.D., Department of Pathology, National Institutes of Health)

Staging of Medullary Thyroid Carcinoma

Once a patient is diagnosed with MTC based on thyroid ultrasound and FNA, a basal serum calcitonin and detailed neck ultrasound should be obtained. The patient should undergo RET mutation testing, and pheochromocytoma should be ruled out using 24-h urine or plasma-free metanephrines and normetanephrines, and adrenal computed tomography (CT) or magnetic resonance imaging (MRI) if there is any uncertainty regarding biochemical screening results. Patients with no clinically appreciable lymph nodes on physical exam and neck ultrasound, and a basal calcitonin level under 400 pg/mL can proceed to surgical management for their MTC. If there are palpable nodes by physical exam, suspicious lymph nodes by ultrasound, or a basal calcitonin level over 400 pg/mL, a full metastatic workup should be initiated.

The metastatic workup for MTC should evaluate the liver using a sensitive imaging modality such as an MRI with contrast. Additionally, a neck and chest CT should be performed to further evaluate the neck compartments and determine whether lung metastases, which can frequently be bilateral, are present. (18 F)-fluorodeoxyglucose positron emission tomography can also be useful in detecting metastatic disease [25].

Staging is then categorized by the American Joint Committee on Cancer (AJCC) tumor, node, metastases (TNM) classification system which has been adapted for all thyroid carcinomas, including differentiated thyroid carcinoma histologies (see Chap. 15 on well-differentiated thyroid cancer).

Prognostic Factors in Medullary Thyroid Cancer

Age, gender, symptoms at presentation, extent of thyroidectomy, and TNM stage have been shown in univariate analysis to be significant prognostic factors in MTC. In a multivariate analysis, increasing age and advanced TNM stage were the only independent negative prognostic factors for survival [21, 26, 27]. Survival decreases dramatically with increasing stage (Table 2). Increased primary tumor size, positive lymph nodes, and distant metastases all decrease survival [28]. Early diagnosis and treatment have been shown to improve outcomes [29]. In patients with early MTC, treatment

Table 2 Ten-year survival in MTC by stage

TNM stage	Overall survival (%)
I	100
II	93
III	71
IV	21

TNM tumor, node, metastases, *MTC* medullary thyroid cancer

with total thyroidectomy and lymph node dissection results in a 95 % cure rate [21].

A preoperative basal calcitonin level over 500 pg/mL is an excellent predictor of failure to achieve biochemical remission after surgery [30]. Biochemically persistent disease following total thyroidectomy is prognostic of decreased survival, likely because this indicates advanced stage and metastases [29]. Likewise, calcitonin doubling time (DT) is a strong and independent predictor of survival. In one series, a DT over 2 years corresponded to a survival of 100 % at 10 years, compared to a DT under 6 months, which had a survival of 8 % at 10 years [31]. In the same series, CEA levels did not always parallel calcitonin levels, and did not correlate with survival. Previous studies have shown CEA is less specific in predicting recurrence and survival, but may correspond to a less-differentiated cell population and worse prognosis when elevated [32–34]. Rapidly increasing tumor marker levels are highly suggestive of distant metastases, hence their ability to predict survival. Distant metastases are the cause of death in half of the patients with MTC. 1-, 5-, and 10-year survival after determining the presence of distant metastases is 51, 26, and 10–20 %, respectively [21].

Some studies of sporadic versus hereditary MTC suggested a difference in survival, while others have not [21, 27, 29]. What has been clearly demonstrated is the specific RET mutation, rather than if it is a somatic or germ-line mutation, has great prognostic significance in MTC because it predicts how aggressively a tumor will behave, which is the basis for the ATA risk stratification guidelines. Among sporadic cases of MTC, the presence of a somatic RET mutation correlates with larger tumors, nodal and distant metastases, advanced stage at diagnosis, worse outcome, and decreased survival [35].

Surgical Management of Medullary Thyroid Carcinoma

The cornerstone of management for all patients with locally contained disease is a total thyroidectomy with central lymph node dissection (complete removal of all lymph nodes from the level VI compartment), and provides the best chance for cure in patients with MTC [25]. The complete central lymph node dissection does increase the risk of hypoparathyroidism postoperatively. Care must be taken to preserve the parathyroid glands and their blood supply, or to remove the glands and perform an autotransplantation. Permanent hypoparathyroidism occurs in 3–4 % of patients who undergo a central neck dissection [36]. The risk of transient or permanent injury to the recurrent laryngeal nerve is also slightly elevated with a lymph node dissection. However, the central compartment dissection is a vital component of appropriate treatment for MTC, and increases the cure rate [37]. Additionally, if any nodes in compartments II, III, IV, or V are suspicious on ultrasound or intraoperatively, or a patient has a calcitonin level over 400 pg/mL, these nodes should be removed [17, 38, 39]. Indeed, undertreated patients with only partial thyroidectomy or incomplete lymph node dissections have worse outcomes [40].

For patients with FMTC, prophylactic thyroidectomy can be considered based on the most recent ATA guidelines. Patients with level A and B germ-line mutations may delay prophylactic thyroidectomy, provided annual surveillance is in place and the family history suggests less aggressive tumor biology. Patients with level C germ-line mutations are recommended to undergo prophylactic thyroidectomy before the age of 5, and patients with level D germ-line mutations are recommended to undergo prophylactic thyroidectomy before the age of 1, although level D germ-line mutations are not generally observed in FMTC [25].

Postoperative Surveillance

Calcitonin and CEA levels should be checked 2 months following a total thyroidectomy with lymph node dissection, and every 6 months afterward. If calcitonin levels are undetectable for 2 years, this interval may be increased to annual surveillance [25].

Patients with detectable calcitonin levels postoperatively are not considered cured. These patients likely had an incomplete surgical resection, or have metastatic disease. In any patient with biochemical recurrence, a neck ultrasound and FNA or biopsy of any suspicious masses is recommended. In the event of biochemical persistence or recurrence, when basal serum calcitonin levels reach above 150 pg/mL, a full metastatic workup is recommended.

Management of Locally Recurrent Medullary Thyroid Carcinoma

For patients found during postoperative surveillance to have a local recurrence, surgical intervention should be considered. Subcentimeter indeterminate lymph nodes can be followed with serial ultrasounds. In one large retrospective study of patients presenting with persistent MTC and serum calcitonin under 1000 pg/mL who previously had no or incomplete neck dissection, reoperation and completion of lymph node dissection lead to biochemical cure in 44% of patients with no prior lymph node dissection, and 18% biochemical cure in patients with incomplete lymph node dissection [41]. While this has not yet been validated in a randomized control trial, this suggests complete lymph node dissections can significantly increase cure rates. External beam radiation therapy (EBRT) may also be used for locoregional control, to relieve pain, and avoid compressive complications [42].

Common toxicities are acute mucositis and dysphagia, and there is no current evidence that EBRT improves survival [43, 44].

Management of Metastatic Medullary Thyroid Carcinoma

Although total thyroidectomy and lymph node dissection will not be curative in patients with distant metastases, palliation of symptoms related to mass effect in the neck, such as pain, tracheal involvement, or esophageal compression, is absolutely indicated. If an R0 resection will not be possible, lymph node dissection can be limited to avoid unnecessary injury to the recurrent laryngeal nerves. However, recently a large retrospective review of a cohort with MTC showed thyroidectomy and lymph node resection improved survival in patients with distant metastases [28]. Given this new information, although the most recent ATA guidelines recommend limited surgery in patients with distant metastatic disease, it may not be in the patient's best interest to rely on medical management alone, or perform an incomplete dissection. The potential survival benefits must be balanced against potentially grave morbidities. If there is extensive compression or invasion of the trachea, a tracheostomy may be required for palliation. Patients with residual gross disease can undergo EBRT to improve locoregional control [45]. However, it is important to appreciate that postradiation fibrosis will make any potential future interventions significantly more technically challenging, and therefore EBRT is best considered in patients who would otherwise not be appropriate surgical candidates.

Isolated brain metastases can be addressed with surgical intervention or EBRT. Patients with multiple distant metastases, such as the liver and lung, do not benefit from having metastases addressed surgically. Additionally, traditional chemotherapies are not particularly efficacious in controlling disease burden or symptoms, in addition to being highly toxic. Recently developed targeted molecular therapies can address metastatic disease in a more refined manner.

Monoclonal antibodies to tyrosine kinase receptors, including RET, can inhibit tyrosine kinase activity, decreasing cell proliferation and other downstream effects of activated tyrosine kinases. The first tyrosine kinase inhibitor (TKI) approved by the Food and Drug Administration (FDA) for use in advanced MTC was vandetanib, an oral multikinase inhibitor of RET, vascular endothelial growth factor receptor (VEGFR), and endothelial growth factor receptor (EGFR), which has been shown to prolong progression-free survival, with a mortality rate not related to progressive disease of 2.2% [46, 47]. Vandetanib has also been shown to control Cushing's syndrome caused by an ACTH-secreting MTC [48]. Since its approval, two other oral multikinase inhibitors have been approved by the FDA for treatment of advanced MTC: sorafenib and cabozantinib.

Sorafenib targets both RET and VEGFR, and has also been shown to increase progression-free survival, cause partial responses in approximately 20% of patients, and stabilize disease in 70% of patients with MTC [49]. In a meta-analysis of all phase II trials of sorafenib for metastatic thyroid cancer of all histologies, the mortality rate not related to progressive disease was 3.7% [50]. Therefore, while sorafenib is quite efficacious in stabilizing disease progression, there are more adverse events compared to vandetanib, and appropriate patient selection is crucial.

Cabozantinib targets RET, VEGF, and hepatocyte growth factor (MET). In a phase III trial conducted on patients with MTC, cabozantinib was shown to prolong progression-free survival as well as overall survival, regardless of RET mutation status [51, 52]. Therefore, it may be particularly useful in patients without an RET mutation who have a weak or no response to vandetanib.

Sunitinib, a TKI currently FDA approved for the use in advanced pancreatic neuroendocrine tumors, has been shown to work synergistically with cisplatin against MTC in vitro, introducing a new potential role for traditional cytotoxic chemotherapy in the treatment of stage IV MTC [53, 54].

Future Directions

Another pathway found to be important in the carcinogenesis of MTC is the mammalian target of rapamycin (mTOR) pathway. Inhibition of mTOR in vitro has been shown to suppress growth in RET mutated MTC cell lines [55, 56]. Therefore, mTOR inhibitors such as everolimus, which have been approved for several other malignancies, may have therapeutic value in MTC. While no phase I, II, or III trials have been completed to evaluate the safety and efficacy of everolimus in MTC, in one study two patients with progressive metastatic MTC showed partial responses [57].

Immunotherapy may also have a role in the treatment of MTC. A phase I trial of a recombinant yeast-CEA vaccine (GI-6207) has shown good safety and tolerance, and one patient with MTC in the trial had a significant inflammatory response at their sites of metastatic disease [58].

Nelfinavir, a protease inhibitor previously used in the treatment of human immunodeficiency virus (HIV), may also have activity against MTC cells by targeting the heat shock protein 90 (HSP90), a chaperone protein required for RET stability. Nelfinavir was able to decrease RET protein levels, block downstream effects of RET, and induce apoptosis in human MTC cell lines in vitro [59].

Recently, the calcium/calmodulin-dependent kinase II (CaMKII) has been shown to be overactive in MTC cells with RET mutations. CaMKII is a serine/threonine protein kinase which among its many signaling functions can activate the MAPK pathway. An endogenous inhibitor of CAMKII, hCamKIINα has also been identified, and an inverse relationship between hCamKIINα expression and local tumor extension as well as lymph node metastases has been observed [60]. This suggests that inhibition of CaMKII can temper tumor behavior. Therefore, CaMKII has the potential to be a very useful target of molecular therapy in patients with stage IV MTC.

The more that is understood about the molecular biology of MTC, the more potential targets can be identified to create new molecular therapies specific to targeting MTC. As with all cancer treatments, the future lies in tailored approaches based on the genetic and cellular abnormalities which cause MTC.

Key Summary Points

- Medullary thyroid cancer originates from parafollicular C cells.
- Hereditary MTC and many forms of sporadic MTC are caused by mutations in the RET proto-oncogene, with a relationship between level of over activation of the RET tyrosine kinase and aggressiveness of tumor behavior.
- Diagnosis of MTC is most accurately made with FNA calcitonin.
- Staging workup includes a metastatic workup for patients with positive lymph nodes on physical exam or ultrasound, and all patients with a calcitonin level above 400 pg/mL.
- Appropriate surgical management of MTC includes a total thyroidectomy, central lymph node dissection, and in patients with clinically concerning lateral nodes or calcitonin level above 400 pg/mL, lateral lymph node dissection.
- Postoperative surveillance includes serum calcitonin and CEA levels to monitor for recurrence and neck ultrasound if there is evidence of biochemical recurrence.
- Local recurrences can be managed by observation, EBRT, or surgical intervention, which may improve cure rates.
- Patients with stage IV disease may still benefit from total thyroidectomy and lymph node dissection for local disease control as well as a potential survival benefit.
- Molecular-targeting therapies, such as TKIs, which can specifically target tumors with a constitutively activated RET mutation, are a promising modality for treating patients with stage IV MTC.
- Future therapies targeting proteins unique to parafollicular C cells and over activated pathways in MTC cells may provide a new and more refined strategy for treating stage IV MTC.

References

1. Williams ED. Histogenesis of medullary carcinoma of the thyroid. J Clin Pathol. 1966;19(2):114–8. (PubMed PMID: 5948665. Pubmed Central PMCID: PMC473198. Epub 1966/03/01. Eng).
2. Dubois PM, Alizon E, David L. [Calcitonin-cells in the thyroid of the human fetus. Immunocytochemical study (author's transl)]. Ann Endocrinol (Paris). 1979;40(1):53–4. (PubMed PMID: 443736. Epub 1979/01/01. Les cellules a calcitonine dans la thyroide du foetus humain. Etude par immunocytochimie. fre).
3. Mian C, Perrino M, Colombo C, Cavedon E, Pennelli G, Ferrero S, et al. Refining calcium test for the diagnosis of medullary thyroid cancer: cutoffs, procedures, and safety. J Clin Endocrinol Metab. 2014;99(5):1656–64. (PubMed PMID: 24552221. Epub 2014/02/21. eng).
4. Chan JK, Tse CH. Parafollicular C-cells do contain carcinoembryonic antigen. Am J Surg Pathol. 1988;12(3):247–8. (PubMed PMID: 3344889. Epub 1988/03/01. eng.)
5. Nakamura T, Ishizaka Y, Nagao M, Hara M, Ishikawa T. Expression of the ret proto-oncogene product in human normal and neoplastic tissues of neural crest origin. J Pathol. 1994;172(3):255–60. (PubMed PMID: 8195928. Epub 1994/03/01. eng).
6. Ichihara M, Murakumo Y, Takahashi M. RET and neuroendocrine tumors. Cancer Lett. 2004;204(2):197–211. (PubMed PMID: 15013219. Epub 2004/03/12. eng).
7. Donis-Keller H, Dou S, Chi D, Carlson KM, Toshima K, Lairmore TC, et al. Mutations in the RET proto-oncogene are associated with MEN 2A and FMTC. Hum Mol Genet. 1993;2(7):851–6. (PubMed PMID: 8103403. Epub 1993/07/01. eng).
8. Mulligan LM, Kwok JB, Healey CS, Elsdon MJ, Eng C, Gardner E, et al. Germ-line mutations of the RET proto-oncogene in multiple endocrine neoplasia type 2A. Nature 1993;363(6428):458–60. (PubMed PMID: 8099202. Epub 1993/06/03. eng).
9. Santoro M, Carlomagno F, Romano A, Bottaro DP, Dathan NA, Grieco M, et al. Activation of RET as a dominant transforming gene by germline mutations of MEN2A and MEN2B. Science 1995;267(5196):381–3. (PubMed PMID: 7824936. Epub 1995/01/20. eng).
10. Figlioli G, Landi S, Romei C, Elisei R, Gemignani F. Medullary thyroid carcinoma (MTC) and RET proto-oncogene: mutation spectrum in the familial cases and a meta-analysis of studies on the sporadic form. Mutat Res. 2013;752(1):36–44. (PubMed PMID: 23059849. Epub 2012/10/13. eng).
11. Romei C, Pardi E, Cetani F, Elisei R. Genetic and clinical features of multiple endocrine neoplasia types 1 and 2. J Oncol. 2012;2012:705036. (PubMed PMID: 23209466. Pubmed Central PMCID: PMC3503399. Epub 2012/12/05. eng).
12. Moura MM, Cavaco BM, Pinto AE, Leite V. High prevalence of RAS mutations in RET-negative sporadic medullary thyroid carcinomas. J Clin Endocrinol Metab. 2011;96(5):E863–8. (PubMed PMID: 21325462. Epub 2011/02/18. eng).
13. Agrawal N, Jiao Y, Sausen M, Leary R, Bettegowda C, Roberts NJ, et al. Exomic sequencing of medullary thyroid cancer reveals dominant and mutually exclusive oncogenic mutations in RET and RAS. J Clin Endocrinol Metab. 2013;98(2):E364–9. (PubMed PMID: 23264394. Pubmed Central PMCID: PMC3565108. Epub 2012/12/25. eng).
14. Trimboli P, Cremonini N, Ceriani L, Saggiorato E, Guidobaldi L, Romanelli F, et al. Calcitonin measurement in aspiration needle washout fluids has higher sensitivity than cytology in detecting medullary thyroid cancer: a retrospective multicentre study. Clin Endocrinol. 2014;80(1):135–40. (PubMed PMID: 23627255. Epub 2013/05/01. eng).
15. Diazzi C, Madeo B, Taliani E, Zirilli L, Romano S, Granata AR, et al. The diagnostic value of calcitonin measurement in wash-out fluid from fine-needle aspiration of thyroid nodules in the diagnosis of medullary thyroid cancer. Endocr Pract. 2013;19(5):769–79. (PubMed PMID: 23757613. Epub 2013/06/13. eng).
16. Machens A, Hoffmann F, Sekulla C, Dralle H. Importance of gender-specific calcitonin thresholds in screening for occult sporadic medullary thyroid cancer. Endocr Relat Cancer. 2009;16(4):1291–8. (PubMed PMID: 19726541. Epub 2009/09/04. eng).
17. Moley JF, DeBenedetti MK. Patterns of nodal metastases in palpable medullary thyroid carcinoma: recommendations for extent of node dissection. Ann Surg. 1999;229(6):880–7 (discussion 7–8. PubMed PMID: 10363903. Pubmed Central PMCID: PMC1420836. Epub 1999/06/11. eng).
18. Scollo C, Baudin E, Travagli JP, Caillou B, Bellon N, Leboulleux S, et al. Rationale for central and bilateral lymph node dissection in sporadic and hereditary medullary thyroid cancer. J Clin Endocrinol Metab. 2003;88(5):2070–5. (PubMed PMID: 12727956. Epub 2003/05/03. eng).
19. Guerrero MA, Lindsay S, Suh I, Vriens MR, Khanafshar E, Shen WT, et al. Medullary thyroid cancer: it is a pain in the neck? J Cancer. 2011;2:200–5. (PubMed PMID: 21509150. Pubmed Central PMCID: PMC3079917. Epub 2011/04/22. eng).
20. Hijazi YM, Nieman LK, Medeiros LJ. Medullary carcinoma of the thyroid as a cause of Cushing's syndrome: a case with ectopic adrenocorticotropin secretion characterized by double enzyme immunostaining. Hum Pathol. 1992;23(5):592–6. (PubMed PMID: 1568756. Epub 1992/05/01. eng).
21. Kebebew E, Ituarte PH, Siperstein AE, Duh QY, Clark OH. Medullary thyroid carcinoma: clinical characteristics, treatment, prognostic factors, and a comparison of staging systems. Cancer 2000;88(5):1139–48. (PubMed PMID: 10699905. Epub 2000/03/04. eng).
22. Farndon JR, Leight GS, Dilley WG, Baylin SB, Smallridge RC, Harrison TS, et al. Familial medullary thyroid carcinoma without associated endocrinopathies: a distinct clinical entity. Brit J Surg. 1986;73(4):278–81. (PubMed PMID: 3697657. Epub 1986/04/01. eng).
23. Eng C, Clayton D, Schuffenecker I, Lenoir G, Cote G, Gagel RF, et al. The relationship between specific RET proto-oncogene mutations and disease phenotype in multiple endocrine neoplasia type 2. International RET mutation consortium analysis. JAMA 1996;276(19):1575–9. (PubMed PMID: 8918855. Epub 1996/11/20. eng).
24. Perry A, Molberg K, Albores-Saavedra J. Physiologic versus neoplastic C-cell hyperplasia of the thyroid: separation of distinct histologic and biologic entities. Cancer 1996;77(4):750–6. (PubMed PMID: 8616768. Epub 1996/02/15. eng).
25. Kloos RT, Eng C, Evans DB, Francis GL, Gagel RF, Gharib H, et al. Medullary thyroid cancer: management guidelines of the American Thyroid Association. Thyroid 2009;19(6):565–612. (PubMed PMID: 19469690. Epub 2009/05/28. eng).
26. Wells SA, Jr., Pacini F, Robinson BG, Santoro M. Multiple endocrine neoplasia type 2 and familial medullary thyroid carcinoma: an update. J Clin Endocrinol Metab. 2013;98(8):3149–64. (PubMed PMID: 23744408. Epub 2013/06/08. eng).
27. Hyer SL, Vini L, A'Hern R, Harmer C. Medullary thyroid cancer: multivariate analysis of prognostic factors influencing survival. Eur J Surg Oncol. 2000;26(7):686–90. (PubMed PMID: 11187027. Epub 2001/02/24. eng).
28. Esfandiari NH, Hughes DT, Yin H, Banerjee M, Haymart MR. The effect of extent of surgery and number of lymph node metastases on overall survival in patients with medullary thyroid cancer. J Clin Endocrinol Metab. 2014;99(2):448–54. (PubMed PMID: 24276457. Pubmed Central PMCID: PMC3913800. Epub 2013/11/28. eng).
29. Rendl G, Manzl M, Hitzl W, Sungler P, Pirich C. Long-term prognosis of medullary thyroid carcinoma. Clin Endocrinol. 2008;69(3):497–505. PubMed PMID: 18331612. (Epub 2008/03/12. eng).

30. Machens A, Schneyer U, Holzhausen HJ, Dralle H. Prospects of remission in medullary thyroid carcinoma according to basal calcitonin level. J Clin Endocrinol Metab. 2005;90(4):2029–34. (PubMed PMID: 15634717. Epub 2005/01/07. eng).

31. Barbet J, Campion L, Kraeber-Bodere F, Chatal JF. Prognostic impact of serum calcitonin and carcinoembryonic antigen doubling-times in patients with medullary thyroid carcinoma. J Clin Endocrinol Metab. 2005;90(11):6077–84. (PubMed PMID: 16091497. Epub 2005/08/11. eng).

32. Busnardo B, Girelli ME, Simioni N, Nacamulli D, Busetto E. Nonparallel patterns of calcitonin and carcinoembryonic antigen levels in the follow-up of medullary thyroid carcinoma. Cancer 1984;53(2):278–85. (PubMed PMID: 6690009. Epub 1984/01/15. eng).

33. Saad MF, Fritsche HA, Jr., Samaan NA. Diagnostic and prognostic values of carcinoembryonic antigen in medullary carcinoma of the thyroid. J Clin Endocrinol Metab. 1984;58(5):889–94. (PubMed PMID: 6707192. Epub 1984/05/01. eng).

34. Gawlik T, d'Amico A, Szpak-Ulczok S, Skoczylas A, Gubala E, Chorazy A, et al. The prognostic value of tumor markers doubling times in medullary thyroid carcinoma—preliminary report. Thyroid Res. 2010;3(1):10. (PubMed PMID: 21047422. Pubmed Central PMCID: PMC2987862. Epub 2010/11/05. eng).

35. Elisei R, Cosci B, Romei C, Bottici V, Renzini G, Molinaro E, et al. Prognostic significance of somatic RET oncogene mutations in sporadic medullary thyroid cancer: a 10-Year follow-up study. J Clin Endocrinol Metab. 2008;93(3):682–7. (PubMed PMID: 18073307).

36. Stamatakos M, Paraskeva P, Katsaronis P, Tasiopoulou G, Kontzoglou K. Surgical approach to the management of medullary thyroid cancer: when is lymph node dissection needed? Oncology 2013;84(6):350–5. (PubMed PMID: 23689063. Epub 2013/05/22. eng).

37. Greenblatt DY, Elson D, Mack E, Chen H. Initial lymph node dissection increases cure rates in patients with medullary thyroid cancer. Asian J Surg. 2007;30(2):108–12. (PubMed PMID: 17475579. Epub 2007/05/04. eng).

38. Dralle H, Machens A. Surgical management of the lateral neck compartment for metastatic thyroid cancer. Current Opin Oncol. 2013;25(1):20–6. (PubMed PMID: 23079930. Epub 2012/10/20. eng).

39. Tamagnini P, Iacobone M, Sebag F, Marcy M, De Micco C, Henry JF. Lymph node involvement in macroscopic medullary thyroid carcinoma. Brit J Surg. 2005;92(4):449–53. (PubMed PMID: 15672437. Epub 2005/01/27. eng).

40. Pelizzo MR, Boschin IM, Bernante P, Toniato A, Piotto A, Pagetta C, et al. Natural history, diagnosis, treatment and outcome of medullary thyroid cancer: 37 years experience on 157 patients. Eur J Surg Oncol. 2007;33(4):493–7. (PubMed PMID: 17125960. Epub 2006/11/28. eng).

41. Machens A, Dralle H. Benefit-risk balance of reoperation for persistent medullary thyroid cancer. Ann Surg. 2013;257(4):751–7. (PubMed PMID: 23023200. Epub 2012/10/02. eng).

42. Fife KM, Bower M, Harmer CL. Medullary thyroid cancer: the role of radiotherapy in local control. Eur J Surg Oncol. 1996;22(6):588–91. (PubMed PMID: 9005145. Epub 1996/12/01. eng).

43. Terezakis SA, Lee KS, Ghossein RA, Rivera M, Tuttle RM, Wolden SL, et al. Role of external beam radiotherapy in patients with advanced or recurrent nonanaplastic thyroid cancer: Memorial Sloan-kettering Cancer Center experience. Int J Radiat Oncol Biol Phys. 2009;73(3):795–801. (PubMed PMID: 18676097. Epub 2008/08/05. eng).

44. Martinez SR, Beal SH, Chen A, Chen SL, Schneider PD. Adjuvant external beam radiation for medullary thyroid carcinoma. J Surg Oncol. 2010;102(2):175–8. (PubMed PMID: 20648590. Pubmed Central PMCID: PMC2908956. Epub 2010/07/22. eng).

45. Schwartz DL, Rana V, Shaw S, Yazbeck C, Ang KK, Morrison WH, et al. Postoperative radiotherapy for advanced medullary thyroid cancer–local disease control in the modern era. Head Neck. 2008;30(7):883–8. (PubMed PMID: 18213725. Epub 2008/01/24. eng).

46. Robinson BG, Paz-Ares L, Krebs A, Vasselli J, Haddad R. Vandetanib (100 mg) in patients with locally advanced or metastatic hereditary medullary thyroid cancer. J Clin Endocrinol Metab. 2010;95(6):2664–71. (PubMed PMID: 20371662. Pubmed Central PMCID: PMC2902067. Epub 2010/04/08. eng).

47. Wells SA, Jr., Robinson BG, Gagel RF, Dralle H, Fagin JA, Santoro M, et al. Vandetanib in patients with locally advanced or metastatic medullary thyroid cancer: a randomized, double-blind phase III trial. J Clin Oncol. 2012;30(2):134–41. (PubMed PMID: 22025146. Pubmed Central PMCID: PMC3675689. Epub 2011/10/26. eng).

48. Nella A, Lodish M, Fox E, Balis F, Quezado M, Whitcomb P, et al. Vandetanib successfully controls medullary thyroid cancer-related Cushing syndrome in an adolescent patient. J Clin Endocrinol Metab. 2014;99(9):3055–9. (PubMed PMID: 24617713. Epub 2014/03/13. Eng).

49. Lam ET, Ringel MD, Kloos RT, Prior TW, Knopp MV, Liang J, et al. Phase II clinical trial of sorafenib in metastatic medullary thyroid cancer. J Clin Oncol. 2010;28(14):2323–30. (PubMed PMID: 20368568. Pubmed Central PMCID: PMC2881718. Epub 2010/04/07. eng).

50. Thomas L, Lai SY, Dong W, Feng L, Dadu R, Regone RM, et al. Sorafenib in metastatic thyroid cancer: a systematic review. Oncologist 2014;19(3):251–8. (PubMed PMID: 24563075. Pubmed Central PMCID: PMC3958462. Epub 2014/02/25. eng).

51. Elisei R, Schlumberger MJ, Muller SP, Schoffski P, Brose MS, Shah MH, et al. Cabozantinib in progressive medullary thyroid cancer. J Clin Oncol. 2013;31(29):3639–46. (PubMed PMID: 24002501. Epub 2013/09/05. eng).

52. Viola D, Cappagli V, Elisei R. Cabozantinib (XL184) for the treatment of locally advanced or metastatic progressive medullary thyroid cancer. Future Oncol. 2013;9(8):1083–92. (PubMed PMID: 23902240. Epub 2013/08/02. eng).

53. Lopergolo A, Nicolini V, Favini E, Dal Bo L, Tortoreto M, Cominetti D, et al. Synergistic cooperation between sunitinib and cisplatin promotes apoptotic cell death in human medullary thyroid cancer. J Clin Endocrinol Metab. 2014;99(2):498–509. (PubMed PMID: 24276455. Epub 2013/11/28. eng).

54. Ravaud A, de la Fouchardiere C, Asselineau J, Delord JP, Do Cao C, Niccoli P, et al. Efficacy of sunitinib in advanced medullary thyroid carcinoma: intermediate results of phase II THYSU. Oncologist 2010;15(2):212–3; (author reply 4. PubMed PMID: 20189981. Pubmed Central PMCID: PMC3227944. Epub 2010/03/02. eng).

55. Gild ML, Landa I, Ryder M, Ghossein RA, Knauf JA, Fagin JA. Targeting mTOR in RET mutant medullary and differentiated thyroid cancer cells. Endocr Relat Cancer 2013;20(5):659–67. (PubMed PMID: 23828865. Epub 2013/07/06. eng).

56. Tamburrino A, Molinolo AA, Salerno P, Chernock RD, Raffeld M, Xi L, et al. Activation of the mTOR pathway in primary medullary thyroid carcinoma and lymph node metastases. Clin Cancer Res. 2012;18(13):3532–40. (PubMed PMID: 22753663. Epub 2012/07/04. eng).

57. Faggiano A, Ramundo V, Dicitore A, Castiglioni S, Borghi MO, Severino R, et al. Everolimus is an active agent in medullary thyroid cancer: a clinical and in vitro study. J Cell Mol Med. 2012;16(7):1563–72. (PubMed PMID: 21883896. Epub 2011/09/03. eng).

58. Bilusic M, Heery CR, Arlen PM, Rauckhorst M, Apelian D, Tsang KY, et al. Phase I trial of a recombinant yeast-CEA vaccine (GI-6207) in adults with metastatic CEA-expressing carcinoma. Cancer Immunol Immunother. 2014;63(3):225–34. (PubMed

PMID: 24327292. Pubmed Central PMCID: PMC3944709. Epub 2013/12/12. eng).

59. Kushchayeva Y, Jensen K, Recupero A, Costello J, Patel A, Klubo-Gwiezdzinska J, et al. The HIV protease inhibitor nelfinavir dowregulates RET signaling and induces apoptosis in medullary thyroid cancer cells. J Clin Endocrinol Metab. 2014;99(5):E734–45. (PubMed PMID: 24483157. Epub 2014/02/04. Eng).

60. Russo E, Salzano M, De Falco V, Mian C, Barollo S, Secondo A, et al. Calcium/calmodulin-dependent protein kinase II and its endogenous inhibitor alpha in medullary thyroid cancer. Clin Cancer Res. 2014;20(6):1513–20. (PubMed PMID: 24449826. Epub 2014/01/23. eng).

John Richard Farndon

1946–2002

Thomas W. J. Lennard

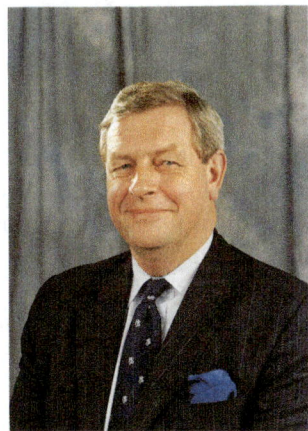

Professor John Richard Farndon

John Richard Farndon's parents were married in 1939 and lived in a rented back-to-back flat in the Tinsley area of Sheffield. This home was destroyed in the blitz of December 1940 and as a consequence they went to live with their parents. John was born on 16 February 1946 and his younger brother was born in 1949. Once the children were born, they moved to a large council estate between Sheffield and Rotherham. This was not far from the Orgreave coking works, which was the site of significant conflict during the miners' strike in 1984. In the 1950s and 1960s in this part of South Yorkshire, coal mining and the steel industry dominated most working lives. Life was very different during their childhood in the 1950s than it is today. There were no cars, telephones, fridges, washing machines, tumble dryers, double glazing, or central heating. The toilets were outside, socks were darned, the baths between the boys were shared and most people in the county supported either Sheffield United or Sheffield Wednesday football teams. Smoking amongst the commu-

nity was almost endemic and all the men drank either mild or bitter beer. John's reflections of his childhood are that it was a happy time and although circumstances were modest, everybody in the community lived in similar homes and shared a common lifestyle. There was no feeling within the Farndon family that they were underprivileged or deprived. The concept of going to university seemed foreign and it was felt that this would not play a part in the children's lives. For holidays, the family usually went on trips to the east coast of England, favourite destinations being Scarborough and Bridlington. One year, Riley's, the local coach operator, took the family to Great Yarmouth and this was considered a really adventurous trip! John's brother Clive, a successful practicing lawyer in Leeds describes their childhood in the 1950s as being "just another couple of lads growing up with their mates on a council estate in South Yorkshire." Time was passed and amusement and entertainment provided, particularly in John's case, by constructing go-karts out of pieces of wood and old pram wheels taken from the local dump. Clive reflects that the steering mechanism had a mind of its own and that brakes were nonexistent. Despite this, he recalls the two of them used to race these carts alongside the main Sheffield to Rotherham road.

For education, the two boys attended the local junior school. This was at a time that the national exam system (called the 11+) was in place, and it was not expected that anyone from John's estate would ever take this test and pass it. This seemed accepted by the local community; families were simply just not academic. There were no role models, icons, or anyone to inspire or stimulate. However, this mould was broken in the summer of 1957 when John passed the 11+ exam and he subsequently attended the Woodhouse Grammar School in Sheffield, a prestigious grammar school with an enviable reputation for both academic and sporting achievement. Clive comments that this must have been a difficult and challenging time for John to adjust, maintaining his connections with those he had grown up with but forging new friendships with a new academic focus in the grammar school. John worked hard, without being a swot, and in this environment his academic abilities flourished. John is remembered in the family as being someone with good

T. W. J. Lennard (✉)
Surgery, Clinical Academic Office, Newcastle University, 3rd Floor, William Leech Building, Framington Place, Newcastle, Tyne and Wear NE2 4HH, UK
e-mail: thomas.lennard@newcastle.ac.uk

J. L. Pasieka, J. A. Lee (eds.), *Surgical Endocrinopathies*, DOI 10.1007/978-3-319-13662-2_14,
© Springer International Publishing Switzerland 2015

humour, a self-effacing demeanour and a complete absence of pomposity, but also someone who had a strong desire to succeed from an early age. He kept these qualities during his time as a medical student and later as a doctor and consultant and his modest beginnings underline the truly remarkable achievements that he had later in life with his global reputation as a successful surgeon.

Following completion of his secondary education at Woodhouse Grammar School Sheffield, John Farndon was admitted to the University of Newcastle upon Tyne in 1964 for the medical course. During his time as a student, he undertook an intercalated degree as a Bachelor of Science in anatomy. Under the direction of Professor Joe Scothorne, Professor of Anatomy, he obtained a first-class honours degree for his dissertation entitled "An investigation of some factors controlling the growth and development of the parathyroid glands in the chick embryo". He was a distinguished medical student during his time in Newcastle and won a number of undergraduate prizes, the most notable of which was the Philipson Scholarship, an award given for the best graduating student. He attained this at the time of his graduation in 1970 when he was also awarded second-class honours. His postgraduate training was also in the northern region of England. After a year as a demonstrator in anatomy, following his house surgical and physician posts, he was appointed to the registrar training program. He conducted a period of research in the Department of Surgery at Newcastle University between 1976 and 1977 and completed his thesis for the degree of doctorate of medicine in 1986, the thesis being entitled "Pheochromocytoma". In January 1979, he was awarded the prestigious Peel Travelling Fellowship and International Research Fellowship in the Department of Surgery, Duke University Medical Centre, Durham, North Carolina. Here, he undertook the seminal work for which he is most remembered on medullary thyroid cancer. Working under the supervision of Dr Sam Wells, John began collecting data on families in whom medullary thyroid cancer had been diagnosed. In addition to those families where this was co-expressed with pheochromatoma and parathyroid disease (MEN II), he found some families where MTC was the sole manifestation of the inherited condition in a given kindred, recording for the first time this familial syndrome (see references [1–8] for Most Significant Publications and see also Chap. 13). In 1981, he was appointed senior lecturer in surgery at Newcastle University and honorary consultant surgeon at the Royal Victoria Infirmary, Newcastle, working under the chairmanship of Professor Ivan Johnston. His international acclaim during his early years as consultant was highlighted by an award of the James IV Travelling Scholarship in 1984 where he visited the Universities of California, Washington, Duke University, Virginia, Michigan, Chicago, Johns Hopkins, and the Memorial Sloan Kettering Hospital. The following year he was awarded the Australian College

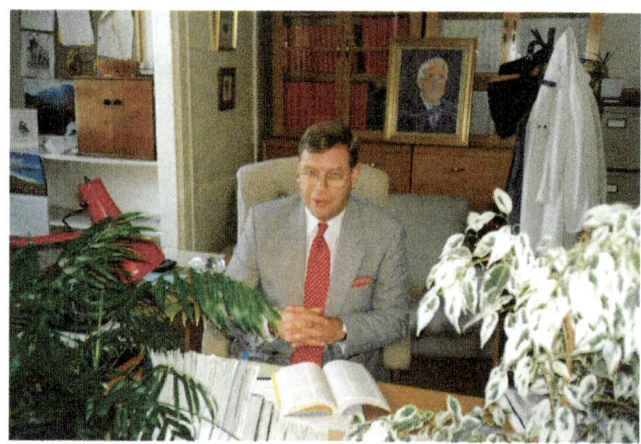

Fig. 1 John in his study at home

of Surgeons Travelling Fellowship and gave lectures in the Universities of Auckland, Christchurch, Sydney, and Melbourne. That same year, in 1985, he was awarded a Hunterian Professorship by the Royal College of Surgeons of England and he gave his Hunterian oration on 6 June 1986 entitled "Parathyroid Transplantation". His reputation as an engaging and informed lecturer grew in the early 1990s during his time as a senior lecturer. He gave talks in Hong Kong, India, Ireland, Adelaide, South Africa, the UK, Malaysia, Hamburg, Athens, Gothenburg, Tokyo, and Boston all at either prestigious meetings or as personal invitations for eponymous lectures (Fig. 1). In 1988, he applied for and was appointed to the Chair of Surgery at the University of Bristol where he was head of the division of surgery and honorary consultant surgeon at the United Bristol Healthcare Trust. His publications numbered nearly 200 and the vast majority of these are in the field of endocrine surgery but also span a wide range of general surgical topics, reflecting the state of UK surgery at the time when specialization was evolving. He was editor of a number of important books, most notably the *Companion to Specialist Surgical Practice* volumes relating to endocrine surgery and he contributed 34 chapters in the leading textbooks of the time, largely on matters relating to endocrine surgery. Up to 2001, he had given 146 papers to learned societies, was in receipt of a further 123 invited talks and meeting chairmanships, and was increasingly recognised as the leading light in endocrine surgery in the UK and internationally. Simply to list his achievements and publications does not give sufficient recognition to the qualities of the man who we remember and respect. As a teacher and a trainer of both undergraduates and postgraduates, he was completely selfless. He would always find time to teach the medical students, was more than willing to hold retractors for surgical trainees and take them through complex operations, no matter what time of day or night and the patient was always the central focus of his attention and motivation. He supervised a large number of research projects leading to higher degrees for his trainees during his time in Newcastle and subsequently in Bristol. For many, this was the launch of their career, and several of his trainees and students have gone on to achieve major roles in the surgical and medical world, influenced and supported by his dedication and commitment. He was a kind and generous man and above all was fun to work with and be around. He had a very good sense of humour and the legendary water fights that used to occur at the end of his operating lists on a Friday evening in theatre 1 at Newcastle's Royal Victoria Infirmary are still remembered! A measure of the respect with which he was held was the fact that he was the surgeon's surgeon and the physician's surgeon. His personal workload, both clinically and academically, was legendary. His reliability and his loyalty were without question. If John said he would do something, it would be done. Most notably, in his later years he undertook editorship of the *British Journal of Surgery*, a post of huge responsibility and workload and he personally reviewed a very significant number of the publications submitted to that journal for consideration. He was president of the British Association of Endocrine Surgeons from 1999 to 2001 and his wisdom, common sense, and leadership skills led him to be involved in a large number of interests outside of medicine and related to medicine in its broadest sense. This included being an assessor for the Commonwealth Universities Scholarship's Commission, an international advisory board member for a number of universities, and an assessor for a number of significant grant awarding bodies. His success in academic surgery led him to being invited to review and advise on the future of academic departments in several international medical schools as well as working for the education committee of the General Medical Council. Within the wider National Health Service in the UK, he was involved in the breast screening committees at the time that this service was being set up nationally, regional and international research training committees and he was governor of one of the local schools in Bristol. As a pioneer in introducing new techniques and advancing the scholarship of surgery, he was without doubt a leading light. This included the establishment of fine needle aspiration biopsy, both in the thyroid gland and in the breast in both Newcastle and the Bristol breast units. Outside medicine, he had a long-standing interest in hockey, a sport that he continued during his under-

graduate career when he was captain and vice president of the medicals hockey club and awarded full colours. He played also for the Tynedale Hockey Club and was interested in gardening, classical music, and of course he was dedicated to the support and development of his family. His untimely, tragic and unexpected sudden death in February 2002 at the very peak of his career left a huge gap not only in the world of breast and endocrine surgery nationally and internationally but also in the hearts of those who were close to him. Undoubtedly, much more was to come from this outstanding, unique, and kind man and those who were lucky enough to work with him and have learned from him remain respectful and in admiration not only for his skill and ability as an academic surgeon but also for his outstanding qualities as a human being that he displayed.

Acknowledgments I would like to give my greatest thanks to Mr. Clive Farndon, John's younger brother, and Mrs. Chris Farndon, John's widow, for the consent to produce this short chapter as well as for their very considerable help in piecing together the life history of John.

References

1. Wells SA, Bayling SB, Leight GS, Dale JK, Dilley WG, Farndon JR. The importance of early diagnosis in patients with hereditary medullary thyroid cancer. Ann Surg. 1982;195(5):595–9.
2. Alderson D, Farndon JR. The effects of transplant mass on insulin release by collagenase dispersed pancreatic fragments in the diabetic dog. World J Surg. 1984;8:598–604.
3. Sainsbury JRC, Farndon JR, Sherbert GV, Harris AL. Epidermal growth factor receptors and oestrogen receptors in human breast cancer. Lancet 1985;325:364–6.
4. Farndon JR, Dilley WG, Bayling SB, Smallridge RC, Harrison TS, Wells SA. Familial medullary thyroid cancer without associated endocrinopathies: a distinct clinical entity. Brit J Surg. 1986;73:278–81.
5. Carlson GL, Farndon JR. Investigation of primary hyperparathyroidism. Current Imaging 1990;2:98–104.
6. Mihai R, Farndon JR. Diagnosis and treatment of adrenal tumours. Surgery 1996;14(7):145–53.
7. Murie JA, Farndon JR. The British Journal of Surgery in the new millennium. Brit J Surg. 2000;87:1–2.
8. Mihai R, Lai T, Schofield G, Farndon JR. Changes in cytoplasmic calcium determine the secretary response to extracellular cations in human parathyroid cells. A confocal microscopy study using FM1–43 dye. Biochem J. 2000;352:253–361.

Well-Differentiated Thyroid Cancer: Papillary, Follicular, and Oncocytic (Hürthle) Cell Cancer

Linwah Yip

Editors' Note: This chapter and the chapter "Update of the Treatment Guidelines for Well-Differentiated Thyroid Cancer" by Dr. Glenn and Wang are excellent companion pieces. We highly suggest reading them together to appreciate the many nuances of therapy for thyroid nodules and thyroid cancer.

In the past decade, the incidence of thyroid cancer in the USA has been increasing at a rate of 5–6 % per year, and mortality rates have been rising at an average of 0.9 % per year [1]. Thyroid cancer is the ninth most commonly diagnosed cancer, and comprises ~4 % of all new cancer cases [1]. The trend in rising thyroid cancer incidence is an international trend, and can be seen in analysis of population-level cancer registries worldwide [2]. Women are threefold more likely to be diagnosed and remarkably, this propensity is observed across different geographic areas and ethnicities [2]. Although the rising rates appear to be coincident with the widespread use of ultrasound and fine-needle aspiration biopsy (FNAB) [3], early detection may not be the only reason for the increased incidence as the trend is observed in men as well as in women, among all ages, in all tumor sizes, and across different racial and ethnic groups [4, 5].

The majority (95–98 %) of thyroid cancers are differentiated (DTC) and include papillary, follicular, and oncocytic (Hürthle) cell carcinomas. All three histologic subtypes arise from the follicular epithelial cells which line the 20–30 million spherical follicles within the thyroid gland that are filled with colloid and can store up to a 3-month supply of thyroid hormone [6]. Papillary thyroid cancer (PTC) represents 80–85 % of diagnosed DTC, and is histologically characterized by neoplastic papillae lined by cuboidal or columnar cells with the cytologic features of clear nuclei, i.e., "Orphan Annie eyes" (80 %), intranuclear inclusions (80–85 %), and nuclear grooves (nearly 100 %). Psammoma bodies are formed from focal areas of infarcted papillae and are only rarely (< 1 %) described in benign thyroid disorders [7]. Fol-

licular thyroid cancer (FTC) represents 4–5 % of DTC, and is rarely occult. The diagnosis of FTC requires capsular and/or vascular invasion, and relies on histologic evaluation. FTC typically is hematogenously disseminated and distant metastases to bone and/or lung are more common than lymph node involvement [8]. Oncocytic (Hürthle) cell thyroid carcinomas (OTC) comprise the final major histologic DTC subtype and are diagnosed in 2–3 % of cases. Hürthle cells were first described in 1894 but not by **Karl Hürthle**. Hürthle cells are now known to be derived from follicular cells and may develop in response to defects in mitochondrial DNA [9]. OTC share many clinical features with FTC particularly a tendency for hematogenous spread and poorer prognosis when compared to PTC. However, unlike FTC, OTC has a higher risk for local recurrence and is less iodine-avid with an overall poorer 10-year survival [10, 11].

Risk Factors

Environmental

Exposure to ionizing radiation is a risk factor for developing DTC, and the risk is dependent on the dose received as well as age at the time of exposure. Radiation to treat benign conditions such as acne, ringworm, and enlargement of the thymus or tonsils used to be common; however, these treatments ended in the 1960s. Other causes of radiation exposure include nuclear accidents, occupational exposures, diagnostic examinations, and therapy for malignant conditions. Although the risk of thyroid cancer after head and neck radiation diminishes when the age at the time of exposure is greater than 15 years, the increased risk can last for up to 40 years [12]. Thus, there has been scrutiny at the increasingly frequent use of computed-tomography (CT) scans and fluoroscopy in pediatric diagnostic imaging. The

L. Yip (✉)
Division of Endocrine Surgery and Surgical Oncology, Department of Surgery, University of Pittsburgh, 3471 Fifth Ave., Suite 101, Pittsburgh, PA 15213, USA
e-mail: yipl@upmc.edu

J. L. Pasieka, J. A. Lee (eds.), *Surgical Endocrinopathies,* DOI 10.1007/978-3-319-13662-2_15,
© Springer International Publishing Switzerland 2015

risks are estimated to be low but current rates of utilized testing will lead to elevated risks of thyroid cancer that are thought to range from 4 to 65 thyroid cancer cases per million people from CT scan use alone [13]. Radiation-induced cancers are often multifocal and carry different molecular alterations. Whether they are phenotypically different from nonradiation-induced tumors is unclear. Although studies of Chernobyl-related thyroid cancer cases suggest a more aggressive clinical course, the younger age at diagnosis and endemic iodine deficiency may have contributed to the cancer aggressiveness [14].

Other environmental risk factors that have been proposed and studied include iodine intake and polybrominated diphenyl ethers found in a widely used flame retardant; however, causal relationships have been difficult to determine. Iodine intake in particular is theorized to play a role in the histologic type of diagnosed DTC but not in the cancer incidence. For example, regions with high iodine intake such as Japan and China have a higher incidence of PTC while areas with endemic iodine deficiency have a higher incidence of FTC [15]. Obesity has also been proposed as a risk factor for thyroid cancer and a number of studies have demonstrated a modest association between body mass index and DTC. The mechanism could be related to either how insulin resistance and subsequent hyperinsulinemia augments pre-activated proliferative pathways, or a result of the pro-invasive effects of leptin and other adipokines [16].

Hereditary

Familial nonmedullary thyroid cancer (FNMTC) is most frequently associated with the familial adenomatosis polyposis (FAP), PTEN hamartoma tumor (PHTS), or **Carney** complex type 1 syndromes (Table 1). Affected members of all three syndromes have a higher incidence of both benign and malignant thyroid disease. FAP is caused by mutations in the *APC* gene and is characterized by > 100 colorectal adenomatous polyps. The diagnosis of the rare cribriform-morular-variant PTC should increase clinical concern, although conventional and follicular-variant PTC are also seen [17]. PHTS was previously known as Cowden's syndrome and is associated with mutations in the *PTEN* tumor suppressor gene. Hashimoto's thyroiditis is seen in up to 40 % of affected patients and there is an overall high 35 % risk of thyroid malignancy [18]. Although FTC comprises a higher proportion of PHTS-associated thyroid cancers, PTC is the most commonly diagnosed histologic DTC type [19]. The risk of thyroid malignancy in Carney complex type 1 is < 5 %, and PTC or FTC are most common [20]. Surveillance for patients who are affected members of a known inherited predisposition syndrome should include yearly thyroid-stimulating hormone (TSH), neck exam, and thyroid ultrasound. Prophylactic thyroidectomy is not indicated although if surgery is directed by cytology findings, then total thyroidectomy is typically recommended [21].

FNMTC can also be diagnosed in the absence of an identified predisposition syndrome or history of radiation

Table 1 Hereditary syndromes associated with DTC

	Familial adenomatosis polyposis	PTEN hamartoma tumor (Cowden's)	Carney complex type 1
Pathognomonic criteria	> 100 colorectal adenomatous polyps	Mucocutaneous lesions and cerebellar tumors	Pigmented skin lesions, i.e., lentigines, cutaneous, and/or mucosal
Major manifestations	–	Breast, endometrial, and thyroid cancer; macrocephaly	Blue nevi, pigmented nodular adrenals, cardiac myxomas
Minor	Extracolonic polyps, congenital hypertrophy of retinal pigment epithelium; soft tissue tumors; desmoids; osteomas	Fibrocystic breast disease, mental retardation, gastrointestinal hamartomas, lipomas; fibromas, renal cell carcinomas, uterine fibroids	Melanotic schawannomas; adrenal, hepatocellular, or pancreatic cancers; pituitary adenomas
Gene	*APC (80 %)*	*PTEN (80 %)*	*PRKAR1A (70 %)*
Prevalence of thyroid disease:			
Benign	40 %	Up to 75 % Hashimoto's thyroiditis in 40 %	Up to 75 %
Cancer	0.4–12 %	35 %	<5 %
Cancer types	CMV-PTC 63 %	PTC 50 %	PTC
	FV-PTC 25 %	FV-PTC 28 %	FTC
	PTC 12 %	FTC 14 %	
Presentation	Possibly more likely in women	Thyroid cancer is earliest presentation	–
Surveillance	Thyroid ultrasound, neck exam, and TSH at diagnosis, then yearly		
Treatment	Total thyroidectomy when surgery indicated		

CMV cribriform-morular variant, *FV* follicular variant, *FTC* follicular thyroid cancer, *PTC* papillary thyroid cancer exposure, and is defined by DTC in at least two first-degree relatives [21]. In a population-level Nordic study, a threefold elevated risk of thyroid cancer was observed even if a single first-degree relative was diagnosed with either PTC or FTC. The risks were more pronounced if the relative was diagnosed at a young age although there was a trend towards concordant age at DTC diagnosis [22]. A number of candidate loci have been identified including *MNG1, TCO, fPTC/PRN, NMTC1, FTEN,* and *FOXE1* [23]. Nonsyndromic FNMTC may be associated with earlier age onset, multifocality, extrathyroidal extension, and lymph node metastasis. Prophylactic thyroidectomy is also not necessary although neck ultrasound is recommended at age 20 or 5–10 years before the proband was diagnosed, and total thyroidectomy is typically performed when surgical intervention is indicated [21].

Genetics of Sporadic DTC

The majority of DTC are sporadic, and the most common genetic alterations implicated in thyroid carcinogenesis involve activating mutations in the mitogen-activated protein kinase (MAPK) and PI3K-AKT pathways that lead to downstream upregulation of tumor-promoting and cancer progression genes [24]. The type of mutation correlates to histologic subtype (Table 2) [24, 25]. For example, FTC are more likely to have mutations in the *RAS* and *PTEN* genes while *BRAF* V600E and *RET/PTC* rearrangements are more common in conventional PTC. Interestingly, follicular-variant PTC

which has morphologic features more consistent with PTC but biologic behavior that is often similar to FTC, shares gene alterations with both histologic types.

BRAF V600E is the most common gene alteration in thyroid carcinogenesis, and can be associated with up to 40–50 % of conventional PTC. *BRAF* mutations may correlate with aggressive tumor characteristics such as extrathyroidal extension, advanced tumor stage at presentation, and lymph node or distant metastases, and may be an independent, age-related predictor of tumor recurrence [26, 27]. In a cohort study, persistent/recurrent disease was most likely in PTC patients who had *BRAF* V600E-positive tumors and who were age ≥65 years [28]. Xing et al. evaluated a multi-institutional and retrospective series of 1840 PTC patients with median follow-up of 33 months, and observed an association between *BRAF* V600E and increased disease-specific mortality. However, in multivariate analysis, the effects of *BRAF* did not appear to be independent of extent of disease at presentation including presence of lymph node metastasis, extrathyroidal extension, and distant metastasis [29].

RAS has a key role in signal transduction from tyrosine kinase and G-protein-coupled receptors to effectors of both the MAPK and PI3K-AKT pathways. Point mutations cause increased affinity of *RAS* to guanosine triphosphate (GTP) or inhibit the autocatalytic GTPase function, and both cause constitutive activation of downstream pathways [30]. *RAS* mutations are the most common gene alterations identified in

Table 2 Correlation between gene alteration and differentiated thyroid cancer subtype

Genetic alteration	Associated DTC
Mutations	
BRAF V600E	Conventional PTC
	Tall-cell-variant PTC
	Follicular-variant PTC, unencapsulated
BRAF K601E	Follicular-variant PTC, encapsulated
RAS	Follicular adenoma
	Conventional PTC
	Follicular-variant PTC
	FTC
	OTC
PTEN	FTC
	OTC
	Conventional PTC (rare)
TSHR	FTC
	Follicular-variant PTC
P53	Conventional PTC
	OTC
PIK3CA	FTC
Rearrangements	
RET/PTC	Conventional PTC
	Follicular-variant PTC (rare)
PAX8-PPARγ	Follicular-variant PTC
	FTC

DTC differentiated thyroid cancer, *PTC* papillary thyroid cancer, *FTC* follicular thyroid cancer, *OTC* oncocytic thyroid carcinoma, *TSHR* thyroid-stimulating hormone receptor indeterminate biopsy specimens, and can include point mutations in *N-*, *K-*, and *H-RAS* hotspots in codons 12/13 and 61 [31]. All three mutant isoforms have been identified in up to 48% of benign follicular adenomas, 50–60% of FTC, and less frequently (20%) in PTC [30]. Although most *RAS*-associated thyroid cancers are indolent, *RAS* mutations have also been identified in medullary, poorly differentiated, and anaplastic thyroid cancers.

RET rearrangements in PTC have been well documented and more than 10 different types of translocations have been described that are identified in 10–20% of PTC [32, 33]. Typically, the 3' tyrosine kinase portion of the *RET* gene fuses with the 5' of a different gene resulting in a ligand-independent dimerization and constitutive activation of effector genes in both the MAPK and PI3-AKT pathways. A higher incidence of *RET/PTC* rearrangements are seen in PTC patients with a previous history of radiation exposure (50–80%) and in younger patients (40–70%) [34, 35]. The two most common fusion proteins are *RET/PTC1* and *RET/PTC3; RET/PTC1*-positive tumors demonstrate either classic papillary architecture or diffuse sclerosing features, while *RET/PTC3* is associated with solid-variant PTC. All of the *RET/PTC* tumor subtypes have a higher rate of lymph node metastases [36].

Less commonly identified gene alterations in PTC and FTC include *BRAF* K601E, thyroid-stimulating hormone receptor (*TSHR*), and somatic *PTEN* mutations in addition to the *PAX8/PPARγ* rearrangement (Table 2). A shift in diagnosed thyroid cancer histologies and molecular profiles was observed in an evaluation of thyroid cancers over four decades at a single institution [37]. In addition to an increased median age at diagnosis, the proportion of classic PTC was observed to decrease over time. Three interesting temporal trends in DTC molecular profiles were observed: (1) The percentage of *BRAF* V600E-positive PTC remained stable although the proportion of classic PTC with *BRAF* V600E mutations increased in the later decades, (2) the prevalence of *RAS* mutations in thyroid cancers increased, and (3) *RET/PTC*-positive PTC decreased over time suggesting that exposure to ionizing radiation may have a diminishing contribution to thyroid carcinogenesis [37].

Mitochondrial DNA mutations have been proposed as an etiology in formation of OTC. Mutations in *GRIM-19*, a regulatory gene involved in apoptosis and mitochondrial metabolism, have been identified in ~15% of oncocytic or Hürthle cell variants of follicular and papillary thyroid carcinoma [38]. Point mutations in *p53, RAS,* and *PTEN* were identified in OTC after evaluation with next-generation sequencing, a method that allows parallel high-volume sequencing, that targets a panel of 284 hot-spot mutations previously reported in DTC [39]. However, 60% of the studied OTC did not have any of the evaluated mutations and further study of the gene alterations that lead to OTC is still needed.

Accumulation of genetic alterations that lead to further dysregulation is one likely trigger for tumor progression, and multiple driver mutations can be found in recurrent/metastatic DTC [24, 39]. Another marker that is associated with aggressive DTC is mutation of the telomerase reverse transcriptase (*TERT*) promoter. Telomerase activation is a marker of malignancy that allows continued cell replication and *TERT* promoter mutations have been identified in other malignancies. *TERT* promoter mutations in thyroid cancers were identified in 7–22% of PTC and ~35% of FTC, were often found in association with *BRAF* or *RAS* mutations, and were more likely in patients with histologically aggressive differentiated thyroid cancer [40, 41]. In a series of 469 thyroid cancer patients of whom 402 had differentiated thyroid cancer, Melo et al. [42] reported that *TERT* promoter mutations were independently associated with an increased risk of disease-specific mortality for both PTC and FTC patients. Other markers of aggressive thyroid cancer have often been synonymous with tumor dedifferentiation and these include mutations in *p53* (25–30%), *PIK3CA* (10–20%), *CTNNB1* (10–20%), and *AKT1* (5–10%) [25].

Clinical Manifestations

Most patients with DTC are asymptomatic. The most common presentation is a thyroid nodule found either on physical exam or incidentally on diagnostic imaging such as CT scan of the chest/neck or carotid duplex imaging. New-onset hypothyroidism may also be an indicator of malignancy, and a careful cervical and thyroid examination should be performed. A clinical history of an enlarging thyroid mass increases the concern for malignancy. On physical exam, an immobile and firm thyroid nodule is also worrisome. Routine evaluation should also assess for dysphagia, positional dyspnea, orthopnea, anterior neck discomfort, hoarseness, tracheal deviation, lymphadenopathy, and the presence of contralateral thyroid nodules. Supine dyspnea that is relieved by positional change, a history of sleep apnea, and/or an inability to palpate the inferior aspect of the thyroid gland should raise concern for a substernal component.

Diagnosis

Neck ultrasound is the gold-standard imaging study used to evaluate thyroid nodule size and nodule characteristics. Suspicious sonographic features include solid consistency, taller-than-wide shape, marked hypoechogenecity, irregular border, intranodular hypervascularity, microcalcifications, and loss of the echogenic halo (Fig. 1a) [43]. Cervical lymphadenopathy should also always be concurrently evaluated on cervical ultrasound. Lymph nodes that are rounded,

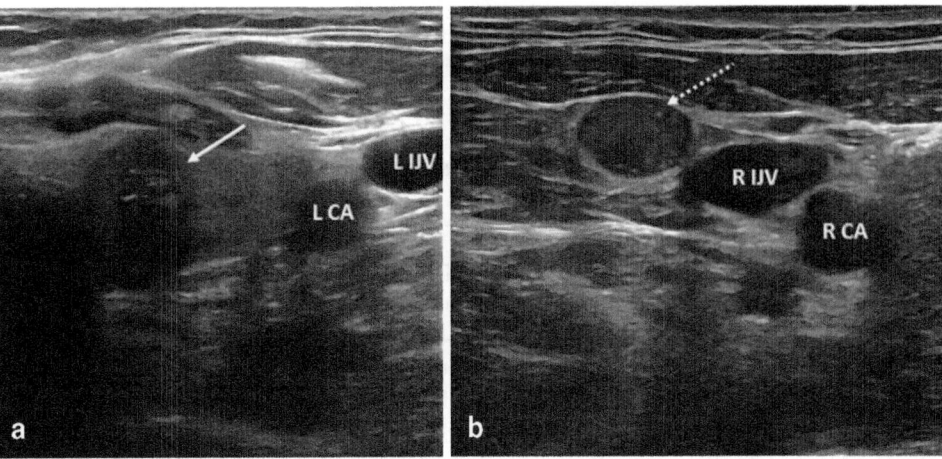

Fig. 1 Preoperative ultrasound images of a left thyroid nodule (**a**, *white arrow*) that has several suspicious sonographic features including taller-than-wide shape, marked hypoechogenecity, microcalcifications, and no well-defined halo. The patient also had a concerning right level 3 lymph node (**b**, *dotted arrow*) that was rounded and lacked a fatty hilum. Histology confirmed multifocal *BRAF* V600E-positive papillary thyroid cancer with metastatic disease in both the central compartment and right lateral neck

have microcalcifications, peripheral vascularization, loss of the fatty hilum, rounded shape, and cystic appearance are concerning and should undergo FNAB (Fig. 1b). A noncontrast CT scan of the neck can be considered if there is clinical concern for substernal extension particularly if the caudal extent of the thyroid gland is not palpable on physical exam as substernal extension below the aortic arch may require a partial sternal split for complete resection.

FNAB is the most sensitive initial diagnostic test and also guides subsequent clinical management. For reporting standardization, cytology results should be classified into one of the six-tiered Bethesda System for Reporting Thyroid Cytopathology categories: inadequate, benign, atypia or follicular lesion of undetermined significance, follicular neoplasm or suspicious for follicular neoplasm, suspicious for malignancy, or positive for malignancy [44]. Thyroidectomy is currently indicated for FNAB results in the indeterminate, positive for malignancy, or persistently inadequate categories. Diagnostic adjuncts may further identify if nodules with indeterminate cytology require surgery, and include (a) molecular testing for somatic mutations/rearrangements that are found in thyroid cancer [31, 45], (b) evaluation of gene expression profiling patterns that may identify nodules at lower risk for malignancy [46], or (c) identification of circulating TSHR messenger RNA (mRNA) that may be a marker of malignancy [47]. Patients with risk factors for thyroid cancer who have a dominant (>1 cm) thyroid nodule, symptomatic thyromegaly, tracheal compression, and/or substernal goiter that are unable to be evaluated completely with FNAB or ultrasound (US) should also be considered for thyroidectomy.

Large nodules (≥4 cm) may have a higher risk of malignancy (7–35%) in addition to a higher likelihood of false-negative benign FNAB results (0.9–20%) [48], and the inability to accurately exclude malignancy in large nodules may be considered another indication for surgery. Banks and colleagues developed a predictor model to aid in the diagnosis of suspicious or indeterminate FNA samples and reported that patient age, nodule size (nodules <1.5 cm and larger nodules ≥3 cm were associated with increased risk), and cytopathology (suspicious for papillary thyroid carcinoma had the greatest risk) were all significant predictors of thyroid cancer. These three variables remained significant on multivariate analysis and, in combination, were predictive with 74% accuracy. The model was then prospectively validated in a separate cohort of 135 thyroidectomy patients, and was able to predict thyroid cancer in ROC analysis with an AUC of 0.85 [49].

Surgical Management

Although PTC can be readily diagnosed on FNAB, the diagnoses of FTC and OTC require further histologic examination of the entire nodule and its capsule in relation to the adjacent thyroid lobe tissue. The decision for initial extent and conduct of thyroidectomy depends on the degree of preoperative concern for DTC, size of the presumptive malignancy, and other clinical features.

Among low-risk DTC patients who undergo lobectomy only, studies suggest a higher rate of local (up to 30%) and contralateral lobe (5–10%) recurrence; however, effects on long-term survival are less clear [50]. For any DTC patient >45 years who also has extrathyroidal extension and/or palpable lymph node metastases (i.e., American Joint Committee on Cancer (AJCC) TNM stage III disease), total thyroidectomy versus thyroid lobectomy improves cause-specific mortality at 30 years (20 vs. 39%) [51]. In a study of >50,000 PTC patients from the National Cancer Data Base, total thyroidectomy compared to lobectomy for PTC≥1 cm was associated with statistically significant improvement in 10-year local recurrence rates (7.7 vs. 9.8%) and 10-year survival (98.4 vs. 97.1%). For PTC <1 cm, the extent of thyroidectomy made no difference in recurrence or survival but the findings of this study are limited by heterogeneity in PTC pathologic subtypes, use of radioactive iodine (RAI) ablation, and variable management with TSH suppression [52].

Thyroidectomy for DTC ≥ 1 cm Diagnosed by Fine-Needle Aspiration

As mentioned previously, DTC diagnosed preoperatively is typically PTC, and thyroidectomy is the initial treatment. The false-negative rate of FNAB that is positive for malignancy is low (1–2%) and patients should be counseled preoperatively about the possibility of false-positive results. Total thyroidectomy or near-total thyroidectomy (which leaves ≤50 mg of tissue at the ligament of Berry) is considered the procedure of choice when the tumor measures ≥ 1 cm on preoperative US. Among experienced thyroid surgeons, initial total thyroidectomy is usually associated with a <1% risk of recurrent laryngeal nerve injury and a <1% risk of permanent hypoparathyroidism [53].

Thyroidectomy for DTC < 1 cm Diagnosed by Fine-Needle Aspiration

FNAB for thyroid nodules <1 cm is typically not performed unless suspicious sonographic features are present. If diagnosed preoperatively, the management of small, papillary thyroid microcarcinomas (PTMC) remains controversial not just in determining the extent of surgery but also in deciding if surgical management should be pursued. Although most studies suggest that PTMC is generally associated with an excellent long-term survival regardless of surgical procedure, there is a small but real percentage of patients who develop lymph node metastasis (up to 35%) and distant metastasis (<1%). In one meta-analysis, recurrent disease from PTMC was associated with multifocality, "nonincidental" disease, age <45 years, and the presence of lymph node disease at presentation [54]. In the absence of these factors, thyroid lobectomy is considered adequate treatment for unifocal PTMC.

Nonoperative management has also been studied by Ito et al. [55]. In a series of 340 patients with PTMC who had observation instead of thyroidectomy, enlargement of the tumor more than 3 mm and lymph node metastasis occurred at 10-year follow-up in 15.9 and 3.4% of the patients, respectively. When compared to patients with PTMC who received immediate thyroidectomy, the rate of lymph node recurrence was the same. Furthermore, most patients who had nonoperative treatment had stable disease even at 10-year follow-up [55]. Nonoperative treatment may be considered for selected patients with intrathyroidal tumors without evidence of lymph node metastasis, although studies with longer follow-up are still needed to determine the natural history of in situ PTMC.

Diagnostic Thyroidectomy

DTC is often first diagnosed on postoperative histology and follicular-variant PTC is now the most common histologic malignancy diagnosed after diagnostic thyroidectomy. For FNAB results in the indeterminate, persistently nondiagnostic, or suspicious categories, diagnostic thyroid lobectomy and isthmusectomy at a minimum is indicated and is associated with histologic DTC in 20, 5–10, and 50% of cases, respectively [56]. The minimum extent of initial diagnostic thyroidectomy is ipsilateral complete lobectomy, and isthmusectomy as the thyroid isthmus is an important anatomic and surgical margin intraoperatively. Partial thyroid lobectomy is an outmoded operation that puts the ipsilateral recurrent laryngeal nerve at unnecessary risk should reoperation be required. Since lobectomy and isthmusthectomy is associated with a 25–40% chance of surgical hypothyroidism requiring chronic replacement levothyroxine therapy, patients should be counseled about this possibility preoperatively.

Extent of Initial Thyroidectomy

The extent of initial thyroidectomy is influenced by a number of clinical factors. For patients with FNAB-proven DTC<1 cm in size or who require diagnostic thyroidectomy, the evidence to date supports initial total thyroidectomy for patients who have: a history of radiation exposure, diagnosed hypothyroidism, a family history of DTC, suspicious sonographic nodule features, a contralateral macronodule (>1 cm), or evidence of lymph node or distant metastasis. A preoperative tumor mutation profile that may be more likely identified in DTC with aggressive histologic features such as *TERT* or *BRAF* V600E may also be an indication for initial total thyroidectomy.

Completion Thyroidectomy

For PTC, completion total thyroidectomy (also termed re-operative contralateral lobectomy) to a thyroid remnant≤1 gm is recommended if total thyroidectomy would have been performed had the diagnosis been known preoperatively, i.e., the tumor is ≥1 cm, high-risk histologic subtype (such as tall cell, sclerosing, or columnar variant), multifocal, non-encapsulated, and/or with apparent nodal involvement [57]. Widely invasive FTC is associated with a worse prognosis and such patients should undergo total thyroidectomy. In the absence of these factors, thyroid lobectomy is usually considered adequate treatment for unifocal PTC or FTC < 1 cm. Because OTC can be multifocal and does not take up RAI as effectively, many support an aggressive surgical approach with total thyroidectomy for all OTC regardless of size.

Lymphadenectomy

Although cervical lymph node involvement is common in DTC and ranges from 20 to 90 % depending on the sensitivity of the detection method, the prognostic significance of lymph node metastasis is controversial. Nodal disease is clinically apparent in < 10 % of patients with PTC or OTC, and most patients have occult micrometastases which likely have little to no prognostic significance for most patients as micrometastatic disease responds well to radioiodine therapy. Metastatic PTC documented in cervical nodes is associated with a risk of local recurrence; however, whether there is also an association with long-term PTC survival has not been clearly demonstrated. In a large Surveillance, Epidemiology, and End Results (SEER) database study evaluating patient outcomes, lymph node metastasis has been shown to be a particularly poor prognostic indicator among FTC and older (> 45 years) PTC patients [58]. Metachronous lymph node metastasis is associated with a higher rate of recurrence and disease-specific mortality and develops in 5–10 % of patients with PTC after thyroidectomy and RAI ablation [59, 60]. In contrast, metachronous nodal disease develops in up to 25 % of patients after thyroidectomy for OTC [61]. Synchronous and metachronous lymph node metastases are rare in FTC and are an indicator of poor prognosis [62]. Whether synchronous or metachronous, the presence of clinically apparent lymph node disease prompts surgical local control to prevent complications related to airway and venous obstruction.

In the preoperative evaluation of DTC, ultrasound is the best test currently used to identify nodal metastases. FNAB with or without thyroglobulin measurement of the aspirate is recommended when clinical or sonographic evidence of nodal metastasis is present. When cervical metastasis is confirmed, a therapeutic function-preserving and compartment-oriented lymphadenectomy is recommended to decrease local recurrence and limit the need for potentially morbid reoperative neck surgery.

DTC, particularly PTC, usually first metastasizes to the central compartment (Level VI) [63]. The central compartment is defined by the boundaries of the hyoid bone (superiorly), carotid arteries (laterally), superficial layer of the deep cervical fascia (anteriorly), and deep layer of the deep cervical fascia (posteriorly). The inferior boundary is defined on the right by the innominate artery and on the left by the equivalent plane. A unilateral central compartment lymph node dissection includes the prelaryngeal (Delphian), pretracheal, in addition to either the right or left paratracheal lymph nodes while a bilateral dissection includes both paratracheal nodal basins. While the data on whether or not prophylactic central neck dissection improves survival is conflicting, routine prophylactic clearance of central compartment nodal tissue has been demonstrated to lower postoperative thyroglobulin levels at 6 months and may decrease recurrence rates in meta-analysis [64]. Prophylactic central neck dissection may also lead to more accurate staging and risk stratification and allow for a selective approach to RAI ablation [65]. However, the risk of hypoparathyroidism appears to be more frequent after thyroidectomy with central compartment neck dissection than after thyroidectomy alone and this risk, as well as the risk of recurrent laryngeal nerve injury, should be considered when deciding whether to perform prophylactic central neck dissection [64].

The lateral compartment is defined by the boundaries of the internal jugular vein (medially), trapezoid muscle (laterally), subclavian vein (inferiorly), and hypoglossal nerve (superiorly). The lymph nodes within the lateral compartment are further separated by anatomic boundaries defining levels I–V. The most common levels involved with metastatic thyroid cancer are II–IV. In the absence of gross involvement, a modified neck dissection which preserves the internal jugular vein, sternocleidomastoid, spinal accessory, and phrenic nerves, is usually performed for metastatic DTC. Prophylactic lateral neck dissection has never been shown to improve long-term outcomes and is not recommended for DTC patients.

Staging

A number of staging systems exist for DTC that incorporate clinical and histologic features including MACIS (metastasis, age, completeness of resection, invasion, size), AGES (age, grade, extent, size), and AMES (age, metastasis, extent, size). The most commonly used is the AJCC TNM staging system currently in its seventh edition which takes into account patient age, tumor size and degree of extrathyroidal extension, nodal metastasis, and distant metastasis (Table 3) [66]. Advanced stage disease is typically classified as AJCC TNM stage III (characterized by large tumor size >4 cm, extrathyroidal tumor extension, and/or central compartment lymph node metastasis) or stage IV (characterized by gross tumor involvement to the adjacent structures, lateral lymph node and/or distant metastasis). Age at diagnosis has a significant effect on prognosis, and elderly patients have a higher risk of disease-related mortality rate compared to younger patients. Unfortunately, older patients present with more aggressive disease with an increased likelihood of extrathyroidal extension, and lymph node and distant metastases, and their cancers tend to be less iodine-avid [67]. In con-

Table 3 American Joint Committee on Cancer (AJCC) 7th Edition, TNM Staging for DTC [66]. (Used with permission of the American Joint Committee on Cancer (AJCC), Chicago, Illinois. The original and primary source for this information is the AJCC Cancer Staging Manual, Seventh Edition (2010) published by Springer Science + Business Media)

Tumor		
Tx Cannot assess	–	–
T0 No evidence of tumor	–	–
T1 Size ≤ 2 cm	–	–
T1a Size ≤ 1 cm	–	–
T1b Size 1–2 cm	–	–
T2 Size 2.1–4 cm	–	–
T3 > 4 cm, or minimal extrathyroidal extension		
T4a Extends beyond capsule to subcutaneous soft tissues, larynx, trachea, esophagus, recurrent laryngeal nerve or recurrent laryngeal nerve		
T4b Invades prevertebral fascia, encases major vessels		
Nodal disease		
Nx Cannot assess	–	–
N0 None	–	–
N1a Level VI (pretracheal, paratracheal, prelaryngeal)		
N1b Lateral cervical or superior mediastinal		
Distant metastasis		
Mx Cannot assess	–	–
M0 None	–	–
M1 Present	–	–
Staging	< 45 years old	≥ 45 years old
I	Any T Any N M0	**T1** N0 M0
II	Any T Any N M1	**T2** N0 M0
III	–	**T3** N0 M0
–	–	T1–3 **N1a** M0
IVa	–	**T4a** Any N M0
–	–	T1–4a **N1b** M0
IVb	–	**T4b** Any N M0
IVc	–	Any T Any N **M1**

trast, patients younger than 45 years of age uniformly have an excellent prognosis and even in the presence of distant metastatic disease cannot have higher than stage II disease. All thyroid clinical scoring systems are imprecise and some patients who are stratified into low-risk groups may still be at risk for disease-related mortality [10].

Other histologic findings can also affect DTC prognosis. FTC, OTC, and FV-PTC are further classified by the degree of invasiveness with minimally invasive tumors having a better prognosis than widely invasive lesions. The majority of postoperative staging systems were devised to stratify DTC patients by mortality risk. However, recurrence can occur in up to 20 % of patients, and the ATA Risk Stratification classifies DTC into low, intermediate, and high risk for recurrence according to degree of extension, histologic subtype, presence of distant metastasis, extrathyroidal I^{131} uptake, and completeness of resection [57]. Adequate surgery is essential for DTC patients as implicit in several DTC staging schema is the information provided by the use of RAI, which in turn depends on complete tumor resection by total thyroidectomy and appropriate lymphadenectomy.

RAI Ablation

The observed results of radioiodine ablation on survival and local recurrence in retrospective studies have been variable. Among DTC patients with low-risk thyroid cancers, the risk of mortality at 10 years is < 2 % and no improvement in survival or local regional recurrence has been consistently demonstrated with RAI ablation [68]. RAI ablation in high-risk DTC patients, e.g., patients with tumors > 1.5 cm, incomplete tumor resection, or AJCC TNM stage III/IV disease, is more likely to be associated with improved disease-specific survival and a lower risk of local recurrence [69]. Among patients with OTC, RAI ablation may also be associated with a longer interval to disease progression and disease specific mortality [70]. Two-stage ablation, i.e., nonoperative destruction of the contralateral lobe after diagnostic lobectomy and isthmusectomy, is occasionally used instead of completion thyroidectomy if there is a major contraindication to reoperation such as vocal cord paralysis.

One role of RAI treatment is to ablate any remaining remnant tissue, which can facilitate surveillance. Thyroglobulin levels in the absence of thyroglobulin antibodies are a sensitive indicator of recurrent or persistent disease and are more likely to be an accurate quantitative measure of tumor burden if all normal thyroid tissue has been ablated. Low-risk DTC such as small FTC (< 1 cm) without vascular invasion, encapsulated FVPTC, or intrathyroidal PTC generally have an excellent overall prognosis and do not need postoperative RAI. As discussed in more detail in another chapter, RAI ablation is generally recommended for all PTC patients with AJCC TNM stage III or IV disease. Recommendations remain mixed for patients with stage II disease and patients with stage I disease who have aggressive pathologic findings such as multifocality, extrathyroidal (either gross or microscopic) or vascular invasion, or concerning histologic subtypes such as tall cell, columnar cell, or insular. Decisions for or against RAI are likely influenced by the accuracy of testing modalities available for long-term surveillance. RAI remnant ablation is recommended for most OTC and FTC patients.

Optimal RAI uptake is achieved through TSH stimulation either by T4 withdrawal or by recombinant human TSH (rhTSH). rhTSH has equivalent efficacy at remnant ablation compared to T4 withdrawal when using standard ^{131}I ablative dose, and provides favorable quality-of-life advantages [71, 72]. A stimulated TSH of > 30 mU/L has been associated with increased tumor RAI uptake; however, no controlled studies have been performed. A low-iodine diet (< 50 μg/day) that restricts intake of iodized or sea salt, dairy products, and seafood for 1–2 weeks prior to RAI ablation can also facilitate thyrocyte iodine uptake.

Prior to the therapeutic ^{131}I dose, a pre-therapy scan can be performed using 1–3 mCi of ^{131}I in order to evaluate the amount of thyroid tissue remaining following thyroidectomy. If inadvertently ablated, large thyroid remnants may cause painful thyroiditis, and thus reoperative surgery is sometimes indicated before RAI administration. Thyroid stunning, or decreased RAI uptake following the pre-therapy scan, is theorized to occur by a mechanism that may be related to downregulation of the sodium-iodide symporter. However, it is controversial and not all studies have demonstrated an associated decrease in thyroid remnant ablation. This effect may be reduced by performing the pre-therapy scan either with the lowest dose of ^{131}I or with ^{123}I.

^{131}I can be administered using three different methods: as an empiric fixed low (30-mCi) or high (100-mCi) dose, by quantitative tumor dosimetry, or by quantitative whole-body dosimetry. Whole-body dosimetry is usually reserved for widespread metastatic disease, and quantitative tumor dosimetry is rarely used as the initial modality. Empiric fixed doses are most commonly utilized but the optimal dose is still somewhat controversial. However, two recent randomized trials demonstrated that for low-risk and selected intermediate-risk DTC patients, low-dose ablation (30 mCi) is associated with lower costs and reduced exposure to radioactivity without any detrimental impact observed on disease-specific survival or recurrence [73, 74]. To evaluate for iodine-avid metastatic disease, a post-therapy whole-body scan (WBS) is frequently obtained 5–8 days after administration of therapeutic ^{131}I, and in ~10 % of patients, the post-therapy scan demonstrates clinically relevant disease which is not seen on the pre-therapy scan and is most often in the neck, chest, and mediastinum.

RAI has been associated with salivary gland dysfunction (sialadenitis, dry mouth, alterations in taste, or salivary duct stones) and premature menopause [69]. Transient testicular failure may develop if large (>300 mCi) doses of ^{131}I are administered. Yet no differences in infertility, miscarriage, or premature births are seen in large long-term studies of women who become pregnant after receiving ^{131}I [75]. In addition to its potentially morbid and long-term side effects, interest at limiting RAI dose is also related to risks of secondary malignancies. One estimation is that 100 mCi of ^{131}I induces 53 solid malignant tumors and 3 leukemias in 10,000 patients over a 10-year follow-up [75, 76]. A causative RAI effect has been difficult to determine and the increased risk for secondary cancers may also be due to an inherent epidemiologic or genetic predisposition to malignancy in DTC patients.

TSH Suppression

In vitro studies demonstrated that thyroid cells are dependent on TSH for differentiation and growth, and this has led to the routine use of levothyroxine to suppress TSH in DTC patients [77]. Retrospective studies have shown that patients treated with TSH suppression may have up to a 25 % reduction in disease recurrence and a 50 % improvement in survival [59]. In meta-analysis, TSH suppression appears to be likely favorable towards preventing disease progression and mortality [78]. Not surprisingly, the benefits of TSH suppression on overall survival and disease-specific survival appear to be more significant for high-risk patients.

The degree to which TSH should be suppressed has been difficult to determine and needs to be balanced against its risks. Even to subclinical levels, TSH suppression is associated with a two- to threefold increased risk of developing atrial fibrillation, impaired cardiac reserve, and postmenopausal osteoporosis [79]. Elderly patients in particular appear to be more susceptible to the associated complications [80]. Surgical treatment and RAI ablation are confounding factors as patients who undergo total or near-total thyroidectomy followed by RAI ablation can be suppressed to a greater degree than those who do not. However, studies have demonstrated that maintaining a higher degree of TSH suppression (<0.1 mU/L) in higher-risk patients may be associated with a lower risk of disease progression although subjecting low-risk patients to this amount of TSH suppression has no advantages [81, 82]. Currently, recommendations support maintaining TSH suppression to <0.1 mU/L for high-risk patients while a TSH of 0.1–0.5 mU/L is considered adequate for low-risk patients [57]. Levothyroxine dosing for TSH suppression is to lean body weight at 2.2–2.5 µg/kg for adults.

Surveillance of DTC Patients

Surveillance includes the selective use of whole-body iodine scanning, serum thyroglobulin (Tg) levels with thyroglobulin antibodies, and neck ultrasound. Risk-adjusted algorithms for surveillance are discussed in another chapter. Among patients with negative post-therapy WBS, the routine use of WBS for surveillance is not a sensitive method to detect recurrent disease. Distant metastases do not always concentrate iodine well which may explain why only 4–10% of patients with distant metastases have a positive surveillance WBS. Once there is suspicion of recurrent or metastatic disease, WBS is only useful to determine if ^{131}I will be a useful treatment adjunct.

When TSH is normal, it has been estimated that a Tg of 1 µg/L corresponds to 1 g of normal thyroid tissue [83]. Approximately 25% of DTC patients have thyroglobulin antibodies which can interfere with the interpretation of the Tg level and should always be obtained simultaneously. When thyroglobulin antibodies do not decrease to normal levels over close follow-up, this can also be a marker of persistent or recurrent disease. Tg levels should be obtained at the same laboratory as there is assay variability that can make comparisons between different laboratories difficult. Elevated Tg levels obtained with TSH stimulation and in the absence of thyroglobulin antibodies has been shown to be highly sensitive in identifying recurrent or persistent DTC. A Tg >2 µg/L can identify metastatic disease with a sensitivity of 89% and a specificity of 96%. Mildly elevated Tg levels (between 0.5 and 2 µg/L) can be seen immediately after thyroidectomy and RAI; however, >90% of these patients have a spontaneous decline of Tg to undetectable levels within 3 years [84].

Cervical US is the surveillance imaging modality of choice, detects nonpalpable local thyroid bed or nodal recurrence with high sensitivity, and can also facilitate pathologic confirmation with FNAB. Metastatic disease can be diagnosed either by the presence of malignant cells seen on cytopathology or by an elevated aspirate thyroglobulin level. The clinical significance of recurrent cervical disease diagnosed by US in patients with undetectable Tg levels is still unclear yet is an increasingly frequent clinical scenario with current use of high-resolution US imaging.

Recurrent Disease

Recurrent disease is often heralded by elevated Tg levels. At the time of remnant ablation, a Tg >30 ng/mL has a 70% positive predictive value for recurrent disease [85]. Persistently elevated Tg levels following thyroidectomy and RAI ablation should prompt further evaluation with cervical US, and levothyroxine should be adjusted to maintain serum TSH <0.1 mU/L.

Structural recurrences in the neck are treated with surgical resection, and a compartment-oriented lymph node dissection is often utilized due to the possibility of microscopic disease that is not visualized radiographically. In patients with recurrent disease in a previously operated field, ultrasound guidance can greatly facilitate focused resection with negligible morbidity and with an observed subsequent decrease in postoperative Tg level [86]. Up to 40% of recurrent disease can be attributed to incomplete surgical resection emphasizing the importance of accurate preoperative imaging prior to initial surgical treatment [87].

^{18}F-FDG PET is only useful in patients with Tg elevations, but no evidence of disease on US or WBS. This is thought to be due to the inverse relationship between loss of iodine avidity and gain of glucose utilization that occurs with tumor dedifferentiation. PET has a sensitivity of 50–70% with an increase in sensitivity as the Tg level increases, and no significant differences appear to occur when the study is obtained with or without TSH stimulation [88]. OTC, in particular, has high avidity for ^{18}F-FDG and the avidity may also have prognostic significance; metastatic OTC lesions with a higher maximum SUV (>10) have been associated with a poorer outcome compared to those with a lower maximum SUV (5-year mortality of 64 vs. 92%) [89].

External beam radiation can be used for locoregional control and palliation of recurrent or persistent disease that is not surgically resectable. There may be benefit for patients who have microscopic noniodine-avid residual disease secondary to extrathyroidal extension or positive surgical margins, and is associated with locoregional control rates at 4 years of up to 70%. Acute toxicity includes mucositis, dysphagia and/or dermatitis requiring placement of a gastrostomy (30%), fatigue, dry mouth, and/or hoarseness requiring placement of a tracheostomy (10%), and the difficulties of reoperation in an irradiated field should it be required subsequently [90].

Distant Metastasis

Among patients with synchronous metastases, age is a strong prognostic indicator; pediatric patients with DTC who present with metastatic disease have a reported 10-year survival of nearly 100% while older patients have a 5-year survival of 35–50% [91, 92]. Pulmonary metastases are the most common especially in PTC and OTC, while bone metastases are more common among FTC patients. Treatment should still include total thyroidectomy and resection of gross cervical disease for local control, prevention of airway and vascular complications, and optimization of ^{131}I ablation. In a study of 169 patients with locoregional and distant metastases, Tg levels obtained with a suppressed TSH correlated to site of metastasis. Tg > 100 ng/mL correlate with lung and/or bone metastasis although lung metastases have been reported in patients with TSH-suppressed Tg levels as low as 2.5 ng/mL. Tg > 300 ng/mL are associated with patients who have at least three metastatic sites [93]. Tg levels in patients with FTC tend to be higher than the levels in comparably sized PTC [94].

Metachronous metastatic lesions that are RAI-avid have a better prognosis. These are usually treated with a maximum cumulative dose of 600 mCi ^{131}I with response and long-term survival related to disease volume. Above this, the risk of leukemia significantly increases. If pulmonary lesions are present, RAI should be administered to limit whole-body retention at 48 h to < 80 mCi in order to prevent pulmonary fibrosis. Surgical metastasectomy of bone lesions has been associated with improved long-term survival in selected patients.

RAI-resistant lesions have a poor prognosis with 10-year survival < 15 %. With improved understanding of the genetic alterations involved in thyroid carcinogenesis, a number of new options for advanced thyroid cancer patients are emerging and include tyrosine kinase and small-molecule inhibitors, and targeted inhibition of upregulated pathways to induce iodine reuptake. The DECISION trial is the only phase III study completed in patients with RAI-refractory progressive thyroid cancer and used sorafenib at 400 mg BID [95]. The trial included 77 centers in 18 countries, and 417 patients were enrolled. Eligibility criteria included adult patients (age ≥ 18) who had locally advanced and/or metastatic RAI-refractory differentiated thyroid cancer, had evidence of progression within 14 months, and had not previously received targeted or cytotoxic therapy. Sorafenib was associated with improved median progression-free survival (PFS) of 10.8 months versus placebo 5.8 months (hazard ratio (HR) 0.59, 95 % confidence interval (CI) 0.45–0.76, $p < .001$), and these improvements were observed in all tumor histologies. Partial responses were observed in 12.2 % in the sorafenib group compared to 0.5 % in the placebo group. Hand/foot syndrome was the most common adverse event, and dose reductions were necessary in 66 % of patients. Secondary malignancies occurred in nine patients who were taking sorafenib (4 %) and included squamous cell carcinomas of the skin, leukemia, and bladder cancer; however, secondary malignancies were also observed in four patients who took placebo [95].

Vemurafenib is a small-molecular and specific inhibitor of *BRAF* V600E. For patients with *BRAF* V600E-positive metastatic melanoma, a phase I trial demonstrated promising clinical efficacy with a 56 % response rate [96]. A phase I trial of vemurafenib was completed in three patients with metastatic PTC and one had a confirmed partial response while the other two patients had stable disease [97]. A unique side effect of vemurafenib is the development of cutaneous squamous cell carcinomas and keratoacanthomas that can occur in up to 30 % of patients who receive selective or non-selective *BRAF* inhibitors [98]. Additional trials are ongoing to further investigate the role of vemurafenib in *BRAF* V600E-positive and RAI-refractory thyroid cancer.

Constitutive activation of the MAPK pathway by *BRAF* V600E resulted in loss of expression of iodide-metabolizing genes in a number of in vitro studies [99–101]. Suppression of the pathway then led to restoration of gene expression [100]. In a mouse model of inducible *BRAF* V600E expression in thyroid follicular cells, treatment with either *MEK* or *BRAF* small-molecular inhibitors led to dramatic increases in RAI uptake [102]. These preclinical findings led rapidly to a trial evaluating the efficacy of selumetinib, a selective *MEK*1 and 2 inhibitor, to induce iodine reuptake in otherwise RAI-refractory metastatic DTC patients [103]. After selumetinib treatment and demonstration of iodine uptake, 40 % (8/20) of study patients were able to receive a therapeutic dose of RAI. Decreases in serum thyroglobulin levels were observed in all treated patients and persisted for up to 6 months. Overall, five patients had partial response and three patients had stable disease. Toxicity related to selumetinib was grade 1 or 2 except in one patient who had a large cumulative prestudy dose of RAI and developed acute leukemia following study treatment [103].

Key Summary Points

- The incidence of thyroid cancer is increasing worldwide, and may not be due to early detection as the trend is observed in both genders, all ages, all tumor sizes, and across racial and ethnic groups.
- A first-degree relative with DTC is a risk factor for developing thyroid cancer, but the predisposition is likely multifactorial and also includes environmental exposures such as radiation exposure, iodine intake, and/or body mass index.
- DTC is most commonly caused by activating mutations in the MAPK and PI3K-AKT pathways. Identification of these genetic alterations has led to improvements in preoperative diagnosis and study of new adjuvant treatment approaches for patients with advanced thyroid cancer.
- DTC patients are typically asymptomatic at presentation, and are diagnosed during workup of a thyroid nodule

identified either on physical examination or incidentally on imaging. Ultrasound characterization and FNAB rarely miss malignancy, although surgical diagnosis is still often necessary.

- The cytologic features of PTC permit diagnosis by FNAB, but the diagnoses of follicular and oncocytic thyroid cancers require histologic examination of the entire nodule and its capsule in relation to the adjacent thyroid lobe tissue. The decision for initial extent and conduct of thyroidectomy depends on the degree of preoperative concern for DTC, size of the presumptive malignancy, and other clinical features.

- RAI administration and degree of TSH suppression are dependent on disease stage that is determined after surgery. High-risk patients receive the most benefit from current postoperative treatment modalities.

- Recurrent structural cervical disease is often treated surgically. When no longer radioactive-iodine-avid, options for advanced thyroid cancer patients include tyrosine kinase and small-molecule inhibitors, and targeted inhibition of upregulated pathways to induce iodine reuptake.

References

1. Howlader N NA, Krapcho M, Garshell J, Miller D, Altekruse SF, Kosary CL, Yu M, Ruhl J, Tatalovich Z, Mariotto A, Lewis DR, Chen HS, Feuer EJ, Cronin KA. editors. SEER cancer statistics review, 1975–2011, National Cancer Institute. Bethesda, MD. Based on November 2013 SEER data submission, posted to the SEER web site, April 2014.

2. Kilfoy BA, Zheng T, Holford TR, Han X, Ward MH, Sjodin A, et al. International patterns and trends in thyroid cancer incidence, 1973–2002. Cancer Causes Control. 2009;20(5):525–31. PubMed PMID: 19016336. Pubmed Central PMCID: 2788231.

3. Davies L, Welch HG. Increasing incidence of thyroid cancer in the United States, 1973–2002. JAMA. 2006;295(18):2164–7. PubMed PMID: 16684987.

4. Chen AY, Jemal A, Ward EM. Increasing incidence of differentiated thyroid cancer in the United States, 1988–2005. Cancer. 2009 Aug 15;115(16):3801–7. PubMed PMID: 19598221.

5. Aschebrook-Kilfoy B, Kaplan EL, Chiu BC, Angelos P, Grogan RH. The acceleration in PTC incidence rates is similar among racial and ethnic groups in the United States. Ann Surg Oncol. 2013;20(8):2746–53. PubMed PMID: 23504142.

6. Junquiera L, Carneiro J. Basic histology: text and atlas. 10th ed. Rio de Janeiro: McGraw-Hill; 2005.

7. LiVolsi VA. Papillary thyroid carcinoma: an update. Mod Pathol. 2011;24(Suppl 2):S1–9. PubMed PMID: 21455196.

8. LiVolsi VA, Baloch ZW. Follicular neoplasms of the thyroid: view, biases, and experiences. Adv Anat Pathol. 2004;11(6):279–87. PubMed PMID: 15505528.

9. Cheung CC, Ezzat S, Ramyar L, Freeman JL, Asa SL. Molecular basis off hurthle cell papillary thyroid carcinoma. J Clin Endocrinol Metabol. 2000;85(2):878–82. PubMed PMID: 10690905.

10. Hundahl SA, Fleming ID, Fremgen AM, Menck HR. A national cancer data base report on 53,856 cases of thyroid carcinoma treated in the U.S., 1985–1995 [see commetns]. Cancer. 1998;83(12):2638–48. PubMed PMID: 9874472.

11. Haigh PI, Urbach DR. The treatment and prognosis of Hurthle cell follicular thyroid carcinoma compared with its non-Hurthle cell counterpart. Surgery. 2005;138(6):1152–7; discussion 7–8. PubMed PMID: 16360403.

12. Schneider AB, Ron E, Lubin J, Stovall M, Gierlowski TC. Dose-response relationships for radiation-induced thyroid cancer and thyroid nodules: evidence for the prolonged effects of radiation on the thyroid. J Clinic Endocrinol Metab. 1993;77(2):362–9. PubMed PMID: 8345040.

13. Mazonakis M, Tzedakis A, Damilakis J, Gourtsoyiannis N. Thyroid dose from common head and neck CT examinations in children: is there an excess risk for thyroid cancer induction? Euro Radiol. 2007;17(5):1352–7. PubMed PMID: 17021703.

14. Sinnott B, Ron E, Schneider AB. Exposing the thyroid to radiation: a review of its current extent, risks, and implications. Endocrine Rev. 2010;31(5):756–73. PubMed PMID: 20650861. Pubmed Central PMCID: 3365850.

15. Pellegriti G, Frasca F, Regalbuto C, Squatrito S, Vigneri R. Worldwide increasing incidence of thyroid cancer: update on epidemiology and risk factors. J Cancer Epidemio. 2013;2013:965212. PubMed PMID: 23737785. Pubmed Central PMCID: 3664492.

16. Pappa T, Alevizaki M. Obesity and thyroid cancer: a clinical update. Thyroid. 2014;24(2):190–9. PubMed PMID: 23879222.

17. Jarrar AM, Milas M, Mitchell J, Laguardia L, O'Malley M, Berber E, et al. Screening for thyroid cancer in patients with familial adenomatous polyposis. Ann Surg. 2011;253(3):515–21. PubMed PMID: 21173694.

18. Milas M, Mester J, Metzger R, Shin J, Mitchell J, Berber E, et al. Should patients with Cowden syndrome undergo prophylactic thyroidectomy? Surgery. 2012;152(6):1201–10. PubMed PMID: 23158187.

19. Ngeow J, Mester J, Rybicki LA, Ni Y, Milas M, Eng C. Incidence and clinical characteristics of thyroid cancer in prospective series of individuals with Cowden and Cowden-like syndrome characterized by germline PTEN, SDH, or KLLN alterations. J Clin Endocrinol Metab. 2011;96(12):E2063–71. PubMed PMID: 21956414. Pubmed Central PMCID: 3232626.

20. Salpea P, Stratakis CA. Carney complex and McCune Albright syndrome: an overview of clinical manifestations and human molecular genetics. Mol Cell Endocrinol. 2014;386(1–2):85–91. PubMed PMID: 24012779. Pubmed Central PMCID: 3943598.

21. Metzger R, Milas M. Inherited cancer syndromes and the thyroid: an update. Curr Opin Oncol. 2014;26(1):51–61. PubMed PMID: 24300902.

22. Fallah M, Pukkala E, Tryggvadottir L, Olsen JH, Tretli S, Sundquist K, et al. Risk of thyroid cancer in first-degree relatives of patients with non-medullary thyroid cancer by histology type and age at diagnosis: a joint study from five Nordic countries. J Med Genet. 2013;50(6):373–82. PubMed PMID: 23585692.

23. Mazeh H, Sippel RS. Familial nonmedullary thyroid carcinoma. Thyroid. 2013;23(9):1049–56. PubMed PMID: 23734600.

24. Xing M. Molecular pathogenesis and mechanisms of thyroid cancer. Nat Rev Cancer. 2013;13(3):184–99. PubMed PMID: 23429735.

25. Nikiforov YE, Nikiforova MN. Molecular genetics and diagnosis of thyroid cancer. Nat Rev Endocrinol. 2011;7(10):569–80. PubMed PMID: 21878896.

26. Tufano RP, Teixeira GV, Bishop J, Carson KA, Xing M. BRAF mutation in PTC and its value in tailoring initial treatment: a systematic review and meta-analysis. Medicine. 2012;91(5):274–86. PubMed PMID: 22932786.

27. Xing M. BRAF mutation in PTC: pathogenic role, molecular bases, and clinical implications. Endocr Rev. 2007;28(7):742–62. PubMed PMID: 17940185.

28. Howell GM, Carty SE, Armstrong MJ, Lebeau SO, Hodak SP, Coyne C, et al. Both BRAF V600E mutation and older age (> / = 65 years) are associated with recurrent PTC. Ann Surg Oncol. 2011;18(13):3566–71. PubMed PMID: 21594703.

29. Xing M, Alzahrani AS, Carson KA, Viola D, Elisei R, Bendlova B, et al. Association between BRAF V600E mutation and mortality

in patients with PTC. JAMA. 2013;309(14):1493–501. PubMed PMID: 23571588.

30. Howell GM, Hodak SP, Yip L. RAS mutations in thyroid cancer. Oncologist. 2013;18(8):926–32. PubMed PMID: 23873720. Pubmed Central PMCID: 3755930.

31. Nikiforov YE, Ohori NP, Hodak SP, Carty SE, LeBeau SO, Ferris RL, et al. Impact of mutational testing on the diagnosis and management of patients with cytologically indeterminate thyroid nodules: a prospective analysis of 1056 FNA samples. J Clin Endocrinol Metabol. 2011;96(11):3390–7. PubMed PMID: 21880806. Pubmed Central PMCID: 3205883.

32. Tallini G, Asa SL. RET oncogene activation in papillary thyroid carcinoma. Adv Anat Pathol. 2001;8(6):345–54. PubMed PMID: 11707626.

33. Nikiforov YE. RET/PTC rearrangement in thyroid tumors. Endocr Pathol. 2002;13(1):3–16. PubMed PMID: 12114746.

34. Nikiforov YE, Rowland JM, Bove KE, Monforte-Munoz H, Fagin JA. Distinct pattern of ret oncogene rearrangements in morphological variants of radiation-induced and sporadic thyroid papillary carcinomas in children. Cancer Res. 1997;57(9):1690–4. PubMed PMID: 9135009.

35. Fenton CL, Lukes Y, Nicholson D, Dinauer CA, Francis GL, Tuttle RM. The ret/PTC mutations are common in sporadic papillary thyroid carcinoma of children and young adults. J Clin Endocrinol Metabol. 2000;85(3):1170–5. PubMed PMID: 10720057.

36. Adeniran AJ, Zhu Z, Gandhi M, Steward DL, Fidler JP, Giordano TJ, et al. Correlation between genetic alterations and microscopic features, clinical manifestations, and prognostic characteristics of thyroid papillary carcinomas. Am J Surg Pathol. 2006;30(2):216–22. PubMed PMID: 16434896.

37. Jung CK, Little MP, Lubin JH, Brenner AV, Wells SA Jr, Sigurdson AJ, et al. The increase in thyroid cancer incidence during the last four decades is accompanied by a high frequency of BRAF mutations and a sharp increase in RAS mutations. J Clin Endocrinol Metabol. 2014 Feb;99(2):E276–85. PubMed PMID: 24248188.

38. Maximo V, Botelho T, Capela J, Soares P, Lima J, Taveira A, et al. Somatic and germline mutation in GRIM-19, a dual function gene involved in mitochondrial metabolism and cell death, is linked to mitochondrion-rich (Hurthle cell) tumours of the thyroid. Brit J Cancer. 2005;92(10):1892–8. PubMed PMID: 15841082. Pubmed Central PMCID: 2361763.

39. Nikiforova MN, Wald AI, Roy S, Durso MB, Nikiforov YE. Targeted next-generation sequencing panel (ThyroSeq) for detection of mutations in thyroid cancer. J Clin Endocrinol Metabol. 2013;98(11):E1852–60. PubMed PMID: 23979959. Pubmed Central PMCID: 3816258.

40. Landa I, Ganly I, Chan TA, Mitsutake N, Matsuse M, Ibrahimpasic T, et al. Frequent somatic TERT promoter mutations in thyroid cancer: higher prevalence in advanced forms of the disease. J Clin Endocrinol Metabol. 2013;98(9):E1562–6. PubMed PMID: 23833040. Pubmed Central PMCID: 3763971.

41. Liu X, Bishop J, Shan Y, Pai S, Liu D, Murugan AK, et al. Highly prevalent TERT promoter mutations in aggressive thyroid cancers. Endocr Relat Cancer. 2013;20(4):603–10. PubMed PMID: 23766237. Pubmed Central PMCID: 3782569.

42. Melo M, da Rocha AG, Vinagre J, Batista R, Peixoto J, Tavares C, et al. TERT promoter mutations are a major indicator of poor outcome in differentiated thyroid carcinomas. J Clin Endocrinol Metabol. 2014;99(5):E754–65. PubMed PMID: 24476079.

43. Moon WJ, Jung SL, Lee JH, Na DG, Baek JH, Lee YH, et al. Benign and malignant thyroid nodules: US differentiation–multicenter retrospective study. Radiology. 2008;247(3):762–70. PubMed PMID: 18403624.

44. Baloch ZW, LiVolsi VA, Asa SL, Rosai J, Merino MJ, Randolph G, et al. Diagnostic terminology and morphologic criteria for cytologic diagnosis of thyroid lesions: a synopsis of the National Cancer Institute Thyroid Fine-Needle Aspiration State of the Science Conference. Diagn Cytopathol. 2008;36(6):425–37. PubMed PMID: 18478609.

45. Yip L WL, Armstrong MJ, Silbermann A, McCoy KL, Stang MT, et al. A clinical algorithm for fine-needle aspiration molecular testing effectively guides the appropriate extent of initial thyroidectomy. Ann Surg, In press. 2013.

46. Alexander EK, Kennedy GC, Baloch ZW, Cibas ES, Chudova D, Diggans J, et al. Preoperative diagnosis of benign thyroid nodules with indeterminate cytology. New Engl J Med. 2012;367(8):705–15. PubMed PMID: 22731672.

47. Milas M, Mazzaglia P, Chia SY, Skugor M, Berber E, Reddy S, et al. The utility of peripheral thyrotropin mRNA in the diagnosis of follicular neoplasms and surveillance of thyroid cancers. Surgery. 2007;141(2):137–46; discussion 46. PubMed PMID: 17263967.

48. Wharry LI, McCoy KL, Stang MT, Armstrong MJ, Lebeau SO, Tublin ME, et al. Thyroid nodules (>/=4 cm): can ultrasound and cytology reliably exclude cancer? World J Surg. 2014 Mar;38(3):614–21. PubMed PMID: 24081539.

49. Banks ND, Kowalski J, Tsai HL, Somervell H, Tufano R, Dackiw AP, et al. A diagnostic predictor model for indeterminate or suspicious thyroid FNA samples. Thyroid. 2008;18(9):933–41. PubMed PMID: 18788917.

50. Mazzaferri EL, Kloos RT. Clinical review 128: current approaches to primary therapy for papillary and FTC. J Clin Endocrinol Metabol. 2001;86(4):1447–63. PubMed PMID: 11297567.

51. Hay ID, Bergstralh EJ, Grant CS, McIver B, Thompson GB, van Heerden JA, et al. Impact of primary surgery on outcome in 300 patients with pathologic tumor-node-metastasis stage III papillary thyroid carcinoma treated at one institution from 1940 through 1989. Surgery. 1999;126(6):1173–81; discussion 81-2. PubMed PMID: 10598204.

52. Bilimoria KY, Bentrem DJ, Ko CY, Stewart AK, Winchester DP, Talamonti MS, et al. Extent of surgery affects survival for papillary thyroid cancer. Ann Surg. 2007;246(3):375–81; discussion 81-4. PubMed PMID: 17717441. Pubmed Central PMCID: 1959355.

53. Sosa JA, Bowman HM, Tielsch JM, Powe NR, Gordon TA, Udelsman R. The importance of surgeon experience for clinical and economic outcomes from thyroidectomy. Ann Surg. 1998;228(3):320–30. PubMed PMID: 9742915. Pubmed Central PMCID: 1191485.

54. Roti E, degli Uberti EC, Bondanelli M, Braverman LE. Thyroid papillary microcarcinoma: a descriptive and meta-analysis study. Euro J Endocrinol. 2008;159(6):659–73. PubMed PMID: 18713843.

55. Ito Y, Miyauchi A, Inoue H, Fukushima M, Kihara M, Higashiyama T, et al. An observational trial for papillary thyroid microcarcinoma in Japanese patients. World J Surg. 2010;34(1):28–35. PubMed PMID: 20020290.

56. Bongiovanni M, Spitale A, Faquin WC, Mazzucchelli L, Baloch ZW. The Bethesda system for reporting thyroid cytopathology: a meta-analysis. Acta Cytol. 2012;56(4):333–9. PubMed PMID: 22846422.

57. American Thyroid Association Guidelines Taskforce on Thyroid N, Differentiated Thyroid C, Cooper DS, Doherty GM, Haugen BR, Kloos RT, et al. Revised American Thyroid Association management guidelines for patients with thyroid nodules and differentiated thyroid cancer. Thyroid. 2009;19(11):1167–214. PubMed PMID: 19860577.

58. Zaydfudim V, Feurer ID, Griffin MR, Phay JE. The impact of lymph node involvement on survival in patients with papillary and follicular thyroid carcinoma. Surgery. 2008;144(6):1070–7; discussion 7-8. PubMed PMID: 19041020.

59. Mazzaferri EL, Jhiang SM. Long-term impact of initial surgical and medical therapy on papillary and follicular thyroid cancer. Am J Med. 1994;97(5):418–28. PubMed PMID: 7977430.

60. Ito Y, Higashiyama T, Takamura Y, Miya A, Kobayashi K, Matsuzuka F, et al. Risk factors for recurrence to the lymph node in papillary thyroid carcinoma patients without preoperatively detectable lateral node metastasis: validity of prophylactic modified radical neck dissection. World J Surg. 2007;31(11):2085–91. PubMed PMID: 17885787.

61. Kushchayeva Y, Duh QY, Kebebew E, Clark OH. Prognostic indications for Hurthle cell cancer. World J Surg. 2004;28(12):1266–70. PubMed PMID: 15517492.

62. Witte J, Goretzki PE, Dieken J, Simon D, Roher HD. Importance of lymph node metastases in follicular thyroid cancer. World J Surg. 2002;26(8):1017–22. PubMed PMID: 12045860.

63. American Thyroid Association Surgery Working G, American Association of Endocrine S, American Academy of O-H, Neck S, American H, Neck S, et al. Consensus statement on the terminology and classification of central neck dissection for thyroid cancer. Thyroid. 2009;19(11):1153–8. PubMed PMID: 19860578.

64. Wang TS, Cheung K, Farrokhyar F, Roman SA, Sosa JA. A meta-analysis of the effect of prophylactic central compartment neck dissection on locoregional recurrence rates in patients with papillary thyroid cancer. Ann Surg Oncol. 2013;20(11):3477–83. PubMed PMID: 23846784.

65. Mazzaferri EL, Doherty GM, Steward DL. The pros and cons of prophylactic central compartment lymph node dissection for papillary thyroid carcinoma. Thyroid. 2009;19(7):683–9. PubMed PMID: 19583485.

66. Edge SB, American Joint Committee on Cancer., American Cancer Society. AJCC cancer staging handbook: from the AJCC cancer staging manual. 7th ed. New York: Springer; 2010. xix, 718 p.

67. Biliotti GC, Martini F, Vezzosi V, Seghi P, Tozzi F, Castagnoli A, et al. Specific features of differentiated thyroid carcinoma in patients over 70 years of age. J Surg Oncol. 2006;93(3):194–8. PubMed PMID: 16482598.

68. Jonklaas J, Cooper DS, Ain KB, Bigos T, Brierley JD, Haugen BR, et al. Radioiodine therapy in patients with stage I differentiated thyroid cancer. Thyroid. 2010;20(12):1423–4. PubMed PMID: 21054207.

69. Jonklaas J, Sarlis NJ, Litofsky D, Ain KB, Bigos ST, Brierley JD, et al. Outcomes of patients with differentiated thyroid carcinoma following initial therapy. Thyroid. 2006;16(12):1229–42. PubMed PMID: 17199433.

70. Lopez-Penabad L, Chiu AC, Hoff AO, Schultz P, Gaztambide S, Ordonez NG, et al. Prognostic factors in patients with Hurthle cell neoplasms of the thyroid. Cancer. 2003;97(5):1186–94. PubMed PMID: 12599224.

71. Pacini F, Ladenson PW, Schlumberger M, Driedger A, Luster M, Kloos RT, et al. Radioiodine ablation of thyroid remnants after preparation with recombinant human thyrotropin in differentiated thyroid carcinoma: results of an international, randomized, controlled study. J Clin Endocrinol Metab. 2006;91(3):926–32. PubMed PMID: 16384850.

72. Taieb D, Sebag F, Cherenko M, Baumstarck-Barrau K, Fortanier C, Farman-Ara B, et al. Quality of life changes and clinical outcomes in thyroid cancer patients undergoing radioiodine remnant ablation (RRA) with recombinant human TSH (rhTSH): a randomized controlled study. Clin Endocrinol. 2009;71(1):115–23. PubMed PMID: 18803678.

73. Mallick U, Harmer C, Yap B, Wadsley J, Clarke S, Moss L, et al. Ablation with low-dose radioiodine and thyrotropin alfa in thyroid cancer. New Engl J Med. 2012;366(18):1674–85. PubMed PMID: 22551128.

74. Schlumberger M, Catargi B, Borget I, Deandreis D, Zerdoud S, Bridji B, et al. Strategies of radioiodine ablation in patients with low-risk thyroid cancer. New Engl J Med. 2012;366(18):1663–73. PubMed PMID: 22551127.

75. Garsi JP, Schlumberger M, Rubino C, Ricard M, Labbe M, Ceccarelli C, et al. Therapeutic administration of 131I for differentiated thyroid cancer: radiation dose to ovaries and outcome of pregnancies. J Nucl Med. 2008;49(5):845–52. PubMed PMID: 18413399.

76. Rubino C, de Vathaire F, Dottorini ME, Hall P, Schvartz C, Couette JE, et al. Second primary malignancies in thyroid cancer patients. Brit J Cancer. 2003;89(9):1638–44. PubMed PMID: 14583762. Pubmed Central PMCID: 2394426.

77. Brabant G. Thyrotropin suppressive therapy in thyroid carcinoma: what are the targets? J Clin Endocrinol Metabol. 2008;93(4):1167–9. PubMed PMID: 18390811.

78. McGriff NJ, Csako G, Gourgiotis L, Lori CG, Pucino F, Sarlis NJ. Effects of thyroid hormone suppression therapy on adverse clinical outcomes in thyroid cancer. Ann Med. 2002;34(7–8):554–64. PubMed PMID: 12553495.

79. Biondi B, Cooper DS. Benefits of thyrotropin suppression versus the risks of adverse effects in differentiated thyroid cancer. Thyroid. 2010;20(2):135–46. PubMed PMID: 20151821.

80. Cappola AR, Fried LP, Arnold AM, Danese MD, Kuller LH, Burke GL, et al. Thyroid status, cardiovascular risk, and mortality in older adults. JAMA. 2006;295(9):1033–41. PubMed PMID: 16507804. Pubmed Central PMCID: 1387822.

81. Pujol P, Daures JP, Nsakala N, Baldet L, Bringer J, Jaffiol C. Degree of thyrotropin suppression as a prognostic determinant in differentiated thyroid cancer. J Clin Endocrinol Metabol. 1996;81(12):4318–23. PubMed PMID: 8954034.

82. Cooper DS, Specker B, Ho M, Sperling M, Ladenson PW, Ross DS, et al. Thyrotropin suppression and disease progression in patients with differentiated thyroid cancer: results from the National Thyroid Cancer Treatment Cooperative Registry. Thyroid. 1998;8(9):737–44. PubMed PMID: 9777742.

83. Spencer CA, LoPresti JS, Fatemi S, Nicoloff JT. Detection of residual and recurrent differentiated thyroid carcinoma by serum thyroglobulin measurement. Thyroid. 1999;9(5):435–41. PubMed PMID: 10365673.

84. Kloos RT, Mazzaferri EL. A single recombinant human thyrotropin-stimulated serum thyroglobulin measurement predicts differentiated thyroid carcinoma metastases three to five years later. J Clin Endocrinol Metabol. 2005;90(9):5047–57. PubMed PMID: 15972576.

85. Kim TY, Kim WB, Kim ES, Ryu JS, Yeo JS, Kim SC, et al. Serum thyroglobulin levels at the time of 131I remnant ablation just after thyroidectomy are useful for early prediction of clinical recurrence in low-risk patients with differentiated thyroid carcinoma. J Clin Endocrinol Metabol. 2005;90(3):1440–5. PubMed PMID: 15613412.

86. McCoy KL, Yim JH, Tublin ME, Burmeister LA, Ogilvie JB, Carty SE. Same-day ultrasound guidance in reoperation for locally recurrent papillary thyroid cancer. Surgery. 2007;142(6):965–72. PubMed PMID: 18063083.

87. Kouvaraki MA, Lee JE, Shapiro SE, Sherman SI, Evans DB. Preventable reoperations for persistent and recurrent papillary thyroid carcinoma. Surgery. 2004;136(6):1183–91. PubMed PMID: 15657574.

88. Shammas A, Degirmenci B, Mountz JM, McCook BM, Branstetter B, Bencherif B, et al. 18F-FDG PET/CT in patients with suspected recurrent or metastatic well-differentiated thyroid cancer. J Nucl Med. 2007;48(2):221–6. PubMed PMID: 17268018.

89. Pryma DA, Schoder H, Gonen M, Robbins RJ, Larson SM, Yeung HW. Diagnostic accuracy and prognostic value of 18F-FDG PET in Hurthle cell thyroid cancer patients. J Nucl Med. 2006;47(8):1260–6. PubMed PMID: 16883003.

90. Terezakis SA, Lee KS, Ghossein RA, Rivera M, Tuttle RM, Wolden SL, et al. Role of external beam radiotherapy in patients with advanced or recurrent nonanaplastic thyroid cancer: Memorial Sloan-kettering Cancer Center experience. Int J Radiat Oncol Biol Phys. 2009;73(3):795–801. PubMed PMID: 18676097.

91. La Quaglia MP, Black T, Holcomb GW, 3rd, Sklar C, Azizkhan RG, Haase GM, et al. Differentiated thyroid cancer: clinical char-

acteristics, treatment, and outcome in patients under 21 years of age who present with distant metastases. A report from the Surgical Discipline Committee of the Children's Cancer Group. J Pediatr Surg. 2000;35(6):955–9; discussion 60. PubMed PMID: 10873043.

92. Sampson E, Brierley JD, Le LW, Rotstein L, Tsang RW. Clinical management and outcome of papillary and follicular (differentiated) thyroid cancer presenting with distant metastasis at diagnosis. Cancer. 2007;110(7):1451–6. PubMed PMID: 17705176.

93. Robbins RJ, Srivastava S, Shaha A, Ghossein R, Larson SM, Fleisher M, et al. Factors influencing the basal and recombinant human thyrotropin-stimulated serum thyroglobulin in patients with metastatic thyroid carcinoma. J Clin Endocrinol Metabol. 2004;89(12):6010–6. PubMed PMID: 15579752.

94. Dralle H, Schwarzrock R, Lang W, Bocker W, Ziegler H, Schroder S, et al. Comparison of histology and immunohistochemistry with thyroglobulin serum levels and radioiodine uptake in recurrences and metastases of differentiated thyroid carcinomas. Acta Endocrinol. 1985;108(4):504–10. PubMed PMID: 3887828.

95. Brose MS, Nutting CM, Jarzab B, Elisei R, Siena S, Bastholt L, et al. Sorafenib in radioactive iodine-refractory, locally advanced or metastatic differentiated thyroid cancer: a randomised, double-blind, phase 3 trial. Lancet. 2014 Jul 26;384(9940):319–28. PubMed PMID: 24768112.

96. Flaherty KT, Puzanov I, Kim KB, Ribas A, McArthur GA, Sosman JA, et al. Inhibition of mutated, activated BRAF in metastatic melanoma. New Engl J Med. 2010;363(9):809–19. PubMed PMID: 20818844. Pubmed Central PMCID: 3724529.

97. Kim KB, Cabanillas ME, Lazar AJ, Williams MD, Sanders DL, Ilagan JL, et al. Clinical responses to vemurafenib in patients with metastatic papillary thyroid cancer harboring BRAF(V600E) mutation. Thyroid. 2013;23(10):1277–83. PubMed PMID: 23489023. Pubmed Central PMCID: 3967415.

98. Boussemart L, Routier E, Mateus C, Opletalova K, Sebille G, Kamsu-Kom N, et al. Prospective study of cutaneous side-effects associated with the BRAF inhibitor vemurafenib: a study of 42 patients. Ann Oncol. 2013;24(6):1691–7. PubMed PMID: 23406731.

99. Durante C, Puxeddu E, Ferretti E, Morisi R, Moretti S, Bruno R, et al. BRAF mutations in papillary thyroid carcinomas inhibit genes involved in iodine metabolism. J Clin Endocrinol Metabol. 2007;92(7):2840–3. PubMed PMID: 17488796.

100. Liu D, Hu S, Hou P, Jiang D, Condouris S, Xing M. Suppression of BRAF/MEK/MAP kinase pathway restores expression of iodide-metabolizing genes in thyroid cells expressing the V600E BRAF mutant. Clin Cancer Res. 2007;13(4):1341–9. PubMed PMID: 17317846.

101. Riesco-Eizaguirre G, Gutierrez-Martinez P, Garcia-Cabezas MA, Nistal M, Santisteban P. The oncogene BRAF V600E is associated with a high risk of recurrence and less differentiated papillary thyroid carcinoma due to the impairment of Na + /I- targeting to the membrane. Endocr Relat Cancer. 2006;13(1):257–69. PubMed PMID: 16601293.

102. Chakravarty D, Santos E, Ryder M, Knauf JA, Liao XH, West BL, et al. Small-molecule MAPK inhibitors restore radioiodine incorporation in mouse thyroid cancers with conditional BRAF activation. J Clin Invest. 2011;121(12):4700–11. PubMed PMID: 22105174. Pubmed Central PMCID: 3225989.

103. Ho AL, Grewal RK, Leboeuf R, Sherman EJ, Pfister DG, Deandreis D, et al. Selumetinib-enhanced radioiodine uptake in advanced thyroid cancer. New Engl J Med. 2013;368(7):623–32. PubMed PMID: 23406027. Pubmed Central PMCID: 3615415.

Karl Hürthle

1860–1945

Kelly L. McCoy and Sally E. Carty

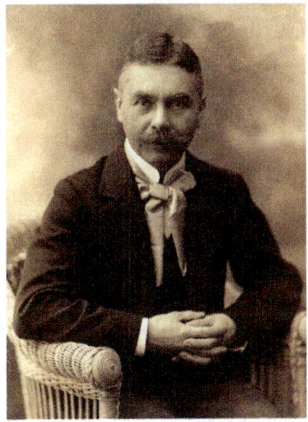

Karl Hürthle (1914), deutscher Physiologe und Kreislaufforscher. Privatbesitz, Dr. Elisabeth Hürthle

Introduction

The cells Karl Hürthle initially described in dogs were actually C cells, i.e., he has long been wrongly credited with the discovery of oncocytic or "Hürthle cells" in the thyroid. In fact, in Germany, these cells are referred to as "Askanazy cells" in protest of the misattributed name, because it was actually endocrine pathologist Max Askanazy who first described the oncocytic cells of the thyroid gland [1, 2]. It was James Ewing who assigned the misnomer in 1919, in his monumental first edition of "Neoplastic Diseases," in which he referred to large cells with abundant pink granular cytoplasm as "Hürthle cells," thus propelling Karl Hürthle into endocrine medical history [3].

K. L. McCoy (✉) · S. E. Carty
Division of Endocrine Surgery, University of Pittsburgh, 3471 Fifth Avenue, Suite 101, Pittsburgh, PA 15213, USA
e-mail: mccoykl@upmc.edu

Early Life and Career

Karl Hürthle was born in Ludwigsburg, Germany on March 16, 1860. He studied Medicine at the University of Tübingen in Tübingen, Germany, one of Europe's oldest universities founded in 1477. Hürthle received his MD in 1884 and was an assistant to Karl von Vierordt and Paul Grützner; the former is known for developing techniques for monitoring blood circulation and pulse oximetry and is considered integral in the development of the modern sphygmomanometer, while the latter is known for his work in circulatory physiology and the physiochemical behavior of pepsin in the digestive system [4, 5].

In 1887, Hürthle moved on to Breslau to become an assistant to Rudolf Heidenhain, who is known for his contributions to the understanding of muscle and nerve physiology. Hürthle then devoted the rest of his long career to his work at the Physiological Institute in Breslau, eventually replacing Heidenhain as professor and director of the Institute in 1898. In 1889, Heidenhain sent Hürthle to represent the city of Breslau at the first International Congress of Physiologists, and it was this scientific meeting that influenced Hürthle to continue in research in physiology [6]. The idea of an International Congress of Physiology had been introduced in 1867 at the first Congress of Medicine, and from September 10 to 12, 1889, Hürthle joined 128 other inaugural members in Basel, Switzerland, and was subsequently appointed to the *Commission International pour unification des appareils enregistreurs,* later known as the Institut Marey. The commission was suggested to the Congress by Étiene-Jules Marey, and it subsequently guided standardization of approved physiological instruments. In 1938, Hürthle wrote a congratulatory message for the 50th anniversary of the International Congress of Physiologists as one of few surviving members at that time [7]. Hürthle retired in 1927 and died in Tübingen in 1945 [6].

Hürthle's primary research interest in hemodynamics led to the study of blood viscosity in different living animals, for example, by measuring carotid flow through a calibrated tube [8]. He was also credited with early recordings of blood pressure in the circle of Willis and performed extensive research in the areas of blood pressure and vasodilation [9].

The Origin of "Hürthle" Cells

The saga of the so-called thyroid Hürthle cell began in 1876 when Baber described what we now know to be the calcitonin-containing C cells in dogs. Evidently unaware of Baber's report, in 1894, also Hürthle published his findings of these same cells in canine thyroid glands [10, 11]. This was Hürthle's sole publication related to thyroid disease. Though it did not actually describe oncocytic cells, his paper, written in German and entitled "Studies on the secretory activity of the thyroid gland" did expand upon some important questions regarding the secretory activity of follicular cells, the mechanism of thyroid hormone secretion, and the formation of thyroid follicles as summarized and translated by Caturegli [6].

In 1898, it was Max Askanazy who was actually the first to describe enlarged epithelial cells with abundant granular and eosinophilic cytoplasm resulting from accumulation of altered mitochondria in a patient with Graves' disease [6, 12]—which today are inaccurately called Hürthle cells. The C cells that Hürthle had described have also been referred to as parafollicular cells, argyrophils, and light cells. C cells are smaller than oxyphil cells and are characterized by their interfollicular position, abundant dense granules, pale cytoplasm, numerous, large mitochondria, and absent Golgi apparatus [13]. Unfortunately, the differing identities were overlooked by James Ewing in his text *Neoplastic Diseases* when he referred to oxphylic cells as "Hürthle cells" [3]. The misapplied Hürthle eponym is used today worldwide except in Germany where these cells are referred to as Askanazy cells in protest.

Askanazy Cells?

Max Askanazy was Hürthle's contemporary (Fig. 1). He was born in Stallupönen, Ostpreussen, which is now Nesterov Russia on February 24, 1865. He trained in Germany at the University of Königsberg and subsequently moved on in 1905 to become a professor of general pathology at the University of Geneva. Askanazy's important work in endocrine pathology extends beyond identifying the controversial Hürthle cell in 1898. In 1904, he also became the first to associate osteitis fibrosa cystica and parathyroid tumors. Nineteen years later, he provided the first description of a gastric carcinoid tumor. He died in 1940 soon after retiring from the University of Geneva [14, 15].

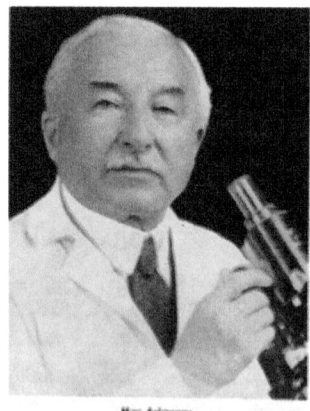

Fig. 1 Max Askanazy (1865–1940). (From the managed family archive of the Franz-Neumann Foundation)

Is Askanazy Alone?

Askanazy does not stand alone as an unintended victim of medical misnomer. Several famous surgeons have been overlooked for their contributions. For example, when the Chicago Medical Society program overran in June of 1894, Lewis L. McArthur was unable to describe his use of a lateral, muscle-splitting abdominal incision. Charles McBurney published a similar technique the following month in *Annals of Surgery*. Though McBurney publicly acknowledged his predecessor, the incision is still taught today as the "McBurney incision." Niels Stenson, a Danish anatomist also known for his description of the parotid duct in 1661, was the first to describe the cardiac anomaly now termed Fallot's tetralogy, but it was Etienne Fallot who did so again two centuries later and earned the famed eponym. Finally, the Charles procedure, named for Sir Richard Henry Havelock Charles, was a procedure for treatment of elephantiasis of the lower limb, but was actually never performed by Dr. Charles; it was wrongly attributed to him in an article by plastic surgeon, Sir Archibald McIndoe in 1950 [16].

Hürthle Cell Lesions

The storied controversial origin of the Hürthle cell fits entirely well with the controversies that still surround the clinical significance of these cells in fine-needle aspirates as well as the diagnosis and clinical behavior of Hürthle cell (oncocytic) neoplasms. Hürthle cell change is a nonspecific finding in the thyroid often seen in benign conditions, but its presence on fine-needle aspiration biopsy (FNAB) can lead to misinterpretation as a Hürthle cell neoplasm [1]. The determination of malignancy among Hürthle cell lesions is based on the presence or absence of vascular or tumor

Fig. 2 **a** Hürthle cells in lymphocytic thyroiditis, **b** Hürthle cell carcinoma, **c** C-cell hyperplasia

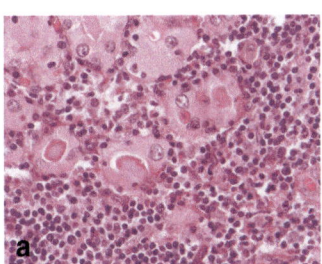 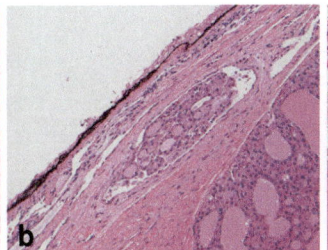 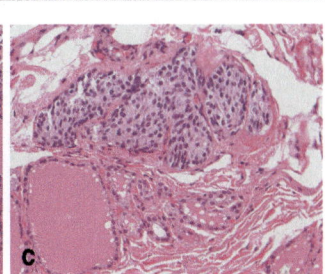

capsular invasion [17]. Welsh described similar cells in the parathyroid glands and referred to them as "oxyphilic cells." Many choose to use the latter term to avoid the more controversial Hürthle eponym (Fig. 2).

References

1. Auger M. Hürthle cells in fine-needle aspirates of the thyroid: a review of their diagnostic criteria and significance Cancer cytopathol. 2014;122:553–4.

2. Askanazy M. Anatomisch Beitrage zur Kenntnis des Morbus Basedowii, insbesondere über die dabei auftretende Muskelerkrankung. Deutsches Arch Klinische Medicin. 1898;61:118–86.

3. Ewing J. Neoplastic diseases: a textbook on tumors. 1st ed. Philadelphia: WB Saunders; 1919.

4. Roguin A. Scipione Riva-Rocci and the men behind the mercury sphygmomanometer. Int J Clin Pract. 2006;60:73–9.

5. Taylor WH. Studies on gastric proteolysis: the secretion of different pepsins by fundic and pyloric glands of the stomach. Biochem J. 1959;71:626–32.

6. Caturegli P. Thyroid history: Karl Hürthle! Now, who was he? Thyroid 2005;15:121–3.

7. Franklin KJ. A short history of the International Congresses of Physiologists. Ann of Sci. 1938;3:241–335.

8. Du Pre Denning A, Watson JH. The viscosity of blood. Proc R Soc Lond B Biol Sci(containing papers of a biological character). 1906;78:328–58.

9. Hill L. Physiology and pathology of the cerebral circulation: an experimental research. London: J & A Churchill; 1866.

10. Baber EC. Contributions to minute anatomy of the thyroid gland of the dog. Phil Transact. 1877;166:557–68.

11. Hürthle K. Beitrage zur Kenntnis des Secretionsvor-gangs in der Schilddrüse. Pflugers Arch Physiol. 1894;56:1–44.

12. Asa SL. My approach to oncocytic tumors of the thyroid. J Clin Pathol. 2004;57:225–32.

13. Roediger WEW. The oxyphil and C cells of the human thyroid gland: a cytochemical and histopathologic review. Cancer. 1975;36:1758–70.

14. Bibliography of Askanazy. Who named it? http://www.whonamedit.com/person_bibliography/2366/.

15. Wang TC, Fox JG, Giraud AS. The biology of gastric cancers. New York: Springer; 2009.

16. Kamath MA. The wrongly famous in medical history. Doctors Lounge Website. http://www.doctorslounge.com/index.php/blogs/page/14102. Accessed 24 Nov 2014.

17. Sandoval MAS, Paz-Pacheco E. Hürthle cell carcinoma of the thyroid. BMJ Case Rep. 2011; Feb 9.

Update of the Treatment Guidelines for Well-Differentiated Thyroid Cancer

Jason A. Glenn and Tracy S. Wang

Introduction

The successful treatment of thyroid malignancy necessitates the collaborative efforts of a multidisciplinary team of endocrinologists, surgeons, radiologists, pathologists, oncologists, and primary care physicians. The overall goal of treatment for well-differentiated thyroid cancer (DTC) is to optimize the initial management of patients in order to minimize the likelihood of developing recurrent disease and/or locoregional or distant metastases. This is best accomplished through timely diagnosis, appropriate preoperative staging, control of locoregional disease through surgery and adjunct therapies (if needed), and long-term surveillance for disease recurrence. In the USA, despite an overall increase in thyroid cancer incidence (5.5 per 100,000 in 1975 vs. 14.7 per 100,000 in 2011), there has been an encouraging trend in 5-year relative survival (92.3 % in 1975 vs. 98.2 % in 2006; Fig. 1) [1]. This difference is likely multifactorial, including improvements in imaging modalities, surgical techniques, and adjunct measures. However, arguably more important is the development and widespread adherence to clinical practice guidelines that have served to help to provide benchmarks for the standard of care for patients with thyroid cancer.

Clinical practice guidelines are an invaluable tool in the successful treatment of not only thyroid malignancy but also virtually every other health disorder. The goals of practice guidelines are to improve patient care by providing consensus on stage-specific therapies, reduce the use of unnecessary or harmful interventions, and to maximize the chance of treatment benefit at an acceptable cost to both the patient and society, as a whole. For guidelines to be successful and widely accepted, they must be based on the best current clinical evidence, be methodologically rigorous, be reproducible, have transparency, and be externally validated. As the literature regarding thyroid cancer treatment has increased exponentially in recent years, for clinical practice guidelines to stay relevant, they should be continuously reassessed and ideally amended every 3–4 years [2].

There are currently no published randomized controlled trials to help guide the surgical management of thyroid cancer, and efforts to answer controversial questions are difficult, given the sample size required for such a study to achieve adequate power [3]. Thus, current clinical practice is largely guided by analysis of relevant large retrospective studies and consensus expert opinion. Several notable organizations such as the American Association of Clinical Endocrinologists (AACE), American Association of Endocrine Surgeons (AAES), American Thyroid Association (ATA), European Thyroid Association (ETA), British Thyroid Association (BTA), and International Association of Endocrine Surgeons (IAES) have developed clinical practice guidelines that standardize treatment within their respective regions. Because some of the available literature falls short of level 1 evidence, none of these recommendations can be considered dogmatic, and no reasonable alternatives can be totally excluded. As such, the adherence to particular recommendations ends up being dependent on the individual practitioner's preference, available surgical expertise, and regional practice habits. In the most recent iteration of the ATA guidelines on the management of patients with DTC, the strength of each recommendation is classified based on the United States Preventive Services Task Force modified schema (Table 1) [4]. In this chapter, our goal is to examine some of the more controversial updates in the treatment of DTC as described by the most recent ATA guidelines, last published in 2009.

Editors' Note: This chapter and the chapter "Well-differentiated Thyroid Cancer" by Dr. Yip are excellent companion pieces. We suggest reading them together to appreciate the many nuances of therapy for thyroid nodules and thyroid cancer.

T. S. Wang (✉)
Division of Surgical Oncology, Section of Endocrine Surgery, Medical College of Wisconsin, 9200 W. Wisconsin Avenue, Milwaukee, WI 53226, USA
e-mail: tswang@mcw.edu

J. A. Glenn
Department of Surgery, Division of Surgical Oncology, Medical College of Wisconsin, Milwaukee, WI, USA

J. L. Pasieka, J. A. Lee (eds.), *Surgical Endocrinopathies*, DOI 10.1007/978-3-319-13662-2_17,
© Springer International Publishing Switzerland 2015

Fig. 1 Incidence, mortality, and 5-year survival for throid cancer in the USA (1975–2011) [1]

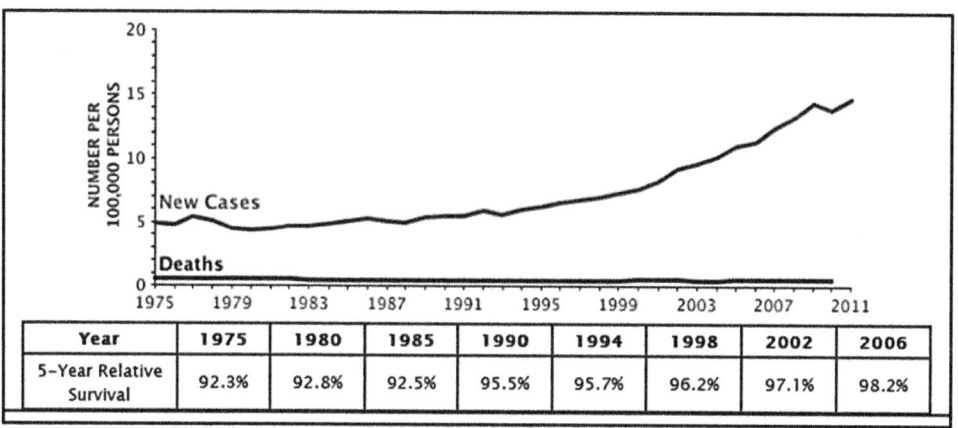

Year	1975	1980	1985	1990	1994	1998	2002	2006
5-Year Relative Survival	92.3%	92.8%	92.5%	95.5%	95.7%	96.2%	97.1%	98.2%

Well-Differentiated Thyroid Cancer (DTC)

According to the National Cancer Institute's Surveillance, Epidemiology, and End Results (SEER) program, as of 2011, there was an estimated 566,700 people in the USA living with thyroid cancer. The incidence has continued to increase each year; approximately 63,000 new thyroid cancers will be diagnosed in 2014 in the USA, a greater than threefold increase since 1973 [1, 5]. Of these, up to 90% are DTC, such as papillary thyroid cancer (PTC) or follicular thyroid cancer (FTC) [5]. In 1996, the ATA published its first version of clinical guidelines on the diagnosis and treatment of DTC [6]. These were subsequently revised in 2006, which particularly sought to outline more authoritative recommendations on the controversial topics of diagnostic evaluation of thyroid nodules, the extent of surgery for small thyroid cancers, the use of radioactive iodine (RAI) ablation following thyroidectomy, the use of thyroxine suppression therapy, and the role of recombinant human thyrotropin (rhTSH) [7]. The 2009 revision offered clarification of prior recommendations, as well as consideration of new information derived from studies published since 2004 [8]. A representative

Table 1 Modified from the US Preventative Task force modified schema for grading strength of recommendations [4]

Rating	Definition
A	Strongly recommends—good evidence suggests that intervention can improve health outcomes
B	Recommends—fair evidence suggests that intervention can improve health outcomes
C	Recommends—expert opinion suggests that intervention can improve health outcomes
D	Recommends against—expert opinion suggests that intervention does not improve health outcomes
E	Recommends against—fair evidence suggests that intervention does not improve health outcomes
F	Strongly recommends against—good evidence suggests that intervention does not improve health outcomes
I	Recommends neither for nor against—evidence is insufficient, conflicting, or of poor quality

group of endocrine surgeons from Europe and head and neck specialists were also included in this iteration of the ATA task force panel in an effort to be more comprehensive in the review of guidelines, especially those related to prophylactic central-compartment neck dissection. An additional revision of the ATA guidelines is in process, as of the publication of this text, which will again clarify current recommendations and focus on less aggressive approaches to small, unifocal, low-risk tumors to help prevent morbidity associated with potential overtreatment.

Thyroid Nodules and the Diagnosis of DTC

It has been estimated that up to 87% of thyroid cancers in the USA are ≤2 cm in greatest diameter [5, 9]. Once a nonpalpable lesion has been incidentally found on imaging or a palpable nodule has first been detected on physical examination, the evaluation for potential malignancy is of the utmost importance for expedient diagnosis, staging, and prevention of disease progression. The goal of this initial evaluation should be to reduce the use of unnecessary or harmful interventions and to maximize the chance of treatment benefit at an acceptable cost. A comprehensive history and physical examination should be performed, including evaluation of risk factors such as head or neck irradiation, endemic goiter, personal or family history of thyroid adenoma or cancer, Cowden disease, Gardner syndrome, or familial adenomatous polyposis. Physical examination should include palpation of the thyroid and cervical neck lymph nodes, including the lateral neck and supraclavicular region. The first recommendation of the 2009 ATA guidelines highlights the next step in the initial evaluation of any thyroid nodule or if thyroidal uptake is seen on fludeoxyglucose (F18)-positron emission tomography (^{18}FDG-PET) scan [7, 8].

Recommendation 1 Measure serum thyroid-stimulating hormone (TSH) in the initial evaluation of a patient with a thyroid nodule. If the serum TSH is subnormal, a radionuclide thyroid scan should be performed using either technetium ^{99m}Tc pertechnetate or ^{123}I. Recommendation rating: A [8].

As serum TSH levels reach the upper limits of normal or higher, there is a direct correlation with increased risk of malignancy [10]. This would suggest that malignancy is rarely seen in a hyperthyroid setting, therefore obviating the immediate necessity for further cytologic evaluation in patients with suppressed TSH levels; in this setting, a radionuclide thyroid scan should be performed [11]. Conversely, an occult malignancy cannot be ruled out in the setting of a euthyroid or hypothyroid state and further cytologic evaluation is indicated [11]. Amended from a "C" rating in the 2006 version, this guideline now carries a recommendation rating of "A," noting that it is strongly recommended based on good evidence [7, 8].

Diagnostic ultrasound (US) of the thyroid and cervical lymph nodes (central and lateral compartments) should be performed for any palpable nodule, thyroid enlargement, or lesion incidentally found on other imaging modalities [7, 8, 12, 13]. This will help to determine how large the nodule is, the location within the gland, the composition of the nodule (solid or cystic), whether there are any additional nodules or associated lymphadenopathy, and whether any nodule or lymph node has benign or malignant features. DTC will involve cervical lymph nodes in up to 50% of patients, with micrometastases reported to be as high as 90% in some series [14]. Characteristics of thyroid nodules that are worrisome for malignancy include hypoechogenicity, hypervascularity, the presence of microcalcifications, and/or irregular borders of the nodule; features of abnormal metastatic lymph nodes include loss of fatty hilum, rounded (not oval) shape, hypoechogenicity, cystic change, calcifications, and peripheral vascularity [11, 14]. Previous studies have examined the importance of preoperative US in patients with a suspicion for malignancy on fine-needle aspiration (FNA), as physical examination alone has a poor sensitivity for identification of central-compartment lymph node metastases and identification of clinically occult lymph node metastases can change the operative management in up to 25% of patients [15–17]. Identification of these lymph nodes allows for a more complete initial operation, possibly decreasing rates of cervical recurrence in patients with PTC [18].

Recommendation 2 Thyroid sonography should be performed in all patients with known or suspected thyroid nodules. Recommendation rating: A [8].

Recommendation 21 Preoperative neck US for the contralateral lobe and cervical (central and especially lateral neck compartments) lymph nodes is recommended for all patients undergoing thyroidectomy for malignant cytologic findings on biopsy. US-guided FNA of sonographically suspicious lymph nodes should be performed to confirm malignancy if this would change management. Recommendation rating: B [8].

Multiple small retrospective studies have demonstrated the incidence of malignancy in incidentally found thyroid lesions to range between 8.6 and 29%, a higher rate than has been reported in palpable nodules [5, 19, 20]. This underscores the importance of evaluation of the thyroid with cervical US in patients with thyroid nodules found incidentally. In the 2009 ATA guidelines, Recommendation 2 carries a rating of "A," previously a "B," noting that it is strongly recommended based on good evidence [7, 8]. For staging purposes and operative planning, if there is US evidence of invasive primary tumor or nodal metastasis, cross-sectional imaging (computed tomography, CT; or magnetic resonance imaging, MRI) should be obtained [8].

FNA is currently the most accurate and cost-effective method for evaluating a suspicious thyroid nodule or lymph node, although its usefulness is dependent on obtaining adequate material for diagnosis. Sub-centimeter thyroid nodules do not routinely require FNA; however, they should be considered in the setting of radiation exposure, personal or family history of thyroid cancer, elevated TSH, Hashimoto's thyroiditis, or US findings of increased central hypervascularity, hypoechoic mass, microcalcifications, or infiltrative margins [8, 11, 12, 14]. US-guided FNA, when compared to palpation guidance, significantly reduces the rate of nondiagnostic and false-negative cytology specimens that would then require repeat FNA [20]. The sensitivity of FNA for detecting malignancy has been demonstrated to be approximately 70–80%; repeat FNA increases the sensitivity of diagnosis on nodules with initially nondiagnostic or indeterminate cytology [21].

Recommendation 5
A. FNA is the procedure of choice in the evaluation of thyroid nodules. Recommendation rating: A
B. US guidance for FNA is recommended for those nodules that are nonpalpable, predominantly cystic, or located posteriorly in the thyroid lobe. Recommendation rating: B [8].

FNA biopsy results were traditionally divided into four categories: nondiagnostic, benign, indeterminate, and malignant (risk of malignancy on final pathology >95%) [8]. The National Cancer Institute Thyroid Fine-Needle Aspiration State of the Science Conference proposed an expanded classification that added two additional categories: follicular lesion of undetermined significance (AFUS; risk of malignancy, 5–10%), and suspicious for malignancy (risk of malignancy, 50–75%) [8]. The Bethesda System for Reporting Thyroid Cytopathology goes on to redefine the "indeterminate" category as "follicular neoplasm or suspicious for follicular neoplasm" [22]. The ATA recommends that histopathologic variants associated with more unfavorable (tall cell, columnar cell, hobnail, variants of PTC; widely invasive FTC, poorly differentiated carcinoma) or more favorable (encapsulated follicular variant without invasion, minimally invasive FTC) outcomes should be identified during evaluation and reporting of FNA results [8, 11].

Use of Molecular Markers in Thyroid Nodules with Indeterminate Cytology

Molecular testing of FNA specimens for possible genetic mutations has emerged as a valuable diagnostic tool in select patients with indeterminate thyroid nodules. Mutations in *BRAF, RET/PTC,* or *RAS* have been identified in over 70 % of papillary cancers and a mutation in PAX8/PPAR gamma in more than 80 % of follicular cancers [23]. Previous studies have shown that because the presence of *BRAF* mutations may be associated with higher rates of cervical recurrence and reoperation, preoperative cytologic identification of BRAF mutations may help to guide the extent of thyroidectomy and lymph node dissection [24]. Molecular markers are available for commercial use, and 2009 ATA guidelines state, with level C evidence, that "use may be considered for patients with indeterminate cytology on FNA to help guide management" [8].

More recently, use of gene-expression classifiers has been described to aid in the diagnosis of a benign thyroid nodule in those nodules with initial indeterminate cytology. In a prospective, double-blind, multicenter study, Alexander et al. utilized a gene-expression classifier that measures the expression of 167 genes in a cohort of 265 cytologically indeterminate nodules with corresponding histological specimens. The gene-expression classifier correctly identified 78/85 malignant nodules as "suspicious" (92 % sensitivity, 95 % confidence interval 84–97; 52 % specificity, 95 % confidence interval 44–59). The negative predictive value for FNA classified as atypical was 95 %, suggesting that the gene-expression classifier may have potential value as a test to "rule out" the presence of malignancy [25]. These initial data have subsequently been verified in a separate study of 339 patients undergoing gene-expression classifier testing; in this cohort, 53 of 121 (44 %) of cytologically indeterminate/gene-expression classifier "suspicious" nodules were malignant, while only 1 of 71 nodules that were gene-expression classifier "benign" have subsequently been found to be malignant [26]. A separate study has questioned the malignancy rate utilizing the gene-expression classifier, however, finding a confirmed malignancy rate of only 16 % in gene-expression classifier "suspicious" lesions [27]. Use of the gene-expression classifier has not yet been discussed in ATA guidelines.

Initial Management of Well-Differentiated Thyroid Cancer

Extent of Surgery for Indeterminate Thyroid Nodules

FNA is diagnostic for PTC, but does not preserve the architecture of the thyroid nodule well enough for accurate diagnosis of FTC, making it better used as a screening test for follicular neoplasms. Some studies report that large indeterminate tumors (>4 cm) have a significantly higher risk of malignancy than smaller tumors (40 vs. 13 % for nodules less than 4 cm), necessitating total thyroidectomy without diagnostic lobectomy [28]. Additional reported factors that carry an increased risk of malignancy include: male gender (43 vs. 16 % for females), patients over age 45 (6 vs. 3 % for age below 45), and when the nodule is judged to be solitary by palpation (25 vs. 6 % for multinodular goiter) [13, 20, 28]. There are other studies, however, that have not demonstrated any of these factors to carry a significant additional risk for malignancy, supporting diagnostic lobectomy with any indeterminate FNA finding [11, 29]. The National Comprehensive Cancer Network (NCCN) guidelines suggest that in the setting of an indeterminate FNA cytology, serum TSH and radionuclide thyroid scan should be done to identify an autonomously functioning nodule that often may be spared from necessitating surgery [11].

After surgical excision, final histology for the majority of indeterminate FNA lesions will turn out to be benign lesions (follicular adenomas, **Hürthle** cell adenomas, adenomatoid nodules, or hyperplastic proliferations of follicular cells). However, there is still an overall risk of malignancy of 15–30 % within this indeterminate category, and given the lack of clarity in true predictive factors of malignancy in cytologically indeterminate thyroid nodules, surgery is currently recommended for definitive diagnosis [28].

Recommendation 24 For patients with an isolated indeterminate solitary nodule who prefer a more limited surgical procedure, thyroid lobectomy is the recommended initial surgical approach. Recommendation rating: C [8].

Recommendation 25

A. Because of an increased risk for malignancy, total thyroidectomy is indicated in patients with indeterminate nodules who have large tumors (>4 cm), when marked atypia is seen on biopsy, when the biopsy reading is "suspicious for papillary carcinoma," in patients with a family history of thyroid carcinoma, and in patients with a history of radiation exposure. Recommendation rating: A [8].

Extent of Surgery for DTC

There has been considerable debate regarding the optimal management and extent of surgical resection for DTC with no evidence of extrathyroidal extension or regional or distant metastases. Earlier recommendations suggested a total or near-total thyroidectomy for cancers >1 cm, even though any difference in survival favoring total thyroidectomy over lobectomy had only been demonstrated in tumors >3 cm [7, 11]. These recommendations were based largely on the possibility of multifocal disease, recurrence, and other practicalities of treatment and follow up. In 2007, Bilimoria et al. utilized the National Cancer Data Base (NCDB) to examine outcomes based on the extent of surgery for PTC; the authors found that the extent of surgery did not impact recurrence or survival in PTC <1 cm. In contrast, patients with a PTC ≥1 cm who underwent thyroid lobectomy alone had significantly higher risks of both recurrence and death [30]. As a result, the current guidelines state that the initial surgical procedure for patients with PTC should be total/near-total thyroidectomy, although thyroid lobectomy alone may be sufficient treatment for low and moderate risk PTC [11].

PTC measuring <1 cm, or papillary thyroid microcarcinomas (PTMC), may be incidentally discovered in up to 10% of all thyroidectomy specimens for benign disease and account for approximately 30% of all PTC [5, 8, 31]. They carry a decreased cancer-specific mortality rate of 0.4%, versus up to 7% seen with tumors >1.5 cm [32]. An occult finding in 5–35% of all autopsies assessed, microcarcinomas rarely progress to clinical disease and likely follow an indolent course [5, 19, 20, 32]. Therefore, the necessity to aggressively treat this finding with total thyroidectomy has come into question and studies have suggested that microcarcinomas may be overtreated. Ito et al. have demonstrated in a cohort of 1235 patients with PTMC that only younger age (<40 years) was an independent predictor of PTMC progression and that older patients may be optimal candidates for observation without any surgical intervention [33]. A recent study examining patients with PTMC in the SEER database showed that, in 29,512 patients, there was no difference in 5- and 10-year disease-specific survival between patients with PTMC who underwent partial versus total thyroidectomy, suggesting that patients may be overtreated with no benefit to overall survival [34].

However, microcarcinomas are found to be multifocal 20% of the time, portending a worse prognosis in this group with higher locoregional recurrence of 20% and early lymph node metastasis in up to 90% of cases [5, 8, 11]. Additional factors that may signify more aggressive behavior of microcarcinomas include: extrathyroidal invasion, solid pattern, absence of capsule, and mutation of oncogenes such as p53 or BRAF [20, 23]. For this subset of patients, total thyroidectomy may be warranted.

Recommendation 26 For patients with thyroid cancer >1 cm, the initial surgical procedure should be a near-total or total thyroidectomy unless there are contraindications to this surgery. Thyroid lobectomy alone may be sufficient treatment for small (<1 cm), low-risk, unifocal, intrathyroidal papillary carcinomas in the absence of prior head and neck irradiation or radiologically or clinically involved cervical nodal metastases. Recommendation rating: A [8].

Role of Central- and Lateral-Compartment Neck Dissections

Regional lymph node metastases are present in 20–90% of patients with DTC [11, 12, 14]. Recent studies have suggested that the risk of locoregional recurrence is higher in patients with lymph node metastases, especially in patients with multiple metastases, extracapsular nodal extension, and patients >45 years [8, 13]. As a result, the role of central- and lateral-compartment neck dissections is critical in the management of patients with DTC. Borders of the central compartment (level VI) are the hyoid bone superiorly, carotid arteries laterally, and the innominate artery inferiorly. The lateral compartment (levels II–V) includes the submandibular and submental nodes (level I); upper, middle, and lower jugular nodes (levels II, III, and IV, respectively); and posterior triangle nodes (level V) (Fig. 2) [35, 36].

Therapeutic central-compartment and lateral-compartment neck dissections for clinically evident lymph node metastasis is well supported in the literature [35, 37, 38]. Therapeutic central-compartment neck dissection should also be performed for any clinical evidence of metastatic disease within the central (level VI) compartment, by either preoperative imaging, physical examination, or intraoperative identification of metastatic disease and for patients with known lateral-compartment metastases [8]. A therapeutic lateral-compartment neck dissection is indicated when there is lateral-compartment (levels II–V) nodal disease on clinical examination or US evaluation, or when there is a high-

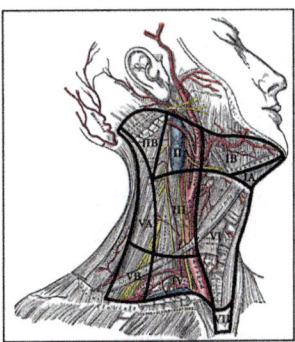

Fig. 2 Lymph node levels with corresponding anatomic landmarks of the neck

risk tumor with significant central neck metastasis [36]. Prophylactic lateral-compartment neck dissections, as well as "berry picking," are not currently recommended, as it has not been shown to improve survival [11, 14, 36].

There is, however, uncertainty with regard to the benefit of routine prophylactic central-compartment neck dissection in patients with DTC. A prophylactic/elective central-compartment neck dissection implies that nodal metastasis is not detectable clinically or by preoperative imaging (clinical N0). Therefore, central-compartment neck dissection may be indicated in the setting of DTC at high risk for nodal metastasis, even without clinically evident nodal disease [36, 38].

Recommendation 27

A. Therapeutic central-compartment (level VI) neck dissection for patients with clinically involved central or lateral neck lymph nodes should accompany total thyroidectomy to provide clearance of disease from the central neck. Recommendation rating: B.

B. Prophylactic central-compartment neck dissection (ipsilateral or bilateral) may be performed in patients with papillary thyroid carcinoma with clinically uninvolved central neck lymph nodes, especially for advanced primary tumors (T3 or T4). Recommendation rating: C [8].

Recommendation 28 Therapeutic lateral neck compartmental lymph node dissection should be performed for patients with biopsy-proven metastatic lateral neck cervical lymphadenopathy. Recommendation rating: B [8].

Role of Completion Thyroidectomy After Initial Thyroid Lobectomy

Completion thyroidectomy after initial thyroid lobectomy is indicated when total or near-total thyroidectomy would have been indicated had the diagnosis of a thyroid malignancy been available before surgery, when remnant ablation is anticipated, or if long-term follow up with thyroglobulin (Tg) or radionuclide imaging is planned. Some studies recommend routine completion thyroidectomy for tumors > 1 cm, as up to 50 % of these patients will have contralateral thyroid disease [39]. While completion thyroidectomy is not currently recommended for incidental PTC < 1 cm in greatest dimension, the role of completion thyroidectomy in the setting of PTMC with incidentally identified micrometastasis to the central-compartment lymph nodes discovered on final pathology is unclear. Factors such as potential complications of reoperative surgery, including hypoparathyroidism and/or recurrent laryngeal nerve injury, need for adjuvant therapy with RAI, and follow-up methods, such as serum thyroglobulin and cervical US, must be considered carefully in these patients. It is reported that up to 30 % of patients experience permanent postoperative complications, such as hypoparathyroidism and recurrent laryngeal nerve injuries following completion thyroidectomy [39, 40].

Recommendation 29 Completion thyroidectomy should be offered to those patients for whom a near-total or total thyroidectomy would have been recommended had the diagnosis been available before the initial surgery. This includes all patients with thyroid cancer except those with small (< 1 cm), unifocal, intrathyroidal, node-negative, low-risk tumors. Therapeutic central neck lymph node dissection should be included if the lymph nodes are clinically involved. Recommendation rating: B [8].

Of note, single-stage total thyroidectomy has been shown to provide a better completeness of resection based on reduced postoperative thyroid remnant RAI uptake when compared to after completion thyroidectomy [40]. If a staged operation for cancer is necessary, surgeon experience may affect the completeness of resection. This should be considered when deciding on extent of surgery at the initial operation.

Postoperative Use of RAI in Patients with DTC

The role of postoperative RAI in patients with DTC includes ablation of normal postsurgical thyroid remnant for easier surveillance and as adjuvant therapy to eliminate suspected micrometastasis. It is generally accepted that patients with DTC at higher risks of recurrent disease (e.g., older age, size > 4 cm, extrathyroidal extension, and regional or distant metastases) should receive RAI postoperatively; in contrast, in patients with low-risk DTC (e.g., younger age and patients with smaller tumors), RAI has not been demonstrated to significantly improve outcomes [8, 11, 12]. Potential side effects of RAI also include radiation thyroiditis, nausea, taste disturbance, sialadenitis, gastritis, bone marrow suppression, transient hypospermia, amenorrhea, and pulmonary fibrosis; patients who received RAI may also be at risk of a RAI-induced second primary malignancy [41, 42]. The optimal dose of RAI to be used is also unclear, as recent data suggest that lower doses (30 mCi) of RAI are as effective as higher doses (100 mCi) when ablating patients with both low-risk and high-risk tumors [42].

Recommendation 32

A. RAI ablation is recommended for all patients with known distant metastases, gross extrathyroidal extension of the tumor regardless of tumor size, or primary tumor size > 4 cm even in the absence of other higher risk features.

B. RAI ablation is recommended for selected patients with 1–4-cm thyroid cancers confined to the thyroid, who have documented lymph node metastases, or other higher risk features when the combination of age, tumor size, lymph node status, and individual histology predicts an intermediate to high risk of recurrence or death from thyroid cancer. Recommendation rating: C [8].

The optimal method for inducing a hypothyroid state prior to RAI therapy also has been controversial. Over the past decade, multiple studies have demonstrated no difference in rates of thyroid bed uptake or local recurrence in patients who have received recombinant thyroid stimulating hormone (rhTSH) prior to RAI, as compared to formal thyroid hormone withdrawal (THW) [43–45]. In some studies, patients who have received rhTSH had similar rates of recurrence, less chance of needing additional therapies after ablation (29.1 vs. 36.8%), and it required less aggressive follow up and TSH suppression [43, 44].

A recent meta-analysis reports an improved quality of life for patients treated with rhTSH, compared to THW, largely due to the absence of hypothyroid symptomatology [32]. Additionally, early resumption of thyroxine following RAI has been advocated to reduce symptom severity and potential hypothyroid complications. In 2007, rhTSH was FDA approved for use as adjuvant treatment with RAI in patients with DTC without evidence of metastatic thyroid cancer [8].

Recommendation 33 Patients undergoing RAI therapy or diagnostic testing can be prepared by LT4 withdrawal for at least 2–3 weeks or LT3 treatment for 2–4 weeks and LT3 withdrawal for 2 weeks with measurement of serum TSH to determine timing of testing or therapy (TSH >30 mU/L). Thyroxine therapy (with or without LT3 for 7–10 days) may be resumed on the second or third day after RAI administration. Recommendation rating: B [8].

Recommendation 34 Remnant ablation can be performed following thyroxine withdrawal or rhTSH stimulation. Recommendation rating: A [8].

Long-Term Management of Well-Differentiated Thyroid Cancer

The primary goal of long-term follow up in patients with DTC is accurate surveillance for detection of recurrent disease. A patient is considered to be disease-free if there is no clinical, radiographic, or biochemical evidence of tumor; the latter is defined as serum Tg levels that are undetectable during TSH stimulation, with no interfering thyroglobulin antibodies [8, 11]. In low-risk patients, initial monitoring for thyroid cancer recurrence includes measurement of serum Tg after TSH stimulation and neck US. Repeat rounds of rhTSH stimulation have not been demonstrated to be useful in patients who had undetectable Tg at the time of initial postoperative follow up. Thus, rhTSH should be repeated only in patients who have had a positive first rhTSH-stimu-

lated Tg and negative imaging; after that time, serum Tg can be measured while on thyroid hormone replacement (suppressed TSH) [46]. There is controversy as to what exactly constitutes a positive or negative stimulated Tg level; it is currently suggested that a single stimulated Tg level >2 ng/mL predicts persistent tumor. Conversely, a single stimulated Tg value of <0.5 ng/mL, without Tg antibody, has up to a 98% likelihood of identifying patients completely free of tumor [47].

Recommendation 43 Serum Tg should be measured every 6–12 months by an immunometric assay. Thyroglobulin antibodies should be quantitatively assessed with every measurement of serum Tg. Recommendation rating: A [8].

Recommendation 45B Low-risk patients who have had remnant ablation, negative cervical US, and undetectable TSH stimulated Tg can be followed up primarily with yearly clinical examination and thyroglobulin measurements on thyroid hormone replacement. Recommendation rating: B [8].

Recommendation 48
A. Following surgery, cervical US to evaluate the thyroid bed and central and lateral cervical nodal compartments should be performed at 6–12 months and then periodically, depending on the patient's risk for recurrent disease and Tg status. Recommendation rating: B.
B. If a positive result would change management, sonographically suspicious lymph nodes greater than 5–8 mm in the smallest diameter should be biopsied for cytology with Tg measurement in the needle washout fluid. Recommendation rating: A [8].

As noted in the ATA recommendation above, routine postoperative surveillance with US of the thyroid bed and central and lateral neck lymph node compartments are an integral part of postoperative management of patients with DTC. Cervical recurrences may be detected in up to 30% of all patients in some studies, attributable in part to improved US technology and serum thyroglobulin assays [14, 20, 48]. The optimal management strategy for recurrence is largely based on relative risk, but may include surgery with comprehensive neck dissection, ^{131}I therapy for RAI-avid disease, external beam radiation, or watchful waiting for stable or slowly progressive asymptomatic disease.

If findings of a malignant lymph node or thyroid bed recurrence would change the management of the patient (i.e., surgical resection versus continued surveillance), FNA is recommended. Obtaining a Tg level in the washout fluid from the needle at the time of FNA may help diagnose metastatic lymphadenopathy [49]. Serum Tg and Tg in FNA needle wash specimens, when combined with US evaluation, each have a >90% sensitivity for correctly identifying nonmalignant cytology [47, 50]. Therefore, an undetectable serum Tg and normal US findings may obviate the necessity of FNA cytology, in the absence of Tg autoantibodies. If persistent or recurrent disease is identified, a comprehensive therapeutic compartment-oriented neck dissection should be performed; a more limited resection may be considered in patients who have previously undergone neck dissection.

Recommendation 50

A. Therapeutic comprehensive compartmental lateral and/or central neck dissection, sparing uninvolved vital structures, should be performed for patients with persistent or recurrent disease confined to the neck. Recommendation rating: B.

B. Limited compartmental lateral and/or central compartmental neck dissection may be a reasonable alternative for patients with recurrent disease having undergone prior comprehensive dissection and/or external beam radiation therapy. Recommendation rating: C [8].

Conclusion

Clinical practice guidelines are important in the management of patients with DTC; they serve as an invaluable reference and provide a standard for all practitioners in patient care. The current guidelines in the management of patients with differentiated thyroid cancer are based on the best available evidence and expert opinion but are not meant to be rigid constructs; interpretation of guidelines require flexibility in order to individualize and optimize patient care, based on personal and institutional capabilities and experiences.

Key Summary Points

- The goal of practice guidelines is to provide consensus for management of patients in order to maximize benefits of treatment and to reduce unnecessary or harmful interventions, at an acceptable cost to patient and society.
- All patients with thyroid nodules should have measurement of serum TSH.
- Thyroid sonography is recommended for all patients with known or suspected thyroid nodules and should include examination of the cervical lymph nodes (central and lateral compartments) for all patients with known or suspected malignancy.
- FNA biopsy is the procedure of choice in the evaluation of thyroid nodules.
- For patients with a differentiated thyroid cancer > 1 cm, total thyroidectomy is the recommended initial surgical procedure. Thyroid lobectomy may be considered in select patients.

- Therapeutic neck dissections should be performed in a compartment-oriented fashion.
- RAI ablation is recommended for all patients with distant metastases, extrathyroidal extension of tumor, or large tumors; it may be recommended in select other patients.

References

1. Howlander N, et al. SEER cancer statistics review, 1975–2011. National Cancer Institute. 2013. http://seer.cancer.gov/csr/1975_2011. Posted to the SEER web site, April 2014.
2. Irani S, et al. Evaluating clinical practice guidelines developed for the management of thyroid nodules and thyroid cancers and assessing the reliability and validity of the AGREE instrument. J Eval Clin Pract. 2011;17(4):729–36.
3. Carling T, et al. American Thyroid Association design and feasibility of a prospective randomized controlled trial of prophylactic central lymph node dissection for papillary thyroid carcinoma. Thyroid. 2012;22(3):237–44.
4. U.S. Preventive Services Task Force Grade Definitions. USPTF. http://www.uspreventiveservicestaskforce.org/uspstf/grades.htm. Accessed 1 May 2014.
5. Davis L, Welch HG. Increasing incidence of thyroid cancer in the United States, 1973–2002. JAMA. 2006;295:2164–67
6. Singer P, et al. Treatment guidelines for patients with thyroid nodules and well-differentiated thyroid cancer. Arch Intern Med. 1996;156:2165–72.
7. Cooper DS, et al. Management guidelines for patients with thyroid nodules and differentiated thyroid cancer. Thyroid. 2006;16(2):109–42.
8. Cooper D, et al. Revised American Thyroid Association Management Guidelines for patients with thyroid nodules and differentiated thyroid cancer. Thyroid. 2009;19(11):1167–214.
9. Grant CS. Papillary thyroid cancer: strategies for optimal individualized surgical management. Clin Ther. 2014;36:1117–26.
10. Boelaert K, et al. Serum thyrotropin concentration as a novel predictor of malignancy in thyroid nodules investigated by fine-needle aspiration. J Clin Endocrinol Metab. 2006;91(11):4295–301.
11. NCCN Clinical Practice Guidelines in Oncology: Thyroid Carcinoma. Version 2. 2013. http://www.nccn.org/professionals/physician_gls/pdf/thyroid.pdf. Accessed 1 May 2014.
12. Gharib H, et al. American Association of Clinical Endocrinologists, Associazione Medici Endocrinologi, and European Thyrois Association Medical Guidelines for Clinical Practice for the Diagnosis and Management of Thyroid Nodules. Endocr Pract. 2010;16(1):1–43.
13. Perros P, et al. Guidelines for the management of thyroid cancer. 2nd ed. British Thyroid Association, Royal College of Physicians; 2007.
14. Conzo G, et al. The current status of lymph node dissection in the treatment of papillary thyroid cancer. A literature review. Clin Ter. 2013;164(4):343–6.
15. Kouvaraki MA, et al. Role of preoperative ultrasonography in the surgical management of patients with thyroid cancer. Surgery. 2003;134(6):946–54.
16. O'Connell K, et al. The utility of routine preoperative cervical ultrasonography in patients undergoing thyroidectomy for differentiated thyroid cancer. Surgery. 2013;154(4):697–701.
17. Stulak JM, et al. Value of preoperative ultrasonography in the surgical management of initial and reoperative papillary thyroid cancer. Arch Surg. 2006;141(5):489–94.

18. Marshall CL, et al. Routine pre-operative ultrasonography for papillary thyroid cancer: effects on cervical recurrence. Surgery. 2009;146(6):1063–72.

19. Chaikhoutdinov I, et al. Incidental thyroid nodules: incidence, evaluation, and outcome. Otolaryngol Head Neck Surg. 2014;150: 939–42.

20. Liebeskind A, et al. Rates of malignancy in incidentally discovered thyroid nodules evaluated with sonography and fine-needle aspiration. J Ultrasound Med. 2005;24:629–34.

21. Sung JY, et al. Diagnostic accuracy of fine-needle aspiration versus core-needle biopsy for the diagnosis of thyroid malignancy in a clinical cohort. Eur Radiol. 2012;22(7):1564–72.

22. Cibas ES, Ali SZ. The Bethesda system for reporting thyroid cytopathology. Am J Clin Pathol. 2009;132(5):658–65.

23. Ahmadieh H, Azar ST. Controversies in the management and followup of differentiated thyroid cancer: beyond the guidelines. J Thyroid Res. 2012; Epub ahead of print.

24. Yip L, et al. Optimizing surgical treatment of papillary thyroid carcinoma associated with BRAF mutation. Surgery. 2009;146(6): 1215–23.

25. Alexander EK, et al. Preoperative diagnosis of benign thyroid nodules with indeterminate cytology. N Engl J Med. 2012;367(8): 705–15.

26. Alexander EK, et al. Multicenter clinical experience with the Afirma gene expression classifier. J Clin Endocrinol Metab. 2014;99(1):119–25.

27. McIver B, et al. An independent study of a gene expression classifier (Afirma™) in the evaluation of cytologically indeterminate thyroid nodules. J Clin Endocrinol Metab. 2014; Epub ahead of print.

28. Tuttle RM, et al. Clinical features associated with an increased risk of thyroid malignancy in patients with follicular neoplasm by fine-needle aspiration. Thyroid. 1998;8(5):377–83.

29. Tamez-Pérez HE, et al. Nondiagnostic thyroid fine needle aspiration cytology: outcome in surgical treatment. Rev Invest Clin. 2007;59(3):180–3.

30. Bilimoria KY, et al. Extent of surgery affects survival for papillary thyroid cancer. Ann Surg. 2007;246(3):375–81; discussion 381–74.

31. Pelizzo MR, et al. High prevalence of occult papillary thyroid carcinoma in a surgical series for benign thyroid disease. Tumori. 1990;76(3):255–7.

32. Yu XM, et al. Current treatment of papillary thyroid microcarcinoma. Adv Surg. 2012;46:191–203.

33. Ito Y, et al. Patient age is significantly related to the progression of papillary microcarcinoma of the thyroid under observation. Thyroid. 2014;24(1):27–34.

34. Wang TS, et al. Papillary thyroid microcarcinoma: an over-treated malignancy? World J Surg. 2014; Epub ahead of print.

35. Carty SE, et al. Consensus statement on the terminology and classification of central neck dissection for thyroid cancer. Thyroid. 2009;19(11):1153–8.

36. Stack BC, et al. American thyroid association consensus review and statement regarding the anatomy, terminology, and rationale for lateral neck dissection in differentiated thyroid cancer. Thyroid. 2012;22(5):501–8.

37. Davidson HC, et al. Papillary thyroid cancer: controversies in the management of neck metastasis. Laryngoscope. 2008;118(12): 2161–5.

38. Mazzaferri EL, et al. The pros and cons of prophylactic central compartment lymph node dissection for papillary thyroid carcinoma. Thyroid. 2009;19(7):683–9.

39. Lee CR, et al. Lobectomy and prophylactic central neck dissection for papillary thyroid microcarcinoma: do involved lymph nodes mandate completion thyroidectomy? World J Surg. 2014;38(4): 872–7.

40. Oltmann SC, et al. Radioactive iodine remnant uptake after completion thyroidectomy: not such a complete cancer operation. Ann Surg Oncol. 2014;21(4):1379–83.

41. Luster M, et al. Guidelines for radioiodine therapy of differentiated thyroid cancer. Eur J Nucl Med Mol Imaging. 2008;35(10): 1941–59.

42. Zaman MU, et al. Controversies about radioactive iodine-131 remnant ablation in low risk thyroid cancers: are we near a consensus? Asian Pac J Cancer Prev. 2013;14(11):6209–13.

43. Hugo J, et al. recombinant human thyroid stimulating hormone-assisted radioactive iodine remnant ablation in thyroid cancer patients at intermediate to high risk of recurrence. Thyroid. 2012;22(10):1007–15.

44. Tu J, et al. Recombinant human thyrotropin-aided versus thyroid hormone withdrawal-aided radioiodine treatment for differentiated thyroid cancer after total thyroidectomy: a meta-analysis. Radiother Oncol. 2014;110(1):25–30.

45. Tuttle RM, et al. Recombinant human TSH-assisted radioactive iodine remnant ablation achieves short-term clinical recurrence rates similar to those of traditional thyroid hormone withdrawal. J Nucl Med. 2008;49(5):764–70.

46. Castagna MG, et al. Limited value of repeat recombinant human thyrotropin (rhTSH)-stimulated thyroglobulin testing in differentiated thyroid carcinoma patients with previous negative rhTSH-stimulated thyroglobulin and undetectable basal serum thyroglobulin levels. J Clin Endocrinol Metab. 2008;93(1):76–81.

47. Kloos RT, Mazzaferri EL. A single recombinant human thyrotropin-stimulated serum thyroglobulin measurement predicts differentiated thyroid carcinoma metastases three to five years later. J Clin Endocrinol Metab. 2005;90(9):5047–57.

48. Tuttle RM, et al. Estimating risk of recurrence in differentiated thyroid cancer after total thyroidectomy and radioactive iodine remnant ablation: using response to therapy variables to modify the initial risk estimates predicted by the new American Thyroid Association staging system. Thyroid. 2010;20(12):1341–9.

49. Boi F, et al. The diagnostic value for differentiated thyroid carcinoma metastases of thyroglobulin (Tg) measurement in washout fluid from fine-needle aspiration biopsy of neck lymph nodes is maintained in the presence of circulating anti-Tg antibodies. J Clin Endocrinol Metab. 2006;91(4):1364–9.

50. Snozek CL, et al. Serum thyroglobulin, high-resolution ultrasound, and lymph node thyroglobulin in diagnosis of differentiated thyroid carcinoma nodal metastases. J Clin Endocrinol Metab. 2007;92(11):4278–81.

Frank Lahey

1880–1953

Kimlynn B. Do, Daniel T. Ruan

Those who knew and loved Frank will remember him as a great leader and a lovable man; a surgeon who seemed at his best when facing the impossible; a friend whose whole-hearted welcome was offered alike to the distinguished visitor and the humble seeker after knowledge. Until the end, he was skillful, kindly, and vital. As such he will remain in our memory.

— Rodney Maingot

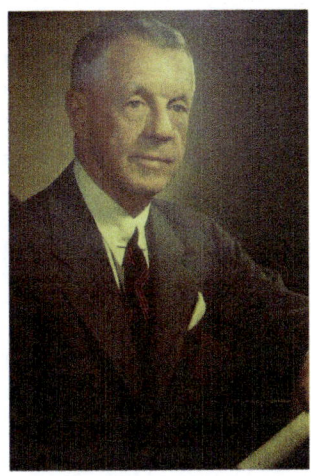

Portrait of Frank Lahey, MD. (Courtesy of Lahey Hospital & Medical Center)

Early Life

Frank Lahey was born in Massachusetts to first-generation Irish immigrants in 1880 [1]. Lahey's grandparents were farmers who immigrated during "The Great Famine" to the town of Stoneham, Massachusetts, located 10 miles north of Boston. In this small New England town, they raised a son, Thomas Lahey, who became a successful businessman. Thomas was an educated man and co-owned the Fletcher and Lahey firm, specializing in the construction of bridges [2].

Thomas married a young woman named Honora, and on June 1, 1880, they had their only child, Frank Howard Lahey. Frank Lahey was a curious child with diverse interests. Howard, as his friends called him, enjoyed the outdoors and sports such as American football, baseball, shooting, and track. As a secondary school student, he partook in track and field competitions with some success.

Thomas Lahey tried to condition his son in the family business, where Frank was employed during his summer vacations. However, despite his father's best efforts, Frank avoided the family firm and had no interest in taking over the family business. Rather, Frank took great interest in Dr. Charles Benson, a progressive local physician. Frank Lahey later admitted that his exposure to Dr. Benson inspired him to become a physician.

Education

Frank Lahey was a diligent and ambitious student. He completed his undergraduate studies at Harvard, graduating at the turn of the twentieth century. He then attended Harvard Medical School, where he received his medical doctorate in 1904 [3]. Following medical school graduation, Dr. Lahey was an intern at the Long Island Hospital. He then returned to Boston to continue his undesignated medical training at the Boston City Hospital, followed by formal surgical training at the Haymarket Square Relief Station [4]. As a surgical trainee, Frank Lahey proved to be well-organized and eager to teach others.

D. T. Ruan (✉)
General and GI Surgery, Endocrine Surgery, Brigham and Women's Hospital, Harvard Medical School, 37 Athelstane Road, Newton Center, Boston, MA 02459, USA
e-mail: druan@partners.org

K. B. Do
Brigham and Women's Hospital, 9541 Duke Dr, Westminster, CA 92683, USA

J. L. Pasieka, J. A. Lee (eds.), *Surgical Endocrinopathies*, DOI 10.1007/978-3-319-13662-2_18,
© Springer International Publishing Switzerland 2015

Early Career and the Lahey Clinic

After completing his surgical training, Frank Lahey had dual appointments at Harvard and Tufts Medical Schools. Although Lahey's schedule was exceedingly demanding, he thrived as a junior faculty member at both institutions. When the USA entered World War I in 1917, Dr. Lahey readily served his country as the director of surgery in the Evacuation Hospital No. 30 in France. Expanding his knowledge as a military surgeon, Dr. Lahey deduced that "asepsis, antisepsis, and anesthesia had created a new surgery" best accomplished by a team. His leadership role in the war influenced his views regarding the organization of health care delivery.

Lahey returned to Massachusetts after his service in World War I. He resumed his appointments at Harvard and Tufts medical schools and started a private practice in Boston's Kenmore Square [5]. Based on his wartime experience, he was convinced that a team-based model could improve the delivery of surgical care. In this paradigm, dedicated and collegial clinicians would collaborate and teach each other. Lahey believed that teamwork was the key to successful surgery, and he began implementing his idea within his newly created private practice, the Lahey Clinic.

Lahey assembled a team of caregivers for his new practice, which included Miss Wallace Blanche, a nurse he met during his years in the war; Dr. Howard Clute, an anesthesiologist; and Dr. Lincoln Sise, a gastroenterologist. For a few years, this team would travel incessantly between Lahey's private practice, the Peter Bent Brigham Hospital, the New England Baptist Hospital, and the New England Deaconess Hospital. The roads were tough and the winters in Boston were unforgiving for frequent travel. Consequently, much time was wasted and the team's morale suffered.

Dr. Lahey frequently spoke of his dream hospital where all aspects of patient care could be provided under a single roof. He envisioned a hospital where patients could acquire multiple consultations from expert physicians working together with a collaborative spirit. Although commonplace today, this idea initially faced great opposition and skepticism from the established Boston medical community. Lahey ended his appointments at Harvard and Tufts to dedicate himself completely to the creation of his dream: a collaborative multidisciplinary clinic.

By 1926, Dr. Lahey had achieved his vision of a multidisciplinary hospital. The Lahey Clinic had integrated waiting rooms, doctors' offices, and examination rooms. Furthermore, Lahey started fellowship programs where young surgeons could further develop their skills and knowledge base under the close guidance of an attending surgeon. The first Lahey fellowship program involved only two trainees, but eventually expanded to approximately 100 fellows.

One of Dr. Lahey's best students was Sara M. Jordan. She first worked with Dr. Lahey as a medical student. Her unique personality captured his attention, so he decided to mentor her after graduation. At first, she was confused about which path of medicine to pursue; Dr. Lahey recognized that she could succeed in any profession and guided her into the rapidly developing field of gastroenterology. Dr. Jordan developed a highly successful career in gastroenterology, and Dr. Lahey later wrote that watching her progress was one of his greatest privileges in his life. As a teacher, Lahey influenced and inspired the careers of many surgeons and nonsurgical specialists [6].

Although Dr. Lahey was a highly skilled surgeon of the gastrointestinal tract, he is best known for his expertise in thyroid surgery. In 1938, he reported over 3000 thyroidectomies with superb outcomes [7]. At that time, many surgeons believed that the recurrent laryngeal nerve should be avoided and undisturbed during thyroidectomy. In contrast, Lahey believed that the intraoperative localization of the recurrent laryngeal nerve allowed for safe removal of the thyroid without nerve injury. In his large series, the recurrent laryngeal nerve was routinely dissected and preserved, which resulted in superior outcomes. This approach is now the standard technique used by endocrine surgical specialists today.

World War II and the Examination of Roosevelt

The USA entered World War II after the attack on Pearl Harbor in December 1941. Dr. Lahey did not hesitate to serve his country again. However, by this time, Lahey had established a reputation as an eminent surgical teacher and innovator. As such, he played an even larger leadership role and was appointed the chairman of the Service for the Procurement and Assignment of Medical Personnel and the chairman of the Medical Consulting Board. This made Dr. Lahey responsible for the hiring of 60,000 doctors for the Army and Navy, and he supervised numerous military clinics and hospitals.

In March of 1944, President Franklin D. Roosevelt (FDR) was 62 years of age and was in poor health [8]. FDR had lost a significant amount of weight and developed a haggard appearance, but his declining health was largely unknown to the public. Although there were rumors that FDR had suffered from a paralytic stroke, heart disease, advanced cancer, and mental illness, FDR likely influenced the Office of Censorship to avoid media scrutiny of his failing health. As a consequence of an adult case of polio, FDR required leg braces and could only walk short distances by moving his torso with the support of a cane. He used a wheelchair for mobility in private, keeping his disability from the public.

At the time, the world was at war with military and civilian casualties on the order of tens of millions and the USA was dealing with an economic depression. FDR's reelection campaign would be compromised if the public knew of his declining health. Defensive of FDR, his personal physician, Ross McIntire, claimed he was in excellent condition for a man of his age and attributed his exhaustion on the war. But the public was skeptical and brushed off McIntire's argument. Worried that the fleeting rumors would compromise FDR's reelection, Dr. Howard Bruenn, a cardiologist from the National Naval Medical Center, was consulted to end the rumors.

However, Dr. Bruenn found that FDR indeed was suffering from advanced heart failure, and he recommended supportive care including digitalis, salt restriction, weight loss, and activity restriction. McIntire, still determined that there was nothing wrong with Roosevelt's health, searched for an additional opinion, which lead to the request for Dr. Lahey.

Dr. Lahey immediately flew to Washington DC where he too diagnosed Roosevelt with end-stage heart failure. Dr. Lahey advocated against serving another term of presidency, believing that Roosevelt could not survive another term in office. But the president and his advisors denied his suggestion. Lahey was conflicted between upholding his integrity as a citizen versus protecting his patient's confidentiality.

Dr. Lahey decided to remain silent about the president's condition, and, consequently, FDR won reelection and continued his next term in the nation's highest office. As Lahey had predicted, FDR did not survive to finish his presidential term. FDR died within a month of Germany's surrender, which shocked the public who was unaware of his illness. Had Dr. Lahey revealed to the public about the true condition of the president, it is unlikely that FDR would have been reelected. As such, Dr. Lahey's decision to remain silent and protect the president's medical information influenced the course of American politics and world history.

Accomplishments

Dr. Lahey's life was replete with accolades and accomplishments [9]. He was surgeon in chief of both the New England Deaconess and New England Baptist Hospitals for over 30 years. He was elected the president of the American Association for the Study of Goiter, the New England Surgical Society, the American Medical Association, and the Interstate Postgraduate Assembly [10]. He founded the American Board of Surgery and was on the executive board of the American College of Surgeons along with numerous other international surgical societies. He took great pride in the Henry Jacob Bigelow Medal in honor of his excellence as a teacher and surgeon, because it was from his peers in the Boston Surgical Society. He was also the recipient of the Medal of Merit presented by the secretary of the US Navy and the Friedenwald Medal given by the American

Gastroenterological Association for his accomplishments in surgery of the digestive tract and the Meritorious Award from the American Goiter Association for his contribution to thyroid disease.

Arguably, Frank Lahey's biggest accomplishment was the creation of the innovative hospital that bears his name. The Lahey Clinic, now a health-care network named the "Lahey Hospital and Medical Center," continues its success as an international center for excellence. Frank Lahey inspired the culture that still exists today, where collaborative specialized teams are directly available to individual patients. As Lahey initiated almost a century ago, every component of a patient's care at the Lahey Medical Center is coordinated under a single roof involving experts across multiple medical and surgical disciplines.

Personal Life

Frank Lahey's athletic spirit from childhood never diminished in his lifetime. He was extremely fond of dog field trials and he brought Lady, his favorite dog, to the office every Sunday. In his younger years, he enjoyed hunting dogs and shooting. In his later years, he played golf with his wife, Ann Wilcox. Similar to how he approached his surgical practice, Dr. Lahey played golf with ambition; he objectively analyzed his golf performance and often consulted golf professionals for technical advice.

Dr. Lahey was noted to be a man of unyielding kindness and generosity by his colleagues and patients. He was a devoted husband and capable outdoorsman. He woke at 6 in the morning every day to read and have breakfast with his Alice. In the afternoon, he would walk home from the hospital to join her for lunch. Mrs. Lahey's tolerance with his busy schedule never wavered, which Frank greatly appreciated. She often accompanied him to his international medical conferences, allowing them to travel the world together. Frank spoke highly of his wife, including the following, "Any doctor's wife who has lived with a doctor as long as Mrs. Lahey has lived with me has to be a fine woman to do it." Frank and Alice cherished their vacations on Lake Winnipesaukee together where they enjoyed the warm weather, fishing, swimming, and golf. Frank Lahey died in 1953 at the age of 73.

References

1. Corman ML. Frank Howard Lahey. Dis Colon Rectum. 1981;24(7):569.
2. Steinberg D. President Franklin D Roosevelt (1882–1945) and Doctor Frank Howard Lahey's (1880–1953) dilemma: the complexities of medical confidentiality with World Leaders. J Med Biogr. 2014 April 15. [Epub ahead of print].

3. Tripod: Lahey Clinic General Surgery Residency Program [Internet]. Frank Lahey Biography (Cited 2014 May). http://lahey_clinic_surgery.tripod.com/laheyclinicsurgery/id15.html.
4. Lahey Hospital & Medical Center [Internet]. The History of Lahey Clinic. (Updated 2014; cited 2014 May). http://www.lahey.org/About_Lahey/The_History_of_Lahey_Clinic.aspx.
5. Beth Israel Deaconess Medical Center [Internet]. c2014. Deaconess Hospital. (Updated 2014; cited 2014 May). http://www.bidmc.org/About-BIDMC/The-History-of-BIDMC/Deaconess-Hospital.aspx.
6. Hunt CJ. Dr. Frank Lahey. Am J Surg. 1953;86(4):361–2.
7. Kaplan EL, Salti GI, Roncella M, Fulton N, Kadowaki M. History of the recurrent laryngeal nerve: from Galen to Lahey. World J Surg. 2009;33:386–93.
8. Steinberg D. Dr. Lahey's dilemma—Boston [Internet]. New York: The New York Times; 2011. (Updated 2011; cited 2014 May). http://www.boston.com/lifestyle/articles/2011/05/29/why_lahey_clinic_founder_frank_lahey_concealed_his_report_on_fdr/?page=5.
9. Maingot R. Frank H. Lahey—the man, the surgeon and the teacher. Lahey Clin Found Bull. 1963;13:80–90.
10. Deaths. JAMA. 1953;152(11):1060.

Thomas Dunhill

1876–1957

Catherine McManus and Orlo Clark

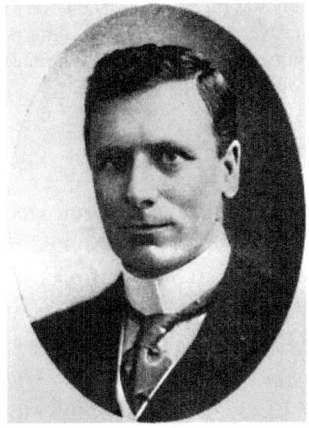

Thomas Peel Dunhill (1876–1957) at the age of 29 when he began his work as physician to outpatients in 1905 at St. Vincent's Hospital. From Thomas Peel Dunhill: Pioneer Thyroid Surgeon, Vellar, 1999. (Reprinted with permission, Copyright © 2002, John Wiley and Sons)

Introduction

In the mid-to-late nineteenth century, the management of severe thyrotoxicosis from exophthalmic goiter was a reflection of the lack of understanding of the disease process and the overall function of the thyroid [1–3]. At this time, exophthalmic goiter was treated medically with a wide range of homeopathic remedies including sodium chloride, sodium phosphate, and morphia, along with bed rest, a diet heavy in milk, and blood from thyroidectomized animals [2, 3]. The rare event of resolution or improvement in a patient's

condition was undoubtedly a result of spontaneous remission rather than such poorly understood medical interventions. In the meantime, patients would enter a state of thyroid crisis and become grossly emaciated, suffering from severe pulmonary and cardiac sequelae, blindness from corneal ulceration, and uncontrollable diarrhea and vomiting [2, 3]. Despite this horrid quality of life, leaders in thyroid surgery, including **Kocher** and Halstead, believed that surgery for patients with thyrotoxicosis placed the patient at too high of a risk to be beneficial [1, 4]. When surgery was attempted, patients suffered from either complications of chloroform anesthesia, postoperative thyroid storm, which was often fatal, or the inevitable recurrence of the thyrotoxicosis secondary to removing an insufficient amount of the thyroid gland [5]. Furthermore, at that time, complications from thyrotoxicosis, including heart failure and atrial fibrillation, were considered relative contraindications to surgery [5]. Although often overshadowed by his contemporaries, Thomas Peel Dunhill was integral in demonstrating the benefits of early surgical intervention for toxic goiter. Through his persistence and ingenuity, as well as his surgical technique, he was able to shift the global consensus towards subtotal thyroidectomy—total resection of one thyroid lobe and subtotal resection of the contralateral lobe.

Thomas Peel Dunhill was born on December 3, 1876, near Kerang in Victoria, Australia, to John Webster Dunhill, the manager of a sheep and cattle station, and his wife Mary Peel [2, 4]. When Thomas was 2 years old, his father died of typhoid fever, at which point Mary Peel brought him and his younger brother, John Webster Dunhill, back to her hometown of Inverleigh [2]. It was there, in 1888, that his mother remarried William Lawry, a local miner [2]. In 1892, Thomas began to study pharmacy, spending his days in a chemist shop at Daylesford and his evenings attending lectures at the Ballarat School of Mines [2]. His dedication to mastering the subject of pharmacology allowed him to become a registered pharmacist in 1898 [2]. By 1899, he had finally made enough money as a pharmacist and was able to enroll at the University of Melbourne to pursue his true passion:

C. McManus (✉)
Department of Surgery, New York Presbyterian Hospital Columbia Campus, Milstein Hospital Building 7GS-313, 177 Fort Washington Ave, New York, NY, 10032, USA
e-mail: cm3304@cumc.columbia.edu

O. Clark
Department of Surgery, University of California San Francisco Medical Center, San Francisco, CA, USA

J. L. Pasieka, J. A. Lee (eds.), *Surgical Endocrinopathies,* DOI 10.1007/978-3-319-13662-2_19,
© Springer International Publishing Switzerland 2015

medicine [2, 6]. During his time there, he was regarded as an "outstanding student" and received first class honors in the subjects of medicine, surgery, and obstetrics [2]. After graduating from the clinical school of the Melbourne Hospital, he started his first resident house appointment at Melbourne Hospital at the age of 27 [6]. During his residency training, he was heavily influenced by his chief William Moore, and this is likely how he became interested in the management of patients who were dying from exophthalmic goiter of the thyroid [3]. In 1905, he had completed his surgical residency training, but, without the financial support from a wealthy family or the proper connections, he left Melbourne Hospital and graciously accepted an invitation from Mother Berchmans Daly (then the Mother Rectress) to join the medical staff at the newly built St. Vincent's Hospital [2,3]. However, there were no surgical positions available at the time, so Dunhill was appointed physician to outpatients and was officially awarded his M.D. in 1906 [2, 6]. It was at this time, with the help of his chief, David Murray Morton, that Dunhill turned his attention to the management of patients with toxic exophthalmic goiter.

At the turn of the twentieth century, physicians, Dunhill included, were giving milk from thyroidectomized animals to thyrotoxic patients in an attempt to provide a factor that would neutralize the thyroid toxin [2, 3]. A similar short-lived practice was to inject a thyroidectomized animal with thyroid extract and then inject that animals' serum into a thyrotoxic patient [3]. By 1907, Dunhill had realized the ineffective results of medical treatment for this disease in the patients suffering from thyrotoxicosis at St. Vincent's Hospital [3]. Inspired by Kocher's report in the *British Medical Journal* of using local anesthesia when operating on the thyroid and having seen the disastrous effects of the general anesthetic at the time (chloroform) on a thyrotoxic patient suffering from cardiac failure, Dunhill took his first step toward making his mark in history [6].

Unfortunately, Dunhill was limited by his position as an outpatient surgeon, and it was only with the assistance of David Murray Morton, who allowed Dunhill the use of a surgical bed, that Dunhill had the opportunity to take on his first patient. Mary Lynch was a 36-year-old Irish servant who had been suffering from exophthalmic goiter for months. She was not only out of work due to her persistent vomiting and emaciation but also so close to death that in the words of Dunhill himself, she "preferred any risk to remaining as she was" [3]. In July 1907, 2 years before **Theodor Kocher** received the Nobel Prize "for his works on the physiology, pathology and surgery of the thyroid gland," Dunhill performed the fourth thyroidectomy ever done at St. Vincent's by removing the right lobe of her thyroid under local anesthesia (Fig. 1) [2, 3, 8]. Mary Lynch not only survived the operation but she also did well postoperatively. After seeing this, other patients

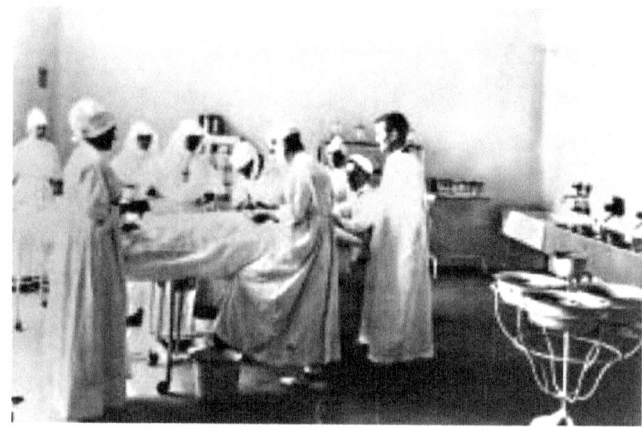

Fig. 1 The operating theater at St. Vincent's Hospital where Dunhill performed his first thyroid surgery in 1907 on Mary Lynch, an Irish servant suffering from severe thyrotoxicosis. From Thomas Peel Dunhill: Pioneer Thyroid Surgeon, Vellar, 1999. (Reprinted with permission, Copyright © 2002, John Wiley and Sons)

who were suffering from severe thyrotoxicosis self-referred to Dunhill for surgery [3, 6]. He operated on six other individuals with severe cases of thyrotoxicosis, including two with atrial fibrillation and cardiac failure, and all recovered well [2]. He published the results of these first seven cases in the *Intercolonial Medical Journal of Australasia* in November of 1907 [2, 3]. Regardless, his medical colleagues still remained wary of surgery as evidenced by the fact that of Dunhill's first 25 patients, only 5 of them were referred by other physicians, and the other 20 were self-referrals after hearing of his success [3].

All of Dunhill's initial patients were severely thyrotoxic and underwent removal of one lobe of the thyroid along with the isthmus. However, of these 25 patients, 6 had a recurrence of thyrotoxic symptoms postoperatively, and required a second operation to remove one half to two thirds of the remaining lobe [2]. Dunhill concluded that in order to cure the disease, it was important to remove a sufficient amount of thyroid tissue. However, at this time, the exact amount of tissue that would be enough to prevent recurrence, but not be so much that the patient developed hypothyroidism and tetany, was unknown [3]. Consequently, other thyroid surgeons including Halstead and **Crile** advocated for removal of one thyroid lobe and a ligation of the superior or inferior thyroid vessels on the other lobe. Dunhill believed that when the remaining lobe was so enlarged, a simple ligation of the vessels did not protect the patient from continuing or recurrent thyrotoxicity and that part of the remaining gland needed to be resected. Unfortunately, at his first attempt to resect one and a half lobes of the thyroid in a thyrotoxic patient with heart failure, the patient died postoperatively from thyroid crisis. Dunhill believed that this patient's death was in part due to the advanced stage of the disease. He argued

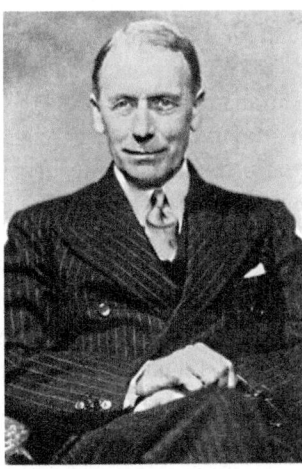

Fig. 2 A portrait of Thomas Peel Dunhill at the age of 59. From Thomas Peel Dunhill: Pioneer Thyroid Surgeon, Vellar, 1999. (Reprinted with permission, Copyright © 2002, John Wiley and Sons)

that if patients were referred at an earlier stage in the disease before cardiac and pulmonary complications occur, they will be better suited to undergo thyroid resection and have a better chance of a full recovery [3]. However, he reasoned that in certain advanced cases it was wise to perform the operation in two stages [2, 5].

In 1909, Dunhill published an article entitled "Remarks on partial thyroidectomy with special reference to exophthalmic goitre and observations on 113 operations under local anesthesia" which detailed his practice of performing the operation in one stage (removal of one lobe and at least half of the other lobe) in the majority of patients and reserving the staged operation only for those who were severely thyrotoxic with advanced disease [2]. He also continued to operate on patients with cardiac manifestations of the disease including heart failure and atrial fibrillation. Specifically, he had operated on eight such patients, half of whom required a staged operation, but all of whom survived and recovered well [2, 3]. Part of Dunhill's success was related to his technique. He carefully dissected the thyroid gland with his fingers and ligated the superior and inferior thyroid arteries early in the operation rather than using a scalpel and forceps through the friable highly vascularized tissue. Consequently, he was often able to achieve a clean dissection and avoid excessive bleeding [2, 3]. He was described as a "meticulous operator with a delicate touch" [6]. Additionally, with the use of local anesthesia, he was able to avoid the complications associated with chloroform including severe nausea and vomiting [2]. In 1910, he was promoted as surgeon to inpatients at St. Vincent's, and, with the help of his colleague Hugh Devine, he helped turn St. Vincent's Hospital into a Clinical School at the University of Melbourne [7].

In 1911, Dunhill set out to England and America to learn from some of the top thyroid centers around the world [6]. He first visited Dr. Frank Hartley in New York, Halsted at Johns Hopkins in Baltimore and the **Mayo** brothers in Rochester, Minnesota, where the operation for thyrotoxicosis consisted of removing one lobe and ligating the superior thyroid vessels in the remaining lobe. Dunhill shared his results with other leaders in thyroid surgery, including Halstead, and emphasized the importance of resecting thyroid tissue bilaterally to successfully treat thyrotoxicosis [2].

From there, he journeyed to England, where the attitude toward surgery for thyrotoxicosis at this time could be summarized by one of England's well-known thyroid surgeons James Berry, who described the operation as "worse than useless" and stated that the risks heavily outweighed the potential benefits [5]. Additionally, the belief that patients tended to get better with conservative treatment persisted. As a result, surgery was viewed a last resort, and patients were not referred until very late in the course of the disease, when generalized anesthesia alone for these emaciated patients with severe cardiac and pulmonary sequelae was often fatal [2]. In February of 1912, Dunhill had the opportunity to present his research in England at the Surgical Section of the Royal Society of Medicine. Unfortunately, he was unable to be in England at the time and James Berry presented Dunhill's results instead [2, 3, 6]. The reaction of most of the surgeons in the audience to Dunhill's 230 cases of thyrotoxicosis with only four deaths was a combination of skepticism and disbelief. Since none of the attendees could compete with Dunhill in terms of volume of cases and low mortality rates, questions were raised regarding Dunhill's honesty in reporting his results and also the accuracy of the diagnosis of thyrotoxicosis and *Graves'* disease in his surgical patients [3, 5].

Despite this criticism, there was a shift in the surgical treatment of thyrotoxicosis in England and America after Dunhill's visit. This cause was aided by the research of his peers whose results confirmed Dunhill's theory. For example, Halstead presented findings in front of the American Surgical Association, in 1913, that in order to cure thyrotoxicosis, it was absolutely necessary to remove part of the second lobe of the thyroid [3, 6]. At the Mayo Clinic, in 1914, nearly 7 years after Dunhill performed his first bilateral resection of the thyroid for thyrotoxicosis, Donald Church Balfour stated that surgery for the thyrotoxic patient entailed removal of one lobe of the thyroid and part of the other lobe and that this technique should be performed "as a rule" [3].

Upon Dunhill's return to St. Vincent's, he was promoted to surgeon to inpatients at the age of 37. He then served in World War I as surgeon to the First Australian General Hospital in 1915, where he was promoted to Lieutenant Colonel in 1917 [2, 3, 6].

Once the war was over, George Gask, one of the surgeons that Dunhill had worked with, was appointed professor of surgery at St. Bartholomew's Hospital in London and invited Dunhill to serve as assistant director [4]. However, upon moving to London, he continued to have to push for early patient referrals and argue for the benefit of surgery in patients who suffered from heart failure and atrial fibrillation as a result of thyrotoxicosis despite all the evidence that had been presented to the contrary [2]. Dunhill reported that atrial fibrillation disappeared after thyroidectomy for toxic goiter but his mortality rate was 7 % (17 of 240 patients) in patients with atrial fibrillation versus about 1 % for other patients with toxic goiter [9]. He worked tirelessly to break the cycle of physicians delaying surgical referrals for thyrotoxic patients for fear of high operative mortality until the patient was at an advanced stage of the disease and consequently was at significant operative risk. With the help of the professor of medicine at St. Bartholomew's Hospital, Francis Fraser, Dunhill was able to persuade referring physicians that if medical management was not improving the condition in the thyrotoxic patient that surgical intervention should be considered sooner rather than later [2, 6].

In 1920, Dunhill altered his technique from lobectomy with removal of the majority of the remaining lobe to a subtotal thyroidectomy, leaving behind the posterior portion of the thyroid gland—a technique first described by Mikulicz in 1885. Charles Mayo and George Crile adopted this technique around the same time [2]. Between the years of 1907 and 1937, he published 29 papers on the surgical treatment of the toxic goiter. In 1928, he was appointed surgeon to the Royal Household and served as surgeon to King George V, Edward VIII, and George VI (Fig. 2) [2]. He retired from St. Bartholomew's in 1935 and continued to have his private practice in England until he stopped operating in 1949. He died in December of 1957 of what was thought to be complications of hemochromatosis.

While Halsted, **Mayo**, **Crile**, **Lahey**, and **Kocher** are often the names that are first mentioned when considering the history of thyroid surgery, Dr. Thomas Peel Dunhill's contributions to the field should not be overlooked. A true pioneer, he championed the efficacy of the subtotal thyroidectomy and challenged his colleagues to see the benefits of early surgical intervention as the optimal treatment for patients with toxic goiter. These principles remain the foundation of surgical management of toxic goiter to the current day.

References

1. Kopp P. Theodor Kocher (1841–1917) Nobel Prize centenary 2009. Arg Gras Endocrinol Metab. 2009;53(9):1176–80.
2. Vellar I. Thomas Peel Dunhill: pioneer thyroid surgeon. ANZ J Surg. 1999;69:375–87.
3. Vellar I. Thomas Peel Dunhill, the forgotten man of thyroid surgery. Med Hist. 1974;18:22–50.
4. Hershman MJ, Campion KM. Thomas Dunhill 1876 1957 Pioneer of thyroid surgery. Ann R Coll Surg Eng. 1985;67(1):33.
5. Hannan S. The magnificent seven: a history of modern thyroid surgery. Int J Surg. 2006;4:187–191.
6. Taylor S. Sir Thomas Peel Dunhill (1876–1957). World J Surg. 1997;21:660–2.
7. Vellar I. Julian Smith: scientific surgeon, photographer, inventor. ANZ J Surg. 2002;72:49–56.
8. Gautschi OP, Hildebrandt G. Emil Theodor Kocher (25/8/1841–27/7/1917)—A Swiss (neuro-) surgeon and Nobel Prize winner. Br J Neurosurg. 2009;234–6.
9. Welbourn R. The history of endocrine surgery. New York: Praeger. 1990; pp. 52–3.

Primary Hyperparathyroidism: Diagnosis and Workup

Cord Sturgeon

Introduction

Primary hyperparathyroidism (PHPT) affects 0.1–0.5% of the adult US population and is more common among women by a factor of 3:1. The incidence of PHPT rises sharply after age 50 and continues to rise with each subsequent decade of age [1]. Recent analysis of a large racially mixed population in southern California indicated that PHPT is more common among African Americans than whites or Asians [1]. Furthermore, the incidence and prevalence of PHPT appear to be rising [1]. The bone and renal effects of long-standing untreated PHPT can have a substantial impact on quality of life and cost of health care [2]. Patients with PHPT also experience a broad spectrum of physical and neurocognitive symptoms that may be difficult to recognize, measure, and quantify. Parathyroid surgeons are first-hand witnesses to the symptom improvement experienced by most patients, even those thought to be asymptomatic prior to surgery [3–5]. Prospective studies have documented the improvements in bone mineral density [6], and cohort studies have demonstrated a reduction in fracture rate [7, 8] and kidney stone formation [9] following curative parathyroidectomy. Despite the clear health and cost benefits [2] to surgical cure of PHPT, approximately only 20–30% of patients are referred for surgery [10, 11]. There is broad agreement among endocrine physicians that patients with symptomatic PHPT or marked hypercalcemia should be referred for surgery [12]. Considerable controversy continues to fuel the debate over which patients with so-called "asymptomatic" PHPT are reasonable to observe. Since 1990, four conferences have been convened with the goal of defining the proper management of asymptomatic PHPT. Although the most recent three conferences have not been conducted under the aegis of a National Institutes of Health (NIH) consensus, and participation among parathyroid surgeons has been limited to a handful of invitees, guidelines from the International Workshop on Asymptomatic Primary Hyperparathyroidism are widely used to direct the care of these patients. Numerous investigators have challenged the recommendations from these guidelines, and many have shown that patients who do not meet the criteria for surgery will still benefit from surgery [4, 5]. Most parathyroid surgeons believe that PHPT is under-recognized, underreported, and undertreated. In this chapter, the diagnosis and workup of PHPT are reviewed. An overarching goal for those physicians who treat PHPT should be to improve the frequency of proper diagnosis and surgical referral for PHPT.

Etiology of Disease

The majority of patients diagnosed with PHPT have no known environmental or genetic risk factors. These patients with sporadic disease comprise approximately 95% of all cases of PHPT. Most cases of sporadic PHPT, approximately 85%, are due to a single parathyroid adenoma. Approximately 15% of sporadic patients have multigland disease, which includes double adenoma and hyperplasia of all parathyroid glands. Less than 1% of patients have PHPT due to parathyroid carcinoma.

A careful family history should be sought for inherited endocrine syndromes in order to detect the clinically relevant potential manifestations of disease. Inherited PHPT syndromes are more likely to be due to multigland disease, and often are associated with additional endocrine and nonendocrine tumors. The predisposition for PHPT may be inherited in patients with multiple endocrine neoplasia (MEN) type I and IIa, hyperparathyroidism-jaw tumor syndrome (HPT-JT), and familial isolated hyperparathyroidism (FIHP) [13, 14]. Patients who inherit MEN-1 (**Wermer's** syndrome) are essentially guaranteed to develop PHPT at some point in life, almost always due to an asymmetric 4-gland hyperplasia. Approximately one third of MEN-2a (**Sipple's**

C. Sturgeon (✉)
Endocrine Surgery, Northwestern University,
676 North Saint Clair St., Suite 650, Chicago, IL 60611, USA
e-mail: csturgeo@nmh.org

J. L. Pasieka, J. A. Lee (eds.), *Surgical Endocrinopathies*, DOI 10.1007/978-3-319-13662-2_20,
© Springer International Publishing Switzerland 2015

syndrome) patients develop PHPT. The relative risk of developing PHPT in MEN-2A can be predicted by knowledge of the exact codon mutation in the rearranged during transfection (RET) oncogene. HPT-JT is characterized by the development of hyperparathyroidism due to single or multiple (occasionally cystic) abnormal parathyroid glands, and osseous fibromas of the maxilla or mandible. Renal cysts, hamartomas, or Wilms' tumors have also been described in HPT-JT. HPT-JT patients have an approximately 10–20 % risk of developing parathyroid carcinoma. Familial isolated hyperparathyroidism (FIHP) is characterized by multigenerational autosomal-dominant inheritance of PHPT in the absence of other manifestations of syndromic disease. No single gene has been identified for FIHP, but candidates have been found in the MEN-1, cell division cycle protein 73 (CDC73), and calcium-sensing receptor (CASR) genes.

PHPT may be acquired due to exposure to radiation or lithium. Patients with a significant head and neck exposure to ionizing radiation, especially at a young age have a higher risk of developing PHPT several decades after exposure. Furthermore, patients with a history of radiation exposure to the head and neck also are at higher risk of developing thyroid cancer. Lithium has been used to treat bipolar disorder, and is still used today, although with a lower frequency than in the past. Prolonged lithium exposure increases the probability of developing PHPT.

Establishing the Diagnosis of PHPT

When PHPT is suspected, the first diagnostic maneuver is to establish that there is a disordered homeostasis between calcium and PTH. Classic hypercalcemic PHPT is diagnosed by demonstrating that the serum calcium and PTH are simultaneously elevated in the absence of hypocalciuria. Some experts routinely measure the 24-h urinary calcium excretion to secure the diagnosis of PHPT and to estimate the severity of disease. The differential diagnosis of hypercalcemia, additional laboratory findings, and the normocalcemic and normohormonal variants of PHPT are discussed in detail below.

Differential Diagnosis of Hypercalcemia When PTH Is Elevated or Inappropriate

Hypercalcemia in an ambulatory setting is usually due to PHPT. In a recent review of a large administrative dataset of outpatients with hypercalcemia, 87 % of cases were due to PHPT [1]. Although the differential diagnosis of hypercalcemia is extensive, checking simultaneous serum calcium and PTH levels as a first maneuver should sort out PHPT from the remainder of the other causes other than benign familial hypocalciuric hypercalcemia (BFHH), thiazide

diuretic-induced hypercalcemia, and the extraordinarily rare phenomenon of ectopic production of PTH by a solid tumor.

In patients with a personal or family history that is concerning for BFHH, a 24-h urine collection for creatinine and calcium should always be ordered. A diagnosis of BFHH is excluded when the 24-h urinary calcium excretion is greater than 100 mg. It is not always necessary to exclude the diagnosis of BFHH through a 24-h urine collection because BFHH is rare compared to PHPT, and patients with BFHH usually have a history that is positive for lifelong mild hypercalcemia in themselves and multiple family members. BFHH is caused by an autosomal-dominant inherited inactivating mutation in the calcium-sensing receptor (CaSR) gene which leads to increased calcium reabsorption by the kidney and an elevated calcium set point. Parathyroidectomy does not restore eucalcemia, and is not helpful in patients with BFHH. In patients with BFHH, the urinary calcium excretion is usually less than 100 mg per day. Also, the calcium to creatinine clearance ratio is usually less than 0.01.

Thiazide diuretics and lithium can both cause hypercalcemia with elevated PTH [15, 16]. Occasionally, the use of thiazides or lithium may unmask or exacerbate a previously subclinical case of PHPT. The treatment for thiazide-induced hypercalcemia is to discontinue the medication and restore euvolemia, and the serum calcium should return to normal. The first step in the management of lithium-induced PHPT is to discontinue the lithium if possible. Some patients will return to a eucalcemic state and be followed. If PHPT persists after discontinuing lithium or thiazides, patients should be offered a parathyroidectomy. In lithium-induced PHPT, there is a higher rate of multiglandular disease [17], but, interestingly, approximately two thirds of cases are due to single adenoma, and focused parathyroidectomy has been used successfully in selected patients [18, 19].

Although very rare, ectopic PTH production by solid tumors has been described. A recent literature review identified reports of ectopic PTH production by solid tumors of the stomach, ovary, uterus, kidney, liver, thymus, pancreas, thyroid, tonsil, and neuroectodermal tissue [20]. This phenomenon is so rare that it has become a diagnosis of exclusion and is not routinely worked up in the evaluation of hypercalcemia.

Differential Diagnosis of Hypercalcemia When the PTH Is Low

When the PTH is very low or undetectable in a patient with hypercalcemia and PHPT has been excluded, other possible causes of hypercalcemia should be explored. Hypercalcemia of malignancy is the second most common cause of hypercalcemia, and is the most likely diagnosis when the PTH is low. Hypercalcemia of malignancy may be due to the secretion of PTH-related peptide (PTH-rP) from the tumor, which mimics the renal and skeletal effects of PTH. The majority of hypercalcemic patients with solid tumors and a substantial percentage of hypercalcemic patients with hematologic malignancy will have elevated serum levels of PTH-rP [21]. There are many solid tumors that secrete PTH-rP, but the most common are squamous cell cancers of the lung, and solid cancers of the kidney, bladder, and ovary. Hematologic malignancies including non-Hodgkin's lymphoma, chronic myeloid/lymphoblastic leukemia, adult T cell leukemia/lymphoma, and multiple myeloma may present with hypercalcemia due to PTH-rP. Hypercalcemia of malignancy may also occur in the absence of measurable PTH-rP, as it frequently does in multiple myeloma or with lytic bone metastases.

There are a number of pharmacologic agents which may cause hypercalcemia. Thiazide diuretics reduce calcium clearance and thereby may lead to hypercalcemia. Vitamin A, vitamin D, lithium, foscarnet, theophylline, aminophylline, estrogens, and antiestrogens have all been associated with hypercalcemia. In cases of drug-induced hypercalcemia, the first step is generally to discontinue the medication, if possible.

Milk-alkali syndrome occurs with the consumption of large amounts of dairy and calcium carbonate. Hypercalcemia may be treated by discontinuing the consumption of calcium. This was originally described when the treatment for peptic ulcer disease included the consumption of large amount of milk and sodium bicarbonate (a.k.a. alkali).

Paget disease of the bone is characterized by excessive bone turnover due to pathologic osteoclastic overactivity and bone resorption with subsequent compensatory osteoblastic overactivity and new bone formation. Hypercalcemia is rare in patients with Paget disease, and, when discovered, PHPT should be ruled out. An association between immobilization and hypercalcemia in Paget disease has been described.

Hypercalcemia can occur after a prolonged period of immobilization and has been described in patients recovering from orthopedic, neurologic, or burn injury.

Granulomatous diseases including sarcoidosis, histoplasmosis, coccidiomycosis, and tuberculosis can cause hypercalcemia. The best-understood granulomatous disease is sarcoidosis. The extra-renal production of 1 alpha-hydroxylase by macrophages in a granuloma can lead to an increased rate of conversion of 25-OH vitamin D to its active form, 1,25-OH vitamin D. Subsequently, calcium absorption is increased in the gastrointestinal tract and calcium resorption is increased in the skeleton leading to hypercalcemia and suppression of PTH.

Hyperthyroidism can cause hypercalcemia by increasing bone turnover, and is effectively treated by reestablishing a euthyroid state. VIPoma (**Verner–Morrison** syndrome) and pheochromocytoma have also been reported to manifest with hypercalcemia, but the cause is not known (secretion of PTH-rP has been suggested). Hypoadrenalism has also been associated with hypercalcemia but the cause is unknown.

Taking the History of a Patient with Hypercalcemia

Patients with hypercalcemia should be questioned about symptoms of disease, personal history, and family history pertinent to the differential diagnosis. Acquired hyperparathyroidism should be suspected when the history is positive for radiation exposure to the head and neck region in childhood or prolonged usage of lithium. Inherited hyperparathyroidism should be suspected when there is a family history of hypercalcemia, hyperparathyroidism, or a syndrome associated with hypercalcemia (MEN-1, MEN-2A, HPT-JT, or FIHP). BFHH should be suspected when the patient reports a lifelong history of mildly elevated calcium, and a family history of hypercalcemia (recalcitrant to parathyroid surgery). Hypercalcemia of malignancy is usually associated with a known advanced cancer rather than an occult malignancy; therefore, a personal history of solid or hematologic malignancies should be obtained. A history of Paget disease of the bone, granulomatous disease, and thyrotoxicosis should be specifically sought. Patients should be asked about consumption of medications or supplements described above that may lead to hypercalcemia.

The duration and severity of disease are established by specifically determining the age or date of onset of hypercalcemia and the highest calcium that the patient has achieved. Significant clinical manifestation seen by the early surgical pioneers like **Mandl** and **Cope** are only seen in 5 % of patients in developed countries. Today, the most common presentation of PHPT is that of mild chronic hypercalcemia without episodes of acute or severe hypercalcemia. Physicians should inquire about objective signs such as declining renal function, kidney stones, osteoporosis, or fragility fracture. The broad spectrum of symptoms and signs of hypercalcemia should be fully explored. Physicians should specifically inquire about a history of hypercalcemic crisis.

The classic pentad of symptoms of PHPT memorized by medical students is "painful bones, kidney stones, abdominal groans, psychogenic moans, and fatigue overtones." Despite this clever mnemonic, the symptoms of hypercalcemia may be insidious and can go unrecognized when the disease has been chronic and mild. Unfortunately, this means that these symptoms are frequently overlooked or attributed to aging by patients and physicians, and the disease may go untreated. Chronic hypercalcemia may be associated with dyspepsia, gastrointestinal reflux disease, constipation, pancreatitis, nephrolithiasis, increased thirst, polyuria, muscle weakness, fatigue, lassitude, bone pain, arthralgia or myalgia, reduced short-term memory, depression, and a decline in cognitive function. Acute severe hypercalcemia presents in a more dramatic fashion and is associated with dehydration, nausea, vomiting, renal failure, mental status changes, cardiac conduction abnormalities, and hypotension. Hypercalcemia of malignancy frequently presents with acute severe hypercalcemia. Parathyroid carcinoma may also present in this more dramatic fashion.

Physical Exam of the Hypercalcemic Patient

Most patients with PHPT will have no specific abnormal findings on physical exam. Parathyroid tumors are almost always impalpable. If a cervical mass is palpated in a patient with known PHPT, the likelihood is that the examiner is feeling a thyroid mass. Likewise, patients are not usually aware of the parathyroid tumor and do not experience compressive or globus symptoms. Parathyroid carcinoma may be the exception to this rule if the tumor is very large, or invasive into the recurrent laryngeal nerve or aerodigestive tract. Recurrent nerve invasion from parathyroid carcinoma may also present with dysphonia, and a paralyzed vocal cord may be present on laryngeal exam.

Other physical exam findings that may accompany PHPT, but are not specific for the disease, include brittle nails and hair, signs of dehydration, diminished deep-tendon reflexes, and proximal muscle weakness. On slit-lamp exam, band keratopathy may be seen. Patients with nephrolithiasis may have tenderness to percussion at the costovertebral angle.

Laboratory Examination

In the evaluation of a hypercalcemic patient, the most germane laboratory examinations to obtain are total serum calcium, serum albumin, serum creatinine, and intact PTH. Many experts also routinely evaluate the vitamin D axis by measuring 25-OH vitamin D levels simultaneously with the calcium and PTH. A 24-h urine collection for creatinine and calcium is helpful to rule out BFHH, and is also used by some experts to estimate severity of disease. It may also be helpful to obtain an ionized calcium level in patients with a total serum calcium that falls within the upper limit of the normal reference range. The diagnosis of classic hypercalcemic PHPT is made by demonstrating that the serum calcium and PTH are simultaneously elevated in the absence of hypocalciuria. The variants of classic hypercalcemic PHPT wherein there is a disordered homeostasis between calcium and PTH, but one or both still fall within the normal reference range, are discussed below.

Patients with PHPT may have low or low-normal serum phosphorous. Alkaline phosphorous may be mildly elevated due to high bone turnover. 25-OH vitamin D is usually at the low end of normal or low, and 1,25-OH vitamin D is usually at the high end of normal or high due to peripheral conversion from the elevated PTH. A 24-h urinary calcium excretion is normal or elevated. The chloride to phosphorous ratio is usually greater than 33. The presence of a mild hyperchloremic metabolic acidosis is sometimes seen. Calcium to creatinine clearance ratio is usually greater than 0.02.

PHPT with Normocalcemia and/or Normal PTH

In patients with hypoalbuminemia, the total serum calcium may be artificially low, and hypercalcemia will only be appreciated when an albumin-corrected calcium level is calculated or an ionized calcium is measured. In addition, some patients with PHPT will have a serum calcium level and ionized calcium level at the upper end of the normal reference range and elevated PTH. When secondary causes of PTH elevation are absent (e.g., renal failure, vitamin D deficiency, malabsorption), this condition has been described as "normocalcemic primary hyperparathyroidism" [22]. Conversely, the condition where the serum calcium is elevated, but the PTH is within the normal reference range but inappropriately high, has been called "normohormonal primary hyperparathyroidism" [23]. These variants of disease are recognized by experts in PHPT, and these patients may have the same symptomology and sequelae as hypercalcemic PHPT [24]. In addition, patients are believed to have similar benefits from parathyroidectomy as those patients with the classic presentation of disease. The trend over the past three decades has been that patients are being diagnosed with less severe disease, including having lower overall serum calcium levels [25]. Because patients are being diagnosed earlier and with milder disease forms, diagnosis is not always simple. Some experts rely upon nomograms that accurately predict disease for those patients with less classic presentations [26].

Imaging Studies in PHPT

The sole purpose of preoperative imaging studies in PHPT is for operative planning. Thus, parathyroid imaging is not performed as part of the diagnostic workup. Additionally, imaging has no role in patients who are not surgical candidates. Institutional accuracy, availability, cost, and radiation exposure should be considered when selecting a preoperative imaging strategy [27]. Parathyroid imaging is plagued by many false-negative and false-positive results, and the interpretation of parathyroid imaging studies is not always straightforward. Consequently, parathyroid imaging should not be used for the confirmation of a diagnosis of PHPT, nor should it be used to exclude or "rule out" the diagnosis. The sole purpose of parathyroid imaging is for the surgeon to plan the operative approach. In the current era, most parathyroid surgeons obtain one or more preoperative imaging studies before parathyroid exploration; however, positive imaging studies are no substitute for a comprehensive understanding of parathyroid anatomy and embryology; therefore, it is wise to consider the famous axiom from John Doppman in 1986: "…the only localization study indicated…is to localize an experienced parathyroid surgeon" [28, 29].

The most commonly used parathyroid localization studies are cervical ultrasound and technetium-99 m methoxyisobutylisonitrile (^{99m}Tc sestamibi) scanning. The sestamibi scan is a functional study for the identification of overactive parathyroid tissue. Overactive parathyroid tissue in either eutopic or ectopic locations may be identified by sestamibi scanning. Unfortunately, only approximately 80 % of patients will have successful localization with sestamibi scanning [30, 31]. False-positive and false-negative results may occur in patients with coexistent benign or malignant thyroid disease. Sestamibi scanning does not yield detailed anatomic information; however, single-photon emission computed tomography (SPECT) sestamibi has advantages over standard planar imaging in this regard, and can identify the depth and location of parathyroid tumors [32]. Cervical ultrasound reveals coexistent thyroid disease, and gives the surgeon precise information about the size, depth, and location of parathyroid tumor(s). Ultrasound is less effective at identifying ectopic parathyroid tumors, and is not able to image parathyroid tumors in the chest. Ultrasound is highly operator dependent, and may be less effective for patients with a large body habitus, kyphosis, goiter, and other head and neck pathologies. The accuracy of ultrasound for parathyroid adenoma is approximately 60–80 % [31, 33, 34]. Ultrasound is considered by many experts to be indispensable because of its superior anatomic definition and the fact that it can be used to identify thyroid pathology that could alter the operative approach, or may be the cause of false-positive sestamibi uptake. When ultrasound and sestamibi are concordant, the sensitivity for single-gland disease at that location has been shown to be 96 % [31].

Cross-sectional imaging, including conventional computed tomography (CT) and magnetic resonance imaging (MRI), have historically been less accurate localization studies than sestamibi scintigraphy or ultrasound with sensitivities of approximately 40–70 % [35–37]. A newer cross-sectional protocol, the 4-D CT, has been used by some experts for preoperative localization [38], and in some centers 4-D CT has been found to have a greater sensitivity than sestamibi scanning or ultrasound for localization of parathyroid adenomas, and identification of multigland disease [38, 39]. To illustrate the relative effectiveness of each modality, a recent meta-analysis demonstrated that ultrasound has a sensitivity and positive predictive value (PPV) of 76 and 93 %, respectively; sestamibi scanning had a sensitivity and PPV

of 79 and 91 %, respectively; and 4-D CT had a sensitivity of 89 and 94 %, respectively [40].

The surgeon should not be dissuaded from an index parathyroid exploration when localization studies fail to identify the location of abnormal parathyroid tissue. Nonlocalizing or "negative" studies neither invalidate the diagnosis of hyperparathyroidism nor should they be a component of the decision to refer the patient to a surgeon. When localization studies fail to reveal the site of a parathyroid adenoma, approximately 75 % of patients will be found to have single-gland disease at bilateral exploration [41]. Because localization studies have many false positives and false negatives, they are highly operator dependent, and interpretation is highly variable between institutions, the results of preoperative imaging should never be used to either confirm or rule out the diagnosis of hyperparathyroidism, and should not be used for the selection of patients fit for surgery.

Conclusion

PHPT is driven by inappropriate autonomous PTH secretion, and is diagnosed by demonstrating that there is a disordered homeostasis between serum calcium and PTH. A 24-h urinary calcium excretion is often measured to rule out BFHH, but may be unnecessary in cases where the patient and family history are clear. Expert guidelines recommend the routine measurement of serum 25-OH vitamin D in patients with PHPT [42]. Localization studies are often obtained by physicians prior to any surgical consultation; however, the purpose of localization studies is for operative planning. Localization studies are not to be used for the confirmation or exclusion of the diagnosis of PHPT [43]. The reason for this is that there are many false-negative and false-positive results. Furthermore, the results of localization studies should not be used as a gating mechanism to determine when or if to send patients for surgical consultation. PHPT is an archetypal surgical disease. Permanent cure is anticipated for nearly all patients with benign sporadic disease. As the US population ages, appropriate use of parathyroidectomy for PHPT may play an important role in increasing health-care value by reducing costly negative health events such as fragility fracture and kidney stone formation through appropriately timed parathyroid surgery instead of chronic medication. Most parathyroid surgeons believe that PHPT is underrecognized, underreported, and undertreated. A broad goal for those physicians who treat PHPT should be to improve the timing and frequency of proper diagnosis and surgical referral for PHPT.

Key Summary Points

- PHPT is the most common cause of hypercalcemia.
- The cause of hypercalcemia can be most easily determined by measuring PTH.
- The majority of cases of hyperparathyroidism are sporadic in nature and due to a single parathyroid adenoma.
- Hyperparathyroidism may be inherited in a syndromic fashion or acquired.
- Normocalcemic and normohormonal variants are now recognized.
- Imaging studies are for the purpose of operative planning and not for confirming or ruling out the diagnosis of PHPT.

References

1. Yeh MW, Ituarte PH, Zhou HC, Nishimoto S, Liu IL, Harari A, et al. Incidence and prevalence of primary hyperparathyroidism in a racially mixed population. J Clin Endocrinol Metab. 2013;98(3):1122–9.
2. Zanocco K, Angelos P, Sturgeon C. Cost-effectiveness analysis of parathyroidectomy for asymptomatic primary hyperparathyroidism. Surgery. 2006;140(6):874–81; discussion 81–2.
3. Quiros RM, Alef MJ, Wilhelm SM, Djuricin G, Loviscek K, Prinz RA. Health-related quality of life in hyperparathyroidism measurably improves after parathyroidectomy. Surgery. 2003;134(4):675–81; discussion 81–3.
4. Sywak MS, Knowlton ST, Pasieka JL, Parsons LL, Jones J. Do the National Institutes of Health consensus guidelines for parathyroidectomy predict symptom severity and surgical outcome in patients with primary hyperparathyroidism? Surgery. 2002;132(6):1013–9; discussion 9–20.
5. Eigelberger MS, Cheah WK, Ituarte PH, Streja L, Duh QY, Clark OH. The NIH criteria for parathyroidectomy in asymptomatic primary hyperparathyroidism: are they too limited? Ann Surg. 2004;239(4):528–35.
6. Rubin MR, Bilezikian JP, McMahon DJ, Jacobs T, Shane E, Siris E, et al. The natural history of primary hyperparathyroidism with or without parathyroid surgery after 15 years. J Clin Endocrinol Metab. 2008;93(9):3462–70.
7. Vestergaard P, Mollerup CL, Frokjaer VG, Christiansen P, Blichert-Toft M, Mosekilde L. Cohort study of risk of fracture before and after surgery for primary hyperparathyroidism. BMJ. 2000;321(7261):598–602.
8. Ogard CG, Engholm G, Almdal TP, Vestergaard H. Increased mortality in patients hospitalized with primary hyperparathyroidism during the period 1977–1993 in Denmark. World J Surg. 2004;28(1):108–11.
9. Deaconson TF, Wilson SD, Lemann J Jr. The effect of parathyroidectomy on the recurrence of nephrolithiasis. Surgery. 1987;102(6):910–3.
10. Yeh MW, Wiseman JE, Ituarte PH, Pasternak JD, Hwang RS, Wu B, et al. Surgery for primary hyperparathyroidism: are the consensus guidelines being followed? Ann Surg. 2012;255(6):1179–83.
11. Wermers RA, Khosla S, Atkinson EJ, Achenbach SJ, Oberg AL, Grant CS, et al. Incidence of primary hyperparathyroidism in Rochester, Minnesota, 1993–2001: an update on the changing epidemiology of the disease. J Bone Miner Res. 2006;21(1):171–7.
12. Bilezikian JP, Khan AA, Potts JT Jr. Third International Workshop on the Management of Asymptomatic Primary H. Guidelines for the management of asymptomatic primary hyperparathyroidism: summary statement from the third international workshop. J Clin Endocrinol Metab. 2009;94(2):335–9.
13. Carpten JD, Robbins CM, Villablanca A, Forsberg L, Presciuttini S, Bailey-Wilson J, et al. HRPT2, encoding parafibromin, is mutated in hyperparathyroidism-jaw tumor syndrome. Nat Genet. 2002;32(4):676–80.
14. Marx SJ, Simonds WF, Agarwal SK, Burns AL, Weinstein LS, Cochran C, et al. Hyperparathyroidism in hereditary syndromes: special expressions and special managements. J Bone Miner Res. 2002;17 Suppl 2:N37–43.
15. Paloyan E, Farland M, Pickleman JR. Hyperparathyroidism coexisting with hypertension and prolonged thiazide administration. JAMA. 1969;210(7):1243–5.
16. Mallette LE, Khouri K, Zengotita H, Hollis BW, Malini S. Lithium treatment increases intact and midregion parathyroid hormone and parathyroid volume. J Clin Endocrinol Metab. 1989;68(3):654–60.
17. Marti JL, Yang CS, Carling T, Roman SA, Sosa JA, Donovan P, et al. Surgical approach and outcomes in patients with lithium-associated hyperparathyroidism. Ann Surg Oncol. 2012;19(11):3465–71.
18. Carchman E, Ogilvie J, Holst J, Yim J, Carty S. Appropriate surgical treatment of lithium-associated hyperparathyroidism. World J Surg. 2008;32(10):2195–9.
19. Wade TJ, Yen TW, Amin AL, Evans DB, Wilson SD, Wang TS. Focused parathyroidectomy with intraoperative parathyroid hormone monitoring in patients with lithium-associated primary hyperparathyroidism. Surgery. 2013;153(5):718–22.
20. Nakajima K, Tamai M, Okaniwa S, Nakamura Y, Kobayashi M, Niwa T, et al. Humoral hypercalcemia associated with gastric carcinoma secreting parathyroid hormone: a case report and review of the literature. Endocr J. 2013;60(5):557–62.
21. Burtis WJ, Brady TG, Orloff JJ, Ersbak JB, Warrell RP Jr., Olson BR, et al. Immunochemical characterization of circulating parathyroid hormone-related protein in patients with humoral hypercalcemia of cancer. N Engl J Med. 1990;322(16):1106–12.
22. Cusano NE, Silverberg SJ, Bilezikian JP. Normocalcemic primary hyperparathyroidism. J Clin Densitom. 2013;16(1):33–9.
23. Wallace LB, Parikh RT, Ross LV, Mazzaglia PJ, Foley C, Shin JJ, et al. The phenotype of primary hyperparathyroidism with normal parathyroid hormone levels: how low can parathyroid hormone go? Surgery. 2011;150(6):1102–12.
24. Lowe H, McMahon DJ, Rubin MR, Bilezikian JP, Silverberg SJ. Normocalcemic primary hyperparathyroidism: further characterization of a new clinical phenotype. J Clin Endocrinol Metab. 2007;92(8):3001–5.
25. Mazzaglia PJ, Berber E, Kovach A, Milas M, Esselstyn C, Siperstein AE. The changing presentation of hyperparathyroidism over 3 decades. Arch Surg. 2008;143(3):260–6.
26. Jin J, Mitchell J, Shin J, Berber E, Siperstein AE, Milas M. Calculating an individual maxPTH to aid diagnosis of normocalemic primary hyperparathyroidism. Surgery. 2012;152(6):1184–92.
27. Kunstman JW, Kirsch JD, Mahajan A, Udelsman R. Clinical review: parathyroid localization and implications for clinical management. J Clin Endocrinol Metab. 2013;98(3):902–12.
28. Brennan MF. Lessons learned…. Ann Surg Oncol. 2006;13(10):1322–8.
29. Doppman J. Reoperative parathyroid surgery; localization procedures. Prog Surg. 1986;18:117–32.
30. Chen H, Mack E, Starling JR. A comprehensive evaluation of perioperative adjuncts during minimally invasive parathyroidectomy: which is most reliable? Ann Surg. 2005;242(3):375–80; discussion 80–3.
31. Arici C, Cheah WK, Ituarte PH, Morita E, Lynch TC, Siperstein AE, et al. Can localization studies be used to direct focused parathyroid operations? Surgery. 2001;129(6):720–9.

32. Lavely WC, Goetze S, Friedman KP, Leal JP, Zhang Z, Garret-Mayer E, et al. Comparison of SPECT/CT, SPECT, and planar imaging with single- and dual-phase (99 m)Tc-sestamibi parathyroid scintigraphy. J Nucl Med. 2007;48(7):1084–9.

33. Siperstein A, Berber E, Barbosa GF, Tsinberg M, Greene AB, Mitchell J, et al. Predicting the success of limited exploration for primary hyperparathyroidism using ultrasound, sestamibi, and intraoperative parathyroid hormone: analysis of 1158 cases. Ann Surg. 2008;248(3):420–8.

34. Siperstein A, Berber E, Mackey R, Alghoul M, Wagner K, Milas M. Prospective evaluation of sestamibi scan, ultrasonography, and rapid PTH to predict the success of limited exploration for sporadic primary hyperparathyroidism. Surgery. 2004;136(4):872–80.

35. Wakamatsu H, Noguchi S, Yamashita H, Yamashita H, Tamura S, Jinnouchi S, et al. Parathyroid scintigraphy with 99mTc-MIBI and 123I subtraction: a comparison with magnetic resonance imaging and ultrasonography. Nucl Med Commun. 2003;24(7):755–62.

36. Ruf J, Lopez Hanninen E, Steinmuller T, Rohlfing T, Bertram H, Gutberlet M, et al. Preoperative localization of parathyroid glands. Use of MRI, scintigraphy, and image fusion. Nuklearmedizin Nucl Med. 2004;43(3):85–90.

37. Harari A, Zarnegar R, Lee J, Kazam E, Inabnet WB 3rd, Fahey TJ 3rd. Computed tomography can guide focused exploration in select patients with primary hyperparathyroidism and negative sestamibi scanning. Surgery. 2008;144(6):970–6; discussion 6–9.

38. Rodgers SE, Hunter GJ, Hamberg LM, Schellingerhout D, Doherty DB, Ayers GD, et al. Improved preoperative planning for directed parathyroidectomy with 4-dimensional computed tomography. Surgery. 2006;140(6):932–40; discussion 40–1.

39. Starker LF, Mahajan A, Bjorklund P, Sze G, Udelsman R, Carling T. 4D parathyroid CT as the initial localization study for patients with de novo primary hyperparathyroidism. Ann Surg Oncol. 2011;18(6):1723–8.

40. Cheung K, Wang TS, Farrokhyar F, Roman SA, Sosa JA. A meta-analysis of preoperative localization techniques for patients with primary hyperparathyroidism. Ann Surg Oncol. 2012;19(2):577–83.

41. Chiu B, Sturgeon C, Angelos P. What is the link between non-localizing sestamibi scans, multigland disease, and persistent hypercalcemia? A study of 401 consecutive patients undergoing parathyroidectomy. Surgery. 2006;140(3):418–22.

42. Eastell R, Arnold A, Brandi ML, Brown EM, D'Amour P, Hanley DA, et al. Diagnosis of asymptomatic primary hyperparathyroidism: proceedings of the third international workshop. J Clin Endocrinol Metab. 2009;94(2):340–50.

43. Udelsman R, Pasieka JL, Sturgeon C, Young JE, Clark OH. Surgery for asymptomatic primary hyperparathyroidism: proceedings of the third international workshop. J Clin Endocrinol Metab. 2009;94(2):366–72.

Sir Richard Owen

1804–1892

William S. Duke and David J. Terris

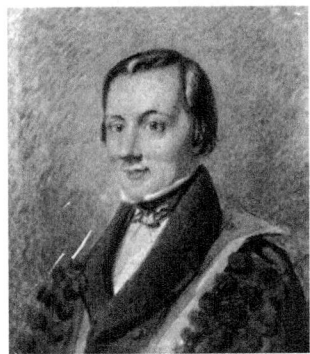

Sir Richard Owen. (Reprinted with permission from Modarari et al. [12]. Courtesy of the Hunterian Museum at the Royal College of Surgeons of England)

Evolution of a Scientist

Richard Owen was born on July 20, 1804, in Lancaster, England, as the son of a West India Merchant father and Huguenot mother [1]. He began his schooling at age six, but did not excel in this environment. He developed an interest in medicine, and in 1820 began an apprenticeship with a local apothecary and surgeon. Over the next few years, Owen worked with several surgeons, eventually obtaining an apprenticeship under James Stockdale Harrison. Through Harrison, Owen had access to the county jail, where he began performing autopsies on deceased criminals and developed an interest in anatomy [1].

Prior to completing his apprenticeship, Owen matriculated at the University of Edinburgh in 1824 [1]. There he studied anatomy under Dr. John Barclay and took courses in both clinical medicine and pharmacology. Owen did not remain

long in Edinburgh, but transferred to St. Bartholomew's Hospital in London in 1825. There, at Barclay's recommendation, he was appointed to prosector for surgical training [1]. He passed his entrance examination for the Royal College of Surgeons in 1826 and established a private practice [1].

In 1827, Owen became assistant conservator to the Hunterian Museum of the Royal College of Surgeons [1]. This museum contained the collections of John Hunter, a famous surgeon of the eighteenth century. Owen would help identify and catalogue more than 10,000 specimens in the collection [2]. He met and attended lectures by other famous anatomists and naturalists, namely Georges Cuvier and Geoffroy Saint-Hilaire, and his interests rapidly shifted from surgery to comparative anatomy. In 1829, he became a lecturer in this field at St. Bartholomew's Hospital, but it was his 1832 *Memoir on the Pearly Nautilus* that vaulted him to the forefront of contemporary anatomists. This work served as a model for subsequent anatomical research publications and is still referenced today when studying these creatures. Owen married the daughter of William Clift, the then chief at the Hunterian Museum, in 1835, and was promoted to head conservator of the museum when Clift retired in 1842 [1].

Owen's academic and scientific résumé grew rapidly. Among his many international accomplishments, in 1836, he was appointed the first Hunterian professor of comparative anatomy and physiology at the Royal College of Surgeons, giving 24 lectures each year until his retirement 20 years later. These lectures were given to large audiences and engendered scientific interest across social classes and professions. He helped establish the Royal Microscopical Society in 1839 and served as its first president. He received honorary degrees from Oxford, Cambridge, and Dublin, and was an honorary or corresponding member of "nearly every scientific society in the world [1]." Owen tutored the royal children at Buckingham Palace, and was given a place of permanent residence at Richmond Park by the queen, where he lived until his death. He was made a knight in the French Legion of Honor by Napoleon III. For reasons unknown,

D. J. Terris (✉) . W. S. Duke
Otolaryngology-Head and Neck Surgery, Georgia Regents University, 1120 15th St., BP-4109, Augusta, GA 30912, USA
e-mail: dterris@gru.edu

J. L. Pasieka, J. A. Lee (eds.), *Surgical Endocrinopathies,* DOI 10.1007/978-3-319-13662-2_21,
© Springer International Publishing Switzerland 2015

he declined his first offer of English knighthood in 1842, though he would ultimately accept this honor in 1883 [1, 3].

During this time, he became more socially and politically active. He was friends with many famous artists and writers of the day, including Charles Dickens and Tennyson. He was a gifted vocalist and played the flute and violoncello, could recite literature and poetry, and loved the theater. In 1845, Owen was elected into "The Club," an exclusive men's dining club composed of authors, artists, scientists, and statesmen. He worked on sewage and public sanitation projects, and in 1847 began service on a government public health commission to influence regulation of abattoirs and the meat production industry [1, 3].

By 1855, Owen had written over 250 scientific papers, including *Descriptive and Illustrative Catalogue of the Physiological Series of Comparative Anatomy,* a five-volume work that described the results of dissection of almost 4000 specimens. To obtain material for this work, he began dissecting animals that died in the gardens of the Zoological Society, a practice that would eventually lead to his identification of new "glandular bodies" in the neck.

It was also during this period that he became very interested in the study of fossils and evolutionary biology, an interest that would both cement his fame in popular history and lead to his academic downfall.

On the Evolution of Natural History

Owen had become very interested in fossilized remains and natural history through his museum work, and by the mid-1830s was one of the world's foremost authorities on osteology, comparative anatomy, and extinct species. In 1842, he published his *Report on British Fossil Reptiles,* in which he proposed the name "Dinosauria" to classify a distinct group of extinct reptiles, and supervised the creation of life-sized models of these creatures for public display at the Crystal Palace, the world's largest glass building, in 1855. He would go on to describe a number of extinct species, including the giant moa and Archaeopteryx, the first known fossilized link between reptiles and birds.

Conflicts over administrative duties at the Royal College of Surgeons led Owen to move to the British Museum in 1856, where he became superintendent of the Natural History Department [1]. He pushed parliament to establish a separate British Museum of Natural History (now known as the Natural History Museum), which was opened in 1881. Museums before this time had been primarily a repository of specimens for scientific research. Owen's revolutionary vision was to create a place of public education, where displays were arranged by subject matter and featured specimens that would most easily convey natural history to the general public [1].

In addition to forever changing the concept of museum design and function, Owen made significant contributions to evolutionary biology. Through his work on comparative vertebrate anatomy, Owen developed the concept of evolutionary homology, whereby structurally similar parts of different species result from the evolutionary differentiation of a corresponding part in a shared ancestor.

Owen believed that the presence of anatomical homologies (such as vertebrate limbs) supported his evolutionary concept of archetypes. He defined his ancestral archetypes as ideas in the mind of the creator, who could foresee all potential modifications of that archetype. Each archetype produced a series of species related by anatomical homologies. Though he initially thought that species were fixed and unchangeable, each uniquely designed by God to be perfectly adapted to its environment and lifestyle, his later anatomical work caused him to concede that species could emerge from an archetype through the influence of divine laws which guided their evolution [4].

1000 Guineas and a Sixpenny Piece

Owen's passion for vertebrate anatomy and his comprehensive examination techniques made him the most popular recipient of exotic animal specimens in the world. He dissected thousands of creatures, and performed dissections of animals that died while housed at the London Zoological Society. These dissections were performed in his house, and often took weeks or months to complete, much to the displeasure of his wife [5].

In 1834, the Zoological Society purchased a great Indian rhinoceros for 1000 guineas (approximately US$ 82,000 today) [6]. When the animal died in November 1849, Owen took the next several months to perform careful dissection of the creature and prepare specimens for preservation. He was excited about the dissection, writing to one of his sisters:

> Amongst other matters time-devouring, and putting out of memory mundane relatives, sisters included, has been the decease of my ponderous and respectable old friend…the rhinoceros…. His anatomy will furnish forth an immortal 'Monograph', and so comfort comes to me in a shape in which it cannot be had by any of my brother Fellows. [5]

The results of his dissection were communicated to the Zoological Society in 1850 and were first published on March 2, 1852 [5, 7]. However, the results are most easily available as part of a four-volume series in the Zoological Society's *Transactions,* which was released over a 10-year period and assigned a final publication date of 1862 [5, 7]. In his 27-page monograph, *On the anatomy of the Indian Rhinoceros,* Owen records in a single sentence during the description of the thyroid gland:

Fig. 1 Specimen of Owen's dissection of the rhinoceros larynx, with the *arrow* indicating the location of the parathyroid gland. (Reprinted with permission from Modarari et al. [12]. Courtesy of the Hunterian Museum at the Royal College of Surgeons of England)

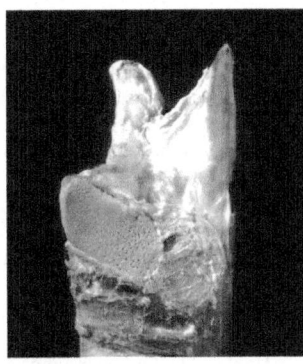

The structure of this body is more distinctly lobular than is usually seen; a small compact yellow glandular body was attached to the thyroid at the point where the veins emerge. [7]

This represents the earliest description of the mammalian parathyroid gland, and the specimen is still housed at the Museum of the Royal College of Surgeons (Fig. 1) [5]. Owen could not have predicted the presence of this gland, so its discovery, partially embedded in the thyroid gland and estimated to be the size of a sixpenny piece (approximately 19 mm), speaks to the thorough nature of his technique and his keen eye for anatomic novelty [5]. Though he did not name this structure, and certainly could not have known its function, he thought it curious and distinct enough to report a second time in 1868 [8]. These structures would be rediscovered in 1877 during a canine dissection by Ivor Sandström, and named the *glandulae parathyroidea*.

Evolution to Extinction

As brilliant, observant, novel, and prolific as he was, many of Owen's "discoveries" unfortunately appear to have been reports of others' findings that were not initially widely published, often with no mention of the original discovery and no acknowledgement of the original source. A spectacular example of this involves his relationship with Gideon Mantell, another naturalist, over the classification and publication of extinct species of giant reptiles. Mantell had discovered many of the earliest known species, but it was Owen who coined the term "dinosauria" and who presented many of the discoveries as his own, with no credit to Mantell. He continued to attack Mantell's scientific credibility and suppress publication of his works until Mantell died, at which time his spine was removed, preserved, and placed in the Royal College of Surgeons' museum under Owen's supervision [9].

Owen was not only frequently accused of plagiarism but also of reproduction and republication of his own previous works, most often without updating the manuscripts to reflect advancements in scientific knowledge since their original publication. This led to some of his later works being perceived as erroneous, which further damaged his scientific reputation [1]. This practice of "double publication" also

makes it difficult to determine the exact date of many of his scientific discoveries [1]. The final blow to Owen's reign as England's premier anatomist, however, came from his very public battles with Darwin and his supporters over the novel concept of natural selection.

Fresh from his voyage on the Beagle, Charles Darwin first met Owen in 1836 when he brought the preeminent anatomist fossils from South America to examine. The two remained cordial for over 20 years, but the evolutionary theories Darwin outlined in *On the Origin of Species* (and possibly Darwin's omission of Owen's own theories from the work) in 1859 seemed to greatly anger Owen.

Though Owen never clearly and completely articulated an independent theory of evolution, he did believe that it must be a divinely ordained process. In an anonymous review of *On the Origin of Species,* universally credited to Owen, the author states that he could not accept the concept of a "selective force exerted by outward circumstances [1]." In particular, Owen vehemently denied that humans could be descended from apes. In support of his position, Owen touted both differences in relative sizes of ape and humans brains as well as the absence of certain structures (primarily the hippocampus minor) in ape brains to prove Darwin and his supporters wrong. Owen's public denouncements of Darwin's theories greatly angered Thomas Huxley, another anatomist and ardent Darwin supporter. Huxley and Owen engaged in a very public battle of personal and scientific integrity, with Huxley ultimately proving the similarities between ape and human brains [10] and winning the war in both the halls of science and the court of public opinion.

Owen retired from active practice at the museum in 1883, but he continued to publish until 1888. He spent his retirement in the company of his grandchildren and documenting findings from his cottage gardens until his death on December 18, 1892.

History is written by the victors, and while many of Owen's original works are available for review in archives, most of what was written about him was published posthumously by Darwin's supporters. While there seems to be little disagreement that he was a man who did not shy from controversy and confrontation, he was likely not the scientific villain he is sometimes characterized to be [2]. Rather, Owen tried to fit the findings of the natural world and fossil record into the religious and social framework of his time, efforts that may have prevented him from appreciating what the evidence was really telling. Additionally, the world was a complex, rapidly changing place during Owen's later career; the animosity afforded him by critics like Huxley may have stemmed as much from a new generation of scientists trying to establish their reputations and ethos as from Owen's own scientific misconceptions and transgressions [11]. Owen's reputation has improved in recent decades, as many contemporary scholars of Victorian paleontology have found sympathy for his complex position [2, 11]. Despite efforts during his time to discredit him, Owen will always be remembered as the man who brought us to the museum, showed us the dinosaurs, and found the parathyroid gland.

References

1. Flower WH. Owen, Richard (1804–1892). In: Lee S, editor. Dictionary of national biography, vol 42. London: Smith, Elder; 1895. p. 1885–900.
2. Rupke N. Richard Owen: biology without Darwin, a revised edition. Chicago: The University of Chicago Press; 2009.
3. Eminent persons. Biographies reprinted from The Times, vol V. London: Macmillan; 1896. p. 1891–2.
4. Carter R. Sir Richard Owen: the archetypal villain [Internet]. c2001 [cited 2014 Mar 3]. http://friendsofdarwin.com/articles/owen/. Accessed 3 Mar 2014.
5. Cave AJE. Richard Owen and the discovery of the parathyroid glands. In: Underwood EA, editor. Science, medicine and history, essays of the evolution of scientific thought and medical practice, written in honour of Charles Singer, vol 2. London: Oxford University Press; 1953. p. 217–22.
6. Nordenström J. The hunt for the parathyroids. Oxford: Wiley; 2013.
7. Owen R. On the anatomy of the Indian Rhinoceros (Rh. Unicornis, L.). Trans Zool Soc Lond. 1862;4:31–58.
8. Owen R. The anatomy of vertebrates, vol III. London: Longmans, Green; 1868.
9. Fairbank JCT. William Adams and the spine of Gideon Algernon Mantell. Ann R Coll Surg Engl. 2004;86:349–52.
10. Huxley TH. On the brain of Ateles Paniscus. PZS of London, Part I.1861;247–60.
11. Desmond AJ. Archetypes and ancestors: palaeontology in Victorian London, 1850–1875. London: Blond & Briggs; 1982.
12. Modarari B, Sawyer A, Ellis H. The glands of Owen. J R Soc Med. 2004;97:494–5.

Fuller Albright

1900–1969

Angela L. Carrelli and Shonni J. Silverberg

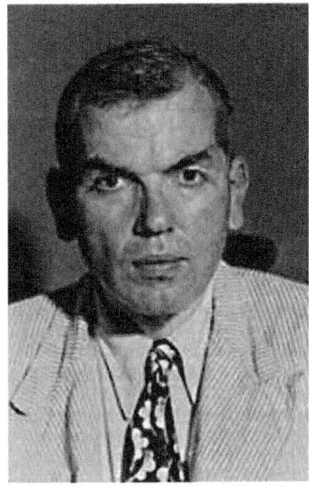

Fuller Albright. (Photograph from March/April 1970 edition of the Harvard Medical Alumni Bulletin)

Fuller Albright was a giant in the field of endocrinology who made landmark contributions to the understanding of many diverse conditions, including postmenopausal osteoporosis, gonadal function, and Cushing's syndrome [1]. However, he is best known for his investigation of calcium metabolism, the primary focus of his earlier career.

Albright was born in Buffalo, NY, on January 12, 1900. He attended Harvard College, followed by Harvard Medical School in 1921, and then completed his medical training in Internal Medicine at The Massachusetts General Hospital. Albright was mentored by Dr. Joseph Aub, a clinical scientist in endocrinology [1]. Between 1928 and 1929, Albright spent 1 year in Vienna studying under the pathologist Dr. Jacob Erdheim, who was credited with establishing the re-

lationship between the parathyroid glands and calcium homeostasis [1]. It may have been during this time that Albright developed his interest in calcium metabolism.

In 1944, Dr. Albright gave the presidential address at the annual meeting of the American Society for Clinical Investigation [2]. He discussed the difficulties of clinical investigation, which he described as "trying to ride two horses—attempting to be an investigator and a clinician at one and the same time." He warned of the "danger on one side that he, as a clinician, be swamped with patients" versus the danger that "he, as an investigator, be segregated entirely from the bedside." Dr. Albright attained success as a clinical investigator by skillfully combining these two roles. In his lifetime, he had 118 scientific publications and was credited with being the first to describe 19 new syndromes or disease manifestations [3].

Dr. Albright offered advice for success in combining practice and the laboratory in his cartoon, which he titled "The Do's and Do-Not's along the road leading to the castle of success in clinical investigation" (Fig. 1) [2, 4]. His list of the ten "Do's" included not only "measure something…make charts…[and] interpret data" but also such key elements as "look from all sides…[and] backing without strings." Importantly, his "Don't" list admonished against being "fooled by numbers" or a "slave to theory." Albright followed these precepts dutifully. Upon his return to the Massachusetts General Hospital in 1929, he began work in the clinical investigation of calcium metabolism. He conducted experiments involving detailed measurements of dietary intake and urinary and fecal output to clarify metabolic pathways [1]. Dr. Albright understood the importance of precise measurements in clinical investigation. His meticulous calcium balance studies shed light on then little known pathways involved in calcium and phosphate metabolism, and on the effects of parathyroid hormone. Albright's accomplishments are even more impressive, given the resources available for his studies in the 1920s. His investigations were limited to the measurement of calcium and phosphorus in blood, urine, and feces, and the use of a parathyroid hormone extract [5]. Assays for mea-

S. J. Silverberg (✉) · A. L. Carrelli
Department of Medicine, Columbia University
College of Physicians & Surgeons, 630 W. 168th St,
PH 8W-864, New York, NY 10032, USA
e-mail: sjs5@cumc.columbia.edu

J. L. Pasieka, J. A. Lee (eds.), *Surgical Endocrinopathies*, DOI 10.1007/978-3-319-13662-2_22,
© Springer International Publishing Switzerland 2015

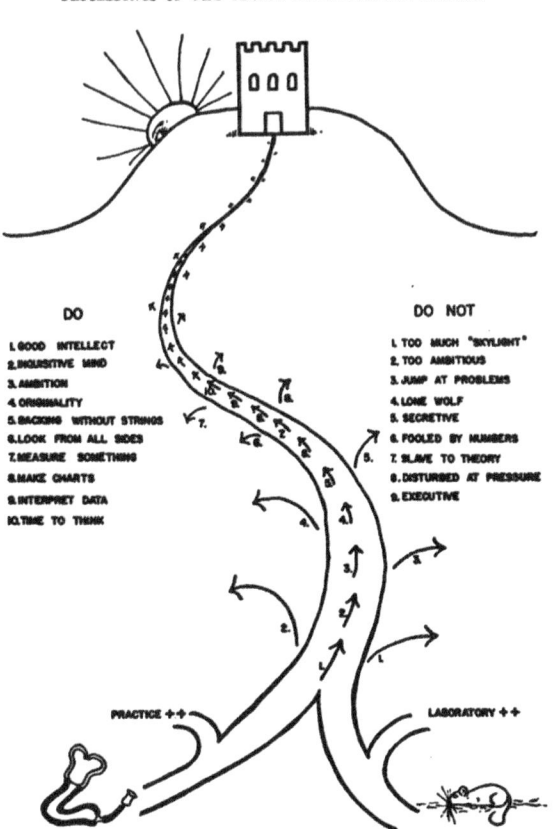

Fig. 1 Fuller Albright's "Do's and Do Nots" for a successful career in clinical investigation. (From [2]. Reprinted with permission from American Society for Clinical Investigation)

these events, and showed that parathyroid hormone effects were evident within the first hour.

In another paper in the series, the effect of parathyroid hormone was explored in normal subjects [8]. Similar techniques were employed as in the prior study. Patients were admitted and maintained on a low-calcium diet. Measurements of calcium and phosphate intake and output were conducted over several days and the response to an infusion of parathyroid hormone extract assessed. The observations were similar: parathyroid hormone increased serum calcium levels, increased urinary calcium and phosphorus excretion, and lowered serum phosphorus levels. They did note that with significant hypercalcemia, a rise in phosphorus can be seen.

Dr. Albright later went on to apply these observations to patients with primary hyperparathyroidism. One of the earliest and surely the best-known cases of primary hyperparathyroidism involved the patient Captain Martell (Fig. 2). The picture highlights the dramatic effect of untreated primary hyperparathyroidism on the skeleton over the course of a decade. Fuller Albright played a key role in the studies on this patient, the results of which provided invaluable insight into the pathophysiology of primary hyperparathyroidism. Captain Martell first presented to Bellevue Hospital in New York City in January 1926 with loss of height and fractures [9]. In 1918, he was a 6-ft 1-in. merchant mariner. Over the course of the year, he lost height and developed a protruding chest. He also complained of muscle weakness and frequent "thick

surement of parathyroid hormone had not yet been developed nor would they be until the work of Berson and Yalow 40 years later [5, 6].

In a series of papers entitled "Studies on the physiology of the parathyroid glands," Dr. Albright and his colleagues described the results of their detailed metabolism studies. One of the papers focused on a case of hypoparathyroidism [7]. Dr. Albright admitted a young man with presumed idiopathic hypoparathyroidism. The report charts measurements for every 8 hours of the 27-day study period. Fluid intake and output were reported along with calcium and phosphorus intake and output. Parathyroid hormone was administered to the patient four times. Dr. Albright and his coinvestigator, Dr. Read Ellsworth, observed that administration of parathyroid hormone led to an increase in serum calcium and a decline in serum phosphorus, and an increase in urinary phosphorus excretion. There was an initial decrease in urinary calcium excretion, followed by a sudden increase in excretion (once the serum calcium level reached approximately 8.5 mg/dL) [7]. Further experiments, with data collection every hour, were conducted to better elucidate the exact time course of

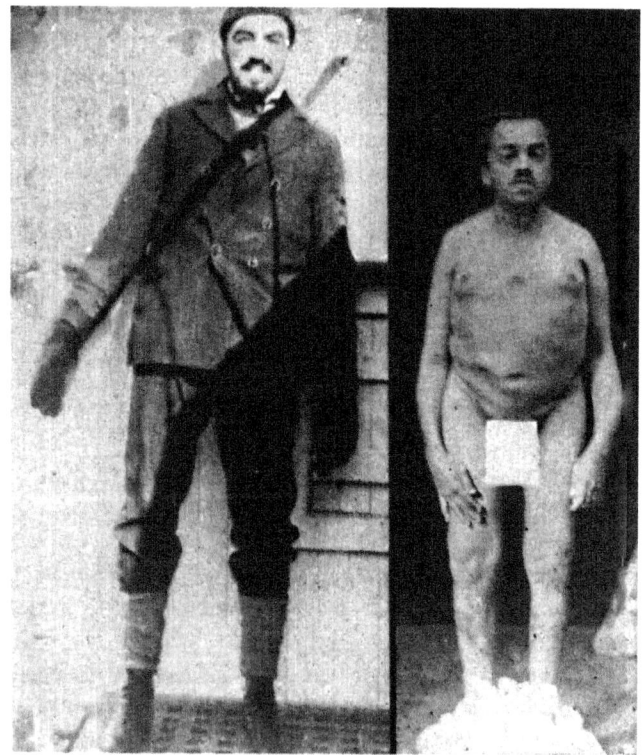

Fig. 2 Patient Captain Martell. (From [9]. Licensed content date 1969. Reprinted with permission from The Endocrine Society)

white gravel" in his urine [10]. By 1926, at age 30, he was 5'6" with the marked kyphosis shown in the right panel of Fig. 2, and he had suffered multiple fractures. He was hospitalized for over 2 months. Testing confirmed an elevated serum calcium, and metabolic studies confirmed excessive calcium excretion, well beyond his intake. Based on prior studies on the effects of administering parathyroid hormone to dogs, hyperparathyroidism was suspected. Dr. Albright noted that "the tentative diagnosis of an overproduction of parathyroid hormone (hyperparathyroidism) was made for the first time in this hemisphere, for the second time in the world" [9]. The patient was referred to Massachusetts General Hospital, where he was first under the care of Dr. Aub and Dr. Bauer, and later Dr. Albright. In 1948, when discussing this case, Albright noted that he did not mention his own name along with those of Aub and Bauer, not "because of modesty" but because he joined Dr. Aub's group after the diagnosis was established [9]. While this may be true, it was Albright's further metabolic studies that were instrumental in expanding the understanding of primary hyperparathyroidism.

In a paper entitled "A case of osteitis fibrosa cystica (osteomalacia?)" with evidence of hyperactivity of the parathyroid bodies," Albright and his colleagues demonstrated that Captain Martell's calcium metabolism, while on a low calcium diet, was similar both "qualitatively and quantitatively" to that of normal subjects receiving parathyroid hormone extract [11]. They concluded that Captain Martell's calcium and phosphorus metabolism was the same as that of normal subjects receiving large doses of **Collip's** extract or parathyroid hormone. Captain Martell went on to have two surgeries to remove two parathyroid glands. Although he was not cured, the metabolic studies described above led Dr. Albright and colleagues to conclude that he did in fact have hyperparathyroidism. The monograph included multiple X-rays of various bones to help characterize the bone disease associated with primary hyperparathyroidism known as osteitis fibrosa cystica. They noted the "mottled" appearance of the skull, generalized "decalcification and coarse trabeculation" in his hands, thinning of the cortex of bones in his shoulder, and the presence of "cysts" in his bones. These features characterize the impact of classic primary hyperparathyroidism on the skeleton. Captain Martell ultimately underwent six unsuccessful surgeries. His seventh parathyroid exploration was successful in finding a parathyroid tumor behind his sternum, but Captain Martell died shortly thereafter [9].

In 1934, Dr. Albright published a seminal case series detailing 17 patients with proven hyperparathyroidism, the largest case series of hyperparathyroidism at that time [12]. He wrote that the purpose of the paper was to clarify the early symptoms of the disease and an approach to its diagnosis. The paper carefully details expected findings, including blood and urinary calcium and phosphorus levels, skeletal and renal imaging, as well as clinical features including the presence of kidney stones. It went on to describe the surgical approach to primary hyperparathyroidism, detailing location and size of the parathyroid adenomas removed, and the "extraordinary" improvement in patients' symptoms following surgery. They also described the risk of postoperative hypoparathyroidism. Through careful study of these patients, they were able to provide one of the earliest and most comprehensive descriptions of classic primary hyperparathyroidism and its effects on the skeleton and kidney.

While this initial case series included mention of hyperparathyroidism due to four-gland hyperplasia, he expanded on this topic a few years later, after having seen six cases of four-gland disease [13]. Dr. Albright and his colleagues (including **Oliver Cope**) concluded that surgery with removal of all parathyroid tissue except "about 200 mg" can lead to a permanent cure, although they acknowledged that the appropriate amount of parathyroid tissue that should be left in place was not yet clear. In 1948, Albright and colleagues published "*The Parathyroid Glands and Metabolic Bone Disease: Selected Studies,*" a book that collects in one place his landmark work on parathyroid gland health and disease. It remained an important resource for many years.

Dr. Albright's understanding of calcium metabolism enabled him to make many other important discoveries in this area. For example, he is credited with first hypothesizing that ectopic hormone production was the cause of the hypercalcemia of malignancy [4]. At a conference in 1941, the case of a 51-year-old man with hypercalcemia and hypophosphatemia was presented. The man underwent a failed parathyroid surgery and was ultimately found to have bony metastasis from renal cell carcinoma. Radiation treatment of his tumor resulted in normalization of serum calcium and phosphorus. Dr. Albright hypothesized that the tumor was producing parathyroid hormone (PTH) [4, 14]. An early assay for PTH was negative. Although this result may be explained by inadequate assay technology, we now know that the hypercalcemia in this patient was due to PTH-related peptide. Albright's concept of ectopic hormone production as the cause was accurate.

Dr. Albright's contributions span multiple different areas of endocrinology. For example, in 1937, he was the first to describe the condition now known as McCune–Albright. Another disease that he described and now carries his name is Albright hereditary osteodystrophy [1]. It was also he who hypothesized that estrogen deficiency plays a key role in the development of postmenopausal osteoporosis [1].

Around 1936, Dr. Albright first noted a hand tremor and soon after he was diagnosed with Parkinson's disease [4]. His disease progressed, and by 1940 he had trouble with writing, followed by gait difficulty. He required assistance with many daily tasks. In the early 1950s, he began to complain of intellectual deficits. He sought treatment from a neurosurgeon, Dr. Irving Cooper, regarding a chemopallidectomy for Parkinson's disease. Although Dr. Cooper and Dr. Albright's other physicians advised him against surgery, he ultimately decided to proceed and underwent a right-sided procedure in June 1956. His symptoms improved immediately postoperatively; however, on the third postoperative day, he had an acute hemorrhage [3]. He was left in a nonfunctional vegetative state until his death in December 1969, at age 69 [1]. While Fuller Albright is remembered as a giant in the field of calcium metabolism as well as for his many other contributions to the field of endocrinology, he is also remembered for his courage in the face of a disabling disease and, as his friend Dr. Henneman wrote, for his "constant sense of gentle humor" [3, 4].

References

1. Kleeman CR, Levine BS, Felsenfeld AJ. Fuller albright: the consummate clinical investigator. Clin J Am Soc Nephrol: CJASN. 2009;4(10):1541–6. doi:10.2215/CJN.03030509.
2. Albright F. Proceedings of the Thirty-Sixth Annual Meeting of the American Society for Clinical Investigation Held in Atlantic City, NJ, May 8, 1044. J Clin Invest. 1944;23(6):921–52.
3. Henneman PH. Fuller Albright, M.D. 1900–1969. Metabolism. 1970;19(3):187–8.
4. Axelrod L. Bones, stones and hormones: the contributions of Fuller Albright. New Engl J Med. 1970;283(18):964–70. doi:10.1056/NEJM197010292831805.
5. Felsenfeld AJ, Levine BS, Kleeman CR. Fuller Albright and our current understanding of calcium and phosphorus regulation and primary hyperparathyroidism. Nefrologia. 2011;31(3):346–57. doi:10.3265/Nefrologia.pre2011.Mar.10774.
6. Berson SA, Yalow RS, Aurbach GD, Potts JT Jr. Immunoassay of bovine and human parathyroid hormone. Proc Natl Acad Sci U S A. 1963;49:613–7.
7. Albright F, Ellsworth R. Studies on the physiology of the parathyroid glands: I. Calcium and phosphorus studies on a case of idiopathic hypoparathyroidism. J Clin Investig. 1929;7(2):183–201. doi:10.1172/JCI100224.
8. Albright F, Bauer W, Ropes M, Aub JC. Studies of calcium and phosphorus metabolism: IV. The effect of the parathyroid hormone. J Clin Investig. 1929;7(1):139–81. doi:10.1172/JCI100218.
9. Albright F. A page out of the history of hyperparathyroidism. J Clin Endocrinol Metab. 1948;8(8):637–57. doi:10.1210/jcem-8-8-637.
10. Hannon RR, Shorr E, McClellan WS, Dubois EF. A case of osteitis fibrosa cystica (osteomalacia?) with evidence of hyperactivity of the para-thyroid bodies. Metabolic study I. J Clin Investig. 1930;8(2):215–27. doi:10.1172/JCI100261.
11. Bauer W, Albright F, Aub JC. A case of osteitis fibrosa cystica (osteomalacia?) with evidence of hyperactivity of the para-thyroid bodies. Metabolic study II. J Clin Invest. 1930;8(2):229–48. doi:10.1172/JCI100262.
12. Albright F, Aub J, Bauer W. Hyperparathyroidism: a common and polymorphic condition as illustrated by seventeen proved cases from one clinic. JAMA. 1934;102(16):1276–87.
13. Albright F, Sulkowitch HW, Bloomberg E. Hyperparathyroidism due to idiopathic hypertrophy (hyperplasia?) of parathyroid tissue. Arch Intern Med. 1938;62(2):199–215. doi:10.001/archinte.1938.0018030020002.
14. Case 27461. In: TB Mallory, editor. N Engl J Med. 1941;225:789–91. doi:10.1056/NEJM194111132252007.

James Bertram Collip

1892–1965

David A. Hanley

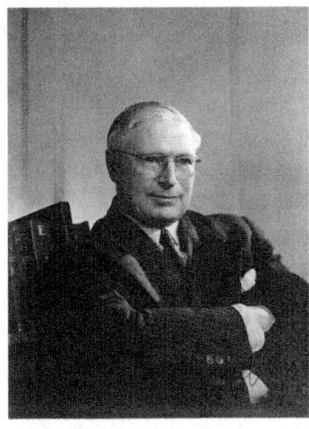

J. B. Collip as Dean of Medicine, in his office at the University of Western Ontario, ca 1950s. (Photo used with permission from Western University, Western Archives, History of Medicine Collection, London, Ontario, Canada)

James Bertram (Bert) Collip was born in Belleville, Ontario, Canada, on November 20, 1892. He had a great interest in chemistry, and must have been an exceptional student, as he entered Trinity College of the University of Toronto at the age of 15. He apparently wanted to study medicine, but was too young to enter medical school. He therefore enrolled in the honours biochemistry and physiology degree program that allowed entry into the later medical years. He excelled there, inspired by A. B. Macallum, the first biochemistry professor in Canada. After graduating at the top of his class, Collip chose to pursue a graduate degree rather than medicine, receiving his PhD in 1916 for studies of hydrochloric acid production by the gastric epithelium (Fig. 1).

D. A. Hanley (✉)
Medicine, Oncology and Community Health Sciences,
Division of Endocrinology and Metabolism, University of Calgary,
Calgary, AB T2T5C7, Canada
e-mail: dahanley@ucalgary.ca

J. B. Collip at the University of Alberta

In 1915, Collip was offered a teaching and research lectureship position in biochemistry in the new medical school at the University of Alberta, in Edmonton. The position there made strong teaching demands on him, but Collip's research program quickly became very productive. He was promoted to assistant professor in 1917 and to associate professor 2 years later. He was also given the opportunity to visit other laboratories, and cultivate new areas of interest—a great start to a research career that was particularly notable for his ability to quickly move from one area of enquiry to another.

Following the First World War, the Rockefeller Foundation awarded large grants to enhance medical education in Canada. In late 1920, Collip received a Rockefeller Foundation Travelling Fellowship, which was to afford him a lengthy (15-month) sabbatical from teaching while he visited three prominent scientists' research laboratories to focus on the biochemistry and physiology of his two main interests: respiration and the "glands of internal secretion" (endocrinology). The initial plan for use of the award was to spend 6 months with Professor J. R. R. Macleod at the University of Toronto; 6 months with Professor D. O. van Slyke, at the Rockefeller Institute in New York; and 4 months with Sir Henry Dale at the National Institute for Medical Research in Hampstead. He chose to first visit Macleod's laboratory at the University of Toronto, to study the effect of acid–base balance on blood sugar. During this time, he met with **Dr. Frederick G. Banting** and **Mr. Charles H. Best** who had begun their studies in Macleod's laboratory, searching for the glucose-active hormone of the pancreas, and offered advice on blood glucose measurements for Banting's planned dog studies. The possibility of an offer of a faculty position at Toronto caused Collip to shorten his planned time in the USA so that he could return to Toronto for the 1921–1922 academic year. He did spend the summer of 1921 at the Centre for Marine Biology at Woods Hole and at the Rockefeller Institute, where he continued his studies of mollusc

J. L. Pasieka, J. A. Lee (eds.), *Surgical Endocrinopathies,* DOI 10.1007/978-3-319-13662-2_23,
© Springer International Publishing Switzerland 2015

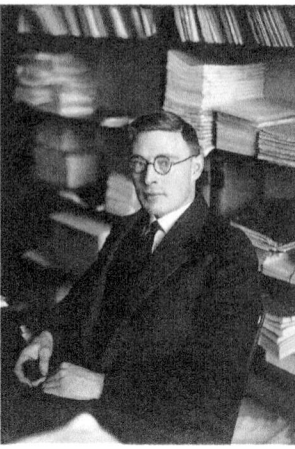

Fig. 1 James Bertram Collip—pioneer of Canadian endocrinology (1892–1965) around the time of his work on the parathyroids. Undated, but probably in the late 1920s, at University of Alberta or not too long after moving to McGill. (Photo used with permission from Western University, Western Archives, History of Medicine Collection, London, Ontario, Canada)

respiration and also acquired expertise in a newer method of blood glucose measurement.

Collip returned to Toronto in the fall of 1921, and the events that followed shaped the rest of his research career. He was invited to become involved in the work that Banting and Best were carrying out with pancreatectomized dogs. They had succeeded in preparing a pancreatic extract that lowered the blood sugar in these newly diabetic dogs. Collip helped the team show that the pancreatic extract increased glycogen stores, and showed that the extract lowered blood glucose in normal rabbits, allowing the establishment of a bioassay to calibrate the potency of the pancreatic extracts. Injections of large doses of the extracts were observed to cause fatal convulsions in the animals. It was Collip who shrewdly deduced that the cause of the convulsions was hypoglycaemia, and the animals could be rescued by glucose administration. Collip then set about improving the yield of insulin in the extraction process and did so by increasing the concentration of ethanol in the extraction solution. The highly purified extract was used in a successful clinical test in January 1922. For a short period of time, Collip lost his ability to purify the extract, as he had broken a biochemist's cardinal rule of keeping an accurate record of his methods, but eventually the technique was recovered. Successful clinical testing of the extracts continued, and a manufacturing agreement with Connaught Laboratories in Toronto and Eli Lilly and Company in Indianapolis allowed a rapid increase in the manufacturing capabilities of insulin, for which there was an immediate huge demand. The research group debated the ethics of whether they should apply for a patent, and finally decided to do so under the names of Collip and Best,

with the patent being assigned to the University of Toronto. The royalties from this patent were to provide significant research support to Collip's laboratory for many years afterward.

During much of his stay in Toronto, Collip was in negotiations with the University of Alberta regarding the nature of his appointment and remuneration there, and he used job offers from other centres as a bargaining chip. The negotiations continued through most of his stay in Toronto, but it was finally agreed that when he returned to the University of Alberta he would have a full professorship, the headship of the soon-to-be-formed Department of Biochemistry, and increased laboratory assistance. The results of the clinical testing of insulin were presented in May of 1922, at the Royal Society of Canada, and Collip returned to Edmonton shortly thereafter.

The discovery of insulin brought the Nobel Prize in Medicine to Banting and Macleod, and immediate fame to all members of the research team. Recognizing the potential clinical importance of glandular extracts, Collip switched his research focus away from respiration and molluscs. The desire to have a more clinical focus to his research probably contributed to his decision to complete a medical degree at the University of Alberta. Because of his PhD in biochemistry and physiology, he was only required to complete the final two clinical years of medicine, obtaining his MD in 1926. Amazingly, he completed these clinical training requirements, while carrying out some of his best research.

Shortly after the success with insulin, and before his work on the parathyroid hormone (PTH), Collip prepared an insulin-like extract from plants, which he named glucokinin. Despite an optimistic paper in the *Journal of Biological Chemistry* [1], and several follow-up studies, glucokinin failed to live up to his hopes. When toxicity problems became apparent, Collip abandoned this line of research in favour of studies of the parathyroid: the extraction of biologically active PTH, and the characterization of its major physiological effects on calcium metabolism.

Why did Collip choose the parathyroid and calcium as his next line of enquiry? His research career was characterized by major directional shifts, but this was not his first venture into calcium metabolism. Prior to his work on insulin in Toronto, in the course of his earlier studies of respiration, he had published experiments in which he correctly identified hypocalcemia as a cause of tetany [2]. Also, in the early twentieth century, hypoparathyroidism and its resultant tetany was becoming a fairly common and occasionally fatal medical complication of the increasing numbers of thyroidectomies performed for goitre, nodular thyroid disease, and hyperthyroidism. Collip's work on hospital wards as a part-time medical student undoubtedly kindled his interest in this important problem.

Considering the success of bovine pancreatic extracts in treating insulin deficiency, it was probably quite logical for Collip to consider a similar approach to the major problem of tetany post thyroidectomy. He soon prepared parathyroid tissue extracts, which he then used to clearly demonstrate the importance of the PTH in regulating extracellular fluid calcium concentrations. He tested his extract in thyroparathyroidectomized dogs, and showed it could prevent or treat tetany by raising the blood calcium [3]. There was an alternate theory for the aetiology of tetany, that the parathyroid was involved in guanidine metabolism and that tetany was the result of guanidine toxicity. However, Collip showed conclusively that the tetany associated with hypoparathyroidism was due to hypocalcaemia and not guanidine toxicity [4].

Unfortunately, although he probably thought so at the time he was doing his experiments, Collip was not the first to describe a biologically active extract from parathyroid tissue. Adolph Hanson, a physician working entirely on his own, had described a nearly identical extraction process, and had published his method in 1923 [5]. A rather bitter conflict arose over who had priority. As a very successful rising star in his field, Collip had a much wider audience for his presentations and publications in this area. Hanson's extract may not have been of as high quality as Collip's, but later patent rulings decided in his favour. For excellent and more detailed accounts of the development of parathyroid extracts, the battles for recognition, and the importance of these battles in the commercial manufacture of parathyroid extracts, the reader is referred to the excellent books by Alison Li [6] and Jörgen Nordenström [7], which I have used as resources for much of the information in this chapter.

Regardless of priority, Collip clearly had by far the best understanding of how to test the parathyroid extract, and he was able to present his findings at meetings of the major scientific societies of the time. He used his extract to make a number of significant advances in our understanding of parathyroid physiology. His extraction method led the way to refinements of the purification steps that allowed the complete amino acid sequencing of PTH 50 years later, and his extract was marketed by Eli Lilly and Company into the latter part of the twentieth century. In addition to clearly demonstrating the primary role of PTH in raising the blood calcium, and preventing tetany, he developed a bioassay/unit system for calibrating doses of the extract. He showed that overdosing dogs with the extract caused hypercalcemia and death [8]. Collip also made the astute observation that, in dogs made hypercalcaemic by large doses of the extract, temporary clinical improvement could be achieved by infusion of fluids: "It has been shown that overdosage phenomena deliberately produced in dogs are favourably influenced by intravenous saline or glucose but this treatment, though helpful, has by no means the virtues of an antidote" [9].

In **Fuller Albright's** presidential address to the annual meeting of the Association for the Study of Internal Secretions in 1947, he detailed the research trail leading to the first North American patient to have parathyroid surgery. He credited Collip's clear demonstration of the hypercalcaemic effects of excess PTH as being instrumental in the decision to proceed with neck surgery in hopes of curing Captain Martell's hyperparathyroidism. As Albright said in his discussion of the preparation of a biologically active extract of parathyroid tissue, "…But Collip did not stop there. The inquiring mind always goes on…" [10].

Collip believed the major effect of PTH was on bone. Later, when Collip had moved to head the biochemistry department at McGill University and had assembled an outstanding research team, his colleague and collaborator, Dr. Hans Selye, performed histologic studies clearly demonstrating the anabolic effect of PTH on bone [11]. This observation seems to have been ignored for many years, but now PTH and its biologically active analogue, teriparatide, are utilized in the treatment of osteoporosis.

By the mid-1920s, Collip was recognized as an outstanding endocrine researcher. In 1925, he was elected president of the Association for the Study of Internal Secretions, which later became the Endocrine Society. His work with PTH cemented his stature in the field, and he received offers to join the Mayo Clinic and McGill University. The offer from McGill was to head the Department of Biochemistry, replacing his mentor, Professor A. B. Macallum, who had wanted to retire from administrative duties. Collip decided in favour of McGill and left the University of Alberta in 1928.

J.B. Collip at McGill University

Collip joined McGill at a time when there was strong support for developing the basic medical sciences in order to regain the prestige McGill had enjoyed in the days of William Osler. His recruitment most certainly met this goal. The medical school constructed a new building for biological sciences, and Collip was given ample space and facilities to expand his research program. His royalties from insulin came with him to McGill and continued to enhance his ability to fund research. McGill supported recruitment to his department, and an important addition was Dr. David Thomson, who collaborated in research, and perhaps more importantly, took on much of the teaching duties, freeing Collip to focus more on research. Collip was able to recruit a number of prominent scientists into the research group, perhaps most notably Hans Selye, and outstanding graduate students such as J. S. L. Browne, who went on to an illustrious career in clinical endocrine research and leadership of the Medical Research Council of Canada.

The 1930s were probably Collip's most productive research years. The work with PTH continued, but initial new research focus was on hormones that could be extracted from the placenta. His laboratory developed two extracts that generated commercial interest. The most important was an oestrogen-like compound they called Emmenin, which was active when taken orally, and with the collaboration of a local pharmaceutical company, Ayerst, McKenna and Harrison, became an important oral oestrogen preparation for clinical use. Emmenin was eventually to be replaced by the more potent oestrogenic agent, Premarin, but was a significant source of royalties, which further aided Collip's research team. The other was an anterior pituitary-like extract which they called APL, and had actions similar to pituitary gonadotropins. Selye proved to be an expert in preparing hypophysectomized rats, which allowed the research group to test APL's effects on gonadal function.

The work with Emmenin and APL facilitated the McGill group's exploration of the hormones of the pituitary gland. Over the decade of the 1930s, the research team, led by Collip and Selye, was able to refine pituitary extracts to obtain reasonably pure components representing growth hormone, thyroid-stimulating hormone (TSH) and adrenocorticotropic hormone (ACTH), which they were able to test in their abundant supply of hypophysectomized rats. During the middle to latter part of the decade, Collip endeavoured to create an institute of endocrine research, similar to Wilder Penfield's Montreal Neurological Institute, but these efforts failed. Toward the end of the decade, the team began to go separate ways, with Selye and Collip disagreeing on the direction the research should take. Selye left the group and joined the Department of Anatomy at McGill in 1941, while Collip left the Department of Biochemistry to take up a new endowed position as the Gilman Cheney Chair of Endocrinology and the head of McGill's new Research Institute of Endocrinology.

As his success grew, so did the demands on Collip's time away from the laboratory. In 1938, he began work with the Canadian National Research Council's Associate Committee on Medical Research, the forerunner of the Medical Research Council of Canada (now the Canadian Institutes of Health Research). This group was chaired by Frederick Banting, and after Banting's death in 1941, Collip replaced him as chairman. The same year, his responsibilities at McGill expanded as he was appointed director of the McGill Institute of Endocrinology. During the Second World War, Collip supervised medical war research at the National Research Council. This included activities such as working to improve the production of the newly discovered penicillin. In 1946, he became the first director of the Division of Medical Research of the National Research Council, a position he held until 1957.

J. B. Collip at the University of Western Ontario

In 1947, Collip was offered the position of Dean of Medicine and head of the Department of Medical Research at the University of Western Ontario (now Western University) in London, which he accepted. During his tenure as dean, the research facilities and activity at Western expanded. His research assistant, Arthur Long, who had been with him since the early 1920s in Edmonton and had come with him to McGill, also followed him to administer the Collip laboratory in London. Others, like Dr. Robert Noble, also followed him to London—a testament to the kind of loyalty Collip could inspire. At Western, Collip did not return to "the bench" himself, but provided leadership and counsel to his younger colleagues. After his retirement as Dean of Medicine in 1961, he continued as head of the Department of Medical Research. He unfortunately did not have a long retirement, passing away shortly after suffering a stroke in 1965.

Collip received many honours during his lifetime. He received 12 honorary degrees from universities in the UK, Canada and the USA. He was made a Commander of the Order of the British Empire in 1943, and for his work as medical liaison officer to Washington during the Second World War, he was awarded the Medal of Freedom with Silver Palm by the US government in 1947. He was nominated for a Nobel Prize six times between 1928 and 1951. His best chance for winning a Nobel Prize was probably for his work with PTH, but the controversy surrounding the assignment of whose extract had priority undoubtedly worked against his candidacy. As a researcher, he was described as someone who went after the big problems, and after grasping the early answers, he would move on to another area of interest, leaving the sorting out of the details to others. His legacy, however, was huge. The four Canadian universities where he carried out his research benefitted tremendously from his presence, while he was there, and he made a lasting contribution to the establishment of a system of government-supported medical research in Canada. In the 1960s, at the entrance to the then-new medical building at the University of Western Ontario is the following tribute to Dr. Collip: "Pioneer in the Biochemistry of the Endocrine System and Dean of the Faculty of Medicine 1947–61. To this great Canadian, in recognition of outstanding service to medical science and the welfare of mankind, the research laboratories of this building are affectionately dedicated."

Acknowledgment In preparing this chapter, I was greatly assisted by having read three excellent works of medical history referenced below: Alison Li's outstanding book on Collip that arose out of her PhD thesis [7]; Jörgen Nordenström's parathyroid history [7] and Professor Michael Bliss' immensely readable history of the discovery of insulin [12]. The two photographs are used with permission from Western University, Western Archives, History of Medicine Collection, London, Ontario, Canada.

References

1. Collip JB. Glucokinin. a new hormone present in plant tissue: preliminary paper. J Biol Chem. 1923;56:513–43.

2. Collip JB. The significance of the calcium-ion in the cell-experimental tetany. Can Med Assoc J. 1920;10(10):935–7.

3. Collip JB. The extraction of a parathyroid hormone which will prevent or control parathyroid tetany and which regulates the level of blood calcium. J Biol Chem. 1925;63:395–438.

4. Collip JB, Clark EP. Concerning the relation of guanidine to parathyroid tetany. J Biol Chem. 1926;67:679–87.

5. Hanson AM. Notes on the hydrochloric x of the bovine parathyroid. Military Surgeon. 1923;53:424.

6. Li AI-S. J.B. Collip and the development of medical research in Canada: extracts and expertise. Montreal: McGill-Queen's University Press; 2003.

7. Nordenström J. The hunt for the parathyroids. Chichester. Wiley; 2013.

8. Collip JB, Clark EP. Further studies on the physiological action of a parathyroid hormone. J Biol Chem. 1925;64:485–507.

9. Collip JB. Clinical use of the parathyroid hormone. Can Med Assoc J. 1925;15(11):1158.

10. Albright F. A page out of the history of hyperparathyroidism. J Clin Endocrinol. 1948;8(8):637–57.

11. Pugsley LI, Selye H. The histological changes in the bone responsible for the action of parathyroid hormone on the calcium metabolism of the rat. J Physiol. 1933;79(1):113–7.

12. Bliss M. The discovery of insulin. Toronto: University of Toronto Press; 1982.

Surgical Management of Hyperparathyroidism

Jacob Moalem and Daniel T. Ruan

Indications for Parathyroidectomy

Parathyroidectomy is indicated for the surgical treatment of many patients with primary, secondary, or tertiary hyperparathyroidism (HPT). Considerable controversy exists regarding the appropriateness of surgery in patients with asymptomatic disease and even regarding the definition of the term "asymptomatic" in this context [1]. With careful questioning, the vast majority of patients with "asymptomatic" primary HPT will report symptoms directly attributable to their disease. Nevertheless, three separate consensus conferences over the past 20 years have largely understated many of the constitutional symptoms known to derive from primary HPT. Not surprisingly, these consensus conferences understated the benefits of parathyroidectomy when they created guidelines for mandatory surgical referral. In the most recent edition of the guidelines for management of patients with asymptomatic primary hyperaparathyroidism [2], only young age (less than 50 years), serum calcium level higher than 1 mg/dL above the upper limit of normal, creatinine clearance less than 60 mL/min, osteoporosis at any site or a previous fracture, and nephrolithiasis were absolute indications for parathyroidectomy.

Unfortunately, these guidelines are often inappropriately used as criteria for referral for parathyroidectomy in symptomatic patients. As a result, many symptomatic patients who might benefit from surgery, but do not meet any of the criteria above, are not referred for surgical consultation. Interestingly, the first line in the consensus manuscript states that "all patients with biochemically confirmed primary hyperparathyroidism who have specific symptoms or signs of their disease should undergo surgical treatment." Additionally, the statement that "surgery is also indicated in patients for whom medical surveillance is neither desired and nor possible" is also often missed. Because of the low surgical morbidity, the high cure rate, the lack of acceptable nonsurgical alternatives, and the improvement in quality of life that most patients realize following parathyroidectomy, many surgeons consider surgery a reasonable option for asymptomatic primary HPT. In our view, the decision to withhold parathyroidectomy should only be made following a detailed discussion of the risks and benefits of the procedure, and therefore should not be made without surgical consultation.

The indications for parathyroidectomy in patients with secondary HPT or tertiary HPT are even less clear. According to the most recent edition of the National Kidney Foundation's consensus statement [3], patients with stage 5D chronic kidney disease (CKD; on dialysis) should maintain their intact parathyroid hormone (PTH) levels in the range of approximately two to nine times the upper limit of normal using a combination of calcitriol, vitamin D analogues, and calcimimetics (recommendations 4.2.3 and 4.2.4). In patients with CKD who fail to respond to pharmacologic therapy, parathyroidectomy is suggested. Other indications for surgery in secondary HPT include renal osteodystrophy, diffuse musculoskeletal pain, calciphylaxis, a calcium × phosphorus product greater than 70, and unrelenting pruritus.

Preoperative Preparation

Biochemical Studies

Surgeons should carefully review the biochemical study results for HPT. As described in detail in Chap. 20, the diagnosis is made by demonstrating inappropriately high PTH level relative to a simultaneously drawn serum calcium level. It is not rare for patients with nonrenal secondary HPT

J. Moalem (✉)
Endocrine Surgery and Endocrinology, Surgery Department, University of Rochester, Rochester, NY, USA
e-mail: Jacob_Moalem@URMC.Rochester.edu

D. T. Ruan
General and GI Surgery, Brigham and Women's Hospital, Boston, MA, USA
Endocrine Surgery, Harvard Medical School, Boston, MA, USA

J. L. Pasieka, J. A. Lee (eds.), *Surgical Endocrinopathies*, DOI 10.1007/978-3-319-13662-2_24,
© Springer International Publishing Switzerland 2015

to be erroneously referred for parathyroidectomy, and it is the surgeon's responsibility to ensure that the preoperative diagnosis is accurate. In our own center, we found that 20 % of patients who were referred for parathyroidectomy were misdiagnosed and did not require surgery. More than half of those patients already had imaging studies that were often falsely positive [4].

Imaging

Once the biochemical diagnosis of primary HPT is confirmed, and the patient is considered to be a candidate for surgery, most surgeons obtain localizing studies. Notably, imaging studies should only be used to localize a tumor and guide a planned surgical exploration. These have no role in making or rejecting the diagnosis of primary HPT. Most commonly, ultrasound and sestamibi are utilized. Both studies are associated with significant false-positive and false-negative rates, and should therefore be interpreted with caution. Even in the case of a positive sestamibi scan, most endocrine surgeons would consider a high-quality ultrasound to be mandatory since it can detect concomitant thyroid pathology in up to 20 or 30 % of patients [5]. Increasingly, endocrine surgeons are performing ultrasound examinations with results that are at least equivalent to those obtained by radiologists [6]. Four-dimensional computed tomography (4D CT) scanning is an emerging technology which combines highly detailed cross-sectional images and an analysis of perfusion characteristics. Reportedly, 4D CT has a higher accuracy than sestamibi or ultrasound [7] but is also operator dependent, as it requires an experienced radiologist to correctly interpret the images. Of note, 4D CT exposes patients to higher radiation doses than methoxyisobutylisonitrile (MIBI), and requires the administration of contrast dye which is relatively contraindicated in patients with renal impairment—a common indication for surgery in primary HPT.

Anesthetic Considerations

Although parathyroidectomy can be safely performed under local/ regional anesthesia with sedation, many surgeons prefer general anesthesia. In our practice, all cases are performed with general anesthesia, supplemented with a bilateral superficial cervical nerve block [8]. This allows the anesthesiologist to decrease the amount of narcotic and antiemetic medications given intraoperatively. If nerve monitoring is planned, an endotracheal tube with surface electrodes should be placed to facilitate this. Since this is a clean case, antibiotics are not required, but experienced endocrine surgeons worldwide differ in their use of antimicrobial prophylaxis [9].

Patient Positioning/Preparation

The patient should be laid on the operating table in the supine position with the neck gently extended, arms tucked, and palms facing up. A shoulder roll is used to achieve neck extension, but care should be taken to avoid hyperextension, particularly in patients with limited range of motion in the neck, as this can contribute to postoperative cervical pain and migraine headaches. The head should be well-supported and stabilized in a foam or gel donut. It is helpful to have the operating table head attachment moved to the foot end of the bed, thus creating a longer, uniform surface and eliminating a potential "gap" in the table into which the shoulder roll can slip during the operation.

While most surgeons prefer the supine position with perhaps slight reverse Trendelenburg tilt, some prefer to refashion the bed into the semi-Fowler's position or the "modified beach-chair" position by tilting the table into the Trendelenburg position, and then flexing the back up and feet down. This may reduce strain to the cervical and lumbar spine. In both positions, the goal is to have the head slightly elevated to reduce venous congestion.

Sequential compression devices are placed and routine chemical thromboprophylaxis is unnecessary. A recent National Surgical Quality Improvement Project (NSQIP) review of thyroid and parathyroid operations demonstrated the risk of deep venous thrombosis (DVT) to be ten times lower than the risk of return to the operating room (0.16 vs. 1.6 %), validating this practice [10]. All joints and contact surfaces are carefully padded. The surgical field, including the mandible, posterior triangles of the neck, and upper chest, is prepped and draped.

Operative Approach

General Principles

Oliver Cope first described the principle that optimal visualization is of paramount importance throughout parathyroidectomy in order to minimize complications. Magnifying loupes should be worn and the field should be brightly illuminated at all times, which is best accomplished with a headlamp. A bloodless surgical field should be scrupulously maintained as bloodstaining can interfere with visualization. Intraoperative efforts to stop bleeding must be tempered, since imprecise maneuvers to stop bleeding can be hazardous. The bleeding vessel must be perfectly visualized and specifically ligated. In a bloody field, attempts to grasp, cauterize, or suture a bleeding vessel could inadvertently injure a nerve or a parathyroid gland (or its blood supply), and so these maneuvers should only be made after the field has been carefully dried and the bleeding site precisely identified. After hemostasis is achieved, gentle irrigation with warm sterile water can often improve an obscured operative field.

Operative Anatomy

Parathyroid Localization

Intimate familiarity with the anatomy and embryology of the parathyroid glands is crucial when performing this operation. The lower parathyroid glands, derived from the third pharyngeal pouch, are known by anatomists as the anterior parathyroids. They are nearly always located in a plane anterior to the recurrent laryngeal nerves, and are most commonly located within 1 cm of the crossing of the nerve with the inferior thyroid artery. Compared with the upper glands, the lower parathyroids have a more lengthy descent to their final resting location, and therefore, are more variable in their final location; ectopic lower glands have been reported as high as the skull base to as low as the anterior mediastinum [11].

It is estimated that in primary HPT, 15% of all lower parathyroid adenomas are located in the thymus gland. In addition, small, clinically insignificant parathyroid rests within normal thymus glands are very common, and likely occur because of the shared embryonic origin of the thymus and lower parathyroids from the third pharyngeal pouch. In conditions like secondary HPT or inherited conditions that lead to parathyroid hyperplasia (e.g., **Wermer's** syndrome MEN-1), these thymic rests become more important and their hypertrophy may be a cause for supranumerary glands and a site for recurrent or persistent disease. Therefore, many surgeons recommend routine cervical thymectomy during parathyroidectomy for secondary HPT or in the context of MEN-1 [12].

Together with the thyroid gland, the upper parathyroid glands are derived from the fourth pharyngeal pouch. These have a shorter migration path than the lower parathyroids, and are therefore more consistent in their location at the posterior aspect of the thyroid gland, usually at the level of the cricoid cartilage. The upper glands are often deep behind the thyroid gland, and require extensive anterior mobilization of the thyroid to be identified [11]. An enlarged upper parathyroid may also descend in the tracheoesophageal groove to assume a final position that is caudal to the level of the lower parathyroid glands; this is a common cause for failed parathyroidectomy, since on imaging studies a descended upper gland can be confused for a lower gland. The most common ectopic locations for upper parathyroid glands include the retroesophageal region or the carotid sheath.

Intrathyroidal parathyroid adenomas occur in approximately 1% of patients with HPT, and tend to be small [13].

The presence of a hypoechoic oval nodule on thyroid ultrasound should alert the surgeon to the possibility of this entity. A preoperative thyroid ultrasound that demonstrates no thyroid nodules allows the surgeon to omit thyroid lobectomy in the search for a missing parathyroid gland.

Operative Philosophy

The "correct" operative approach to primary HPT is highly controversial. While many centers have adopted a focused approach to this disease and make efforts to restrict the operation to one gland that is identified preoperatively as abnormal, other surgeons continue to routinely dissect all four parathyroid glands. The focused approach can be done via a central or lateral approach; both are described below.

Incision Placement

Central Approach

An anterior cervical incision is made in a skin crease in close proximity to the patient's cricoid cartilage. Great care should be paid to ensure that the incision is symmetric, perpendicular to the skin surface, and created in the deepest recess of a skin crease. The length of the incision should be influenced slightly by the size of the patient, the size of their thyroid gland, and by the anticipated difficulty in finding the parathyroid gland(s). In some cases, an incision 3 cm or shorter suffices. It is a fallacy that a lengthy, unsightly incision is required for a four-gland exploration; most endocrine surgeons routinely "convert" from a planned focused parathyroidectomy to a bilateral exploration without lengthening the incision. On the other hand, safe visualization should never be compromised for a shorter incision length. In patients who do not have an optimally located skin crease, a longer incision in a skin crease is preferred over a shorter one in an area without natural folds.

Flap Elevation, Dissection of Strap Muscles

Once the skin is incised, the superior and inferior skin edges are elevated with skin hooks. This facilitates the identification and division of the platysma muscle, which is easily lifted with the skin and subcutaneous tissues from the underlying strap muscles that remain taut at the depth of the incision. Once the platysma muscle is divided, the subplatysmal plane is raised superiorly to the level of the thyroid cartilage and inferiorly to the level of the sternal notch. The skin hooks can be used to elevate the skin/platysma complex while a Kittner dissector is used to retract the strap muscles cephalad for the development of the inferior flap, and caudad for the development of the inferior flap. Occasionally, large anterior

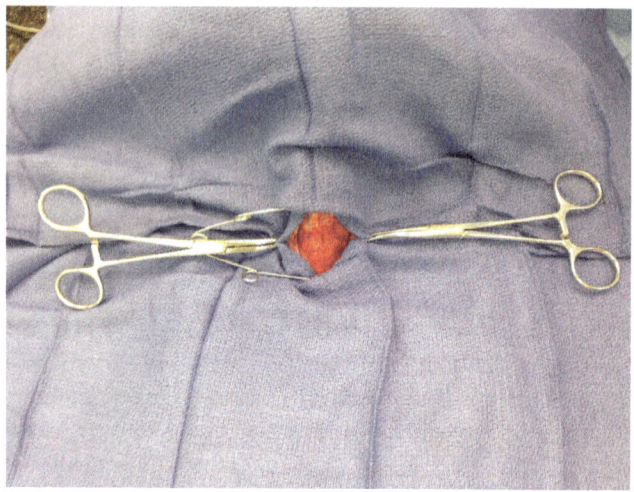

Fig. 1 Initial setup for parathyroidectomy—sublpatysmal plane having been developed, the skin edges are protected under edges of a surgical towel kept in place by a simple spring retractor

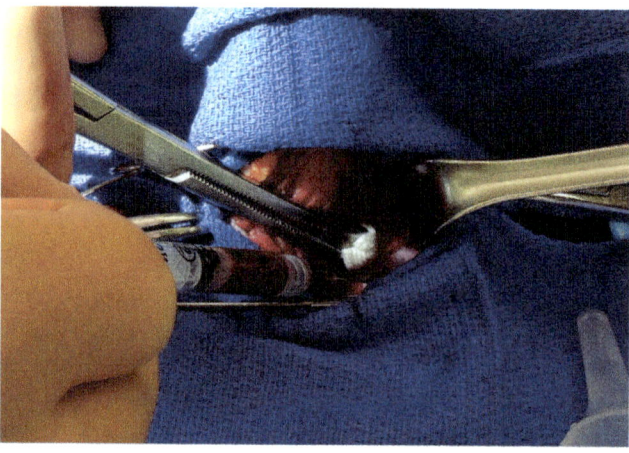

Fig. 2 With sternohyoid muscle retracted laterally (to *left*), and sternothyroid muscle and thyroid gland retracted medially under a Kitner dissector, PTH level is drawn from the *left* internal jugular vein

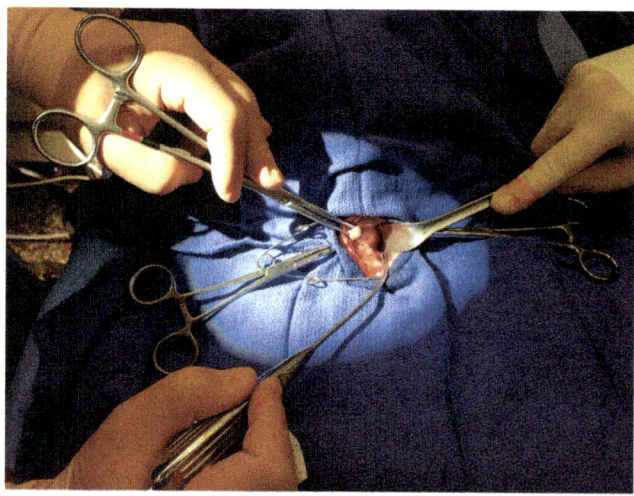

Fig. 3 As the thyroid gland is being elevated and rolled over the trachea, and the strap muscles are retracted laterally, a pediatric suction cannula is used to bluntly and atraumatically dissect the filmy attachments off of the lateral and posterior aspect of the thyroid capsule

jugular vein branches are seen in this plane, and their ligation and division may facilitate the complete development of this plane.

After the subplatysmal plane is developed, a self-retaining retractor is placed. To protect the incised skin edges from inadvertent cautery injury, one may tuck the straight edge of a surgical towel under the skin edges, which can be secured with a low-profile retractor (Fig. 1). Next, the median raphe between the sternohyoid muscles is incised from the level of the thyroid cartilage down to the sternal notch using electrocautery. Occasionally, the median raphe is difficult to identify—it is noteworthy that it is wider and therefore easier to identify caudally, near its sternal origin.

The sternothyroid muscle is then elevated off of the sternohyoid, in a relatively avascular plane requiring minimal or no electrocautery. When the plane between the strap muscles is difficult to identify, it is helpful to elevate the medial border of the sternohyoid muscle while retracting the thyroid isthmus medially with a Kittner dissector. This accentuates the groove between the two strap muscles and facilitates their separation, which should proceed laterally until the internal jugular vein is identified. In cases where nerve monitoring is used, it is recommended to stimulate the vagus nerve at this stage of the operation to ensure the baseline functional integrity of the nerve monitoring circuit and of the nerve itself [14]. The vagus is identified deep, between the jugular vein and common carotid artery.

Intraoperative parathyroid hormone (IOPTH) monitoring is required to achieve the lowest risk of persistent or recurrent HPT after minimally invasive parathyroidectomy. We obtain the samples by direct venipuncture of the jugular vein using a 22-gauge needle (Fig. 2). Usually, this venipuncture site does not require suture repair if direct pressure is applied for a short time. Other surgeons prefer to

have the levels drawn from a large-bore indwelling intravenous (IV) line or an arterial line. However the sample is obtained, care should be taken to avoid hemolysis from vigorous negative pressure or during transfer or handling of the sample, as this results in a substantial artificial decrease in the PTH value [15, 16].

Next, the sternothyroid muscle, which does not extend to the midline, is elevated off of the thyroid gland. The thyroid gland is retracted over the anterior surface of the trachea while dissecting the sternothyroid muscle off of the thyroid capsule while an assistant retracts the strap muscles laterally (Fig. 3). Often, careful and complete mobilization of the sternothyroid muscle is all that is required to identify the parathyroid glands—they will usually "find themselves" as the thyroid is elevated further and further onto the anterior surface of the trachea (Fig. 4).

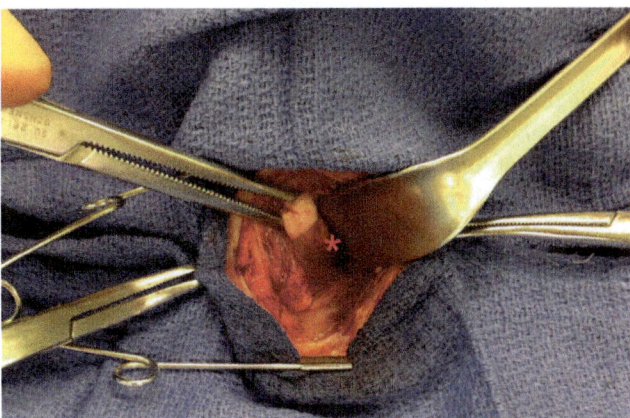

Fig. 4 A parathyroid adenoma (*red asterisk*) is visualized deep to the posterior aspect of the thyroid capsule

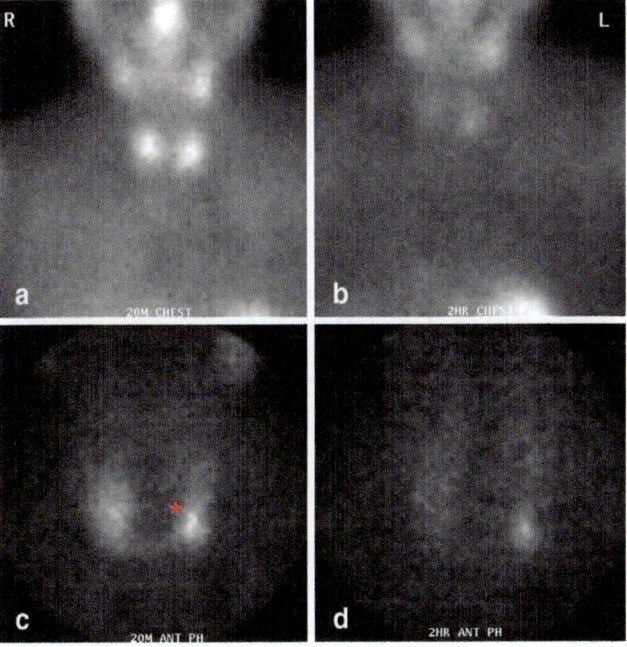

Fig. 5 Immediate (**a**, **c**) and delayed (**b**, **d**) sestamibi images (global views (**a**, **b**) and pinhole images (**c**, **d**)) demonstrating a left upper parathyroid adenoma (*red asterisk*). Note the relatively medial position of the parathyroid mass on image **c** and **d**

Parathyroid Localization

The sequence of intraoperative maneuvers used to identify the parathyroid gland depends on whether the upper or lower gland is the target. Upper glands, which on sestamibi scan often appear medial to the upper pole of the thyroid (Fig. 5), tend to lie quite deep behind the upper and midpole regions of the thyroid. Their identification and removal often requires extensive medial mobilization of the thyroid gland, and, rarely, the blunt opening of Reeve's space between the upper pole of the thyroid and the cricothyroid muscle. On occasion, division of superior thyroid vessels or the middle thyroid vein can facilitate sufficient mobilization of the upper pole of the thyroid to identify these glands.

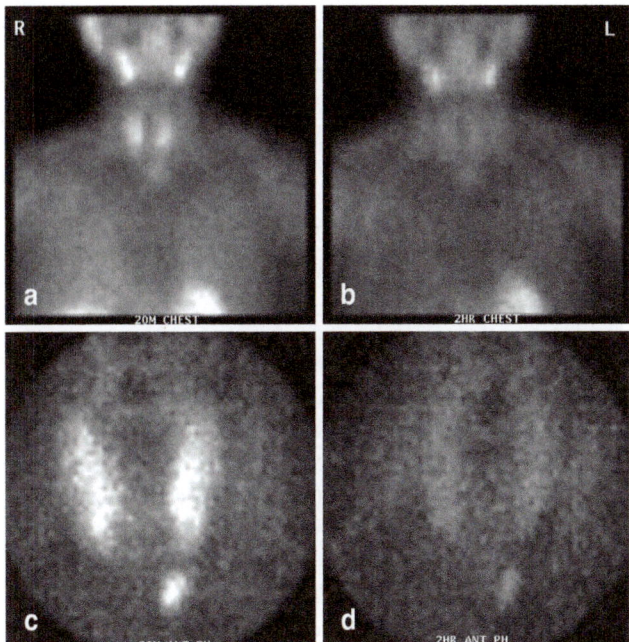

Fig. 6 Immediate (**a**, **c**) and delayed (**b**, **d**) sestamibi images (global views (**a**, **b**) and pinhole images (**c**, **d**)) demonstrating a left lower parathyroid adenoma. At surgery, the adenoma was identified within the thymus gland

The lower glands (Fig. 6) generally require less mobilization of the thyroid gland to identify. They are sometimes visible immediately upon reflecting the sternothyroid muscle off of the thyroid gland. If no gland is identified, I search lower in the anterior mediastinum. If thymectomy is required, I divide the thyrothymic ligament, and grasp and retract the cervical portion of the thymus cephalad as the loose areolar tissues are pushed down. Occasional perforating vessels are clipped or divided using bipolar cautery. Usually, the cervical thymus will thin out and cleave itself. Otherwise, especially if sufficient thymic tissue has been mobilized to include the entire parathyroid, it may be ligated or clipped, and divided.

In cases where a parathyroid gland remains elusive, it is often helpful to reflect on the gland that has already been found on that side and its relationship with the recurrent laryngeal nerve. If the gland that was already identified was in a location anterior to the nerve, then a more comprehensive search is undertaken for the upper gland concentrating on the region of the tracheoesophageal groove, with extension of the field to include the carotid sheath, retropharyngeal, and retroesophageal spaces extending both above and below the thyroid gland. In cases where the lower gland is missing (i.e., the identified gland was posterior to the nerve), the search focuses on the thyrothymic ligament and thymus, and the accessible portion of the superior mediastinum are also explored. In all cases of a missing parathyroid, the carotid sheath should be opened and explored from the root of the neck to the skull base. If thyroid nodules are present on ultrasound, thyroid lobectomy should be done. Proximal ligation of the inferior thyroid artery has not been demonstrated to be curative, but may devascularize the missing parathyroid gland. Median sternotomy is not indicated unless the operation is being performed for life-threatening hypercalcemia. In the majority of revision parathyroidectomies, the "missing parathyroid" will eventually be found in a normal anatomic position. Therefore, following this progression, even if the gland has not been found, the operation should be concluded, and the patient should be reimaged and planned for revisional surgery [17].

Lateral Approach

The lateral approach to the parathyroids can be taken either through a **Kocher**-type skin incision or through a lateral incision centered on the anterior border of the sternocleidomastoid (SCM) muscle. Regardless of the skin incision, the subplatysmal plane is developed, and following this, the anterior border of the SCM is dissected. The plane between the anterior border of the SCM and the strap muscle and thyroid complex is then entered, retracting the SCM and carotid artery laterally and the strap muscles and thyroid gland medially. It is imperative to keep the dissection medial to the carotid artery, which may slip medially from under the retractor and confuse the dissection field. This approach, which offers direct access to the posterior tracheoesophageal groove, is most useful in redo cases involving an upper gland.

The main advantage of this approach is also its greatest weakness: The direct access to the tracheoesophageal groove means that the parathyroid can be identified more directly, but it also means that the recurrent laryngeal nerve is encountered more directly than when the central approach is used. Because this approach leads to the deep aspect of the tracheoesophageal groove, it takes extra effort to expose and remove a lower parathyroid, which is located in a more anterior plane. Additionally, this approach is useful for a planned unilateral exploration.

Radioguidance

Some surgeons utilize radioguidance to facilitate the intraoperative localization of parathyroid adenomas. For this technique, 10 mCi of technetium (Tc-99 m sestamibi) is injected 1–3 h prior to surgery. Background counts are obtained at the level of the thyroid isthmus, and the parathyroid gland is then localized, and a small transverse incision is made over it. Subplatysmal planes are raised and the straps are separated in the midline. Gamma probe can be used to guide dissection trajectory, recognizing that the heart and salivary glands also concentrate Tc-99m sestamibi, and lead to falsely positive results with deep probing. When the adenoma is identified, in vivo counts are obtained; these are usually 150% above the background counts. The parathyroid adenoma is then meticulously removed and placed on the tip of the gamma probe to obtain ex vivo counts. Counts greater than 20% of background confirm the presence of parathyroid tissue in the resected specimen [18].

Intraoperative PTH Monitoring

While there are at least six published criteria for IOPTH use during parathyroidectomy [19], all rely on a precipitous decline in PTH following resection of a solitary adenoma. The most commonly used criterion is the Miami criterion [20]—a 50% decline from baseline 10 min post excision. Some experts also require normalization of the PTH level—this increases the sensitivity (likelihood of cure), but also increases the likelihood of unnecessarily "converting" to a bilateral neck exploration in the event of a slower decline in the PTH following removal of an adenoma. Most surgeons make an effort to avoid manipulating the neck and stimulating the remaining parathyroid glands during the waiting periods between PTH draws, although, theoretically, manipulation of normal and suppressed glands should not result in significant release of PTH.

It should be noted that the published guidelines should not be regarded as absolute requirements. The operating surgeon should consider the change in PTH as one factor in the context of the risk that the patient may have multigland disease. Other intraoperative factors should include the size and consistency of the resected parathyroid gland and whether or not the ipsilateral parathyroid has been identified and its size. The absolute value of the final PTH level is also a factor; a final level greater than 40 has been suggested to be associated with a higher risk of recurrence. Preoperative risk factors for multigland disease include a family history of primary HPT, a history of lithium use, or a history of multiple endocrine neoplasia.

Closure

Following the extraction of the specimen, the field is inspected for hemostasis. A recent study suggested that positional maneuvers, such as the Valsalva maneuver or placing the patient in the Trendelenburg position, can identify bleeding points that were otherwise not suspected [21]. The use of topical hemostatic agents has not been shown to reduce the incidence of hematoma, but these can be used. The routine use of drains is unnecessary after parathyroidectomy [22].

The strap muscles are closed using simple interrupted absorbable suture with care to leave the gaps between sutures, and also at the caudal aspect of the decussation so as to allow a potential hematoma, a means of egress to the more superficial layers of the neck. While some surgeons close the straps in layers, others omit reapproximating the sternothyroid muscle. Platysma is closed, again using interrupted suture, and a subcuticular suture is placed for the skin edges. I use Dermabond™ as a sterile dressing, and often remove the subcuticular stitch, but this is purely a matter of preference.

Postoperative care instructions include elevation of the head to decrease venous pooling in the neck, ice to the neck to induce vasoconstriction, and frequent exams of the neck to ensure that no hematoma is forming. The required length of stay following parathyroidectomy remains controversial. Practices vary from immediate discharge [23], to a required observation period prior to same-day discharge, to required overnight stay [24].

Post-parathyroidectomy discharge instructions include routine wound care instructions, observation for hematoma, and instructions regarding the signs and symptoms of hypocalcemia. Most patients are prescribed calcium supplements, although there is no evidence that this improves bone density after surgery.

Conclusions

Parathyroidectomy is the second most commonly performed endocrine operation. There are considerable variations among surgeons and practices in the indications for parathyroidectomy, the conduct of the operation, and in postoperative care. Minimally invasive parathyroidectomy with IOPTH monitoring can achieve excellent results with minimal morbidity in selected patients. With high-quality data from prospectively collected, robust databases, our management of patients with primary HPT should become less variable and outcomes should continue to improve.

Key Summary Points

- Parathyroidectomy should be considered in patients with biochemically confirmed primary HPT, even in the absence of classic symptoms.
- Parathyroid imaging studies should be used for surgical guidance, not to diagnose HPT.
- Although their craniocaudal position can vary, the upper and lower parathyroid glands are consistently located posterior and anterior to the recurrent laryngeal nerve, respectively.
- When searching for an ectopic parathyroid gland, the location of the ipsilateral parathyroid should guide a strategic dissection.

References

1. Eigelberger MS, Cheah WK, Ituarte PH, et al. The NIH criteria for parathyroidectomy in asymptomatic primary hyperparathyroidism: are they too limited? Ann Surg 2004;239(4):528–35.
2. Bilezikian JP, Khan AA, Potts JT Jr. Guidelines for the management of asymptomatic primary hyperparathyroidism: summary statement from the third international workshop. J Clin Endocrinol Metab 2009;94(2):335–9.
3. Uhlig K, Berns JS, Kestenbaum B, et al. KDOQI US commentary on the 2009 KDIGO Clinical Practice Guideline for the diagnosis, evaluation, and treatment of ckd-mineral and bone disorder (CKD-MBD). Am J Kidney Dis. 2010;55(5):773–99.
4. Iannuzzi JC, Choi DX, Farkas RL, et al. Surgeon beware: many patients referred for parathyroidectomy are misdiagnosed with primary hyperparathyroidism. Surgery. 2012;152(4):635–40; discussion 640–2.
5. Adler JT, Chen H, Schaefer S, Sippel RS. Does routine use of ultrasound result in additional thyroid procedures in patients with primary hyperparathyroidism? J Am Coll Surg. 2010;211(4):536–9.
6. Milas M, Stephen A, Berber E, et al. Ultrasonography for the endocrine surgeon: a valuable clinical tool that enhances diagnostic and therapeutic outcomes. Surgery. 2005;138(6):1193–201.
7. Mortenson MM, et al. Parathyroid exploration in the reoperative neck: improved preoperative localization with 4D-computed tomography. J Am Coll Surg. 2008;206(5):888–95.
8. Udelsman R, Donovan PI. Open minimally invasive parathyroid surgery. World J Surg. 2004;28(12):1224–6.
9. Moalem J, Ruan DT, Farkas RL, et al. Patterns of antibiotic prophylaxis use for thyroidectomy and parathyroidectomy: results of an international survey of endocrine surgeons. J Am Coll Surg; 210(6):949–56.
10. Roy M, Rajamanickam V, Chen H, Sippel R. Is DVT prophylaxis necessary for thyroidectomy and parathyroidectomy? Surgery. 2010;148(6):1163–9.
11. Lal G, Clark OH. Thyroid, para thyroid, and adrenal. In: Charles Brunicardi F, editor. Schwartz's principles of surgery. New York: McGraw-Hill, 2010.
12. Uno N, Tominaga Y, Matsuoka S, Tsuzuki T, Shimabukuro S, Sato T, et al. Incidence of parathyroid glands located in thymus in patients with renal hyperparathyroidism. World J Surg. 2008;32(11):2516–9.
13. Mazeh H, Kouniavsky G, Schneider DF, Makris KI, Sippel RS, Dackiw AP, et al. Intrathyroidal parathyroid glands: small, but mighty (a Napoleon phenomenon). Surgery. 2012;152(6)1193–200.
14. Randolph GW, Dralle H, Abdullah H, Barczynski M, Bellantone R, Brauckhoff M, et al. Electrophysiologic recurrent laryngeal nerve monitoring during thyroid and parathyroid surgery: international standards guideline statement. The Laryngoscope. 2011;121(S1):S1–16.
15. Moalem J, et al. Hemolysis falsely decreases intraoperative parathyroid hormone levels. Am J Surg. 2009;197(2):222–6.
16. Moalem J, et al. Prospective evaluation of the rate and impact of hemolysis on intraoperative parathyroid hormone (IOPTH) assay results. Ann Surg Oncol. 2010;17(11):2963–9.
17. Udelsman R, Donovan PI. Remedial parathyroid surgery: changing trends in 130 consecutive cases. Ann Surg. 2006;244(3):471.
18. Pitt SC, Chen H. Minimally invasive parathyroidectomy: gamma probe guided. In: Duh QY, Clark OH, Kebebew E, editor. Atlas of

endocrine surgical techniques. Philadelphia: Elsevier Health Sciences, 2010.

19. Carneiro DM, Solorzano CC, Nader MC, Ramirez M, Irvin GL III. Comparison of intraoperative iPTH assay (QPTH) criteria in guiding parathyroidectomy: which criterion is the most accurate?. Surgery. 2003;134(6):973–9.

20. Irvin GL, Solorzano CC, Carneiro DM. Quick intraoperative parathyroid hormone assay: surgical adjunct to allow limited parathyroidectomy, improve success rate, and predict outcome. World J Surg. 2004;28(12):1287–92.

21. Moumoulidis I, Martinez Del Pero M, Brennan L, Jani P. Haemostasis in head and neck surgical procedures: Valsalva manoeuvre versus Trendelenburg tilt. Ann R Coll Surg Engl. 2010;92(4):292–4.

22. Morrissey AT, Chau J, Yunker WK, et al. Comparison of drain versus no drain thyroidectomy: randomized prospective clinical trial. J Otolaryngol Head Neck Surg. 2008;37(1):43–7.

23. Irvin GL III, Sfakianakis G, Yeung L, Deriso GT, Fishman LM, Molinari AS, Foss JN. Ambulatory parathyroidectomy for primary hyperparathyroidism. Arch Surg. 1996;131(10):1074.

24. Stavrakis AI, Ituarte PH, Ko CY, Yeh MW. Surgeon volume as a predictor of outcomes in inpatient and outpatient endocrine surgery. Surgery. 2007;142(6):887–99.

Felix Mandl

1892–1957

Scott M. Thompson and Geoffrey B. Thompson

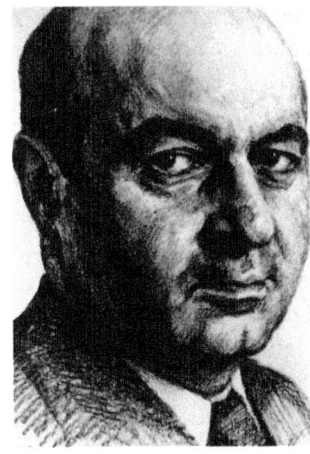

Felix Mandl. (Reprinted from [15], Copyright 2000, with permission from Elsevier)

Early Life and Training

Felix Mandl M.D. son of industrialist Emil Mandl and Linda Basch Mandl, was born on November 8, 1892, in the city of Brno (Brünn in German) located in the modern-day Czech Republic [2]. After graduating from his local German high school, Mandl entered the medical school of the University of Vienna in 1910 [2]. His medical training was disrupted

---

With this daring operation and his monumental thesis entitled "Clinical and Experimental Studies in Localized and Generalized Osteitis Fibrosa," Mandl laid the foundations for parathyroid surgery. Hanoch Milwidsky, 1957 [1]

S. M. Thompson (✉)
Medical Scientist Training Program, College of Medicine, Mayo Clinic, Rochester, MN, USA
e-mail: thompson.scott@mayo.edu

G. B. Thompson
Surgery, College of Medicine, Mayo Clinic, Rochester, MN, USA
e-mail: thompson.geoffrey@mayo.edu

during World War I when he served in the Austro-Hungarian army from 1914 to 1919 [2]. Shortly thereafter, he received his M.D. degree in 1919 and entered surgical residency under Julius Von Hochenegg in the Department of Surgery II at Vienna General Hospital [1]. He worked as a surgical trainee assuming the position of chief resident in 1923 and was promoted to lecturer in surgery at the University of Vienna in 1928. In 1932, he became the director of the surgery department at the S Canning-Childs Hospital and Research Institute in Vienna [3].

Albert Jahne and the First Parathyroidectomy

It was during his early surgical training that Felix Mandl made surgical history by performing the first successful parathyroidectomy for a patient suffering from osteitis fibrosa cystica (von Recklinghausen's disease of the bone). In 1924, Albert Jahne, a 34-year-old streetcar conductor in Vienna, was admitted to the Department of Surgery II, University of Vienna. Jahne had begun developing progressive lower-extremity weakness and bone pain in 1919. By October 1924, the 38-year-old Jahne required crutches to ambulate and roentgen (X-ray) analysis demonstrated cystic lesions in his pelvis and femurs [3]. The prevailing hypothesis for Jahne's bone lesions at that time was based on Viennese pathologist Jacob Erdheim's (1874–1937) theory that osteitis fibrosa cystica was due to a deficiency of parathyroid hormone and that parathyroid hyperplasia was secondary to increased calcium metabolism in bone [4]. Erdheim first recognized an association between the parathyroid glands and calcium levels in 1906. Experimentally, he determined that cauterization of the parathyroid glands of laboratory rats resulted in both tetany and defective mineralization of teeth. Additionally, he observed devascularization and destruction of the parathyroid glands at postmortem examination in three patients who died of postoperative tetany following thyroidectomy for goiter and later identified parathyroid hyperplasia in patients with osteomalacia [3].

J. L. Pasieka, J. A. Lee (eds.), *Surgical Endocrinopathies,* DOI 10.1007/978-3-319-13662-2_25,
© Springer International Publishing Switzerland 2015

Given Erdheim's prevailing hypothesis of compensatory parathyroid hyperplasia in response to osteitis fibrosa cystica, Albert Jahne was initially treated with "parathyreoidin tablets," a concentrate of parathyroid extract [3]. However, his symptoms continued to worsen, and he developed a pathologic fracture of his left femur on December 12, 1924. His fracture healed by February 1925 but over the next 4 months he became cachectic, was no longer able to ambulate due to lower-extremity pain, and he developed a white precipitate in his urine. On June 22, 1925, he was readmitted to the hospital. On July 2, 1925, still operating under Erdheim's hypothesis of compensatory parathyroid hyperplasia, Mandl transplanted four parathyroid glands from a patient who died from trauma into Jahne's preperitoneal space [3]. Although Jahne's symptoms did not improve, Mandl had directly tested Erdheim's hypothesis in a patient, thereby providing evidence against the theory of compensatory parathyroid hyperplasia in the pathophysiology of osteitis fibrosa cystica.

Consequently, Mandl hypothesized that Jahne's bone lesions were not compensatory due to a deficiency of parathyroid hormone but rather due to an excess of parathyroid hormone. On July 30, 1925, Mandl set out to test his hypothesis by taking Jahne to the operating room to perform a cervical exploration for a parathyroid tumor [3]. In the operating room, Mandl discovered that "in the rim between larynx and esophagus, a dark, partly grayish nodule separate from the thyroid was located in the inferior parathyroid position close to the inferior thyroid artery and between its branches, adhering to the left recurrent nerve." The $2.5 \times 1.5 \times 1.2$-cm grayish-white nodule was surgically removed, and further exploration of the neck revealed that the remaining three parathyroid glands were macroscopically normal [3]. Pathologic analysis by Erdheim and his colleagues concluded that

> the cell structure is typical for parathyroid tissue…it is most likely a so-called 'atypical (fetal) adenoma' of the parathyroid gland with polymorphous cell structure which may be a 'malignant degeneration.' In one part of the tumor there is a hyaline round-shaped patch with numerous pigmented cells (remnants of a previous hemorrhage). There is no evidence of a rim of normal parathyroid tissue. [3]

Subsequently, Jahne's urinary calcium excretion decreased from a preoperative level of 54–7.6 mg% by postoperative day 11 and he did not develop tetany [3]. He was discharged from the hospital on August 7, 1925, and made a rapid recovery: His strength improved, his body weight increased, his lower-extremity pain subsided, he was able to begin ambulating with a cane, and X-rays of his bones demonstrated healing of his cystic lesions and an increase in his bone density. In effect, Mandl had performed the first successful parathyroidectomy. He presented the case at the Vienna Congress of Physicians on December 4, 1925, and subsequently published his findings [4–8]. At clinical follow-up in 1929, Jahne remained asymptomatic and biochemical

analysis demonstrated "blood calcium levels between 13 and 14 mg/100 mL (normal range, 8.4 to 10.4 mg/100 mL) and urinary calcium excretions between 264 and 300 mg/100 mL (normal range, <200 mg%)" [3]. Ultimately, Mandl had demonstrated that Jahne's osteitis fibrosa cystica was secondary to a hyperfunctioning parathyroid gland, thereby disproving Erdheim's compensatory parathyroid hyperplasia hypothesis that had stood for nearly 20 years.

Unfortunately, Jahne's symptoms began to return in 1931, and, by January 1933, he was bedridden. He was diagnosed clinically and biochemically with recurrent hyperparathyroidism and on October 18, 1933, Mandl took Jahne to the operating room for a repeat cervical exploration to examine for another parathyroid tumor. According to Mandl, "there was neither a local recurrence nor another adenoma in the entire neck and in the mediastinum explored through the neck" [3]. Jahne's symptoms and biochemical parameters did not improve over the next 3 years and in February 1936, he passed away from uremia. Postmortem examination demonstrated generalized cystic fibrosis with brown tumors in multiple bones and bilateral hydronephrosis with nephrocalcinosis [3]. Ultimately, Jahne's clinical course raised the question of parathyroid carcinoma but no metastatic parathyroid tissue was found at autopsy [4]. An excellent and detailed English translation of the operative, pathology, and clinical reports regarding the case of Albert Jahne was published by Niederle et al. in 2006 [3].

Professional Rise and Exile to Jerusalem

Throughout the 1920s, Mandl's contributions to the fields of surgery and experimental endocrinology were prolific. In December 1926, he applied for the Venia Legendi for Surgery having authored more than 50 scientific publications on topics including surgery of the stomach and rectum, treatment of sports injuries, and the diagnostic and therapeutic uses of the anesthetic procaine hydrochloride [2]. He submitted his thesis titled *Clinical and Experimental Studies in Localized and Generalized Osteitis Fibrosa* which demonstrated the causative role of parathyroid hyperplasia in generalized osteitis fibrosa cystica, thereby laying the foundation for the surgical management of primary parathyroid disorders [7, 8]. He presented his thesis on December 10, 1927, and was awarded the Venia Legendi for Surgery by the Medical Faculty at the University of Vienna on December 14, 1927. He continued his prolific surgical career at the Vienna General Hospital until 1932 when he became the director of the surgery department at the S Canning-Childs Hospital and Research Institute in Vienna.

Unfortunately, the rise of Nazism during the 1930s significantly impacted Mandl's surgical career. In 1938, Mandl was on a lecture tour in England when the political situation in

Austria decompensated under the Nazis [3]. Because Mandl was Jewish, he was expelled from the University of Vienna on April 22, 1938, and he lost his position at the hospital [9]. Unable to return to Vienna, he immigrated to Jerusalem. He was appointed head of the Surgical Department B at the Hadassah University Hospital and was made a full professor in 1939 [2]. Hanoch Milwidsky, Mandl's colleague at Hadassah, described him as "not only an excellent clinician and surgeon but an extremely gifted teacher dedicated to his patients and pupils alike…he possessed a highly developed clinical judgment and self criticism, freely admitting his own errors, always ready to discuss and accept other opinions even of his pupils and students" [1]. In Israel, Mandl helped to found the medical journal *Acta Medica Orientalia* [10].

Return to Vienna and Death

Mandl returned to Austria in 1947 and was appointed director of the Emperor Franz-Josef Hospital in Vienna. The hospital was heavily damaged during World War II and was rebuilt under Mandl's direction [2, 3]. Additionally, his lectureship rights were reinstated, and he was appointed to the academic rank of associate professor. Since the Nazis had stripped him of his professional accomplishments, he had to submit for renewal of his Venia Legendi of Surgery, this time with more than 230 scientific publications to his name.

Additionally, Mandl had become involved in several national and international surgical associations and scientific societies. He was a member of the Vienna Medical Association, the Viennese Association of Surgeons, and Austrian Cancer Society, and an honorary member of the surgical societies of Venice, Padua, and Piedmont. He was a member of the International Society of Surgeons. Furthermore, he helped to found the Austrian section of the International College of Surgeons (ICS) and served as vice president of the ICS [3, 11]. In 1956, the ICS awarded Mandl its highest distinction, the rank of master surgeon. Moreover, the ICS had planned to honor Mandl with a special issue of the *Journal of the International College of Surgeons,* known as a *Festschrift,* dedicated to him in November 1957 [1, 3]. Unfortunately, Mandl came down with a particularly bad case of the grippe in the fall of 1957. He unexpectedly passed away at the age of 65 from acute heart failure on October 15, 1957 [2, 3]. Mandl had not lived to see his *Festschrift* and instead it appeared as a memorial issue [1, 12]. The "Last Message of Felix Mandl" was read at the opening session of the Austrian Federation Meeting by his assistant, Dr. R. Gottlob [11].

Legacy

Felix Mandl was a pioneer in numerous areas of surgery, medicine, and science, having made significant contributions to the fields of general and endocrine surgery, traumatology, regional anesthesiology, and endocrine physiology, to name a few. As a young surgical resident, his bold willingness to challenge Erdheim's hypothesis of compensatory parathyroid hyperplasia in osteitis fibrosa cystica resulted in the first successful parathyroidectomy, thereby establishing certain fundamental principles of parathyroid pathophysiology and laying the foundation for the modern surgical management of parathyroid disorders [13, 14]. Despite his tremendous success, including the rank of master surgeon, he was remembered by many who knew him as modest and warmhearted [1, 2, 10, 12]. Ernst Israel, Mandl's colleague from Jerusalem, writing at the time of Mandl's death, wrote,

> Three weeks before his death I visited him in Vienna and we spent many hours together. Although in the meantime he had become one of the great in the surgical world, highly respected and honored, he was as modest as ever…I shall always remember Felix Mandl, his brilliant mind, his courage in action, his sympathy and understanding for the sufferings of the sick—a faithful friend, lonely and shy, and always hiding a great tenderness of heart. [10]

References

1. Milwidsky H. In memoriam: Professor Felix Mandl. Acta Med Orient. 1957;16(11–12):247–8.
2. Schonbauer L. Prof. Dr. Felix Mandl; 1892–1957. J Int Coll Surg. 1957;28(5 Pt 1):706–7.
3. Niederle BE, Schmidt G, Organ CH, Niederle B. Albert J and his surgeon: a historical reevaluation of the first parathyroidectomy. J Am Coll Surg. 2006;202(1):181–90.
4. Zeiger MA, Shen WT, Felger EA, editors. The supreme triumph of the surgeon's art: a narrative history of endocrine surgery. San Francisco: University of California Medical Humanities Press; 2013.
5. Mandl F. Therapeutischer Versuch bei Ostitis fibrosa generalisata mittels Exstirpation eines Epithelkörperchentumors. Wien Klin Wochenschr. 1925;38:1343–1344.
6. Mandl F. Therapeutischer Versuch bei einem Fall von Ostitis fibrosa generalisata mittels Exstirpation eines Epithelkörpchentumors. Zbl Chir. 1926;53:260–4.
7. Mandl F. Klinisches und Experimentelles zur Frage der lokalisierten und generalisierten Ostitis fibrosa (Unter besonderer Berücksichtigung der Therapie der letzteren). Teil 1. Arch Klin Chir. 1926;143:1–48.
8. Mandl F. Klinisches und Experimentelles zur Frage der lokalisierten und generalisierten Ostitis fibrosa (unter besonderer Berücksichtigung der Therapie der letzteren). Teil 2. Arch Klin Chir. 1926;143:245–8.

9. Mandl F. University of Vienna [updated 20 Sep 2012]. Available from: http://gedenkbuch.univie.ac.at/index.php?gedenkbuch=1&id=435&no_cache=1&L=2&person_single_id=34442&person_name=felixmandl&person_geburtstag_tag=not_selected&person_geburtstag_monat=not_selected&person_geburtstag_jahr=not_selected&person_fakultaet=not_selected&person_kategorie=not_selected&person_volltextsuche=&search_person_x=1&result_page=1. Accessed: 12 April 2014.

10. Israel E. Felix Mandl: an appreciation. Acta Med Orient. 1957;16(11–12):249–50.

11. LAST MESSAGE of Felix Mandl. J Int Coll Surg. 1957;28(5 Pt 1):704–5.

12. Grana F. Felix Mandl: a tribute. J Int Coll Surg. 1957;28(6 Pt 1):835–6.

13. Mandl F. The development of parathyroidectomy during the last fifteen years. J Int Coll Surg. 1940;3(4):297–311.

14. Mandl F. Diseases of the parathyroids. J Int Coll Surg. 1957;27(4):520–7.

15. Organ CH. The history of parathyroid surgery, 1850–1996: the Excelsior Surgical Society 1998 Edward D Churchill Lecture. J Am Coll Surg. 2000;191(3):284–99.

Oliver Cope

1902–1994

Sareh Parangi

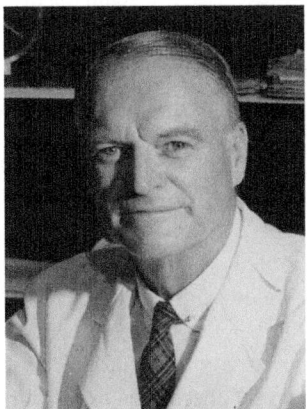

Oliver Cope in 1964. (Courtesy of the MGH Archives)

Introduction

Oliver Cope is known to many as one of the fathers of endocrine surgery and for his seminal work on the anatomy and surgical treatment of parathyroid disorders. The "Oliver Cope Meritorious Achievement Award" is the highest honor bestowed upon members of the American Association of Endocrine Surgeons for lifetime achievement in the field, which has only been awarded six times in 30 years. In reality, Oliver Cope's life and achievements go beyond endocrine surgery and showcase a meticulous surgeon who devoted his entire life to caring for his patients. He has a wide range of achievements related to the surgical practices for burns and breast cancer, as well as diseases of the thyroid and parathyroid glands. This underlines his unique ability to combine detailed biologic and physiologic knowledge with passionate care of patients.

S. Parangi (✉)
Department of Surgery, Harvard Medical School, Massachusetts General Hospital, Boston, MA, USA
e-mail: sparangi@partners.org

Oliver Cope Early Work

Oliver Cope was born in Germantown, Pennsylvania in 1902. His mother was a pacifist and active in the suffrage movement. She insisted that Oliver learn multiple languages and forbade the use of English at the dinner table. She also wanted him to pursue music, and he played the fiddle almost every day of his life. His father was a Quaker architect and the tenets of this religion, including simple living, permeated Oliver Cope's entire life. He attended Haverford College for 1 year before transferring to Harvard University, where he majored in chemistry. In college, he was involved with the Glee club and the Liberal Club where he led a successful campaign to admit Jewish students to Harvard. Along the way, he developed a deep interest in medicine and was admitted to Harvard Medical School. During his second year of medical school, he travelled to China where he worked as a news correspondent and interestingly was the first westerner to interview Chiang Kai-Shek, which he did in secret in 1924 [1].

After his graduation, he became a surgical resident at the Massachusetts General Hospital (MGH) in 1928. He arrived at MGH during a remarkable transformation of the American surgical scene. Around this time, MGH had begun a "full time" surgical service propelled by Edward P. Richardson to do research, which meant that surgeons joining would have full-time appointments at Harvard Medical School, yet they would retain the ability to be in private practice. This fusion of practice and research allowed a deepening of the investigative work performed by surgeons, especially since a modest monetary support was provided [2] (Fig. 1).

During his time as a resident, he clearly impressed the surgical staff and was named administrative assistant to Dr. Edward D. Churchill, who became the chief of The West Service at MGH in 1931 and later chief of surgery. Dr. Churchill's assignment as chief was critical to Oliver Cope's transformation into a surgeon–scientist; Dr. Churchill believed "that integration of research oriented full time staff" was necessary to allow a depth of understanding of surgical

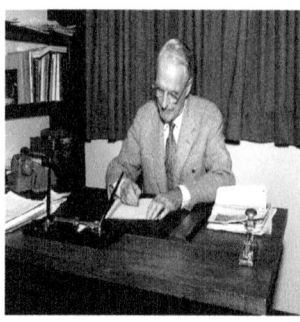

Fig. 1 Oliver Cope at work at the Massachusetts General Hospital. (Courtesy of the MGH Archives)

diseases that did not exist prior to that in Boston. This was also when the concept of "surgical specialization" was developed, which went against the more prominent concept among other surgical leaders of the time: the general surgeon. Dr. Churchill's general concept was that, as chief of surgery, he could see the landscape and needs of the department and the field of surgery better than most. He would then assign the most pressing issues to be addressed to his most promising surgical staff and residents. Dr. Churchill's mandate that each faculty study one or two areas was supplemented by monetary support. Oliver Cope was assigned to work on burns and then parathyroid disorders where knowledge was still sparse when he began his research [2].

Dr. Cope had shown himself to be driven and exceptionally bright. He spoke multiple languages fluently including German and French, thus in 1933, he was chosen as The Moseley Traveling Fellow at MGH. He embarked on a trip to Europe to study the pathophysiology of the endocrine glands with Ludwig Pick in Berlin and then with Sir Henry Dale in London the following year [1].

Cope's Work on Parathyroid Disorders

Cope's work on parathyroid disorders is truly a testament to his meticulous nature and remarkable ability to insightfully tie together vast amounts of information from a minute amount of clinical material. During the time he was putting together a mental story about the diagnosis and surgical treatment of hyperparathyroidism, it was quite difficult to even read the works of others on the subject. Ivar Sandstrom first described the parathyroid glands in Uppsala, Sweden, as a medical student in 1880. The work was published in Swedish and barely noticed elsewhere, until study of its function began in the 1890s, and surgeons started focusing on preserving the parathyroid glands during thyroid surgery as a way to prevent tetany. Hyperparathyroidism was first described in 1925, and was basically thought to be a disease caused by a single enlarged gland or "adenoma" and that removal of this

adenoma would result in a cure of the condition. The exact relation of the bony disease to the parathyroid gland was not yet understood.

In July of 1925, **Dr. Mandl** in Vienna treated Albert J. Herr who was suffering from advanced osteitis fibrosa (also known then as von Reckinghausen's disease) with parathyroid extract. When that failed to improve things, Mandl actually grafted fresh parathyroid tissue from a victim of a streetcar accident, which significantly worsened the patient's bone loss and increased calcium levels in his urine. Dr. Mandl then performed a neck exploration and removed a 21-mm parathyroid gland, which resulted in rapid clearing of urinary calcium and improved bone health. Simultaneously in the USA, a team of medical doctors at MGH were using parathyroid hormone (PTH) in the form of parathyroid extract, to treat lead poisoning, and they noted the effects on the bones. Dr. Aub, a physician in New York City (NYC) whose laboratory Dr. Cope had worked in, noted a similar bone disease in the sea captain Charles Martell who had lost 7 in of height rapidly. Aub referred him to Boston where it was confirmed that his calcium metabolism resembled what had been seen in the lead poisoning patients treated with PTH extract. This patient was then referred to the chief of surgery at MGH, Edward Richardson, who without any knowledge of Mandl's work in Vienna performed two operations in the neck where he was only able to find and remove normal parathyroid tissue. By 1931, there had been some more activity on both sides of the Atlantic, and the British surgeons Walton and Hunter had removed a handful of parathyroid adenomas from patients' necks and one from the mediastinum. In 1931, Dr. Churchill, who had by then become the chief of surgery at MGH, was asked to reoperate on Charles Martell who had one more unsuccessful operation in NYC (right thyroid lobectomy) in the meantime [3]. Four additional patients also diagnosed with hyperparathryoidism were also hospitalized at MGH by the medical service and were awaiting surgical cure. Dr. Churchill recognized he had already performed one successful operation, yet many other good surgeons had failed, and his future success would depend on

> the ability of the surgeon to know a parathyroid gland when he saw it and to know the distribution of the glands, where they hide, and also be delicate enough in technique to be able to use his knowledge. [4]

Cope, who was by then a senior surgical resident under Dr. Churchill, was assigned the task of learning about the parathyroids and told simply that he would not "have the privilege of operating on the first patient," until Churchill was satisfied with his understanding of parathyroid gland anatomy. Cope made quick friends with Dr. Benjamin Castleman, a resident in pathology at the MGH, and together they performed 30 postmortem exams of the neck and mediastinum. They microscopically examined every "little piece of fat" to try and tell what was parathyroid. At that time, there was no other person in the pathology department who could recognize these glands. Eventually, they no longer needed to microscopically examine everything because they routinely recognized parathyroid tissue. Shortly after, they recognized the wide anatomic variation and the location of these glands in the thymus and mediastinum. Cope also learned from the pathologist that glands with adenomas might also suffer from hyperplasia and cancer, both of which he was later able to recognize and diagnose. By 1932, Churchill was satisfied with Cope's understanding of the anatomy of the parathyroids, and he supervised Cope in his first parathyroid operation. Cope found the parathyroid adenoma successfully in his first operation, but he was scolded by Churchill for being "too rough," as well as leaving "the field too bloody" from using the wrong scissors and instruments for traction of the thyroid. Cope realized he had been taught to be quick thus far in his residency, but now he had to learn to slow down and be more precise for this particular type of surgery to be successful. Cope then performed two other operations; by his third operation, Churchill was finally satisfied with his new work ethic. By this time, Cope was able to operate independently without Churchill "dropping in" and proceeded with operating on Captain Martell; he performed a total of three more neck operations between June and October of 1932, but he found no parathyroid tissue in the neck of the sea Captain. Dr. Churchill, then satisfied that there was no tumor in the neck, took over in November of 1932, and found the tumor in the anterior mediastinum, removing it with a partial sternal split. Unfortunately, this patient ultimately passed away in December from tetany, larygneal spasm, and renal failure, and was reported as "Case Number 6" in Cope and Churchill's paper describing the first 30 patients treated at MGII in *Annals of Surgery* in 1936. Cope reported being very grateful to the lessons that were taught to him by this patient [4].

By early 1934, Drs. Churchill and Cope had seen three unusual cases of hyperparathyroidism in which each patient had recurrent disease and kidney stones. Despite removal of one enlarged gland successfully, they were requiring removal of multiple other glands to be cured; he recognized this and reported it as "clear cell hyperplasia". By 1935, a mere 2 years after he went to England to "learn about endocrine surgery" from the European experts, Oliver Cope wrote a *New England Journal of Medicine* paper on the subject of parathyroidectomy, describing in detail the lessons learned by him and his colleagues Drs. Churchill, **Albright**, and Castleman after treating 27 patients with parathyroid disorders [5]. From this relatively small cohort of patients, Cope inferred a large amount of important information, all of which endocrine surgeons follow and use to this day. It is a true testament to his clinical acumen and detail-oriented nature that he integrated these critical lessons from this early cohort of patients. In his paper, he outlined principles that remain important in the care of parathyroid patients today:

1. Parathyroid surgery is not the same as thyroid surgery. He discovered that gentle handling of parathyroid tissue was paramount, and devascularization of healthy tissue could lead to life-threatening tetany. He wrote, "surgery of the parathyroid glands involves, naturally, many of the same anatomical considerations common to thyroid surgery. The identification of parathyroid tissue is, however, so much more difficult, that although the anatomical considerations may be the same, the surgical technique must be considerably different". He smartly wrote that"every surgeon versed in thyroid surgery realizes the difficulty of recognizing parathyroid tissue. It is one thing, however, to avoid the removal of parathyroid tissue in performing a thyroidectomy and quite another to expose and identify all of the parathyroid tissue present." He clearly understood that "Infinite care, a bloodless technique, time and patience are required to solve, satisfactorily, the problems of parathyroid surgery."

2. He recognized that parathyroid adenomas and hyperplasia should be treated differently; a subtotal parathyroidectomy was needed for hyperplasia, followed by a complete parathyroidectomy at a later date if need be.

3. He documented that the removal of all parathyroid tissue resulted in tetany and possibly death, and there was no hormone replacement therapy that was effective.

4. He also recognized that the size of the resected gland was not the most important factor. He saw that one patient had a 6.5-cm tumor that weighed 53 g, but a different patient with a 10-mm tumor had much worse osteoporosis and incapacitating spinal deformities, which were dramatically cured after surgery and removal.

5. He described the difficulties with redo parathyroid surgery in lessons he learned in four of these patients that were referred to him after failure to cure them at other hospitals, and describes the wide range of locations of the parathyroids "from the pharynx to the mediastinum", including tumors "buried in the thyroid." His findings described his depth of understanding of the disease. He wrote

"Hyperparathyroidism is a more common disease than usually suspected; that its treatment is surgery; that to accomplish surgical results the problem is not only one of exposing parathyroid tissue but equally of one knowing how much to remove. Overzealous removal of too much tissue may end in graver disabilities than the disease itself…and that difficulty of the operative procedure lies in the evaluation of how much tissue to leave behind with no set rule as to how many milligrams should be left." [5]

Cope's Work on Burns

While Cope's work on the parathyroids is known best to endocrine surgeons, his contributions to the field of surgery are much wider. Dr. Cope's work on the care of burn patients is a true testament to his willingness to rigorously test therapies instead of following medical dogma. While the majority of his work in burns was initiated after his work on the parathyroids, he actually became interested in this area much earlier. Oliver Cope's first experience with burn victims was instrumental to his understanding that serious burns caused many more problems than those visible to the naked eye. As a medical student, he was in the MGH Emergency Ward (EW) when 30 burn victims from a devastating fire at Beacon Oil in Everett were brought in [2]. Cope would write "Staff, house officers, and surgical students were down in the EW, stripping the burns of the dead epidermis and squirting the wounds, soaking the patients in tannic acid. As the tannic acid was being applied, the patients were dying because of the ignored signs of developing dehydration. It was evident that the priorities were off balance". In the early 1940s, Dr. Churchill assigned Oliver Cope, Bradford Cannon, a plastic surgeon, and Francis Moore, then a first-year surgical resident, to improve the treatment of burns. Cope and Bradford started a series of animal experiments testing various regimens for burns, including the standard practice of applying tannic acid to tan the wound. Their work demonstrated that contrary to popular belief and the surgical doctrine, prompt removal of all dead tissue, application of gauze treated with bland ointments, such as boric acid gauze, and immediate repair of the wound, not tannic acid, was most effective. The simplest treatment and the easiest to administer resulted in the fastest healing [6]. A thorough analysis of their own burn victims convinced them that fluid resuscitation and management of a burned airway were keys to survival and infection-free healing.

Almost immediately after reporting his research findings, Oliver Cope found himself and his team using their treatments on victims of the horrific Cocoanut Grove Night Club Fire in 1942. A rapidly spreading fire began in the basement of the Cocoanut Grove where 1000 football fans were celebrating in a space legally meant for 600. Overcrowding, and locked emergency doors, spelled disaster when a match was lit by a young bus boy to change a light bulb, igniting hanging gauze decorations, and then rapidly spreading. With only one working revolving door serving as an exit, the night club became a death trap and ultimately 492 people died, making this the second largest fire in the history of the USA, and hundreds of victims were brought within minutes to the MGH. During the 2 h following the fire, 114 burn victims were brought to the MGH; the majority were dead or died within minutes, but 39 lived to be treated at MGH. Cope wrote a few papers describing the tragedy, and in a remarkable feat of triage, clearly influenced by training

for World War II, all patients were settled in an "isolation ward" specifically made on the spot for burn victims within 3 h of arrival [7]. They were treated rapidly with oxygen, intravenous fluids, and fresh-frozen plasma for shock. Surface burns were treated without debridement but with bland boric ointment gauze and pressure dressings with no attempts at cleansing or debridement and morphine and antibiotics, essentially, all the elements of modern day burn treatment. Seven patients died within the first 3 days, all due to severe lung injury and pulmonary edema; even these patients yielded useful information to Cope, who described the bronchial and airway changes seen during postmortem examination of three of the patients. The results of the simplified and systematic treatment of the burns were evident almost immediately and many of the wounds healed within 2 weeks as Cope had shown in his earlier research. Oliver Cope undertook extensive metabolic study of the patients in the hospital, measuring nitrogen balance, and steroid secretion, thus trying to understand the metabolic response to burns. He became a proponent of organizing a prearranged plan for disasters, including having access to a classified list of required personnel. Cope became instrumental in the developing interest of The Shriner's organization to start a hospital specializing in burns adjacent to MGH. In the early 1960s, he mounted a plan to get federal funding for burn research to teach the next generation of surgeons the most effective care for burn victims, especially children.

Cope's Work on Breast Cancer

As Cope's career progressed, he became more involved in the care of breast cancer patients. He became one of the earliest proponents of lumpectomy and radiation, and he questioned the standard of care at that time, which was the radical mastectomy. He first came to think of this nontraditional treatment when a patient refused to have her breast removed in 1958; this patient led him to look at his own mastectomy results, and to his horror, he discovered that "75 % of the women who undergo mastectomy ultimately die of cancer." In 1967, his thoughts were published in Vogue and Women's Day; he became known in his own words as "a staunch supporter of women to protect themselves from unnecessary mutilation." While he tried publishing this work in medical journals as early as 1972, it was rejected by many surgical journals; Dr. Austen, the chief of surgery at MGH, had to mediate for him even among his colleagues at the hospital because of the radical nature of his proposed procedures [1]. He wrote what was probably the first book on breast cancer for the lay audience, *The Breast,* in which Cope admonished other doctors who felt that he was too "sentimental" when women complained about losing their breasts. He wrote "I ask in return if they had cancer of the penis, and there were two treatments, each equally good in the care of the cancer, one irradiation and the other surgical excision of the penis, which would they choose?" Decades later, Cope's unorthodox views were proven in the seminal randomized trials that showed lumpectomy and radiation to be equivalent to mastectomy. His deep appreciation for the emotional welfare of breast cancer patients undergoing mutilating mastectomies also led him to ruminate on the difficulty convincing the "male medical profession, that a women's desires should be considered." This was personal and deeply introspective for Cope, which concluded in him saying "I had not realized how chauvinistic I have been" [8]. No doubt that his appreciation for the plight of breast cancer patients also played a role in him being a proponent of women in surgery. Patricia Numann, a recent president of the American College of Surgeons, recalls fondly when she was a young surgeon, she met Oliver Cope at a dinner of the American Surgical Association in 1983, when she was not yet a member and he had already been the president. She remembers how influential her conversations about breast surgery and being a woman surgeon were to her career and his kindness in quickly mailing her a copy of his work and a personal letter encouraging the young female surgeon (personal communication, Dr. Numann).

Conclusion

Oliver Cope was a remarkable man and those who knew him at the height of his career called him "brilliant, innovative, a real biologist" who was known for the precision of his work. He was quite reserved in his demeanor. Later in life, as he turned to breast conservation, his patients called him a "Quaker reformer." Yet, Cope had remarkable insight into his own psyche and that of his patients. When he was 44, he went into psychiatric analysis with the psychiatrist Dr. Bibring, the first full female professor at Harvard Medical School and a student of Freud, for at least 3 years. This experience left him with a deep appreciation of a patient's emotional response, and he thought patients often understand "the emotional roots of their illnesses," but doctors, who are too "chemically minded," (himself included) are often too busy to listen, since they find "it's quicker to order an X-ray" "instead of listening" [1, 9]. This belief in the psychiatric nature of many diseases led to some interesting theories and discussions surrounding the basis of Graves' disease. Cope had a strong opinion that the pathogenesis of Graves' disease was due to psychic trauma. He often cited outstanding experiences in his own practice, noting the possibility of cure of Grave's by appropriate psychotherapy. Later in his career when it was discovered that Grave's disease was a

disorder of the immune system, Cope still stuck with his theory, quoting ample evidence of the importance of the central nervous system to immune system health. At weekly rounds when residents presented patients with **Grave's** disease, if they did not detail the emotional background of the patient, including past traumas, they were severely scolded. In fact, Dr. Cope managed for 2 years to persuade an able psychiatrist Dr. Quarton to join the MGH Thyroid Unit to study the causative role of psychic trauma in Graves' disease [10]. In fact, in 1966 he put together the first conference on behavioral science in medicine to "fill in the gaps," going on to publish a monograph entitled "Man, Mind, and Medicine" in 1968. He thought overall that this monograph was the "most important contribution" he had made, which is truly remarkable for a man who made so many varied contributions to the care of surgical patients [1].

All of Cope's thoughts on the education of surgeons was ahead of his time; he became a full professor of surgery in 1963 and adopted a radical view that surgeons should focus less on technique and more on the biology and pathology of disease, really emphasizing the need for the parallel education of surgeons and medical doctors. This concept was of course entirely pleasing to endocrine surgeons or surgical endocrinologists who are staunch proponents of surgeons learning the entire spectrum of molecular/physiologic/pathologic nature of the diseases they treat. Dr. Cope passed away in 1994 at age 91, 1 day after his wife Alice. He left behind an incredible legacy that all surgeons must strive to live up to.

References

1. Austen WG, et al. Oliver Cope: 1902–1994. The Harvard University Gazette. Boston: Harvard University; 1997.
2. Bull W, Bull M. Something in the ether. Vol. 1. Beverly: Memoirs Unlimited; 2011. p. 527.
3. Welbourn RB. The history of endocrine surgery. New York: Praeger; 1990.
4. Cope O. The study of hyperparathyroidism at the Massachusetts General Hospital. N Engl J Med. 1966;274(21):1174–82.
5. Cope O. The surgery of subtotal parathyroidectomy. New Engl J Med. 1935;213:470–4.
6. Cannon B, Cope O. Rate of epithelial regeneration: a clinical method of measurement, and the effect of various agents recommended in the treatment of burns. Ann Surg. 1943;117(1):85–92.
7. Cope O. Care of the victims of the coconut grove fire at the Massachusetts General Hospital. New Engl J Med. 1943;229:138–47.
8. Boston Globe. 30 July 1981. Boston.
9. Bibring GL. Psychoanalysis: a personal view [Interview]; Summary. 1975. WGBH Media Library & Archives. http://openvault.wgbh.org/catalog/e731ef-psychoanalysis-a-personal-view. Accessed: 21 May 2014.
10. Stanbury JB. A constant ferment. Ipswich: Ipswich Press; 1991. p. 201.

Parathyroidectomy: Postoperative Considerations/Complications

Adrian Harvey

Introduction

The parathyroid glands were discovered in the 1800s, by **Sir Richard Owen** in a rhinoceros and subsequently by Ivor Sandstrom in human cadavers [1, 2]. Subsequent observations by astute clinicians and scientists led to the understanding of their important function in calcium homeostasis. Eventually, the observation of parathyroid tumors in association with significant bone and kidney disease led to the hypothesis that parathyroid tumors may be causative and surgical removal could potentially result in cure [1, 3].

The work of surgical pioneers such as **Felix Mandel**, E. J. Lewis, Isaac Olch, **Oliver Cope**, and Edward Churchill helped to define the role of surgery in the treatment of hyperparathyroidism [1, 3, 4]. The intervening period of time has seen significant changes in presentation, diagnosis, and treatment of parathyroid disease. The indications for surgery have been refined, and additional surgical techniques and adjuncts have been developed and studied. Currently, approximately 20,000 parathyroid surgeries are performed each year in the USA [5]. The modern parathyroid surgeon must be an expert diagnostician, familiar with the full spectrum of parathyroid disease including secondary and tertiary hyperparathyroidism, familial syndromes, and mild, less clinically apparent forms of primary hyperparathyroidism. He/she must be an astute decision maker and a meticulous surgeon with expertise in the various surgical techniques and use of adjuncts. Finally, the surgical management of parathyroid disease demands a familiarity with the potential postoperative issue or complications faced by these patients. This chapter outlines important postoperative considerations in parathyroid surgery.

A. Harvey (✉)
Department of Surgery, Surgery and Oncology, Foothills Medical Center 1403-29th St NW, University of Calgary, Calgary, AB T2N2T9, Canada
e-mail: adrian.harvey@albertahealthservices.ca

Complications/Considerations

Hypocalcemia/Hungry Bone Syndrome

The importance of the parathyroid glands after thyroid surgery was illustrated early via Dr. William Halstead's observations of the divergent patterns of postoperative complications between two prominent European surgeons, **Kocher** and Billroth [6]. While Kocher was a meticulous surgeon known for careful dissection, complete removal of the thyroid and preservation of surrounding structures in a "bloodless field," Billroth's surgeries were conducted at a more rapid pace with remnant thyroid tissue and more likely injury to adjacent anatomy. Interestingly, while Kocher's patients commonly developed hypothyroid myxedema, they rarely developed tetany, an almost inverse pattern to that seen in Billroth's practice (Table 1).

Similarly, the potential for hypocalcemia following parathyroid surgery was demonstrated in early clinical experience. The first "successful" parathyroidectomy was performed by Isaac Olch in 1929 [1, 3]. The patient had significant bone disease with cystic tumors and a palpable parathyroid gland. Postoperatively, the patient developed tetany and was treated with calcium. Postoperative hypocalcemia in these patients may be related to intentional or accidental removal or devascularization of all functional parathyroid tissue. In addition, the clinical picture may be contributed to by suppression of the remaining normal glands or by an abrupt change in the balance of bone remodeling. Prolonged, significant hypocalcemia due to this latter mechanism is referred to as hungry bone syndrome.

The presumed pathophysiology of hungry bone syndrome results from the impact of a prolonged period of excess parathyroid hormone (PTH) on the process of bone remodeling [7]. Crucial to normal bone health, remodeling consists of osteoclast-mediated bone resorption coupled 2–3 weeks later with osteoblast-mediated bone formation. The portion of bone in this "in-between" phase is referred to as the remodeling space. In the preoperative state, PTH elevation tips

J. L. Pasieka, J. A. Lee (eds.), *Surgical Endocrinopathies*, DOI 10.1007/978-3-319-13662-2_27,
© Springer International Publishing Switzerland 2015

Table 1 Postoperative complications after parathyroidectomy

Complication	Incidence	Reference(s)
Hypocalcemia (HBS)		
Primary	5–100% (0–75%)	[7, 13–33]
Secondary	80–100% (27–95%)	[24, 38–42]
RLN injury		
Initial	0.1–1.5%	[8, 28, 29]
Reoperation	2.3–6%	[35, 36, 45, 46]
Wound		
Hematoma	<1%	[28, 47, 48]
Infection	0.02–0.3%	[49, 51]
Other		
VTE	0.1–0.25%	[29, 49, 52]
Pseudogout	Rare	[59]
Cardiac	0.08–0.11%	[11, 12, 29, 49, 53]
Pulmonary	0.13–0.29%	[29, 49, 53]
Pneumothorax	Rare	[56, 57]
Tetraplegia	Rare	[58]
Hyperthyroidism		
Biochemical	33%	[54]
Clinical	Rare	[55]

HBS hungry bone syndrome, *RLN* recurrent laryngeal nerve, *VTE* venous thromboembolism

the balance in favor of osteoclastic resorption resulting in an expansion of the remodeling space and an overall depletion in bone mineralization. Following successful parathyroidectomy, bone resorption abruptly decreases tipping the balance in favor of formation. The drop in remodeling space requires increased skeletal usage of minerals and may result in the abrupt drop in plasma levels of calcium and phosphate. While most hypocalcemia following surgery is mild and self-limiting, the term hungry bone syndrome is typically reserved for those requiring significant supplementation, often in the form of intravenous (IV) calcium over a prolonged period of time.

Hypocalcemia may present with perioral or extremity paresthesias and/or muscle cramping. Clinical assessment can be performed with **Chvostek's** or **Trousseau's** signs [8]. Chvostek's sign is elicited by tapping over the proximal facial nerve with resultant muscle twitching at the corner of the mouth. While simple to perform, this test is lacking in both specificity, as it is present in 10% of the normal population, and sensitivity, being absent in 30% of those with hypocalcemia [9, 10]. The Trousseau sign is tested by inflating a blood pressure cuff above the systolic pressure for 2–3 min. The resultant hypoxia and acidosis are then observed to elicit carpo-pedal spasm in the setting of hypocalcemia-related nerve irritability. This test is more sensitive than Chvostek's but is more arduous and painful to perform. Thus, some authors have suggested that its practice be abandoned [8]. More profound hypocalcemia can result in seizures, tetany, and in rare cases cardiac failure, which is reversible with treatment [11, 12].

Hypocalcemia: Primary Hyperparathyroidism

Reported rates of hypocalcemia following surgery for primary hyperparathyroidism vary widely in the literature. This likely reflects the heterogeneity in patients, the duration of disease, and surgical practice across publications. Early reports of transient postoperative hypocalcemia in the 1980s quoted rates in the 20–50% range [7, 13, 14]. The higher side of this range appeared to be associated with the practice of routine biopsy of all parathyroids found during bilateral exploration. While larger contemporary series tend to quote lower rates, a wide range continues to be reported in the literature. This variability appears to be due to a wide number of factors related to: (1) the patient, (2) the disease, and (3) surgical findings and techniques (Table 2).

Conflicting reports exist regarding the impact of age on the risk of postoperative hypocalcemia. Some reports have found an association with older age [15, 16]. Conn et al. found that postoperative hypocalcemia was significantly more common in older patients and in those with hypertension [16]. In contrast, Zuberi et al. reported that younger patients seem to be at higher risk [17]. Gender, however, does not appear to have a significant, independent impact [18]. Preoperative medications have also been linked to the risk of postoperative hypocalcemia. Schnieder et al. reported a series of 281 patients undergoing surgery for primary hyperparathyroidism [19]. On multivariate analysis, the authors

Table 2 Factors predicting hypocalcemia after parathyroidectomy

Factor	↑/↓	References
Primary hyperparathyroidism		
Age	↑(↓)	[15–17]
Gender	No effect	[18]
Preoperative calcium	↑	[16, 22]
Preoperative PTH	↑	[16, 21]
Preoperative vitamin D	↑	[20, 21]
Bone disease	↑	[22, 26, 27]
Preoperative ALP	↑	[15, 30]
Calcium-lowering meds	↑	[19]
Extensive exploration/bx	↑	[13, 16, 22, 31, 32]
# Glands removed	↑	[17, 22, 24]
Adenoma weight	↑	[7, 14, 15]
PTH drop >85%	↑	[23, 33]
Secondary hyperparathyroidism		
Age	↓	[39]
Pre-op calcium	↓	[41]
Pre-op ALP	↓	[41]
Pre-op PTH	↑	[42]
Calcium-lowering meds	↑	[40]
Weight removed	↓	[41]

PTH parathyroid hormone, *ALP* alkaline phosphatase, *bx* biopsy, ↑ decreased level of factor linked to greater risk, ↑ increased level of factor linked to greater risk found that patient taking two or more calcium-lowering medications were significantly more likely to encounter postoperative hypocalcemia.

The role of the patient's vitamin D status has also been suggested to influence postoperative calcium levels. Stewart et al. reported a higher incidence of symptomatic hypocalcemia following parathyroid surgery in vitamin D-deficient patients [20]. Lang et al. noted similar findings in a series of 80 patients treated with minimally invasive parathyroidectomy [21]. However, the authors noted that these patients also tended to have a higher preoperative PTH bringing into question the mechanism of this effect. In contrast, Press et al. in a series of more than 1700 patients noted no difference in oral calcium intake and postoperative, symptomatic hypocalcemia between groups of patients with markedly different vitamin D levels. Potentially, the routine use of supplementation in these patients may have masked smaller differences. In all three aforementioned series, 25-hydroxy vitamin D3 was measured.

As one might expect, certain disease factors seem to be linked to the risk of postoperative hypocalcemia. Higher levels of both PTH and calcium have been linked to increased risk [16]. Using multivariate analysis on a series of 6000 patients undergoing parathyroidectomy for primary hyperparathyroidism, Vasher et al. found preoperative calcium was independently predictive of postoperative hypocalcemia [22]. At their center, the authors utilize the preoperative calcium level as part of the protocol to determine upfront the level of post parathyroidectomy calcium supplementation. Similarly, Lang et al. found preoperative PTH levels to be significantly higher in patients requiring postoperative calcium supplementation [21]. These findings are certainly not universal with several additional series failing to observe a significant link between preoperative laboratory values and hypocalcemia in the postoperative period [17, 20, 23–25].

Given the proposed role of increased skeletal mineral usage in the etiology of postoperative hypocalcemia, it would seem reasonable to hypothesize that more advanced bone disease would portend a higher risk. Certainly, series that report a substantial rate of skeletal manifestations tend to have high rates of postoperative hypocalcemia [26, 27]. Gopal et al. reported a series of 79 patients treated for primary hyperparathyroidism in western India [27]. In this patient population, radiographic evidence of skeletal manifestations was evident in 75% of the patients. In this series, all patients were started on immediate postoperative oral calcium. Despite this, 60% of patients developed transient hypoparathyroidism and 30% showed evidence of significant hungry bone syndrome. Similarly, Agarwal et al. reported symptomatic hypocalcemia despite routine oral calcium and vitamin D supplementation in 46/52 patients with osteitis fibrosa cystica following surgery. All 46 patients required treatment with IV calcium gluconate. In comparison, large studies

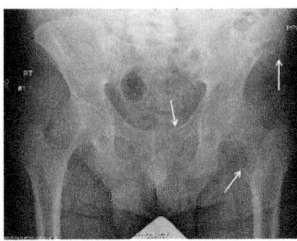

Fig. 1 Radiograph showing advanced bone disease with osteitis fibrosa cystica in a patient with hyperparathyroidism. *Arrows* indicate osteolytic bone lesions

from more developed countries in which most patients have asymptomatic hyperparathyroidism and advanced bone disease is rare report significantly lower rates of hypocalcemia and rarely mention IV calcium infusion [22, 28, 29].

Radiologic evidence of skeletal manifestations may include osteitis fibrosa cystica, lytic lesions, browns tumors, subperiosteal erosions, and fractures [7, 26, 27] (Fig. 1) In addition, Vasher et al. found that a bone mineral density t score of < 3.0 was predictive of postoperative hypocalcemia on multivariate analysis. Alkaline phosphatase has also been suggested as a serum marker of more advanced bone disease. Multiple series have demonstrated that elevated levels of alkaline phosphatase were associated with the need for postoperative calcium [15, 30]. Additional serum bone markers are not used in routine clinical practice.

Intraoperative factors have also demonstrated a clear impact. In general, hypocalcemia has been associated with more extensive removal or manipulation of parathyroid tissue [13, 14, 16, 17, 22, 24, 25, 31, 32]. The practice of routine biopsy of all parathyroid glands during a bilateral exploration was largely abandoned in the 1980s after it was shown to result in higher rates of postoperative hypocalcemia with similar cure rates compared to a more conservative strategy [13]. Even in the absence of biopsies, it appears that more extensive exploration may result in a greater degree of hypoparathyroidism [16, 22, 31, 32]. In a randomized controlled trial of unilateral versus bilateral exploration, Bergenfelz et al. reported that patients undergoing the more extensive operation required more oral calcium supplementation, and had lower postoperative calcium levels and more frequent episodes of symptomatic hypocalcemia [31]. In a subsequent review of a large-scale national database, including more than 2700 patients, the same author demonstrated lower rates of postoperative hypoparathyroidism associated with the use of preoperative localization and intraoperative PTH [32].

Given the aforementioned reports, it is not surprising that postoperative hypocalcemia is more common when a greater number of glands require removal at surgery [17, 22, 24]. Even when a single gland is removed, the weight of the parathyroid adenoma appears to be correlated with the need for calcium supplementation [7, 14, 15]. In addition, the magnitude of the drop in intraoperative PTH is predictive of the postoperative course [23, 33]. Crea et al. found that an 85% drop in intraoperative PTH was reliably predictive of postoperative hypocalcemia in patients with primary hyperparathyroidism.

Perhaps the final factor contributing to the wide range of quoted rates in the literature lies in the evolution and variability of postoperative care. In particular, there has been a shift toward short-stay or same-day discharge after parathyroid surgery in many centers. As postoperative issues have the potential to delay discharge, many centers now practice routine calcium supplementation following parathyroidectomy. In the series of 6000 patients reported by Vasher et al., routine postoperative oral calcium supplementation was tailored to the patients' risk for postoperative hypocalcemia [22]. In that report, less than 8% of patients reported hypocalcemic symptoms and just 0.1% required return to the emergency department for IV calcium. Thus, it is likely that oral supplementation is given to many patients in sufficient quantities to avoid hypocalcemia that would have been reported in earlier series during which this practice was less common.

Permanent hypoparathyroidism is exceedingly rare (<1%) following initial surgery. While significantly higher rates have been reported following multiple explorations, more recent studies have demonstrated that reoperative parathyroid surgery in experienced hands can be performed with minimal morbidity [34–37].

Hypocalcemia: Renal Hyperparathyroidism

Rates of hypercalcemia following surgery for renal hyperparathyroidism are significantly higher than those seen in the primary hyperparathyroidism literature [24, 38-42]. Certainly, this should not come as a surprise when the initial etiology in this population is linked to hypocalcemia. Virtually all patients undergoing operation for secondary hyperparathyroidism require postoperative oral calcium supplementation. In addition, more profound hypocalcemia related to hungry bones is significantly more common. Goldfarb et al. reported that 27% of 79 patients undergoing subtotal parathyroidectomy for secondary hyperparathyroidism required postoperative IV calcium [39].

Similar to the literature on primary hyperparathyroidism, several authors have examined the risk factors for significant postoperative hypocalcemia and hungry bone syndrome following parathyroidectomy. Contrary to the aforementioned literature, young age and low preoperative calcium and alkaline phosphatase levels appear to be linked to the development of severe hypocalcemia. The data on preoperative PTH are less clear with some reports showing no link [39–41] while others associate a high PTH with postoperative hypocalcemia [42]. Preoperative use of cinecalcet has also been linked to hungry bone syndrome [40]. Interestingly, Torer et al. reported that lower weight of resected parathyroid tissue was associated with postoperative hypocalcemia opposite of what has been observed in primary hyperparathyroidism [41].

Postoperative Care

At our institution, patients are followed up postoperatively with twice-daily serum calcium (albumin corrected) and phosphate levels. Magnesium levels are obtained in cases of difficult-to-correct hypocalcemia or suspected hungry bone disease. Routine oral calcium supplementation is not routinely given in cases of primary hyperparathyroidism as we do not practice same-day discharge. Oral calcium supplementation may be started at the surgeons' discretion if a high likelihood of significant postoperative hypocalcemia is suspected. Mild postoperative hypocalcemia in patients with primary hyperparathyroidism is typically manageable with oral calcium and vitamin D supplementation alone. Patients with secondary hyperparathyroidism are followed up for a longer period of time, as patients with hungry bone syndrome may not reach the nadir of their serum calcium level for several days after surgery [39]. The patients are placed on oral calcium supplementation and resume their 1,25-dihydroxy vitamin D3 supplements. Close coordination with the dialysis team is important as alterations of calcium concentration in the dialysate are often utilized to control serum levels in those with hungry bone syndrome. When required, IV calcium gluconate infusion is instituted. Prolonged infusions or more concentrated solutions are given through a peripherally inserted central catheter (PICC) or central venous line.

Hypocalcemia Summary

Considerable variability in the rates of postoperative hypocalcemia is quoted in the literature. Significant, prolonged hypocalcemia is uncommon in primary hyperparathyroidism without bone involvement. When this does occur, it can typically be managed with oral calcium supplementation. In contrast, hypocalcemia is more common following surgery for secondary hyperparathyroidism. These patients are more likely to require IV calcium infusion and more prolonged in-hospital observation. Specific risk factors have been identified which increase the risk of significant hypocalcemia following surgery. Many of these risk factors are specific to either primary or secondary disease.

Other Complications

RLN Injury

Injury to the recurrent laryngeal nerve (RLN) is uncommon in parathyroid surgery. Nonetheless, careful dissection is warranted given the proximity of the parathyroid glands to the nerve. Untch et al. examined the proximity of the parathyroid glands to the RLN in 136 patients undergoing parathyroid surgery. The authors noted the median distance to the nerve was 5 mm, with the superior glands on average lying closer than the inferior glands [43]. Large series from centers with experienced endocrine surgeons typically report rates between 0 and 1.5% for initial surgery [8, 28, 29]. However, the association between surgeon experience and complications in endocrine surgery has been well documented and may limit the generalizability of these findings [44]. Early studies suggested that reoperative exploration carried a significantly higher risk. Patow et al. reported a 6.6% rate of nerve injury in 163 patients undergoing reoperative surgery [45]. However, more recent series, utilizing preoperative localization algorithms and performed by experienced parathyroid surgeons, have reported injury rates closely approximating those seen in initial surgery [35, 36, 46].

Wound Complications

Postoperative hematoma is a rare complication of parathyroid surgery. Most series quote rates of less than 1% [28, 47, 48]. Regardless, this complication is potentially life-threatening and should be managed with expedient exploration and evacuation. Similarly, surgical site infection is quite rare after parathyroid/thyroid surgery. Gupra et al. examined 30-day mortality and morbidity following thyroid and parathyroid surgeries using the National Surgical Quality Improvement Program database over a 2-year period. In a sample of 6154 parathyroid surgeries, superficial and deep neck infections were seen in just 0.3 and 0.02%, respectively [49]. As parathyroid surgery is considered a "clean" procedure, routine preoperative antibiotic prophylaxis is not mandated [50]. In a randomized, controlled trial of 500 patients undergoing thyroidectomy, Aveia et al. failed to show any difference in surgical site infection between those given routine antibiotic prophylaxis and those who were not [51]. While evidence does not exist to support the routine use of antibiotics in these operations, practice appears to vary between centers and surgeons. Moalem et al. surveyed 518 members of the American Association of Endocrine Surgeons (AAES) and the International Association of Endocrine Surgeons (IAES) [50]. Of the 57.1% who responded, 62% reported that they "never" administer preoperative antibiotics and 26.2% responded that they "always" do.

Rare Complications

Additional complications have been reported following parathyroid surgery but are exceedingly rare. Deep venous thrombosis and pulmonary embolism are seen in 0.1–0.25% [29, 49, 52]. Roy et al. compared the incidence of deep vein thrombosis/pulmonary embolism (DVT/PE) in 16,022 patients who underwent thyroid and parathyroid surgery with a total cohort of almost 350,000 patients undergoing any surgical procedure [52]. They found that the risk of DVT/PE (0.16%) was significantly lower than in the larger population of surgical patients. In addition, given that the likelihood of return to the operating room for a neck hematoma was ten times that of DVT/PE, the authors recommended that pharmacologic prophylaxis be reserved for patients at higher risk of venous thromboembolism.

Postoperative cardiac events are rare as is pneumonia and respiratory failure requiring intubation and admission to the intensive care unit [29, 49, 53]. Biochemical evidence of hyperthyroidism can be seen in up to a third of patients [54] but is rarely clinically significant [55]. Postoperative pneumothorax has been reported typically associated with mediastinal dissection [56, 57]. Tetraplegia following parathyroidectomy for secondary hyperparathyroidism has been reported as well [58]. These cases were thought to be a consequence of extreme neck positioning, potentially in the setting of bone involvement of the cervical spine. One final complication that deserved mention is the development of postoperative pseudogout [59]. This rare complication is likely related to release of calcium pyrophosphate crystals from the articular cartilage as a result of decreased solubility in the face of falling serum calcium. Pseudogout can affect any joint but is most commonly seen in the knee [59].

The overall morbidity of parathyroid surgery is quite low. In addition to hypocalcemia, a range of other complications/postoperative issues have been described that the parathyroid surgeon must be aware of. As hospital stays decrease for these surgeries, patients may present following discharge. Young et al. examined the 30-day postoperative incidence of presentation to the emergency department in 570 patients following thyroid or parathyroid surgeries [60]. The rate of emergency department visits was 11% and not significantly different between thyroid and parathyroid procedures. The most common presenting complaint was paresthesias. Most patients with paresthesias were found to have no electrolyte abnormalities or mild deficiencies that were corrected in the emergency department (ED) and then were discharged home.

Recurrence/Persistence

In experienced hands, parathyroid surgery is highly successful. However, a small proportion of patients will present with persistent or recurrent disease. Persistent disease is defined by hypercalcemia occurring within 6 months of surgery, while recurrent disease is characterized by initial eucalcemia with hypercalcemia developing beyond 6 months [8]. Most operative failures are persistent disease. The rate of persistent/recurrent disease is approximately 1–5% [29, 48, 61–64]. Potential causes of operative failure include: (1) failure to locate an adenoma; (2) inadequate resection in multigland hyperplasia, double adenoma, or unrecognized familial disease; and (3) rare cases of parathyromatosis or recurrence of parathyroid cancer.

A number of factors may show recurrence/persistence following parathyroid surgery. Surgeon experience plays a significant role in operative failure. A number of series have found preventable causes of reoperation to be significantly more common in patients operated on at low-volume centers [65, 66]. Chen et al. found that reoperations on patients initially operated on at low-volume centers more often found a missed adenoma in a normal anatomic position (89%) compared to those from high-volume centers (13%) [65]. Most series have not suggested a difference in persistent or recurrent disease with focused versus bilateral exploration [29, 31, 48, 63]. However, more recent data have suggested a trend toward increased late recurrence in focused surgery [62, 67]. Interestingly, operative failure may be higher following resection of double adenoma [61]. A potential explanation for this phenomenon is that a proportion of these cases represent unrecognized four-gland hyperplasia. Finally, the shape of the intraoperative PTH curve may predict recurrence. Schnieder et al. found that patients with PTH levels showing a "rebound" after reaching the >50% drop criteria had double the chance of recurrence compared to those that did not [68].

Recurrence after surgery for renal hyperparathyroidism appears to be slightly higher. In secondary hyperparathyroidism, the recurrence rate may be related to the extent of initial surgery [69–71]. In general, total parathyroidectomy has lower recurrence rates than total with autotransplant or subtotal resections [69–71]. In addition, supranumerary glands are found in 13% of patients with secondary hyperparathyroidism. Most commonly, these are located in the thymus. In an analysis of 95 patients undergoing neck reexploration for recurrent secondary hyperparathyroidism, Schneider et al. found intrathymic parathyroid glands in 28.4% [72]. On the basis of this data, the authors suggested that bilateral cervical thymectomy should be routine in the initial operative treatment of secondary hyperparathyroidism. Similarly, recurrence in patients with tertiary hyperparathyroidism may be linked to the extent of initial operation [73–76]. Total parathyroidectomy ± autotransplant and subtotal appear to have similar results [73, 74, 76, 77]. However, the argument that not all glands necessarily develop autonomous function has led some surgeons to consider more limited resections [75]. Kebebew et al. found that patients undergoing reoperation were more likely to have undergone initial one- or two gland resections [74]. In contrast, Pitt et al. compared recurrence in 140 patients who underwent limited versus subtotal parathyroidectomy for tertiary hyperparathyroidism [75]. The authors found that recurrence/persistence was independent of the extent of operation on logistical regression. In addition, postoperative hypocalcemia was more common after subtotal resection.

Reoperation

Given the potential for increased perioperative morbidity, patients with recurrent or persistent hyperparathyroidism should be evaluated by an experienced parathyroid surgeon [8, 35–37, 45]. Careful assessment of the patient should follow an organized approach to determine if another operation is appropriate. All previous records should be reviewed and a careful history taken. As failed exploration may result from an error in diagnosis, care should be taken to confirm that the patient does indeed have primary hyperparathyroidism. Secondary hyperparathyroidism and familial hypocalciuric hypercalcemia must be excluded. Evidence of familial disease should be sought on history as these patients are more prone to recurrence [78–80]. If appropriate, patients should be referred for genetic testing. All previous documentation including biochemical testing, imaging, operative reports, and histology should be reviewed. This should give the surgeon a sense of whether recurrence is likely related to multigland disease or a missed adenoma.

The decision to proceed to reoperation should balance the benefits against the increased difficulty, and potential morbidity of surgery in a previously operated field. While no specific guidelines exist for reoperative surgery, indications can be extrapolated from those published for the initial procedure [81]. Patients with mild, asymptomatic hyperparathyroidism may be better served with observation. Once the decision to explore reoperation has been made, the focus should shift to localization. Reexploration in the absence of localization is rarely indicated. Noninvasive tests should be utilized initially. These may include ultrasound, Tc99 sestamibi scan with single-photon emission computed tomography (CT), 4-D CT, and magnetic resonance imaging (MRI). When noninvasive tests fail to localize the abnormal parathyroid tissue, selective venous sampling for PTH can be utilized. If an equivocal finding is noted on cross-sectional imaging, this can be clarified with ultrasound-guided fine-needle aspiration with PTH assay of the needle wash. Preoperative laryngoscopy is mandatory prior to any reoperative parathyroid surgery.

A full description of reoperative parathyroid surgery is beyond the scope of this chapter. Needless to say, the parathyroid surgeon should be familiar with the principles of reoperative neck surgery and have extensive knowledge of parathyroid anatomy including the locations of potential ectopic glands. The surgeon may take advantage of an alternate operative approach, lateral to the strap muscles in order to minimize dissection in previously operated planes. Finally, he/she should be prepared to alter the operative plan in the face of unexpected findings. In experienced hands, and in appropriately selected patients, reoperative parathyroid surgery can be performed safely, with cure rates approximating those seen at initial exploration [35, 36, 46, 74, 81–83].

Conclusion

While generally an effective procedure with low morbidity, parathyroid surgery has some important postoperative considerations with which the experienced endocrine surgeon should be familiar. The most common postoperative issue encountered is hypocalcemia. Following surgery for primary hyperparathyroidism, hypocalcemia is typically mild and manageable with oral calcium supplementation, often as an outpatient. Several risk factors related to the patient, the disease, and the surgical procedure have been identified which may predict the occurrence of more severe hypocalcemia. In rare patients with more marked disease, particularly those with skeletal involvement, hungry bone syndrome may result in more profound and prolonged hypocalcemia, potentially requiring IV calcium infusion. Hungry bone syndrome is more common following surgery for renal hyperparathyroidism. These patients are inappropriate for same-day/early discharge surgery and require more careful postoperative observation. Parathyroid surgeons should be aware of additional, more rare complications which include but are not limited to: (1) RLN injury, (2) wound hematoma or infection, (3) venous thromboembolism, (4) and general postoperative cardiopulmonary complications.

Following initial surgery for primary hyperparathyroidism, persistent or recurrent disease occurs in less than 5%. Outcomes and morbidity are both linked to surgeon experience. Recurrence is more common following surgery for renal hyperparathyroidism and may be linked to the extent of initial resection. In secondary hyperparathyroidism, supranumerary and ectopic glands are common. These are often found in the thymus. Several authors suggest that bilateral cervical thymectomy be routine in these patients. When recurrent or persistent disease is encountered, referral to an experienced parathyroid surgeon is critical. A thorough history and review of previous documentation and testing should be undertaken. The surgeon must confirm the diagnosis, determine the likely cause of recurrence, and weigh the benefits of reoperation with potential morbidity. Localization is paramount to safe reoperative surgery and blind exploration is rarely, if ever, indicated. Noninvasive studies are utilized first with invasive tests reserved for unclear or discordant imaging. In experienced hands, outcomes of reoperative surgery approximate those seen at initial exploration with acceptable morbidity.

Key Summary Points

- In addition to diagnostic knowledge, astute decision making, and surgical skill, the modern parathyroid surgeon must be familiar with the full range of potential postoperative issues.

- Postoperative hypocalcemia may be related to removal/devascularization of all parathyroids, suppression of remaining glands, or abrupt changes in bone metabolism.
- Significant/prolonged postoperative hypocalcemia is more common in patients with renal hyperparathyroidism.
- Risk factors for hypocalcemia have been identified that may help the clinician anticipate the need for more prolonged/inpatient calcium supplementation.
- The RLN injury is low but may be more common in reoperative surgery.
- Wound infections are rare, and convincing evidence for prophylactic antibiotic use is lacking.
- Recurrent or persistent disease following surgery for primary hyperparathyroidism occurs in 1–5%, (may be higher in renal hyperparathyroidism).
- Assessment of patients requiring reoperative parathyroid surgery should be left to an experienced surgeon with a high-volume practice.

References

1. Lew JI, Solorzano CC. Surgical management of primary hyperparathyroidism: state of the art. Surg Clin North Am. 2009;89:1205–25.
2. R O. On the anatomy of the Indian Rhinoceros. Tran Zoo Soc Lon. 1862;4:31–58.
3. Barr DP, Bulgar HA, Dixon HH. Hyperparathyroidism. JAMA. 1929;92:951–2.
4. Cope O. The study of hyperparathyroidism at the Massachusetts General Hospital. N Engl J Med. 1966;274:1174–82.
5. Sosa JA, Wang TS, Yeo HL, et al. The maturation of a specialty: workforce projections for endocrine surgery. Surgery. 2007;142:876–83.
6. R M, A R, G R. The history and evolution of tecniques for thyroid surgery. In: D T, CG, editors. Thytroid and parathyroid disease: medical and surgical management. New York: Thieme Medical; 2009. p. 1–35.
7. Witteveen JE, van Thiel S, Romijn JA, Hamdy NA. Hungry bone syndrome: still a challenge in the post-operative management of primary hyperparathyroidism: a systematic review of the literature. Eur J Endocrinol. 2013;168:R45–53.
8. Carty SE. Prevention and management of complications in parathyroid surgery. Otolaryngol Clin North Am. 2004;37:897–907, xi.
9. Fonseca OA, Calverley JR. Neurological manifestations of hypoparathyroidism. Arch Intern Med. 1967;120:202–6.
10. Meneret A, Guey S, Degos B. Chvostek sign, frequently found in healthy subjects, is not a useful clinical sign. Neurology. 2013;80:1067.
11. Aguiar P, Cruz D, Ferro Rodrigues R, Peixoto L, Araujo F, Ducla Soares JL. Hypocalcemic cardiomyopathy. Rev Port Cardiol. 2013;32:331–5.
12. Hurley K, Baggs D. Hypocalcemic cardiac failure in the emergency department. J Emerg Med. 2005;28:155–9.
13. Kaplan EL, Bartlett S, Sugimoto J, Fredland A. Relation of postoperative hypocalcemia to operative techniques: deleterious effect of excessive use of parathyroid biopsy. Surgery. 1982;92:827–34.
14. Zamboni WA, Folse R. Adenoma weight: a predictor of transient hypocalcemia after parathyroidectomy. Am J Surg. 1986;152:611–15.

15. Brasier AR, Nussbaum SR. Hungry bone syndrome: clinical and biochemical predictors of its occurrence after parathyroid surgery. Am J Med. 1988;84:654–60.

16. Conn CA, Clark J, Bumpous J, Goldstein R, Fleming M, Flynn MB. Hypocalcemia after neck exploration for untreated primary hyperparathyroidism. Am Surg. 2006;72:1234–7.

17. Zuberi KA, Urquhart AC. Serum PTH and ionized calcium levels as predictors of symptomatic hypocalcemia after parathyroidectomy. Laryngoscope. 2010;120(4):192.

18. Mazeh H, Sippel RS, Chen H. The role of gender in primary hyperparathyroidism: same disease, different presentation. Ann Surg Oncol. 2012;19:2958–62.

19. Schneider DF, Day GM, De Jong SA. Calcium-lowering medications in patients with primary hyperparathyroidism: intraoperative findings and postoperative hypocalcemia. Am J Surg. 2012;203:357–60; discussion 360.

20. Stewart ZA, Blackford A, Somervell H, et al. 25-hydroxyvitamin D deficiency is a risk factor for symptoms of postoperative hypocalcemia and secondary hyperparathyroidism after minimally invasive parathyroidectomy. Surgery. 2005;138:1018–25; discussion 1025.

21. Lang BH, Lo CY. Vitamin D3 deficiency is associated with late-onset hypocalcemia after minimally invasive parathyroidectomy in a vitamin D borderline area. World J Surg. 2010;34:1350–5.

22. Vasher M, Goodman A, Politz D, Norman J. Postoperative calcium requirements in 6,000 patients undergoing outpatient parathyroidectomy: easily avoiding symptomatic hypocalcemia. J Am Coll Surg. 2010;211:49–54.

23. Crea N, Pata G, Casella C, Cappelli C, Salerni B. Predictive factors for postoperative severe hypocalcaemia after parathyroidectomy for primary hyperparathyroidism. Am Surg. 2012;78:352–8.

24. Mittendorf EA, Merlino JI, McHenry CR. Post-parathyroidectomy hypocalcemia: incidence, risk factors, and management. Am Surg. 2004;70:114–9; discussion 119.

25. Strickland PL, Recabaren J. Are preoperative serum calcium, parathyroid hormone, and adenoma weight predictive of postoperative hypocalcemia? Am Surg. 2002;68:1080–2.

26. Agarwal G, Mishra SK, Kar DK, et al. Recovery pattern of patients with osteitis fibrosa cystica in primary hyperparathyroidism after successful parathyroidectomy. Surgery. 2002;132:1075–83; discussion 1083.

27. Gopal RA, Acharya SV, Bandgar T, Menon PS, Dalvi AN, Shah NS. Clinical profile of primary hyperparathyroidism from western India: a single center experience. J Postgrad Med. 2010;56:79–84.

28. Allendorf J, DiGorgi M, Spanknebel K, Inabnet W, Chabot J, Logerfo P. 1112 consecutive bilateral neck explorations for primary hyperparathyroidism. World J Surg. 2007;31:2075–80.

29. Udelsman R, Lin Z, Donovan P. The superiority of minimally invasive parathyroidectomy based on 1650 consecutive patients with primary hyperparathyroidism. Ann Surg. 2011;253:585–91.

30. Heath DA, Van't Hoff W, Barnes AD, Gray JG. Value of 1-alpha-hydroxy vitamin D3 in treatment of primary hyperparathyroidism before parathyroidectomy. Br Med J. 1979;1:450–2.

31. Bergenfelz A, Lindblom P, Tibblin S, Westerdahl J. Unilateral versus bilateral neck exploration for primary hyperparathyroidism: a prospective randomized controlled trial. Ann Surg. 2002;236:543–51.

32. Bergenfelz AO, Jansson SK, Wallin GK, et al. Impact of modern techniques on short-term outcome after surgery for primary hyperparathyroidism: a multicenter study comprising 2,708 patients. Langenbecks Arch Surg. 2009;394:851–60.

33. Shoman N, Melck A, Holmes D, et al. Utility of intraoperative parathyroid hormone measurement in predicting postparathyroidectomy hypocalcemia. J Otolaryngol Head Neck Surg. 2008;37:16–22.

34. Karakas E, Muller HH, Schlosshauer T, Rothmund M, Bartsch DK. Reoperations for primary hyperparathyroidism–improvement of outcome over two decades. Langenbecks Arch Surg. 2013;398:99–106.

35. Prescott JD, Udelsman R. Remedial operation for primary hyperparathyroidism. World J Surg. 2009;33:2324–34.

36. Udelsman R, Donovan PI. Remedial parathyroid surgery: changing trends in 130 consecutive cases. Ann Surg. 2006;244:471–9.

37. Udelsman R. Approach to the patient with persistent or recurrent primary hyperparathyroidism. J Clin Endocrinol Metab. 2011;96:2950–58.

38. Conzo G, Perna A, Candela G, et al. Long-term outcomes following "presumed" total parathyroidectomy for secondary hyperparathyroidism of chronic kidney disease. G Chir. 2012;33:379–82.

39. Goldfarb M, Gondek SS, Lim SM, Farra JC, Nose V, Lew JI. Postoperative hungry bone syndrome in patients with secondary hyperparathyroidism of renal origin. World J Surg. 2012;36:1314–9.

40. Meyers MO, Russell CP, Ollila DW, Yeh JJ, Kim HJ, Calvo BF. Postoperative hypocalcemia after parathyroidectomy for renal hyperparathyroidism in the era of cinacalcet. Am Surg. 2009;75:843–7.

41. Torer N, Torun D, Torer N, et al. Predictors of early postoperative hypocalcemia in hemodialysis patients with secondary hyperparathyroidism. Transplant Proc. 2009;41:3642–6.

42. Viaene L, Evenepoel P, Bammens B, Claes K, Kuypers D, Vanrenterghem Y. Calcium requirements after parathyroidectomy in patients with refractory secondary hyperparathyroidism. Nephron Clin Pract. 2008;110:c80–5.

43. Untch BR, Adam MA, Danko ME, et al. Tumor proximity to the recurrent laryngeal nerve in patients with primary hyperparathyroidism undergoing parathyroidectomy. Ann Surg Oncol. 2012;19:3823–6.

44. Stavrakis AI, Ituarte PH, Ko CY, Yeh MW. Surgeon volume as a predictor of outcomes in inpatient and outpatient endocrine surgery. Surgery. 2007;142:887–99; discussion 887.

45. Patow CA, Norton JA, Brennan MF. Vocal cord paralysis and reoperative parathyroidectomy. A prospective study. Ann Surg. 1986;203:282–5.

46. Richards ML, Thompson GB, Farley DR, Grant CS. Reoperative parathyroidectomy in 228 patients during the era of minimal-access surgery and intraoperative parathyroid hormone monitoring. Am J Surg. 2008;196:937–42; discussion 942.

47. Carty SE, Roberts MM, Virji MA, Haywood L, Yim JH. Elevated serum parathormone level after "concise parathyroidectomy" for primary sporadic hyperparathyroidism. Surgery. 2002;132:1086–92; discussion 1092.

48. Udelsman R. Six hundred fifty-six consecutive explorations for primary hyperparathyroidism. Ann Surg. 2002;235:665–70; discussion 670.

49. Gupta PK, Smith RB, Gupta H, Forse RA, Fang X, Lydiatt WM. Outcomes after thyroidectomy and parathyroidectomy. Head Neck. 2012;34:477–84.

50. Moalem J, Ruan DT, Farkas RL, et al. Patterns of antibiotic prophylaxis use for thyroidectomy and parathyroidectomy: results of an international survey of endocrine surgeons. J Am Coll Surg. 2010;210:949–56.

51. Avenia N, Sanguinetti A, Cirocchi R, et al. Antibiotic prophylaxis in thyroid surgery: a preliminary multicentric Italian experience. Ann Surg Innov Res. 2009;3:10.

52. Roy M, Rajamanickam V, Chen H, Sippel R. Is DVT prophylaxis necessary for thyroidectomy and parathyroidectomy? Surgery. 2010;148:1163–8; discussion 1168.

53. Gupta PK, Gupta H, Natarajan B, et al. Postoperative respiratory failure after thyroid and parathyroid surgery: analysis of national surgical quality improvement program. Head Neck. 2012;34:321–7.

54. Stang MT, Yim JH, Challinor SM, Bahl S, Carty SE. Hyperthyroidism after parathyroid exploration. Surgery. 2005;138:1058–64; discussion 1064.

55. Parker G, Brand WW, Dyess E, Webster SA. Acute thyroiditis complicating parathyroidectomy. Am J Med Sci. 2010;339:491–2.

56. Guerrero MA, Wray CJ, Kee SS, Frenzel JC, Perrier ND. Minimally invasive parathyroidectomy complicated by pneumothoraces: a report of 4 cases. J Surg Educ. 2007;64:101–7; discussion 113.

57. Slater B, Inabnet WB. Pneumothorax: an uncommon complication of minimally invasive parathyroidectomy. Surg Laparosc Endosc Percutan Tech. 2005;15:38–40.

58. Mercieri M, Paolini S, Mercieri A, et al. Tetraplegia following parathyroidectomy in two long-term haemodialysis patients. Anaesthesia. 2009;64:1010–3.

59. Doshi J, Wheatley H. Pseudogout: an unusual and forgotten metabolic sequela of parathyroidectomy. Head Neck. 2008;30:1650–3.

60. Young WG, Succar E, Hsu L, Talpos G, Ghanem TA. Causes of emergency department visits following thyroid and parathyroid surgery. JAMA Otolaryngol Head Neck Surg. 2013;139:1175–80.

61. Alhefdhi A, Schneider DF, Sippel R, Chen H. Recurrent and persistence primary hyperparathyroidism occurs more frequently in patients with double adenomas. J Surg Res. 2014;190(1):198–202.

62. Norman J, Lopez J, Politz D. Abandoning unilateral parathyroidectomy: why we reversed our position after 15,000 parathyroid operations. J Am Coll Surg. 2012;214:260–9.

63. Schneider DF, Mazeh H, Chen H, Sippel RS. Predictors of recurrence in primary hyperparathyroidism: an analysis of 1386 cases. Ann Surg. 2014;259:563–8.

64. Sosa JA, Powe NR, Levine MA, Udelsman R, Zeiger MA. Profile of a clinical practice: thresholds for surgery and surgical outcomes for patients with primary hyperparathyroidism: a national survey of endocrine surgeons. J Clin Endocrinol Metab. 1998;83:2658–65.

65. Chen H, Wang TS, Yen TW, et al. Operative failures after parathyroidectomy for hyperparathyroidism: the influence of surgical volume. Ann Surg. 2010;252:691–5.

66. Mitchell J, Milas M, Barbosa G, Sutton J, Berber E, Siperstein A. Avoidable reoperations for thyroid and parathyroid surgery: effect of hospital volume. Surgery. 2008;144:899–906; discussion 906.

67. Schneider DF, Mazeh H, Sippel RS, Chen H. Is minimally invasive parathyroidectomy associated with greater recurrence compared to bilateral exploration? Analysis of more than 1,000 cases. Surgery. 2012;152:1008–15.

68. Schneider DF, Ojomo KA, Mazeh H, Oltmann SC, Sippel RS, Chen H. Significance of rebounding parathyroid hormone levels during parathyroidectomy. J Surg Res. 2013;184:265–8.

69. Conzo G, Perna AF, Sinisi AA, et al. Total parathyroidectomy without autotransplantation in the surgical treatment of secondary hyperparathyroidism of chronic kidney disease. J Endocrinol Invest. 2012;35:8–13.

70. Gagne ER, Urena P, Leite-Silva S, et al. Short- and long-term efficacy of total parathyroidectomy with immediate autografting compared with subtotal parathyroidectomy in hemodialysis patients. J Am Soc Nephrol. 1992;3:1008–17.

71. Rayes N, Seehofer D, Schindler R, et al. Long-term results of subtotal vs total parathyroidectomy without autotransplantation in kidney transplant recipients. Arch Surg. 2008;143:756–61; discussion 761.

72. Schneider R, Bartsch DK, Schlosser K. Relevance of bilateral cervical thymectomy in patients with renal hyperparathyroidism: analysis of 161 patients undergoing reoperative parathyroidectomy. World J Surg. 2013;37:2155–61.

73. Hsieh TM, Sun CK, Chen YT, Chou FF. Total parathyroidectomy versus subtotal parathyroidectomy in the treatment of tertiary hyperparathyroidism. Am Surg. 2012;78:600–4.

74. Kebebew E, Duh QY, Clark OH. Tertiary hyperparathyroidism: histologic patterns of disease and results of parathyroidectomy. Arch Surg. 2004;139:974–7.

75. Pitt SC, Panneerselvan R, Chen H, Sippel RS. Tertiary hyperparathyroidism: is less than a subtotal resection ever appropriate? A study of long-term outcomes. Surgery. 2009;146:1130–37.

76. Sadideen HM, Taylor JD, Goldsmith DJ. Total parathyroidectomy without autotransplantation after renal transplantation for tertiary hyperparathyroidism: long-term follow-up. Int Urol Nephrol. 2012;44:275–81.

77. Schlosser K, Endres N, Celik I, Fendrich V, Rothmund M, Fernandez ED. Surgical treatment of tertiary hyperparathyroidism: the choice of procedure matters! World J Surg. 2007;31:1947–53.

78. Burgess JR, David R, Parameswaran V, Greenaway TM, Shepherd JJ. The outcome of subtotal parathyroidectomy for the treatment of hyperparathyroidism in multiple endocrine neoplasia type 1. Arch Surg. 1998;133:126–9.

79. Hessman O, Stalberg P, Sundin A, et al. High success rate of parathyroid reoperation may be achieved with improved localization diagnosis. World J Surg. 2008;32:774–81; discussion 782.

80. Salmeron MD, Gonzalez JM, Sancho Insenser J, et al. Causes and treatment of recurrent hyperparathyroidism after subtotal parathyroidectomy in the presence of multiple endocrine neoplasia 1. World J Surg. 2010;34:1325–31.

81. Bilezikian JP, Khan AA, Potts JTJ. Guidelines for the management of asymptomatic primary hyperparathyroidism: summary statement from the third international workshop. J Clin Endocrinol Metab. 2009;94:335–9.

82. Akerstrom G, Rudberg C, Grimelius L, Johansson H, Lundstrom B, Rastad J. Causes of failed primary exploration and technical aspects of re-operation in primary hyperparathyroidism. World J Surg. 1992;16:562–8; discussion 568.

83. Caron NR, Sturgeon C, Clark OH. Persistent and recurrent hyperparathyroidism. Curr Treat Options Oncol. 2004;5:335–45.

František Chvostek

1835-1884

Dawn M. Elfenbein and Herbert Chen

František Chvostek (1835–1884) was born in Frýdek-Místek, Moravia on May 21, 1835. The historical country of Moravia occupied most of the eastern part, which is now known as the Czech Republic. It shared a border and history with Austria as part of the Austro-Hungarian Empire that was ruled for centuries by the Hapsburg family. After World War I, Moravia became a part of Czechoslovakia. It officially ceased to exist as a political entity in 1949 when the Communist party rearranged the land into regions with borders that were very different than those that existed historically. With the fall of the Soviet Union and the breakup of Czechoslovakia in 1993, the land formerly known as Moravia became a part of the Czech Republic.

Chvostek moved from Moravia to Vienna, Austria and studied medicine at Josephinum, where he received his doctorate in 1861. The school, also called Josephs-Akademie, was an academy for the training of military doctors. It was founded in 1782 by Joseph II, Holy Roman Emperor and ruler of the Habsburg lands at the time. Joseph II was a subscriber to the reform movement of the time known as the Age of Enlightenment. This new way of thinking emphasized reason and rationality over tradition, and sought to advance knowledge through the scientific method. In addition to founding the Josephinum Medical School, Jospeh II attempted to centralize medical care in Vienna through the establishment of a single, large hospital—Allgemeines Krankenhaus—which was developed from already-existing buildings that were used as a home for the poor and invalid. This was rededicated for use as a hospital on August 16, 1784. Although revolutionary in its design and its intent to centralize medical care for all those requiring medical services whether or not they could pay, including mental health services, it was

plagued by poor sanitation that caused epidemics and a 20% death rate [1]. It is in this very hospital in 1847 that Dr. Ignaz Philipp Semmelweis made his famous discovery that hand disinfection between patients on an obstetrical ward drastically reduced the incidence of puerperal fever. The hospital still exists today and is the largest university hospital in Europe, and is the site of the Medical University of Vienna.

Chvostek served at Garnisonspital Nr. 1 (English: "military hospital") in Vienna for 2 years after his graduation, then served at his medical school as the assistant of Dr. Adalbert Duchek, a favorite teacher at Josephinum. He developed an interest in electrotherapy, and began lecturing on this topic in 1868 at the school. When Duchek left in 1871, Chvostek took over as the director of the medical clinic until the academy closed in 1874. Today, the Josephinum Academy is home to the Institute for the History of Medicine of the Medical University of Vienna.

In 1876, he published the paper describing what is now known as Chvostek's sign, "Beitrag zur Tetanie" (English: "An article about Tetany") in the Vienna medical press. He described increased mechanical irritability of peripheral nerves in tetany. The sign consists of the rapid contraction of the facial muscles supplied by the seventh cranial nerve elicited by tapping on the nerve itself. Chvostek described percussing the seventh nerve in front of the external auditory meatus, and claimed that the muscle contraction evoked was not a reflex, but was due to direct stimulation of the facial nerve [2]. A few years later, in 1882, Schultze elicited the same response by tapping a region between the zygomatic arch and the corner of the mouth, and debate ensued about whether this was direct stimulation of muscle fibers, nerve, reflex, or some combination of mechanisms [3]. Figure 28.1 shows the two points over which to percuss to elicit the response. Medical students today are taught to perform this maneuver when examining a patient with hypoparathyroidism or with suspected hypocalcemia, but it is interesting to note that Chvostek's original publication happened before parathyroid glands were even discovered in humans. Ivar Viktor Sandström, a Swedish medical student, first described

H. Chen (✉)
Division of General Surgery, K3-705 Clinical Science Center, University of Wisconsin, 600 Highland Ave, Madison, WI 53792 USA
e-mail: chen@surgery.wisc.edu

D. M. Elfenbein
Department of Surgery, University of Wisconsin, Madison, WI, USA

J. L. Pasieka, J. A. Lee (eds.), *Surgical Endocrinopathies,* DOI 10.1007/978-3-319-13662-2_28,
© Springer International Publishing Switzerland 2015

the gland in humans 4 years after Chvostek's description of his sign in 1880 [4], and it was not until many years later that the glands were known to regulate calcium metabolism. Chvostek was describing something he observed in patients with tetany; it was only later that we fully understood the underlying pathophysiology of tetany and only later that Chvostek's sign became associated with hypocalcemia.

Chvostek's sign has been reported to be positive in many diseases: tetany in the newborn, hypoparathyroidism, alkalosis, rickets, diptheria, measles, scarlet fever, alcoholism, whooping cough, typhoid fever, tonsillar diseases, myxedema, joint neuralgia, and tuberculosis. The common pathway in many of these states seems to be hypocalcemia, but many published papers report a positive Chvostek's sign in 5–50 % of normal healthy people, particularly children, giving it a fairly poor specificity. In 20 % of patients with a positive Chvostek's sign, this is a unilateral finding, and is a transient finding in other patients. Additionally, it can be negative in up to 30 % of patients who do have hypocalcemia, making its sensitivity poor, as well [5]. Dr. Chvostek had a son who followed in his father's footsteps and became a physician. Franz Chvostek, Jr. published numerous papers describing the sign first described by his father, and was one of the first to associate the sign with derangement of the parathyroid glands. He concluded one article written in 1907 (31 years after his father originally described the sign) with the following

> We believe that the mechanical hyperexcitability of the nerves, especially the facial, is an easily elicited and important symptoms of diseases of the parathyroids, a delicate test which reveals to us a disturbance in the functions of these organs. [6]

In addition to his discovery of the sign that eventually was linked to hypocalcemia and hypoparathyroidism, he was a prolific writer and was very interested in the use of electricity as medical therapy. Chvostek published at least 163 articles on various medical subjects, mostly related to pathology and treatment of diseases of the nervous system, but at least six on the therapeutic use of electricity in medicine [7]. Interestingly, what seemed to capture his attention for many years was the treatment of another endocrine disorder, goiter.

In 1835, **Robert James Graves** described a disease that presented with goiter and exophthalmos. Today, we know Graves' disease as hyperthyroidism caused by circulating autoantibodies, but during Chvostek's time, exophthalmic goiter was thought to be caused by derangement of the sympathetic nervous system. Specifically, Chvostek himself thought the main pathology of exophthalmic goiter was the medulla oblongata, and that cervical chain ganglia and the cervical vagus nerve were involved in what was thought to be primarily a neurologic problem. Because Chvostek believed that neurologic pathologies were amenable to electric therapy, he treated and published his results of over 30 women with the affliction. He describes placing one electrode over

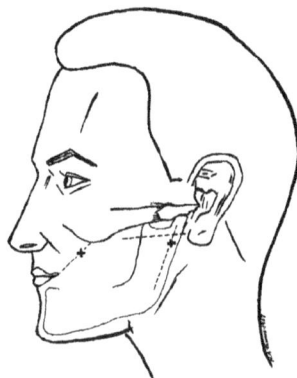

Fig. 28.1 Chvostek's sign. (From [3]. Reprinted with permission from Elsevier Limited.)

the position of the cervical sympathetic ganglion and one on either the goiter or the eyelids. He reports that the electric current had a direct effect on the medulla oblongata, the cervical sympathetic chain, and the vagus nerves. He kept the current going just sufficient to produce a sensation of burning, and noted that "strong currents have not seldom been followed by patients getting worse." He noted decrease in the pulse rates of women treated with electrotherapy, as well as improvement in exophthalmos and shrinking of the goiter in all 30 women [8].

A few years later, news of Chvostek's electrolysis technique made it across the Atlantic Ocean to Baltimore. In one 1886 article, it is reported that Chvostek cured nine cases of gonorrheal orchitis, one traumatic infiltration in the leg, six indolent inguinal buboes (inflamed lymph nodes), 30 goiters, and improved one patient with a large pannus by passing electrical current through patients. Chvostek's method is described in more detail: "Ordinary sponge electrodes are attached to the skin and then to a battery of thirteen Seimens-Halske cells, passing the current in sittings of 5 min and changing the location of the electrodes every minute or two. If no improvement is seen after 15 sittings, the treatment need not be further pursued." The author goes on to write that he personally tried the method on one woman and the goiter diminished somewhat after three sittings, but then the patient mysteriously left the city and had not yet returned at the time of publication. The author expressed that he received a letter from her affirming her belief in the method and stating that she wished to resume treatment upon her return to Baltimore, but the reader is left to wonder if the woman shared her doctor's enthusiasm for electrolysis, despite the unit that housed the battery cells having the added bonus that it was "beautiful as a piece of office furniture" (Fig. 28.2) [9].

Chvostek died in 1884, the same year as the famous geneticist, Gregor Mendel, who also was born in Moravia. Ten years after his death, Robert Newman called Chvostek "a

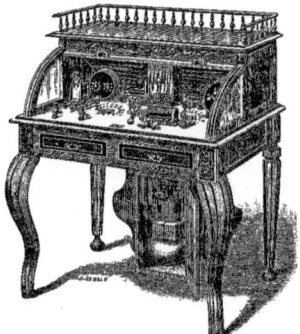

Fig. 28.2 Furniture that housed batteries for electrotherapy in Baltimore. (From [9])

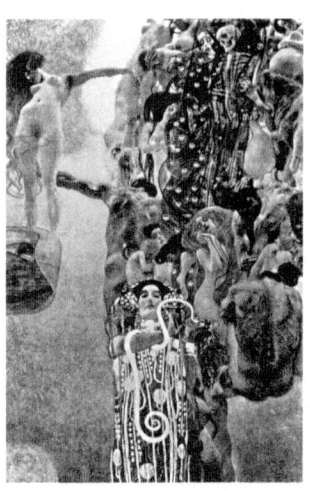

Fig. 28.3 Medicine, Gustav Klimt

pioneer" in the observation and treatment of exophthalmic goiter in an article in the *Journal of the American Medical Association* (JAMA) [10]. Fifteen years after Chvostek's death, his accomplishments were lauded in an editorial that heavily criticized the work of the famous artist, Gustav Klimt. Klimt was commissioned to decorate the ceiling of the Great Hall of the University of Vienna. The most controversial of the grouping, *Medicine,* was unveiled in 1901. A massive river of chaotically arranged naked figures flows around a figure of death, represented as a skeleton. Life, represented as a nude young female with an infant at her feet, floats nearby. The female figure Hygieia holds the cup of Lethe (oblivion) with the Aesculapian snake around her arm (Fig. 28.3). Critics and university officials despised the work, saying that the painter emphasized the powerlessness of the healing arts at a time when Vienna was leading the world in medical research, thanks, in part to the pioneering work of Frantisek Chvostek. A journalist of the time, Karl Krauss, sarcastically likened the chaotic confusion of decrepit bodies to the situation in a state hospital, and the painting was never affixed to the ceiling of the Great Hall. In May, 1945, the painting was destroyed as retreating German SS forces set fire to Schloss Immendorf, the castle in which it was being stored [11].

Acknowledgment The authors would like to gratefully acknowledge Micaela Sullivan-Fowler, Curator/History of Health Sciences Librarian, Ebling Library at the University of Wisconsin for her research assistance in obtaining the historical documents for this chapter.

References

1. http://www.sciencemuseum.org.uk/broughttolife/people/allgemeineskrankenhaus.aspx. Accessed: 15 May 2014.
2. Kugelberg E. The mechanism of Chvostek's sign. AMA Arch Neur Psych. 1951:65(4):511–7.
3. Hoffman E. The chvostek sign. Am J Surg. 1958;96;33–7.
4. Breimer L, Sourander P. The discovery of the parathyroid glands in 1880: triumph and tragedy for Ival Sandstrom. Bull Inst Hist Med. 1981;5:558–63.
5. Cooper MS, Gittoes NJ. Diagnosis and management of hypocalcaemia. BMJ. 2008;336:1298–302.
6. Bass MH. Chvostek's sign and its significance in older children. Am J Med Sci. 1912;144:64. (Within this, Bass cites Chvostek's quoted work: Wein. klin. Woch., 1907, No. 17).
7. Nature. 1935 Apr 20: 611–12.
8. Amort R. A treatise on electrolysis and its applications to therapeutical and surgical treatment in disease. New York: William Wood; 1886. http://archive.org/stream/treatiseonelectr00amorrich/treatiseonelectr00amorrich_djvu.txt. Accessed 15 May 2014. (Within the book, Amort cites Chvostek's method in an article published in Die Therapie der Basedowschen Krankheit. Zt'schr. F. Ther. Mit Einbzhung der Elektro. und Hydrotherapie, 1:81–83.)
9. Rohe GH. Electrolysis and some of its applications in medicine and surgery. Maryland Med J. Nov 1886.
10. Newman R. Electricity in the treatment of exophthalmic goitre. JAMA. 1895;XXV(23):975–8.
11. Bistori M, Galanakis E. Doctors versus artists: Gustav Klimt's medicine. BMJ. 2002;325:1506–8.

Armand Trousseau

1801–1867

Maureen Daly Moore and Thomas J. Fahey

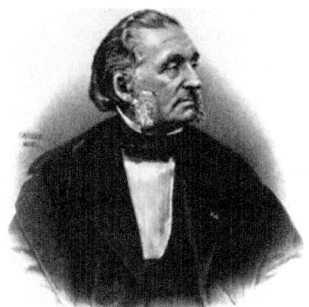

Illustation of Armand Trousseau

History of Armand Trousseau

Born in Tours, France in 1801, Armand Trousseau (1801–1867) studied medicine under the apprenticeship of the knowledgeable Pierre Bretonneau in Paris [1, 2]. Dr. Trousseau began his studies in his hometown, eventually moving to Paris to pursue clinical observations (Medicine) at the Hôpital Générale during the infamous diphtheria epidemic [1, 2]. Receiving his doctorate in 1825, he quickly progressed to Agrégé in 1827, the highest teaching post on the faculty [2]. A year later, Trousseau was assigned by the French government to probe the causes of epidemics occurring in the south of France [2]. After completing his assignment, Trousseau traveled to Gibraltar to investigate the causes of yellow fever, which at that time had claimed the lives of many French people [2]. His research led to the published work entitled, *Anatomical, Pathological, and Therapeutic Researches of the Yellow Fever of Gibraltar* [2].

In addition to gaining notoriety for his work on yellow fever, Trousseau wrote a monograph on laryngeal tuberculosis that also garnered him widespread recognition [2]. He received the top honor from the French Academy of Medicine, in 1837, for his monologue discussing laryngeal tuberculosis. Trousseau succeeded his mentor, Bretonneau, becoming one of the first in France to perform a tracheotomy in patients suffering from croup and diphtheria; 25 % of his cases were successful [2]. He wrote a monograph on the procedural elements of tracheostomy as well as intubation in 1851, noting that tracheostomy was the only way to save a patient from succumbing to diphtheria-related laryngo-pharyngeal swelling and suffocation [2].

Regarding his academic appointments, Trousseau was appointed physician at the Hôpital St. Antoine in 1839 [2]. As his accomplishments and publications mounted, Trousseau went on to become the chair of therapy and pharmacology. His work as a distinguished chair demonstrated his exemplary teaching and diagnostic capabilities [2]. In 1850, he assumed the chair of clinical medicine working at the Hôtel-Dieu [2]. After 6 years as chair of clinical medicine, Trousseau was once again distinguished for his accomplishments by being elected as a member of the prestigious French Academy of Medicine [2].

Trousseau eloquently described the presentation of many disease states and in doing so allowed the reader to draw a vivid sketch of the patient's complaints in his/her mind. As the author of many great medical dissertations, including Clinique Medicale de l'Hotel Dieu de Paris, he allowed his students to learn about certain diseases using a case description basis. In his monographs, he described well-known medical eponyms such as Addison's disease, Graves' disease and what is now known as Trousseau's sign of latent tetany—being the first to describe this sign.

T. J. Fahey (✉)
Division of Endocrine Surgery, General Surgery, New York Presbyterian/Weill Cornell Medical Center, 1300 York Avenue, New York, NY 10065, USA
e-mail: tjfahey@med.cornell.edu

M. D. Moore
General Surgery, New York Hospital Weill-Cornell Medical Center, New York, NY, USA

J. L. Pasieka, J. A. Lee (eds.), *Surgical Endocrinopathies,* DOI 10.1007/978-3-319-13662-2_29,
© Springer International Publishing Switzerland 2015

Trousseau's Sign and Its Significance in Endocrinology

...I describe to you the phenomena which characterize contractions, I shall show you that compression of the affected limb brings them on very rapidly and without fail. I discovered this influence of pressure [on tetany of upper extremities] by chance. I was present when a woman suffering from contractions was being bled from the arm at the Necker Hospital, and I saw a paroxsym return in the hand on the same side when the bandage was applied round the arm. I at first thought it was brought on by the venous congestion caused by the pressure on the vein; but on trying to account for the phenomenon, I found in other patients that by compressing the arteries, the same results were produced. I have often since repeated the experiment, and as the contractions cease as soon as the pressure is removed, and the patient is therefore not much troubled...In the upper limbs, the thumb is forcibly and violently adducted; the fingers are pressed closely together, and semi-flexed over the thumb in consequence of the flexion of the metacarpo-phalangeal articulation; and the palm of the hand...assumes a conical shape. [3]

Trousseau described how this "mild form of tetany" might last 5 min to several hours without interruption, upon which the sensation of formication returns yielding termination of the spasm [3]. He also described how pain, tingling and numbness, anesthesia, and impaired touch accompany the convulsions [4]. Regarding the pathophysiology of the tetany, Trousseau hypothesized that both arterial and venous compression resulted in vascular congestion [3]. He went on to report that cold temperatures seem to hinder the contractions when applied to the affected area, yet when normal temperature returns, the convulsions are short to follow [3]. Trousseau also offered an explanation as to the etiology of latent tetany, and believed that the mild convulsions were rheumatic in nature, dismissing the notion that serious "organic lesions" could be the culprit [3]. He also attributed pregnancy, lactation, diarrhea, and emotional disturbance as causes of latent tetany, describing many cases with the aforementioned ailments he personally witnessed on the hospital wards [3]. Today, Trousseau's sign of latent tetany is used as a clinical diagnostic tool for hypocalcemia usually following thyroid or parathyroid surgery. Though he did not know it at the time, Trousseau's sign would prove to be clinically useful for the detection and treatment of hypocalcemia after thyroid and parathyroid surgeries.

In most patients, signs of hypocalcemia such as tetany and paresthesias, are manifested through neuromuscular hyperexcitablity as classically displayed in Trousseau's sign [5]. Observed in 94 % of patients with hypocalcemia and in only 1 % of people with normal calcium levels, Trousseau's sign is regarded as a more specific physical exam finding than other tests such as **Chvostek**'s sign of masseter muscle contractions on tapping the facial nerve [6]. In order to elicit Trousseaus sign, the clinician inflates a blood pressure cuff on an upper extremity of the patient such that the pressure in the cuff is greater than or equal to the patients' systolic blood pressure

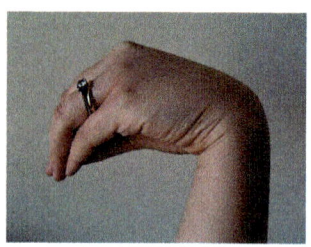

Fig. 1 The elicitation of Trousseau's sign

for about 3–5 min [5, 6]. A positive Trousseau's sign is documented if there is spasm of the hand musculature such that the thumb is adducted, metacarpohalagneal joints are flexed, the proximal and distal interphalagenal joints are extended, and the wrist is flexed [5, 6]. The spasms of the hand are due to temporary ischemia of the vasculature and hyperexcitable nerves [6]. The sign was described by Trousseau as a posture of opposition (main d'accoucheur). Trousseau's sign can be seen with serum calcium levels ranging between 7.5 and 8.5 mg/dL or less [5] (Fig. 2). Trousseau's sign was likely not routinely used after thyroid or parathyroid surgery until the mid-twentieth century, as the first parathyroid surgery did not occur until 1925 [7]. Postoperative tetany, however, was described in 1879 by Anton Wolfer in a patient who underwent a total thyroidectomy performed by **Dr. Theodor Billroth** [7]. Initially, the posteroperative tetany was felt to be secondary to hyperemia of the brain rather than hypocalcemia. It was not discovered until approximately 25 years after Dr. Billroth's first total thyroidectomy that hypocalcemia was in fact the cause of the tetany, rather than hyperemia of the brain [7]. Through multiple animal experiments, pathologist Dr. William MacCallum demonstrated that post-parathyroidectomy tetany could indeed be resolved by either injection of pure parathyroid hormone extract or by injection of calcium itself [7].

Trousseau's Other Contributions to the Field of Endocrinology

In addition to his contribution describing ways to elicit latent tetany, Trousseau was responsible for renaming *Basedow*'s disease to Graves' disease, a well-known endocrine disorder of the time [8]:

Gentleman: You may have noticed at No. 34, in St. Bernard Ward, a young woman who has a somewhat strange phyisognomy. Her face has a savage expression, her eyeballs are prominent, and her complexion pale. She complains of palpitation of the heart; her pulse at the wrist is frequent...you could see that her thyroid gland was considerably hypertrophied. The coexistence of these three pathological phenomena—palpation, hypertrophy of the thyroid gland, and prominence of the eyeballs—constitutes a morbid entity...Basedow's disease. Although ophthalmologists, like Demours, Mackenzie, Sichel, and Desmarres, had already mentioned this complaint, which is so remarkable from its three prominent symptoms, **Graves** was the one who called attention to it, and afterwards, from **Basedow** giving a fuller description of it, it was known after his name...the credit of priority belonged to Graves in a great measure. [8]

In the same fashion of proposing to change "*Basedow*'s disease" to "*Graves*' disease," Trousseau suggested to name Addison's disease after the English physician who discovered it, **Dr. Thomas Addison** [8]. "I propose then, to give the name of 'Addison's Disease' to that singular cachexia which is specially characterized by the decoloration, or rather the peculiar coloration—the bronzed tint—of the skin, which obtained for the malady the name under which Addison described it, viz., *bronzed disease*." In his monologue, Trousseau goes on to describe how Dr. Addison described 11 cases associating *bronzed disease* with lesions on the suprarenal capsules, known today as the adrenal glands. Trousseau's naming and renaming of Addison's and Graves' disease may seem trivial; however, since the nineteenth century, medicine has recognized these two common diseases by these names [8].

Discussion of Trousseau's contributions to endocrinology would not be complete without differentiating Trousseau's sign from Trousseau's syndrome (Trousseau's sign of malignancy). Trousseau described the relationship between venous thromboembolism and visceral malignancy, now known as Trousseau's syndrome. Trousseau observed migratory thrombophlebitis, also referred to by Trousseau as "phelgmasia alba dolens," in patients with cancer who had painful edema in their upper or lower extremities [9]. He associated this edema with painful cord-like structures [9]. The essentials of diagnosing Trousseau's syndrome are erythema, induration, and tenderness along a superficial vein [10]. Trousseau had the foresight to associate malignancy with a hypercoagulable state as he described the characteristic change in the hemodynamic system itself [9]. Ironically, on January 1, 1867, Trousseau noticed the same phlebitis in his own upper extremity that he at one time had diagnosed in his own patients. Upon noticing the phlebitis in his arm, he remarked to one of his students that he then knew he had cancer and death was upon him. A mere few months later, Trousseau succumbed to gastric cancer [9]. Trousseau was his own final diagnostician.

Conclusions

Among many other accomplishments, Trousseau contributed greatly to the field of endocrinology through his description of latent tetany and the naming of Graves' disease and Addison's disease. Perhaps most impressive of all, is the way in which Trousseau eloquently described the pathogenesis and clinical presentation of diseases by intertwining specific cases of patients in hospital wards with his prior medical knowledge. While we now favor (if not demand) large clinical trials to provide level I evidence to support new findings, the observations and accomplishments of Armand Trousseau continue to be an outstanding example of how close observation of a single patient by a keen observer can provide detailed information that leads to advances in medicine and surgery.

References

1. Medvei VC. The history of clinical endocrinology: a comprehensive account of endocrinology from earliest times to the present day. Carnforth: Parthenon; 1993.
2. Firkin BG, Whitworth JA. Dictionary of medical eponyms. Carnforth: Parthenon; 1987.
3. Trousseau A. Lectures on clinical medicine, delivered at the Hôtel-Dieu, Paris. 3rd. ed. [Translated by Cormack Sir John., translator.]. London: New Sydenham Society; 1872. (I), pp. 817–19.
4. Pearce J. Armand Trousseau—some of his contributions to neurology. J Hist Neurosci. 2002;11(2);125–35.
5. Shoback D, Sellmeyer D, Bikle DD. Chapter 8. Metabolic Bone Disease. In: Gardner DG, Shoback D. eds. New York: McGraw Hill; 2007.
6. Jesus JE, Landry A. Chvostek's and Trousseau's signs. New Engl J Med. 2012;367(11):e15.
7. Organ CH. The history of parathyroid surgery, 1850–1996: the excelsior surgical society 1998 Edward D Churchill lecture. J Am Coll Surg. 2000;191(3):284–99.
8. Trousseau A. Lectures on clinical medicine, delivered at the Hôtel-Dieu, Paris. 3rd. ed. [Translated by Cormack Sir John., translator.]. London: New Sydenham Society; 1872. (II), pp. 158–9, 772–3.
9. Wakefield TW, Rectenwald JR, Messina LM. Chapter 35. Veins & Lymphatics. In Doherty GM, Editors. Current diagnosis & treatment: surgery. New York: Lange Medical Books/McGraw-Hill; 2010. p. 13e.
10. Khorana AA. Malignancy, thrombosis and Trousseau: the case for an eponym. J Thrombosis Haemostasis. 2003;1(12):2463–65.

Theodor Billroth

1829–1894

Wen T. Shen

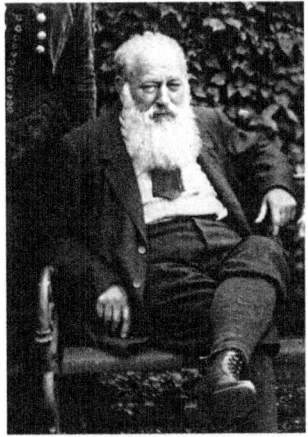

Theodor Billroth. Eigenbesitz, (Auschnitt) Salkammergut 1892, fotograf Erich Conrad

The second half of the nineteenth century was a period of tremendous advancement in surgery and a transition of the profession into the modern age. Leading this charge was the legendary Theodor Billroth. In an illustrious career spent in Berlin, Zurich, and Vienna, Billroth pioneered the field of gastrointestinal surgery, making innumerable technical and scientific contributions and training many future leaders who would go on to spread his teachings worldwide. Several of the principles and techniques he first put forth are still taught today, and the standard reconstruction after gastrectomy still bears his name. Despite his many triumphs in gastrointestinal surgery, an area that bedeviled Billroth for much of his career was surgery of the thyroid gland. The modern-day endocrine surgeon can learn much from the negative experiences of one of the true giants of surgery.

Christian Albert Theodor Billroth was born in 1829 in the town of Bergen auf Rügen, in the Kingdom of Prussia [1].

He attended medical school in Germany, at the University of Greifswald, and remained in Germany for his first surgical faculty position at the University of Berlin [1]. He became professor of surgery in short order, joining the faculty at the University of Zurich in 1860 and assuming the position of director of the surgery department there [1]. Billroth's greatest surgical successes would come during his nearly three decades at the University of Vienna, where in 1867 he was appointed chair of surgery (at the ripe old age of 38) [1]. An impressive list of surgical "firsts" transpired during Billroth's Austrian tenure; in a single decade, he performed the first successful esophagectomy (1871), laryngectomy (1873), and gastrectomy (1881) [1, 2]. In addition to distinguishing himself as both a surgeon and scientist, Billroth was prominent in the cultural arena. He was an accomplished pianist and violinist, and a longtime friend and colleague of the composer Johannes Brahms [3]. Billroth even attempted to apply some of his scientific methods to the study of musicality, devoting time towards the end of his career to defining the cognitive abilities necessary for the appreciation of music.

In the area of thyroid surgery, however, Billroth's record was largely one of ignominy. While Billroth was able to push the boundaries of surgery in other areas of the body, his attempts at safe resection of the thyroid gland were decidedly in keeping with other surgeons of the era: fraught with complications and an exceedingly high mortality rate. Writing in 1866, US surgeon Samuel Gross referred to thyroid surgery as "horrid butchery" and stated emphatically that "no sensible man" would even attempt it [4]. Billroth had set out early in his career to pioneer the removal of goiter. During his time in Zurich, in the 1860s, he noted the high incidence of endemic goiter in the local population and began performing operations to remove these enlarged thyroid glands [2]. Of the first 20 patients in whom he attempted resection, 8 died,

W. T. Shen (✉)
Department of Surgery, UCSF/ Mt. Zion Medical Center,
University of California, 1600 Divisadero Street, C349,
San Francisco, CA 94115, USA
e-mail: wen.shen@ucsfmedctr.org

J. L. Pasieka, J. A. Lee (eds.), *Surgical Endocrinopathies,* DOI 10.1007/978-3-319-13662-2_30,
© Springer International Publishing Switzerland 2015

mostly from sepsis [2, 5]. In addition, many suffered tetany, a perhaps unsurprising result since the presence and function of the parathyroid glands had yet to be established [6]. Disheartened by these poor results, Billroth stopped performing thyroidectomies and only resumed several years later, once he had established himself in Vienna. He wrote honestly and unflinchingly about his negative initial attempts at thyroidectomy:

> On carefully reviewing the results of my experience, I have come to the following conclusions…much less favorable in its results is the operation for completely removing deep-seated substernal or unilateral [goiters] accompanied by a high degree of dyspnea; even in cases in which the operation is immediately successful in saving life, the ultimate result is frequently unfavorable. [7]

When Billroth later resumed thyroid operations after moving to Vienna, he was able to eventually reduce the mortality rate from the initial 40 % seen in Zurich; between 1877 and 1881, he performed 48 thyroidectomies with a more acceptable mortality rate of 8.3 % [2, 4]. He never gained renown for this operation, however, and would remain in the shadow of his former protégé **Theodor Kocher** of Bern; Kocher would serve as the true founding father of modern thyroid surgery, eventually receiving the Nobel Prize in 1909 for his contributions (the first surgeon ever awarded this honor) [2].

Billroth was able to successfully perform new, revolutionary operations throughout the gastrointestinal tract; why did surgery of the thyroid gland pose such a challenge for this master technician? The devil, as in so much of endocrine surgery, lay in the details. Safe resection of the thyroid gland, as we now know quite well, requires a level of technical refinement and attention to surrounding anatomic structures that are in many ways worlds removed from the techniques that can be safely employed in surgery of other areas of the body. The methods that had served Billroth well in his other operations were likely disadvantageous when he faced the thyroid gland. Perhaps the best description of Billroth's technical approach to the thyroid came from William Halsted, who had traveled to Vienna to observe Billroth and made note of his techniques. In Halsted's mind, Billroth's operative style for thyroidectomy paled in comparison to that of Theodor Kocher, whom Halsted had also observed. In his landmark 1920 book on the history of thyroid surgery, *The Operative Story of Goitre*, Halsted remarked:

> Notwithstanding much speculation on the subject by various authors, it has not been made clear why Kocher's cases of cachexia strumipriva should have been so free from tetany, nor why Billroth's total extirpations should have been so frequently followed by tetany and should have so seldom manifested symptoms of thyroid deprivation. I have pondered this question for many years and conclude that the explanation probably lies in the operative methods of the two illustrious surgeons. Kocher,

neat and precise, operating in a relatively bloodless manner, scrupulously removed the entire thyroid gland, doing little damage outside of its capsule. Billroth, operating more rapidly and, as I recall his manner (1879 and 1880), with less regard for the tissues and less concern for hemorrhage, might easily have removed the parathyroids or at least have interfered with their blood supply, and have left fragments of the thyroid. Surprising, however, is the fact that the function of the parathyroids was so seldom interfered with by Kocher, notwithstanding his careful procedure; for these little bodies were entirely disregarded by surgeons until years after the discoveries of Gley (1891) and, Vassale and Generali (1896). [8]

In retrospect, Billroth's most lasting contribution to endocrine surgery may have been in his mentorship of future leaders in the field. As mentioned, Theodor Kocher was one of his early protégés and would become the first true giant of thyroid surgery in the modern era. One of Billroth's other acolytes, Anton Wölfler, made a seminal contribution to the practice of thyroid surgery when he provided detailed descriptions of postoperative tetany in a patient who had undergone thyroidectomy [6]. Wölfler, however, incorrectly attributed the signs and symptoms of hypocalcemia he observed to brain edema, and it would not be until many years later that the true function of the parathyroid glands would be delineated [6]. Another of Billroth's trainees, Jan Mikulicz-Radecki, developed the technique for subtotal thyroidectomy, which helped preserve parathyroid function and reduced the rates of hypothyroidism, and became a standard operation for many surgeons during the first half of the twentieth century [9].

Theodor Billroth's legacy is undoubtedly one of the most important in the history of modern surgery, but his contributions to the operative treatment of goiter are perhaps best viewed now in more negative terms: the modern surgeon can learn from Billroth the potential pitfalls of indelicate thyroid surgery. Regardless of new technologies, minimally invasive approaches, and other advancements that have emerged in the century and a half since Billroth's initial attempts at thyroidectomy in the 1860s, the principles of the operation remain the same: keep the field as bloodless as possible, and avoid injury to the parathyroid glands and recurrent laryngeal nerves. Billroth, with his reported rapid pace of operating and apparent disregard for tissue preservation and hemostasis, paid the price for improper technique in the form of poor outcomes, especially when compared to his counterpart Kocher. The history of surgery is all too often spent focused on triumphs and heroic figures. In the case of Theodor Billroth and surgery of the thyroid gland, we can also learn a great deal from the shortcomings of even our most legendary predecessors.

References

1. Fong ZV, Lavu H, Rosato EL, Yeo CJ, Cowan SW. Christian Albert Theodor Billroth, M.D., founding father of abdominal surgery (1829-1894). Am Surg. 2012;78:280–1.
2. Hannan SA. The magnificent seven: a history of modern thyroid surgery. Int J Surg. 2006;4:187–91.
3. Rutledge RH. A medical musical friendship: Billroth and Brahms. J Surg Educ. 2007;64:57–60.
4. Lee K, Martha AZ. William Stewart Halsted and Goiter: from "Horrid Butchery" to "Supreme Triumph". In: Zeiger MA, Shen WT, Felger EA, Editors. "The Supreme Triumph of the Surgeon's Art": a narrative history of endocrine surgery. Oakland: University of California Press; 2013.
5. Rogers-SJ, Kauffman GL, Jr . A historical perspective on surgery of the thyroid and parathyroid glands. Otolaryngol Clin North Am. 2008;41:1059–67.
6. Schulte K-M, Hans-DR. History of thyroid and parathyroid surgery. In: Oertli D, Udelsmans R, Editors. Surgery of the thyroid and parathyroid glands. London: Springer; 2012.
7. Billroth T. Clinical surgery: extracts from the reports of surgical practice between the years of 1860–1876. London: The New Sydenham; 1881.
8. Halsted W. The operative story of goitre. Baltimore: The Johns Hopkins Hospital Reports; 1920.
9. Barczynski M, Cichon S, Konturek A, Cichon W. Mikulicz's innovative achievements in the field of thyroid surgery. World J Surg. 2005;29:1090.

Adrenal Physiology

Jessica Furst and Salila Kurra

Embryology

The development of the adrenal glands explains the physiologic differences between the diverse endocrine functions of the layers of the gland. The adrenal cortex and the adrenal medulla have distinct embryologic precursors, which is why the adrenal cortex is responsible for the production of various steroid hormones while the medulla functions as part of the sympathetic nervous system [1]. The fetal adrenal gland is first detected at the 8th week of gestation [2].

Adrenal Cortex

The adrenal cortex develops from the mesenchymal cells of the posterior abdominal wall (mesoderm) [3]. The adrenal cortex is composed of a fetal zone and a definitive zone in fetal and early postnatal life and then goes on to have regression of the fetal zone and differentiation of the definitive zone over the first year of life [2, 3]. At birth, the cortex is quite large and the fetal adrenal gland is actually 10–20 times larger than the adult adrenal gland when measured relative to total body weight [4]. The definitive zone develops into the zona glomerulosa and zona fasciculata by birth, while the zona reticularis develops during the first year of life [4]. Ectopic cortical tissue can be found along the path of migration of structures arising from the urogenital ridge such as the epididymis, ovary, testicle, or broad ligament of the uterus as well as in locations outside the normal migration pattern of renal or pelvic structures [5]. Adrenal cortical development

is influenced by a host of genes that are not only vital for normal development but also implicated in oncogensis in children and adults. Wnt signaling, a member of the "wingless-like mouse mammary tumor virus integration site" family of morphogens which is responsible for the differentiation of the layers of adrenal cortex may be implicated in abnormal cell growth in the adult adrenal cortex [6]. Steroidogenesis, a key function of the adrenal cortex is influenced by steroidogenic factor-1 (SF-1), a nuclear receptor vital for normal development [7]. Overexpression of SF-1 has been frequently found in adrenocortical tumors [8].

Adrenal Medulla

The medulla develops from the neural crest cells [3]. At 6 weeks' gestation, the neural crest cells migrate from the spinal ganglia along the central vein into the adrenal cortex where they form the adrenal medulla, detectable by week 8 of gestation [3]. The neural crest cells transform into sympathogonia and pheochromocytes that go on to develop storage granules by 12 weeks gestation [4]. Pheochromoblasts and pheochromocytes also form on both sides of the abdominal aorta to form paraganglia [3]. Most paraganglionic cells are at the level of the inferior mesenteric artery and aortic bifurcation where they fuse anteriorly in the fetus to form the organ of **Zuckerkandl**, a major source of catecholamines in the developing fetus [3]. The adrenal pheochromoblasts mature into chromaffin cells [3]. The adrenal medulla is quite small at birth and develops into an adult form by 6 months of age [3]. Ectopic medullary tissue can be found along the path of migration of neural crest cells anywhere along the abdominal aorta, the para-aortic sympathetic chain, the celiac plexus, or the urinary bladder [4]. This can have implications later in life if ectopic medullary tissue becomes malignant causing paragangliomas along the path of neural crest cell migration [9].

S. Kurra (✉)
Department of Medicine, Columbia University Medical Center, 161 Fort Washington Avenue, 8th Floor, Room 827, New York, NY 10023, USA
e-mail: sk850@columbia.edu

J. Furst
Endocrinology, Department of Medicine, Columbia University Medical Center, 630 West 168th St., PH 8W, Room 864, New York, NY 10032, USA

J. L. Pasieka, J. A. Lee (eds.), *Surgical Endocrinopathies,* DOI 10.1007/978-3-319-13662-2_31,
© Springer International Publishing Switzerland 2015

Fig. 1 Adrenal anatomy and blood supply

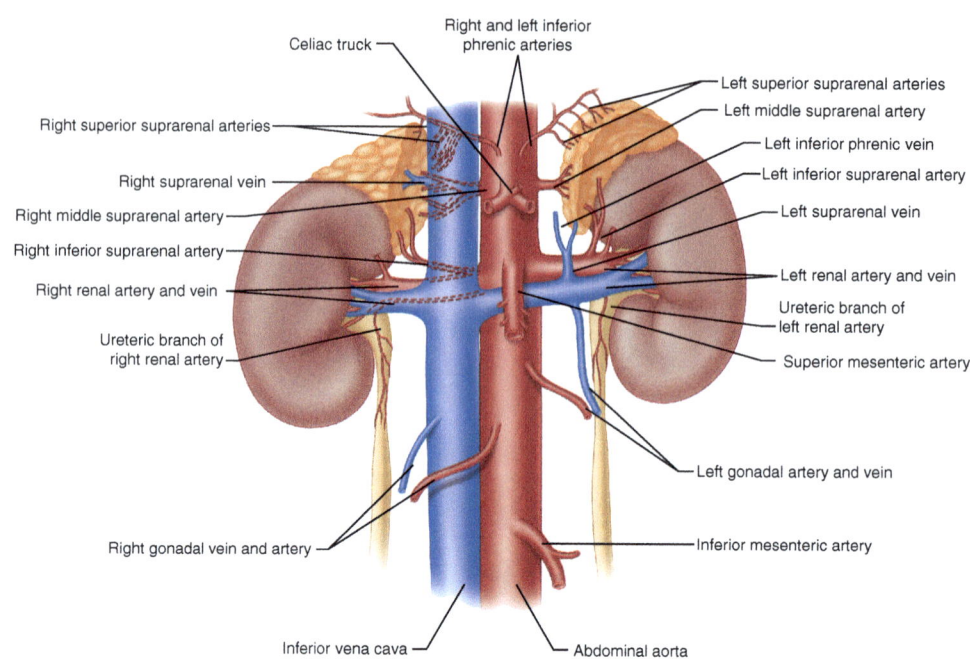

Anatomy

Location

The right adrenal gland is located above the right kidney, between the liver and the diaphragm [10]. The left adrenal gland is between the kidney and the aorta close to the pancreatic tail and splenic artery [10].

Gross Anatomy

The adrenal glands weigh 4–5 g each and are located in the retroperitoneum above the upper poles of the kidneys as seen in Fig. 1 [10]. They can increase by 50% during times of stress such as critical illness or pregnancy [4]. The adrenal cortex surrounds the adrenal medulla [11]. The gland is separated from adjacent structures by pararenal fat and Gerota's fascia [1]. The adrenal cortex is golden yellow in color and accounts for 80–90% of the volume of the entire adrenal gland [1]. The adrenal medulla is dark brown in color and is 10–20% of the volume of the entire adrenal gland [1].

Blood Supply

Arteries

The adrenal gland has three main groups of arteries carrying oxygenated blood to the cortex and medulla [10]. The superior adrenal arteries also known as superior suprarenal arteries (which originate from the inferior phrenic arteries), the middle adrenal arteries also known as middle suprarenal arteries (which originate from the aorta), and the inferior adrenal arteries also known as inferior suprarenal arteries (which originate from the right and left renal arteries) [10]. The arteries branch to form a plexus within the adrenal capsule to supply the cortex [10]. There are numerous minor branches that supply the gland such as branches from the intercostal arteries, the left ovarian artery and the left internal spermatic artery [10]. Some arterial vessels penetrate the medulla, which obtains additional blood supply from branches of arteries that supply the central vein and cortical tissue around this vein [10].

Veins

Each adrenal gland is drained by a major adrenal vein [10]. The left adrenal vein (2–3 cm) is longer than the right adrenal vein [4].

Left adrenal vein: drains into the left renal vein typically after joining the left inferior phrenic vein [4].

Right adrenal vein: drains directly into the inferior vena cava as it exits the adrenal gland [4].

Lymphatic Drainage

There are two lymphatic plexuses, one in the cortex and one in the medulla [4]. Most lymphatic drainage from the adrenal glands goes to the lateral aortic lymph nodes and the para-aortic nodes and a minority of the lymphatic drainage terminates in the thoracic duct [4]. These lymphatic drainage patterns help explain the spread of malignant adrenal tumors [4] which commonly invade the inferior vena cava, para-aortic lymph nodes, liver, and lungs [9].

Nervous Innervation

Visceral afferent innervation from the celiac plexus, aorti-corenal ganglia, and renal autonomic ganglia as well as the posterior vagus nerve, phrenic nerve, and greater and lesser splanchnic nerves are the main nervous system components that supply the adrenal glands [10]. These nerve fibers travel through the adrenal cortex and terminate in the medulla, where they function as postsynaptic sympathetic nerves, essentially enabling the adrenal medulla to function under neuroendocrine control in the secretion of catecholamines [10].

Microscopic Anatomy

Adrenal Cortex

The zona glomerulosa is approximately 15% of the adrenal cortex and is responsible for aldosterone production [4]. It is composed of small, lipid-poor cells beneath the adrenal capsule. The zona fasciculata makes up 75% of the cortex and is responsible for cortisol production [4]. It is composed of more lipid-rich cells than the zona glomerulosa, known as clear cells [4]. The zona reticularis makes up 10% of the cortex, and is primarily responsible for androgen production, and has cells containing lipofuscin granules [4]. Both the zona fasciculata and zona reticularis are under the control of adrenocorticotropic hormone (ACTH) [4].

Adrenal Medulla

The adrenal medulla is composed of chromaffin cells [4]. These are large columnar cells with neurosecretory granules composed of catecholamines (epinephrine and norepinephrine) as well as proteins, lipids, chromogranins, neuropeptides, and proopiomelanocortin [4]. These cells are arranged in cords around a network of venous sinusoids that drain blood from the cortex [4].

Physiology

As the adrenal cortex develops from the mesoderm lining the abdominal wall and the adrenal medulla develops from neural crest cells, they develop distinct endocrine functions despite being one gland [1]. The unique functional aspects of

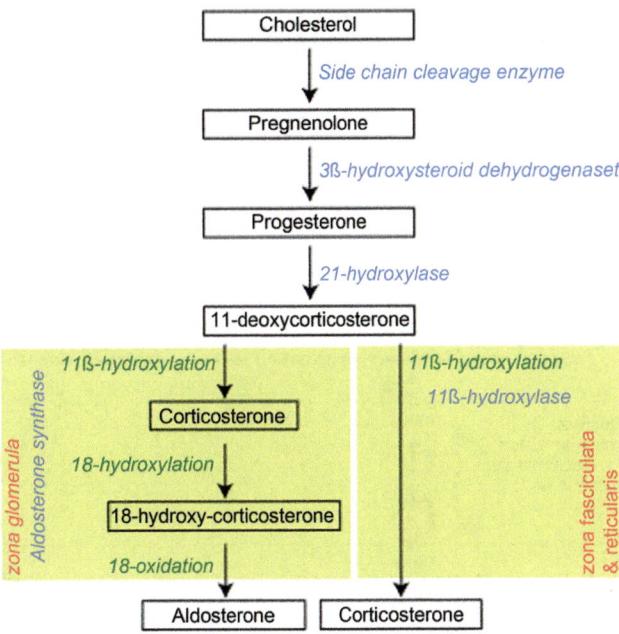

Fig. 2 Biosynthesis of aldosterone and cortisol. (Author: Jean-Iteinne Poirrier. Date: February 9, 2007. License: CC BY-SA 2.5, Creative Commons)

each component layer of the adrenal gland will be explored in this section.

Adrenal Cortex

The adrenal cortex secretes three major hormones: aldosterone, cortisol, and adrenal androgens [4]. These are produced from cholesterol through complex biochemical pathways with numerous intermediate steps as outlined in Fig. 2. Low-density lipoprotein is the major source for the cholesterol supplied to the adrenal gland [4].

The zona glomerulosa produces aldosterone, which is under the regulation of the renin–angiotensin system [4]. The zona fasciculata and zona reticularis produce cortisol and adrenal androgens, respectively, under the regulation of ACTH [4]. Because the zona glomerulosa lacks the enzyme, 17α-hydroxylase, it cannot produce 17-hydroxypregnenolone, the precursor for adrenal androgens or 17-hydroxyprogesterone, the precursor for cortisol [5]. The zona fasciculata and reticularis have 17α-hydroxylase activity; therefore cortisol and adrenal androgens are produced exclusively by the zona fasciculata and reticularis [5]. The zona glomerulosa, by contrast, is the only part of the adrenal cortex in humans that has 18-hydroxycorticosterone activity, a key step in aldosterone production [12].

Renin-angiotensin-aldosterone system

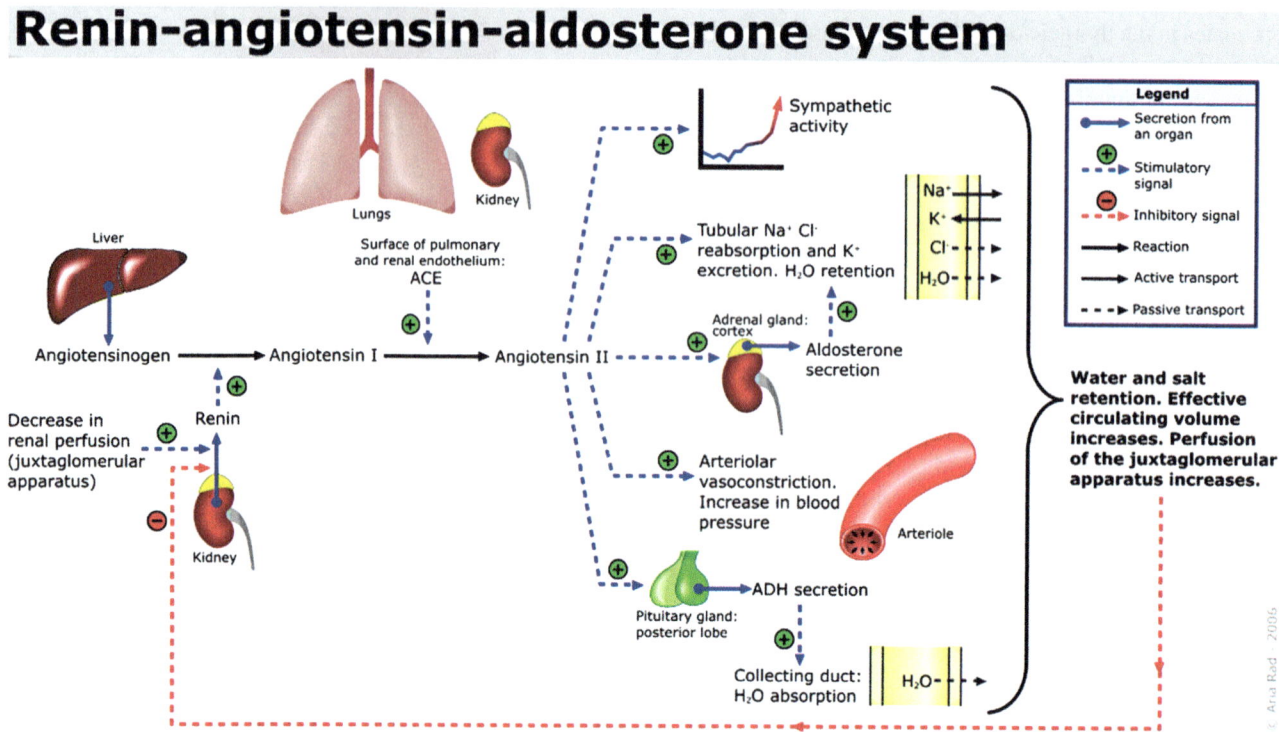

Fig. 3 Renin–angiotensin–aldosterone system. (Author: A. Rad. Date: February 2, 2006. License: GFDL-self Created using XaraX[1], Creative Commons)

Zona Glomerulosa

Synthesis, Circulation, Action, Inhibition

Aldosterone, the predominant mineralocorticoid is produced by the zona glomerulosa and involves a close feedback loop with the renin–angiotensin system of the kidneys (Fig. 3) [13]. Stimuli for aldosterone secretion include elevated serum potassium levels, sympathetic stimulation, decreased pressure sensed by the renal afferent arteriole, a part of the tubuloglomerular feedback mechanism, and ACTH [14]. Hypotension or decreased blood flow is sensed by the macula densa, specialized cells in the distal convoluted tubule, which stimulates the juxtaglomerular apparatus to release renin, which causes angiotensinogen to be converted to angiotensin I [1]. Renin is produced by the juxtaglomerular cells of the kidney, which are microscopic structures located between the vascular pole of the renal corpuscle and the distal convoluted tubule of the same nephron, surrounding the glomerular afferent arterioles [15]. Next, angiotensin I is converted to angiotensin II by the enzyme, angiotensin-converting enzyme (ACE), an enzyme primarily found in the pulmonary vasculature [1]. Angiotensin II stimulates the adrenal glands to produce aldosterone, triggers the release of epinephrine and norepinephrine from the adrenal medulla, promotes the release of vasopressin or antidiuretic hormone, which increases water absorption by the kidney collecting duct and also functions as an arterial smooth muscle constrictor [1].

Once aldosterone is released into the circulation, it has several effects that result in enhanced absorption of sodium and water and secretion of potassium and hydrogen ions [12]. Aldosterone binds to the mineralocorticoid receptor within cells of the renal cortical collecting ducts [16]. Aldosterone acts within 1 h of secretion to increase sodium channel activity on the apical membranes of cells in the cortical collecting tubule, increasing apical membrane permeability for sodium [12]. Via a sodium potassium adenosine triphosphatase (ATPase) pump, aldosterone acts on the principal cells to promote sodium absorption and potassium excretion. At the intercalated cell of the kidney's cortical collecting tubule, aldosterone promotes the secretion of protons via an ATPase pump [16]. These effects augment the difference in electrical potential across the renal tubule, making the lumen more negative and thus more favorable for aldosterone-induced secretion of potassium and hydrogen ions, which carry a positive charge [4].

Aldosterone secretion is inhibited by dopamine directly at the level of the adrenal gland [9]. Atrial natriuretic factor also directly inhibits dopamine and also blocks the stimulatory effects of angiotensin II, potassium, and ACTH [9]. Somatostatin inhibits aldosterone secretion by inhibiting angiotensin II [9].

Metabolism and Excretion

Hepatic metabolism reduces and conjugates aldosterone, which is then excreted in the urine [9]. People with impaired hepatic function from cirrhosis or congestive heart failure can have elevated aldosterone levels from decreased clearance [9].

Zona Fasciculata/Zona Reticularis

The zona fasciculata is the site of cortisol and the zona reticularis is the site of adrenal androgen production [1]. Cortisol is the major glucocorticoid but other glucocorticoids such as cortisone are produced by the adrenal cortex. Aldosterone, while a mineralocorticoid, does also exert some glucocorticoid effects [9].

Cortisol

Synthesis, Circulation, Action, Inhibition

The process leading to cortisol secretion by the adrenal cortex starts at the level of the hypothalamus in the midbrain. Corticotropin-releasing hormone (CRH), produced in the hypothalamus is secreted to the anterior pituitary gland where it stimulates the formation and secretion of ACTH from the precursor proopiomelanocortin [17].

ACTH secretion is pulsatile and is governed by circadian rhythms whereby ACTH secretion is high during the morning hours and becomes lower in the late evening through the early part of sleep, reaching its trough around 3–4 a.m. ACTH levels start to climb as people awaken in the early morning leading to a corresponding increase in cortisol levels in the early daytime [18]. This pattern can be disrupted by shift work where people change their sleep/wake cycles, by changes in physical stress such as starvation, exercise, critical illness, psychiatric illnesses, and illnesses that affect cortisol production, such as Cushing's syndrome, or cortisol binding, such as liver disease [4]. ACTH binds to receptors throughout the zona fasciculata and zona reticularis through a G protein mechanism, whereby ACTH binding triggers a cascade of events involving an increase in cyclic adenosine monophosphate (cAMP) and activation of protein kinase A, which leads to more cortisol production from cholesterol [4]. ACTH controls the rate-limiting step of cortisol synthesis, the conversion of cholesterol to pregnenolone [1]. This allows feedback regulation where low cortisol levels trigger increased production of cortisol from cholesterol by upregulation of ACTH [4].

Most cortisol (~80%) circulates bound to corticosteroid-binding globulin (CBG), which is produced by the liver [19]. About 10–15% is bound to albumin and 10% of circulating cortisol is free but this percentage can increase rapidly with stress [4, 20]. CBG also binds to progesterone, aldosterone, and 11-deoxycorticosterone [20]. CBG levels can increase, especially when estrogen levels are high such as during pregnancy or with oral contraceptive use [4]. Diabetes and hyperthyroidism will also increase CBG and thus increase circulating cortisol levels [4]. CBG levels decline with chronic steroid use and with various disease states including cirrhosis [20]. CBG binds to cortisol in a 1:1 ratio and controls the delivery of cortisol to organs and tissues [20].

Cortisol Function

Cortisol affects all major organ systems and biological processes. Free cortisol is the biologically active form [21]. The glucocorticoid receptor is present in nearly all cells and is a member of the steroid hormone receptor family of proteins [21]. Like all steroid receptors, once cortisol binds to the glucocorticoid receptor, it translocates to the cell nucleus and initiates transcription [21]. The steroid–receptor complex must dimerize to bind the glucocorticoid response elements, specific DNA sequences that control regulatory processes [9]. The glucocorticoid-responsive genes are regulated based on a complex interplay between the cortisol–glucocorticoid receptor complex and other transcription factors as well as through membrane-associated receptors and second messengers [21]. While glucocorticoids increase transcription of many genes, they suppress transcription of others [9].

At the level of the embryo, surfactant production is stimulated by glucocorticoids [9]. Glucocorticoids promote differentiation of neural crest cells into chromaffin cells in the developing adrenal medulla [9].

In the central nervous system, many cells are directly influenced by glucocorticoid binding. Mood, behavior, sleep patterns, and reception of sensory input are all modulated by glucocorticoids [22].

In the immune system, glucocorticoids block many inflammatory pathways including the number of T and B lymphocytes in the peripheral circulation [9], the phagocytic and cytotoxic functions of macrophages [9], and synthesis of arachidonic acid, a mediator of the vasodilatory inflammatory response that leads to the production of prostaglandins and thromboxanes [21]. Glucocorticoids inhibit fibroblasts and cause loss of connective tissue, thin skin, easy bruising, and delayed wound healing [1].

In the kidney, glucocorticoids enhance renal sodium retention, which leads to increased water absorption [21]. Additionally, glucocorticoids have weak mineralocorticoid activity and induce the angiotensin II receptor which results in increased aldosterone levels and sodium and water retention [21]. By contrast, atrial natriuretic factor also contains glucocorticoid-responsive elements and atrial natriuretic factor will increase in the presence of glucocorticoids [9]. This leads to greater excretion of salt and water [9].

In bone, glucocorticoids inhibit osteoblast function, which decreases new bone formation [9]. In children, glucocorticoids reduce chondrocyte proliferation and induce apoptosis, which is vital for longitudinal growth as chondrocytes take up calcium, secrete calcium phosphate and hydroxyapatite, and form mineralized bone [23]. In adults, glucocorticoids inhibit osteocalcin, an extracellular matrix protein that causes bone mineralization [23]. Glucocorticoids exert indirect effects on bone by decreasing intestinal calcium absorption and decreasing renal calcium reabsorption [24].

In the metabolism of lipids and glucose, glucocorticoids play a crucial role. They are responsible for both glycogen synthesis and hepatic gluconeogenesis [22]. They inhibit glucose transport into cells [25] to inhibit glucose utilization by peripheral tissues and promote lipolysis in adipose tissue [22, 26]. Food intake increases the glucocorticoid response and glucocorticoids may also regulate leptin, a hormone produced by adipose cells that regulates food intake at the central nervous system level [27]. Glucocorticoids promote leptin secretion by adipocytes and this may be one mechanism for increased body fat when people take oral glucocorticoids [28]. Glucocorticoids increase protein breakdown and urinary nitrogen excretion [1].

Glucocorticoids inhibit their own production by feedback inhibition at the pituitary level to block further ACTH secretion and they act at the hypothalamus to block CRH secretion [29]. If cortisol levels remain elevated due to exogenous glucocorticoid use, ACTH levels will decrease to a point where they are no longer responsive to stimulation [29]. This leads to suppression of CRH and ACTH release and atrophy of the adrenal cortex, which can be apparent on adrenal imaging such as computed tomography (CT) scan or magnetic resonance imaging (MRI) [29]. In addition to physiologic suppression, exogenous steroid use will also suppress the hypothalamic–pituitary–adrenal (HPA) axis and stop CRH and thus, ACTH secretion [29].

Metabolism and Excretion

Cortisol is metabolized in both the liver and the kidney with conversion to cortisone by 11ß-hydroxysteroid dehydrogenase [9]. Conjugated cortisol and cortisone metabolites are then excreted in the urine [4].

Adrenal Androgens

Synthesis, Circulation, Action, Inhibition

The major adrenal androgens are dehydroepiandrosterone (DHEA), dehydroepiandrosterone sulfate (DHEAS), and androstenedione [9]. DHEA and DHEAS are formed in the zona reticularis from 17-α-hydroxypregnenolone by 17,20-hydroxylase [30]. Androstenedione is formed by cleavage of 17-α-hydroxyprogesterone and then is convert-

ed to testosterone, of which a small amount is converted to estradiol [4]. Estradiol is also formed directly from androstenedione [4]. Peripheral tissues, especially in women, use the enzyme 5α-dihydrotestosterone to convert DHEA and DHEAS to testosterone [9] and peripheral tissues also interconvert DHEA and DHEAS [9]. In women, adrenal androgens are responsible for axillary and pubic hair development and may also contribute to libido [1]. In men, most testosterone is produced by the testes and the adrenal contribution is minimal [9].

The secretion of androgens, similarly to cortisol is governed by ACTH with pulsatile increases in DHEA and androstenedione occurring in concert with ACTH pulses [4]. However, there are probably other factors that control adrenal androgen release as chronic steroid administration, which suppresses ACTH and suppresses cortisol production, does not completely suppress androgen production [9]. Prolactin and insulin-like growth factor (IGF)-1 may serve as stimulators of adrenal androgen release [9].

Metabolism and Excretion

DHEA is metabolized by adrenal, hepatic, or renal conversion to DHEAS, which is excreted by the kidneys or further metabolized by oxidation to androstenedione [4, 9].

Androstenedione can be converted to testosterone or reduced further to etiocholanediol and androstanediol [4, 31]. All adrenal androgen metabolites are conjugated to sulfates or glucuronides and ultimately excreted in urine[4].

Adrenal Medulla

The adrenal medulla and surrounding paraganglia are part of the sympathetic or autonomic nervous system [1]. Sympathetic preganglionic nerves exit the central nervous system from the thoracic and lumbar spinal nerves and terminate in the preganglionic and paravertebral nerve ganglia [10]. From here, postganglionic fibers originate and supply the pheochromocytes of the adrenal medulla [10]. The neurotransmitter of the preganglionic fibers is acetylcholine and the postganglionic fibers release catecholamines and chromogranins from preformed storage granules [4]. The adrenal medulla is a unique structure in that it is a sympathetic ganglion itself since it releases hormones directly into the circulation [4].

Catecholamines

Synthesis, Circulation, Action, Inhibition

Catecholamines are synthesized from tyrosine, which comes from food (meats) or is made in the liver from phenylalanine [4]. Tyrosine is converted to L-dihydroxyphenylalanine (L-DOPA) by the enzyme tyrosine hydroxylase, which is the rate-limiting step in catecholamine synthesis [4]. L-DOPA is then converted to dopamine which enters granulate storage vesicles and is hydroxylated to norepinephrine and stored within the vesicle [4]. Norepinephrine can diffuse into the cytoplasm from these storage granules where it is converted to epinephrine, a reaction catalyzed by the enzyme phenylethanolamine-N-methyltransferase (PNMT) [4]. The adrenal medulla has high levels of cortisol due to blood flow from the surrounding adrenal cortex [4]. This leads to high levels of PNMT and significantly higher epinephrine than norepinephrine content in the medulla [4]. Stimuli for catecholamine secretion include both physiologic and pathophysiologic processes such as exercise, stress (both emotional and pathophysiological), and hypoglycemia [1].

Once catecholamines are released, they bind to their receptors with rather low affinity. In fact, 85% of secreted catecholamines are reabsorbed by the very nerves from which they were released [32]. Fifteen percent of norepinephrine leaves the adrenal medulla and enters the systemic circulation [32].

Norepinephrine and epinephrine bind to receptors on organs, muscles, and nerves throughout the body causing a range of physiologic actions to promote sympathomimetic activity, which is commonly known as the "fight or flight response" [33]. Adrenergic receptors are classified as α and β and include subtypes α_{1A}, α_{1B}, α_{1C}, α_{2A}, α_{2B}, α_{2C} and β_1, β_2, β_3, β_4 [33]. Norepinephrine is a more potent agonist of α-adrenergic receptors and epinephrine is a more potent agonist of β-adrenergic receptors [33]. $\alpha2$-Receptors are unique in that they are located on presynaptic sympathetic nerve endings and binding of norepinephrine or epinephrine causes feedback inhibition of their release [33]. Dopamine receptors have four subtypes D_1–D_4 [33].

Both α-adrenergic and β-adrenergic receptors are transmembrane proteins with areas of homology and areas of specificity where only certain guanylyl nucleotide binding proteins (G proteins) can attach [33]. Once a catecholamine binds to an α receptor, a G-protein-bound subunit activates an intracellular G-protein-coupled pathway that includes activation of phospholipase C, release of inositol 1,4,5-trisphosphate (IP3), increase in intracellular calcium concentrations and terminates with activation of calcium-dependent protein kinases, which phosphorylate and activate their substrates [33]. Once a catecholamine binds to a β-receptor, a G-protein-bound subunit activates adenylyl cyclase, which raises intracellular production of cAMP [33]. cAMP binds to cAMP-dependent protein kinases, which leads to phosphorylation and activation of their substrates [33].

Norepinephrine

Norepinephrine is made not just in the adrenal medulla but also in the sympathetic paraganglia and central nervous system [4]. It exerts its action mainly on α-adrenergic receptors to cause contraction of skeletal muscles and vasoconstriction of vascular smooth muscle [4]. For example, it stimulates α-adrenergic receptors in arterial smooth muscle to cause increased blood pressure [4]. α-adrenergic receptor stimulation of hepatocytes increases glycogenolysis and gluconeogenesis and α-adrenergic receptor stimulation of the ciliary muscle in the eye causes pupil dilation [4]. Norepinephrine is also active at β_1-adrenergic receptors, which increases cardiac contractility and heart rate [4]. Norepinephrine activation of β_3-adrenergic receptors on fat cells causes lipolysis and increased serum levels of free fatty acids [4].

Epinephrine

Epinephrine is made in the adrenal medulla from norepinephrine by the enzyme PNMT [4]. It stimulates β-receptors with greater affinity than norepinephrine [33]. Epinephrine acts on β_1-receptors in the heart to cause increased cardiac contractility [33]. β_1-receptors are also important for salt and water balance in the kidney as the juxtaglomerular apparatus has β_1-receptors which when stimulated increase the release of renin to activate the renin–angiotensin system, increase aldosterone secretion, and cause secretion of potassium and hydrogen ions and retention of sodium [33]. Epinephrine acts on β_2-receptors, which are responsible for skeletal and smooth muscle vasodilation, glycogenolysis, increased release of insulin and glucagon from the pancreas and increased peripheral conversion of levothyroxine (T4) to triiodothyronine (T3) in the liver and kidney [33]. Epinephrine also acts on β_3-adrenergic receptors on fat cells to cause lipolysis [33].

Dopamine

Unlike norepinephrine and epinephrine, dopamine is not a significant catecholamine in the systemic circulation but rather has an important role as a central neurotransmitter. It inhibits prolactin release and suppresses TSH at the hypothalamic–pituitary level and has many nonendocrine functions such as its activity in the brain's reward pathways [4, 31]. In systemic circulation, dopamine's actions are most notable for renal artery dilation through D1 receptors [33].

Some examples of specific types of catecholamine receptors and their actions at specific locations are detailed below in Table 1.

Metabolism and Excretion

Both epinephrine and norepinephrine are metabolized by catechol-O-methyltransferase (COMT), which converts epinephrine to metanephrine, which is further metabolized by

Table 1 Catecholamine effects. (Adapted from [4])

Receptor	Receptor subtype	Dominant catecholamine	Organ/tissue	Effect
Alpha	α_1	Norepinephrine	Smooth muscle	Vasoconstriction
			Eye	Pupillary dilation
			Skin	Piloerection
			Liver	Promote glycogenolysis, gluconeogenesis
–	α_2	Norepinephrine	Smooth muscle	Vasoconstriction
			Adipose tissue	Inhibit lipolysis
			Pancreas	Decrease insulin release
			Presynaptic fibers in CNS	Inhibit norepinephrine release (feedback inhibition)
Beta	β_1	Epinephrine	Myocardium	Increased contractility, increase heart rate
			Juxtaglomerular apparatus	Increased renin release
			Adipose tissue	Increased lipolysis
–	β_2	Epinephrine	Smooth muscle	Decrease intestinal motility, bronchodilation
			Striated muscle	Increased muscle mass and contractions
			Pancreas	Increase insulin and glucagon release
			Liver, kidney	Increase peripheral conversion of T4→T3
–	β_3	Epinephrine	Adipose tissue	Lipolysis
			Skeletal muscle	Thermogenesis
Dopamine	D_1	Dopamine	Renal smooth muscle	Vasodilation to dilate renal artery
–	D_2–D_4	Dopamine	CNS	Controls emotion and cognitive function

CNS central nervous system

phenol-sulfotransferase (PST) to metanephrine sulfate and by monoamine oxidase (MAO) to vanillylmandelic acid (3-methoxy-4-hydroxymandelic acid) [1]. Norepinephrine also undergoes initial metabolism by COMT to normetanephrine, which is further metabolized by PST to normetanephrine sulfate and by MAO to vanillymandelic acid [1]. COMT is widely distributed throughout the body and can be found specifically in blood cells, liver, kidney, and smooth muscle [1]. Metabolized catecholamines are excreted in the urine [1].

Chromogranin A, Adrenomedullin, and Opioid-Like Peptides

In addition to catecholamines, the postsynaptic secretory granules of the adrenal medulla contain other important chemical messengers [4].

Chromogranin A
Chromogranin A is found ubiquitously throughout the body including in the pituitary gland, parathyroid gland, and pancreatic islet cells [4]. In the adrenal medulla, chromogranin A is an important prohormone responsible for vasostatin I and II, amino terminal fragments that inhibit vasoconstriction [4]. It is also the prohormone for catestatin, a blocker of acetylcholine receptors and thus an inhibitor of adrenosympathetic activity [4].

Adrenomedullin
Adrenomedullin is produced both by the zona glomerulosa and the adrenal medulla. It is a cleavage product of the preproadrenomedullin, a prohormone and it suppresses aldosterone secretion in the adrenal gland [34]. In other organs such as the heart, it is a natriuretic peptide [34]. It is found in tumors such as pheochromocytomas where it stimulates tumor growth and survival [34].

Enkephalins
Chromaffin cells secrete met- and leu-enkephalin, which are opiate-like peptides stored in the same granules as catecholamines [4]. They play important roles in mood regulation and cell growth based on their binding to various opioid receptors [4].

Key Summary Points
- The adrenal cortex develops from cells of the posterior abdominal wall whereas the adrenal medulla develops from neural crest cells leading to diverse physiology between the cortex and medulla.
- There are two adrenal glands located in the retroperitoneum with a rich arterial supply from three major groups of arteries.
- Lymphatic drainage from the adrenal glands goes to the lateral aortic lymph nodes and the para-aortic nodes and a minority of the lymphatic drainage terminates in the thoracic duct.

- The adrenal cortex is composed of three zones. The zona glomerulosa produces aldosterone. The zona fasciculata and reticularis produce cortisol and adrenal androgens, respectively.
- Aldosterone promotes the retention of sodium and the secretion of potassium and hydrogen ions by the kidneys.
- Stimuli for aldosterone secretion include elevated serum potassium levels, sympathetic stimulation, decreased pressure sensed by the renal afferent arteriole, and adrenocorticotrophic hormone (ACTH).
- Cortisol, the predominant glucocorticoid is produced by the zona fasciculata within a tightly regulated feedback loop with ACTH, which is released in a pulsatile manner and closely linked with circadian rhythms.
- Cortisol has pleiotropic effects on all organ systems including the central nervous system, the immune system, the kidneys, and the skeletal system.
- The major adrenal androgens are DHEA, DHEAS, and androstenedione, and they are produced in the zona reticularis.
- The adrenal medulla is part of the sympathetic nervous system and is responsible for the synthesis of catecholamines: epinephrine, norepinephrine, and dopamine and for the production of chromogranin A, adrenomedullin, and enkephalins.
- Epinephrine and norepinephrine are responsible for sympathetic responses throughout the body such as pupillary dilation, increased heart rate and contractility, vasodilation, and breakdown of glycogen and lipids.

References

1. Niewoehner CB. Endocrine pathophysiology. 2nd ed. pathophysiology series. Raleigh: Hayes Barton. xi; 2004. p. 414.
2. Else T. Hammer GD. Genetic analysis of adrenal absence: agenesis and aplasia. Trends Endocrinol Metab. 2005;16(10):458–68.
3. Moore KL, Persaud TVN. Before we are born: essentials of embryology and birth defects. 6th ed. Philadelphia: Saunders. xv; 2003. p. 448.
4. Shoback D. Greenspan's basic and clinical endocrinology. New York: McGraw-Hill Medical; 2011. p. 1. (online resource (p. 880))
5. Ishimoto H, Jaffe RB. Development and function of the human fetal adrenal cortex: a key component in the feto-placental unit. Endocr Rev. 2011;32(3):317–55.
6. Kim AC, et al. Targeted disruption of beta-catenin in Sf1-expressing cells impairs development and maintenance of the adrenal cortex. Development. 2008;135(15):2593–602.
7. Ozisik G, et al. SF1 in the development of the adrenal gland and gonads. Horm Res. 2003;59(1):94–8.
8. Fassnacht M, Kroiss M, Allolio B. Update in adrenocortical carcinoma. J Clin Endocrinol Metab. 2013;98(12):4551–64.
9. Williams RH, Wilson JD, Foster DW. Williams textbook of endocrinology. 8th ed. Philadelphia: W.B. Saunders. xxii, 1992. p. 1712.
10. Boglione L, et al. The development of the suprarenal gland: surgical and anatomical considerations. Panminerva Med. 2001;43(1):33–7.
11. Mesiano S Jaffe RB. Developmental and functional biology of the primate fetal adrenal cortex. Endocr Rev. 1997;18(3):378–403.
12. Williams JS Williams GH. 50th anniversary of aldosterone. J Clin Endocrinol Metab. 2003;88(6):2364–72.
13. Augustin M, et al. Plasma renin activity (PRA) and plasma aldosterone in the adrenal cortex hyperactivity. Studies on 50 hypertensive patients. Endocrinologie. 1984;22(1):37–45.
14. White PC. Disorders of aldosterone biosynthesis and action. N Engl J Med. 1994;331(4):250–8.
15. Moore KL, Dalley AF, Agur AMR. Clinically oriented anatomy. 5th ed. Philadelphia: Lippincott Williams & Wilkins. xxxiii, 2006. p. 1209.
16. Summa V, et al. Short term effect of aldosterone on Na, K-ATPase cell surface expression in kidney collecting duct cells. J Biol Chem. 2001;276(50):47087–93.
17. Arlt W, Stewart PM. Adrenal corticosteroid biosynthesis, metabolism, and action. Endocrinol Metab Clin North Am. 2005;34(2):293–313, viii.
18. Krieger DT, et al. Characterization of the normal temporal pattern of plasma corticosteroid levels. J Clin Endocrinol Metab. 1971;32(2):266–84.
19. Zhou A, et al. The S-to-R transition of corticosteroid-binding globulin and the mechanism of hormone release. J Mol Biol. 2008;380(1):244–51.
20. Cizza G, Rother KI. Cortisol binding globulin: more than just a carrier? J Clin Endocrinol Metab. 2012;97(1):77–80.
21. Rhen T, Cidlowski JA. Antiinflammatory action of glucocorticoids–new mechanisms for old drugs. N Engl J Med. 2005;353(16):1711–23.
22. Rousseau GG, Baxter JD. Glucocorticoid hormone action. Monographs on endocrinology, V. New York: Springer-Verlag. 1979. p. 638.
23. van der Eerden BC, Karperien M, Wit JM. Systemic and local regulation of the growth plate. Endocr Rev. 2003;24(6):782–801.
24. Canalis E. Mechanisms of glucocorticoid action in bone. Curr Osteoporos Rep. 2005;3(3):98–102.
25. Weinstein SP, et al. Glucocorticoid-induced insulin resistance: dexamethasone inhibits the activation of glucose transport in rat skeletal muscle by both insulin- and non-insulin-related stimuli. Diabetes. 1995;44(4):441–5.
26. Livingston JN, Lockwood DH. Effect of glucocorticoids on the glucose transport system of isolated fat cells. J Biol Chem. 1975;250(21):8353–60.
27. Friedman JM, Halaas JL. Leptin and the regulation of body weight in mammals. Nature. 1998;395(6704):763–70.
28. Leal-Cerro A, et al. Influence of cortisol status on leptin secretion. Pituitary. 2001;4(1–2):111–6.
29. Van den Berghe G. Neuroendocrine pathobiology of chronic critical illness. Crit Care Clin. 2002;18(3):509–28.
30. Endoh A, et al. The zona reticularis is the site of biosynthesis of dehydroepiandrosterone and dehydroepiandrosterone sulfate in the adult human adrenal cortex resulting from its low expression of 3 beta-hydroxysteroid dehydrogenase. J Clin Endocrinol Metab. 1996;81(10):3558–65.
31. Haugen BR. Drugs that suppress TSH or cause central hypothyroidism. Best Pract Res Clin Endocrinol Metab. 2009;23(6):793–800.
32. Vincent S, Robertson D. The broader view: catecholamine abnormalities. Clin Auton Res. 2002;12(1):I44–9.
33. Katzung BG. Teton data systems (firm), basic & clinical pharmacology, in STAT!Ref electronic medical library. Jackson: Teton Data Systems; 2002.
34. Hinson JP, Kapas S, Smith DM. Adrenomedullin, a multifunctional regulatory peptide. Endocr Rev. 2000;21(2):138–67.

Thomas Addison

1793–1860

William F. Young

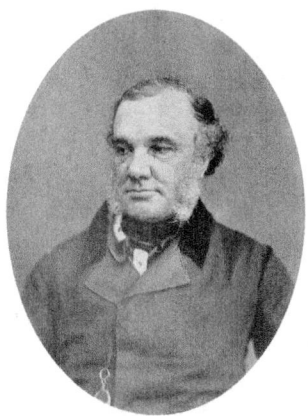

Thomas Addison was a remarkably astute clinician at Guy's Hospital, who recognized an association between skin hyperpigmentation and diseased adrenal glands at autopsy—he pursued this association and convinced the medical world of the critical role of intact adrenal glands. (Author: H. Watkins, date unknown. Creative Commons Attribution 4.0 International license)

Addison: The Man

Thomas Addison (1793–1860) is recognized for the two conditions that bear his name—Addison's disease (frequently referred to as primary adrenocortical failure) and Addison's anemia (now known as pernicious anemia). Addison was born in Newcastle upon Tyne, where he attended the Royal Free Grammar School and excelled in Latin. He entered medical school in 1812 at the University of Edinburgh and graduated in 1815—his M.D. thesis was entitled: "Concerning Syphilis and Mercury" [1]. He moved to London to become a house surgeon at Lock Hospital and a pupil at the Carey Street Public Dispensary, where a dermatologist (Thomas Bateman, 1778–1821) inspired an interest in dermatologic disorders.

In 1824, Addison founded the Department of Dermatology at Guy's Hospital. He obtained his diploma of Licentiate of the Royal College of Physicians (LRCP) in 1819 and in 1827 he was appointed lecturer of Materia Medica. In 1837, Addison was advanced to full physician at Guy's Hospital. Addison was a brilliant diagnostician and his uniquely coherent lectures were very popular. He was observed to have an uncanny clinical intuition and he was remarkably persistent to seek a unifying diagnosis. Addison recognized the key role for autopsy and correlating the pathology findings with signs and symptoms.

Addison was investigating an atypical anemia and was intrigued by pathological findings in the adrenal glands in some of the patients. On March 15, 1849, Addison delivered a paper before the South London Medical Society, where he was the first to describe pernicious anemia [2]. Six years later, he published his classic monograph: "On the Constitutional and Local Effects of Disease of the Suprarenal Capsule" [3] (Fig. 1). Although Addison's work was debated in Scotland and England and many were quite skeptical, the syndrome of primary adrenal failure was confirmed by **Trousseau** in 1856 and he gave it the eponym "Addison's disease."

Addison was a bedside diagnostician. Thomas Wilks wrote:

> Possessing unusually vigorous perceptive powers, being shrewd and sagacious beyond the average of men, the patient before him was scanned with a penetrating glance from which few diseases could escape detection. He never reasoned from a half discovered fact, but would remain at the bedside with a dogged determination to track out the disease to its very source for a period which often wearied his class and his attendant friends. To those who knew him best his power of searching into the complex framework of the body and dragging the hidden malady to light, appeared unrivalled, but that great object being accomplished, the same energetic power was not devoted to its alleviation or cure. [4]

Addison was described in the medical press [5] as follows:

> He is a fine, dashing, big, burly, busting man, proud and pompous as a parish beadle in his robe of office. Dark, and of sallow

W. F. Young (✉)
Division of Endocrinology, Diabetes, Metabolism, and Nutrition, Mayo Clinic College of Medicine, 200 First Street SW, Rochester, MN 55905, USA

J. L. Pasieka, J. A. Lee (eds.), *Surgical Endocrinopathies*, DOI 10.1007/978-3-319-13662-2_32,
© Springer International Publishing Switzerland 2015

ON THE

CONSTITUTIONAL AND LOCAL EFFECTS

OF

D I S E A S E

OF THE

S U P R A - R E N A L   C A P S U L E S.

BY

T H O M A S   A D D I S O N, M.D.,

SENIOR PHYSICIAN TO GUY'S HOSPITAL.

L O N D O N :
SAMUEL HIGHLEY, 32 FLEET STREET.
1855.

Fig. 1 Title page from Thomas Addison's classic monograph: [3]. (Used with permission Pickering & Chatto 144–146 New Bond Street, London)

complexion, an intelligent countenance and noble forehead, he is what the ladies would renounce a fine man. He had mentally and physically a tall idea of himself. Every sentence is polished, is powerful: he prefers the grandiloquent. Slow and studied are his opening sentences, studied the regularity of his intonations. The advantages of his tall and graceful person are artfully employed to add to the favourable impression; his attitudes, tones and manner are studied and systematic.

It was speculated that, in addition to gallstones and jaundice, endogenous depression led to his retirement from medicine in 1860 [6]. In a letter dated March 17, 1860, he wrote to E. Galton, one of his students: "A considerable breakdown in my health has scared me from the anxieties, responsibilities and excitement of my profession, whether temporarily or permanently cannot yet be determined; but whatever may be the issue, be assured that nothing was better calculated to soothe me than the kind interest manifested by the pupils of Guy's Hospital during the many trying years devoted to that Institution" [6]. Later that year (June 19, 1960), Addison committed suicide. His death was reported in the Brighton Herald of June 30, 1860:

Dr Addison, formerly a physician to Guy's Hospital, committed suicide by jumping down the area (i.e. the space between the front of the house and the street) of 15 Wellington Villas, where he had for some time been residing, under the care of two attendants, having before attempted self-destruction. He was 72 yrs of age (sic), and laboured under the form of insanity called melancholia, resulting from overwork of the brain. He was walking in the garden with his attendants, when he was summoned in to dinner. He made as if towards the front door, but suddenly threw himself over a dwarf-wall into the area—a distance of nine feet—and, falling on his head, the frontal bone was fractured, and death resulted at one o'clock yesterday morning.

Addison's Disease: The Monograph

Addison's monograph (Fig. 1) on disease of the suprarenal capsules [3] is one of the most remarkable medical books of the nineteenth century. The monograph text is 39 pages in length and contains 11 color plates. Written before the invention of color photography, the patient images in the book were drawn by artists. He starts his monograph with: "It will hardly be disputed that at the present moment, the functions of the supra-renal capsules, and the influence they exercise in the general economy, are almost or altogether unknown" [3]. Addison reported the clinical presentations and autopsy findings in 12 patients. He wrote:

The discoloration pervades the whole surface of the body, but is commonly most strongly manifested on the face, neck, superior extremities, penis, scrotum, and in the flexures of the axillae and around the navel…. The leading and characteristic features of the morbid state to which I would direct your attention, are, anaemia, general languor and debility, remarkable feebleness of the heart's action, irritability of the stomach, and a peculiar change of the colour in the skin, occurring in connexion with a diseased condition of the "supra-renal capsules." [3]

Addison's 12 cases are summarized in Table 1 and included 8 men and 4 women, aged from 22 to 60 years, having the clinical manifestations of this disease. The clinical presentations were dominated by recurrent vomiting, skin hyperpigmentation, and weak pulse. The adrenal glands at autopsy showed tuberculosis/infection ($n=5$), metastatic disease ($n=4$), apparent autoimmune disease ($n=1$), probable bilateral adrenal hemorrhage ($n=1$), and unknown ($n=1$). Several cases are particularly instructive.

Addison's case III was a 26-year-old carpenter who had been well up to 6 months before presentation. His first symptoms were right leg and low back pain. He had noticed darkening of his lips and face. He developed light-headedness, especially with standing. He slowly became more disabled and had to discontinue work. On physical examination, the patient had a "highly strumous appearance" with patchy facial hyperpigmentation. He had marked tenderness over the upper three lumbar vertebrae. His heart rate was 80 beats per minute and "small and weak." During the hospitalization, the patient developed intractable hiccups and he became "more

Table 1 Clinical and autopsy findings in Addison's 12 cases

Case	Age	Sex	Presenting symptoms	Adrenal pathology at autopsy	2015 Perspective on probable etiology of adrenal failure
I, James Wootten	32	M	Cough and increasing skin pigmentation	"The supra-renal capsules were diseased on both sides, the left about the size of a hen's egg…" "Both capsules were as hard as stones"	Uncertain -? old hemorrhage
II, James Jackson	35	M	Headaches, nausea, vomiting, increasing skin pigmentation	"The supra-renal capsules contained both of them compact fibrinous concretions, seated in the structure of the organ; superficially examined they were not unlike some forms of strumous tubercle"	Probable tuberculosis
III, Henry Patton	26	M	Leg and back pain; hyperpigmentation	"Each supra-renal capsule was completely destroyed and converted into a mass of strumous disease, the latter of all degrees of consistency"	Tuberculosis
IV, John Iveson	22	M	Recurrent vomiting, facial hyperpigmentation	"The two supra-renal capsules together weighed 49 grains; they appeared exceedingly small and atrophied; the right one was natural, firm; the left deformed by contraction; each adherent to surrounding parts by dense areolar tissue. The section gave a pale and homogeneous aspect; it presented a fibrous tissue, fat and cells about the size of white blood-corpuscles"	Autoimmune
V, Ann Roots	?	F	Breast mass, parotid swelling, recurrent vomiting, skin pigmentation	"The only marked disease was in the renal capsules, both of which were enlarged, lobulated, and the seat of morbid deposits apparently of a scrofulous character; they were at least four times their natural thickness, feeling solid and hard; on the left side one part had gone into suppuration, containing two drachms of yellow pus. The kidneys themselves healthy"	Infectious
VI, R.H., Esq	"Middle age"	M	Weight loss, fatigue, recurrent vomiting, hyperpigmentation, vitiligo	"…both the renal capsules were enlarged, (the united weight of the two being one and a half ounce,) of rather irregular surface and considerably indurated. When cut into, instead of exhibiting the ordinary appearance of combination of dark and yellow substances, they seemed to consist of a firm, slightly transparent reddish basis, interspersed with irregular spots of opake yellow matter, the whole bearing a strong resemblance to an enlarged mesenteric gland, mottled with tubercular deposit"	Tuberculosis/ autoimmune
VII, M.T.	60	F	Breast cancer, skin hyperpigtation	"Both supra-renal capsules contained a considerable amount of cancerous deposit, invading their entire structure, and almost obliterating their cavities"	Metastatic breast cancer
VIII, Elizabeth Hannah Lawrence	53	F	Recurrent vomiting, emaciation, hyper pigmentation	"The left supra-renal capsule was infiltrated with malignant material, and closely adherent to the vessels of the kidney"	Metastatic stomach cancer
IX, Thomas Clouston	58	M	Nausea, sweats, blindness left eye, debility, dark skin	"Tubercular deposit was likewise found in one of the supra-renal capsules"	Tuberculosis

Table 1 (continued)

Case	Age	Sex	Presenting symptoms	Adrenal pathology at autopsy	2015 Perspective on probable etiology of adrenal failure
X, Jane Roff	28	F	Uterine cancer, hyperpigmentation	"…left capsule…. A malignant tumor had developed at that precise point, where the large vein escapes from the organ;…pro-jected into the interior of the vein, so as almost or entirely to obstruct it, and had moreover led to rupture and effusion into, or a sort of apoplexy of the capsule itself"	Metastatic uterine cancer and adrenal hemorrhage
XI, William Godfrey	Not reported	M	Lung cancer and facial hyperpigmentation	"…extensive disease of one of the supra-renal capsules; the organ being very much enlarged, and converted into a hard mass of apparently carcinomatous disease"	Metastatic lung cancer
Mr. S (presented under case VI)	60	M	Anemia, extreme feeble-ness of heart action, irri-tability of the stomach, and hyperpigmentation	Autopsy refused	Autoimmune

feeble, pulse scarcely perceptible, lies in a torpid and ty-phoid state." The patient died on the 6th hospital day. At au-topsy, "each supra-renal capsule was completely destroyed and converted into a mass of strumous disease, the latter of all degrees of consistency. The left supra-renal capsule had formed at the upper part a close connexion with the outer coat of the stomach. The upper part of this capsule seemed fluid, and of the colour of pus; the lower firmer; and of the consistency of putty." These findings are demonstrated in the color drawings (Fig. 2). In addition, autopsy confirmed find-ings consistent with pulmonary tuberculosis and tuberculous spondylitis (Pott's disease) of the lumbar spine and thus ex-plaining his initial symptoms of back and leg pain.

Addison's case IV was a 22-year-old man who presented with recurrent vomiting, dingy facial discoloration. Based on the autopsy findings of atrophic adrenal glands, Addison concluded: "It is, moreover, of some significance and impor-tance to observe, that in the present instance, the diseased condition of the supra-renal capsules did not result as usual from a deposit either of a strumous or malignant character, but appears rather to have been occasioned by an actual in-flammation—that inflammation having destroyed the integ-rity of the organs, and finally led to their contraction and atrophy" [3]. With this case, Addison was describing (for the first time) autoimmune primary adrenal failure. The most common cause of primary adrenal failure has evolved over time, from tuberculosis in 1855 to autoimmune disease in the twenty-first century (in approximately 80% of cases).

Addison's case VI was a middle-aged man who presented with weight loss, fatigue, recurrent vomiting, hyperpigmen-tation, and vitiligo. Addison noted: "With universal dinginess of the surface, there were, especially about the neck, hands and arms, several well-defined patches of a deeper, or some-what chestnut-brown hue, interspersed here and there with blanched or almost dead-white portions of integument, con-trasting in a very remarkable manner with both the general

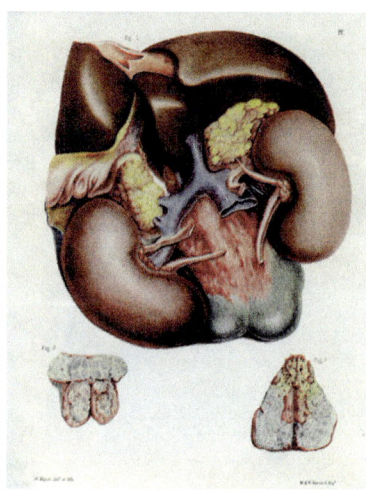

Fig. 2 Color drawing (plate IV) of Henry Patten in November of 1854. This patient presented with symptoms related to tuberculous involve-ment of the lumbar spine (Pott's disease) and progressive primary ad-renal failure, which at autopsy was shown to be caused by the spread of tuberculosis to the adrenal glands. The legend from Addison's monograph states: "*Fig. 1.* The liver of Henry Patten, with the diseased supra-renal capsules in situ. *Figs. 2 & 3.* Sections of the diseased supra-renal capsules." (Used with permission Pickering & Chatto 144–146 New Bond Street, London)

dinginess and deeper brown patches; and what is very re-markable, wherever the integument presented the blanched or dead-white appearance, the hairs upon its surface were observed to have turned completely white" [3]. Although ad-renal tuberculosis deposits were found in this patient, it may be that, in view of the vitiligo, the true nature of adrenal fail-ure was autoimmune in nature. Addison was unable to pro-vide a colored drawing of this patient. However, he had seen a patient (Mr. S) in March of 1855 (the year his monograph was published) with an identical presentation. Although the family of Mr. S refused an autopsy to confirm Addison's

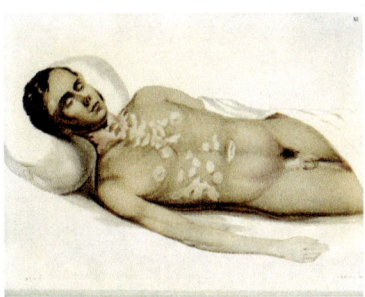

Fig. 3 Color drawing (plate XI) of "Mr. S" in March of 1855. This patient had an identical presentation to Addison's case VI. Although the family of Mr. S. refused an autopsy to confirm Addison's suspicion of primary adrenal disease, they did agree to have a sketch made of the discolored skin. This color drawing shows typical skin hyperpigmentation of Addison's disease in a patient with vitiligo—thus, this patient very likely had autoimmune primary adrenal failure. The legend from Addison's monograph states: "Head, neck, and trunk of Mr. S., exhibiting peculiar discolorations and white patches of the integument, similar to those observed in CASE VI." (Used with permission Pickering & Chatto 144–146 New Bond Street, London)

suspicion of primary adrenal disease, they did agree to have a sketch made of the discolored skin. Addison wrote: "Of course this representation does not carry along with it such authority and conviction as one taken from a subject actually proved to have had diseased capsules. Nevertheless I entertain no doubt whatever that the capsules were diseased; and even if they were not, I hold myself answerable for the most perfect resemblance between the two cases, so far as the affection of the integument was concerned." The color drawing of this patient (Fig. 3) shows typical skin hyperpigmentation of Addison's disease in a patient with vitiligo—thus, this patient very likely had autoimmune primary adrenal failure. Approximately, one half of patients with autoimmune adrenal failure have one or more other autoimmune endocrine disorders. In such patients, the etiology of their findings may be autoimmune polyglandular syndrome type II. Affected patients typically present between the ages of 20–40 years with primary adrenal insufficiency as the main manifestation. Autoimmune thyroid disease (e.g., *Hashimoto* thyroiditis, *Graves'* disease), vitiligo, and type 1 diabetes mellitus are common in patients with autoimmune polyglandular syndrome type II [7].

In discussing case VII, a 60-year-old woman with metastatic breast cancer, Addison concludes:

> I have already expressed my belief that the urgency of the symptoms, and the quick or slow progress of the disease, are determined by the activity or rapidity of the morbid change going on in the capsules, and by the actual amount or degree of that change; and that universal disease of both capsules will in all probability be found to prove uniformly fatal. [3]

Conclusion

Thomas Addison was a remarkably astute clinician who recognized an association between skin hyperpigmentation and diseased adrenal glands at autopsy. In the absence of twentieth- and twenty-first-century medical technology, he pursued this association and convinced the medical world of the critical role of intact adrenal glands.

Acknowledgment Background information and original works of Thomas Addison were provided by the courtesy of Mayo Clinic Libraries History of Medicine Collection.

References

1. Addison T. Dissertatio medica inauguralis quaedam de syphilide et hydrargyro complectens—Concerning Syphilis and Mecury, Doctoral thesis, University of Edinburgh, 1815
2. Addison T. Anaemia—disease of the suprarenal capsules in which the disease is not distinctly separated from a new form of anaemia. Lond Med Gaz. 1849;43:517–18.
3. Addison T. On the constitutional and local effects of disease of the supra-renal capsules. London 1855. London: Samuel Highley of 32 Fleet Street; 1855. (Reprinted in facsimile, 1968, by Dawsons of Pall Mall (copyright: Pickering & Chatto 144–146 New Bond Street, London)).
4. Wilks S, Daldy TM, editors. "Biography" prefixed to the New Sydenham Society's A collection of the published writings of Thomas Addison, M.D. London: 8vo; 1868, p. xii.
5. Pearce, JMS. Thomas Addison (1793–1860). J Royal Soc Med 2004;97:297–300.
6. Stanford, E. Thomas Addison and his times: the tragic last year: 1859–1860. History Med 1973;5:3–10.
7. Amerio P, Di Rollo D, Carbone A, Auriemma M, Marra ME, De Remigis P, Feliciani C, Tracanna M, Tulli A. Polyglandular autoimmune diseases in a dermatological clinical setting: vitiligo-associated autoimmune diseases. Eur J Dermatol. 2010 May–Jun;20(3):354–8.

Primary Aldosteronism

Konstantinos P. Economopoulos and Carrie C. Lubitz

Epidemiology

Hypertension (HTN; Table 1) affects 76 million Americans and 1 billion people worldwide and is the leading cause of heart disease, stroke, and death. The Joint National Committee (JNC) on prevention, evaluation, and treatment of high blood pressure recommends medical treatment of patients with HTN and guidelines target modifiable lifestyle risk factors, treatment of end-organ damage, and identification of cause as primary goals for treatment. Currently, workup for identifiable secondary causes is recommended in cases when blood pressure control is not achieved [1–4].

Primary aldosteronism (PA) is the most common cause of secondary HTN. Detection and, therefore, reported prevalence have increased with education and screening. The prevalence of PA in the hypertensive population is estimated to be more than 10% in recent studies, correlating with increased use of screening aldosterone–renin ratio (ARR) [5]. Furthermore, PA is correlated with the severity of hypertension, with upwards of 23% prevalence in the resistant hypertension population and resultant worse cardiovascular outcomes [3, 6–8]. In comparison to primary hypertensive patients matched for blood pressure, patients with PA have four times increased odds of stroke, seven times increased odds of nonfatal myocardial infarction, and 12 times increased odds of atrial fibrillation [9].

PA is characterized by autonomous, inappropriately elevated plasma aldosterone. Unlike primary HTN, the hyperaldosteronism is nonsuppressible with sodium loading and can result in hypernatremia, hypokalemia, metabolic alkalosis, and suppression of renin [10]. There is a slight preponderance of males and no difference in incidence between race/ethnicities, and the mean age for diagnosis is 52 years for PA [11]. HTN alone is frequently the only sign of PA. In rare cases, patients can present with signs and symptoms of hypokalemia (i.e., muscle cramping, weakness) or patients may be diagnosed during biochemical evaluation of a nodule found on imaging as aldosterone-producing adenomas (APA) constituting 1% of adrenal incidentalomas [12].

PA is most commonly caused by an APA (also known as **Conn's** syndrome) or bilateral adrenal hyperplasia (BAH) [9, 10, 13–16]. In the largest prospective study to date, 1180 consecutive unselected hypertensive patients at 14 hospitals were assessed for PA. They found that 4.8% had an APA and 6.4% had BAH [8]. Furthermore, a higher proportion of APA among PA patients is reported at centers that perform adrenal venous sampling (AVS), suggesting a significant rate of underdiagnosis of unilateral disease within the PA population with imaging alone [5, 8, 17]. A small subset of patients, less than 3%, has unilateral hyperplasia which is diagnosed and treated using the same algorithm as APA with similar success rates [18]. Aldosterone-secreting adrenocortical carcinoma (ACC) occurs in 10.6% of ACC [19].

Familial Hyperaldosteronism

Familial hyperaldosteronism (FH) is a group of autosomal dominant inherited diseases, consisting of three subtypes: (1) type I or glucocorticoid-remediable aldosteronism (GRA) is due to a CYP11B1/CYP11B2 chimeric gene at chromosome 8q22, (2) type II is due to an unknown mutation at chromosome 7p22, and (3) type III is due to mutations in the KCNJ5 gene at chromosome 11 which encodes a G-protein-gated potassium channel.

Type I FH or GRA has a prevalence of 0.66% in patients with PA [20] and is the only form of PA in which aldosterone hypersecretion can be suppressed with glucocorticoids [21]. The CYP11B1 gene encodes for the 11-β hydroxylase isozyme that converts 11-deoxycorticosterone to corticosterone in the zona glomerulosa and CYP11B2 encodes for

C. C. Lubitz (✉)
Department of Surgery, Harvard Medical School,
Massachusetts General Hospital, Boston, MA, USA
e-mail: clubitz@partners.org

K. P. Economopoulos
Department of Surgery, Massachusetts General Hospital, Boston,
MA, USA

J. L. Pasieka, J. A. Lee (eds.), *Surgical Endocrinopathies,* DOI 10.1007/978-3-319-13662-2_33,
© Springer International Publishing Switzerland 2015

Table 1 Frequently used abbreviations

Frequently used abbreviations	
AACE	American Association of Clinical Endocrinologists
AAES	American Association of Endocrine Surgeons
AHA	American Heart Association
APA	Aldosterone-producing adenoma
ARR	Aldosterone–renin ratio
AVS	Adrenal venous sampling
BAH	Bilateral adrenal hyperplasia (a.k.a. bilateral idiopathic hyperplasia, idiopathic hyperaldosteronism)
FH	Familial hyperaldosteronism
GRA	Glucocorticoid-remediable aldosteronism
HTN	Hypertension
JNC	Joint National Committee
PA	Primary hyperaldosteronism

the 11-β hydroxylase isozyme that converts 11-deoxycortisol to cortisol [18, 22]. The mutation in patients with GRA fuses the promoter of CYP11B1 with the exon sequences of CYP11B2, resulting in a chimeric CYP11B1/CYP11B2 gene leading to: (1) an adrenocorticotropic hormone (ACTH)-dependent activation of the aldosterone synthase that converts corticosterone to aldosterone, and (2) an increase in the production of 18-oxocortisol and 18-hydroxycortisol [18, 22]. Normokalemia is characteristic in more than 50 % of GRA patients as aldosterone release is primarily under the influence of ACTH and not potassium [23]. Diagnosis of GRA should be made by genetic testing of selective PA patients who have the following criteria: (1) onset at a young age (e.g., <20 years old), (2) family history of PA, and (3) cerebrovascular complications (e.g., hemorrhagic strokes due to ruptured intracranial aneurysms) at a young age (e.g., <40 years old) [24]. Exogenous administration of glucocorticoids (e.g., dexamethasone) is considered the optimum therapy, while treatment with mineralocorticoid-receptor antagonists (MRA; e.g., eplerenone) is considered an effective alternative with less potential adverse effects [25].

Type II FH is the most common form of FH with 6 % prevalence in the PA populations [20]. Type II FN is an autosomal dominant inherited disease thought to be due to mutations located in chromosome 7p22 [26, 27]. Type II FH is clinically and biochemically indistinguishable from sporadic PA and as a result the diagnosis should be suspected in patients with a positive family history of PA [28]. There is no genetic test for type II FH available, and the same treatment protocols for PA patients should be followed. Blood-related family members should be screened for PA.

Type III FH is a rare condition, first described in 2008, associated with a number of mutations in the KCNJ5 gene encoding the G-protein-gated potassium channel Kir 3.4 [29–34]. These mutations lead to increased sodium conductance, which causes depolarization of glomerulosa cells and subsequent increased calcium [30]. Calcium entry signals aldosterone production and cellular proliferation, leading to

hyperaldosteronism and massive hyperplasia of the adrenal glands. The clinical spectrum of the disease is broad, ranging from mild hypertension responsive to antihypertensive medications [31] to severe and resistant hypertension that requires bilateral adrenalectomy [34]. Certain mutations in the KCNJ5, as G151R, may be implicated with the more severe forms of type III FH [33]. Commercially available genetic testing is available for type III FH and patients presenting at a very young age or with family members with PA should be referred for screening. As with type II FH, the same treatment protocols for type III PA patients should be followed for the mild and moderate forms of type III FH. However, bilateral laparoscopic adrenalectomy may be required for severe forms of type III FH.

Diagnosis

Consensus guidelines vary on who should be referred for screening. While it is under debate, there are no current recommendations to screen all patients with hypertension for PA [11, 14, 15, 35]. Experts agree that patients with resistant hypertension (patients who remain above target blood pressure on three antihypertensive medications of which one is a diuretic) should be referred to a hypertension specialist to be assessed for secondary causes of hypertension [2–4]. Alternate forms of secondary hypertension and subtype differentiation should be considered (Table 2). Patients with hypertension with hypokalemia should be screened for both Cushing's syndrome as well as PA. Lastly, patients who present with an incidentaloma found on abdominal imaging should undergo a functional workup. In rare cases, patients may present with a family history of PA or early-onset HTN or cerebrovascular accident.

While serum potassium level (K^+) has been cited historically as a screening blood test for PA, K^+ alone is inadequate as a screening test. In a recent study, hypokalemia only occurred in 9–38 % of a PA-confirmed population,

Table 2 Physiological patterns of differential diagnoses

Disease	Potassium	Aldosterone	Renin
Aldosterone-producing adenoma	50% ↓↓	↑↑	↓
Bilateral adrenal hyperplasia	17% ↓	↑↑	↓
Loop-diuretic therapy	↓	↓	↑
Renal artery stenosis	↓	↑	↑
Congenital adrenal hyperplasia	↓	↓	↓
Cushing's syndrome	↓	↓	↓
Familial hyperaldosteronism			
Type I or GRA	Normal	↑↑	↓
Type II	↓	↑	↓
Type III	↓	↑	↓

Table 3 Consensus guideline recommendations for PA screening

Guidelines	Criterion for screening	Suggested ARR threshold	Confirmatory test	Imaging	AVS
AACE/AAES guidelines for the management of adrenal incidentalomas [12]	Incidental adrenal nodules + HTN, new HTN, HTN + hypokalemia, resistant HTN	ARR ≥ 20 + Plasma aldosterone ≥ 15 ng/dL	Oral salt loading or saline infusion testing	CT	Yes, in all except age < 40+ unilateral 1-cm nodule on CT (directly to surgery)
American Heart Association guidelines for resistant hypertension [3]	Resistant hypertension	ARR 20–30 (using minimum renin 0.5 ng/mL/h) ± plasma aldo ≥ 15 ng/dL	–	–	–
Endocrine Society clinical practice guidelines [4]	JNC 7 [2] stage 2, resistant HTN, hypokalemia, incidentalomas, family history	ARR 20–40	Oral sodium, saline infusion, captopril, or fludrocortisone suppression testing	CT	Yes, in all surgical candidates
ESH/SSC guidelines for the management of arterial hypertension	Incidental adrenal nodules + HTN, new HTN, HTN + hypokalemia, resistant HTN	ARR ≥ 20 + Plasma aldosterone ≥ 15 ng/dL	Oral salt loading or saline infusion testing	CT	Yes, in all except age < 40 + unilateral 1-cm nodule on CT

AACE American Association of Clinical Endocrinologists, *AAES* American Association of Endocrine Surgeons, *ARR* plasma renin to aldosterone ratio, *ESH* European Society of Hypertension, *ESC* European Society of Cardiology

more commonly in patients with an APA [5]. The Endocrine Society, European Society of Hypertension, American Association of Endocrine Surgeons (AAES), American Association of Clinical Endocrinologists (AACE), and the American Heart Association (AHA) all advocate the use of the plasma ARR as the initial serological screening test for PA in hypertensive patients; however, threshold ratios and next steps in management differ (Table 3) [2–4, 36]. Some experts recommend use of a combination of tests. The AHA and AAES/AACE guidelines use an absolute serum aldosterone level ≥ 15 ng/dL in addition to an elevated ARR for diagnosis of PA. An ARR > 30 and a serum aldosterone > 20 ng/dL were shown to have both sensitivity and specificity > 90 % in diagnosing APA [37]. Rossi et al. developed a model using the combination of plasma renin activity (PRA), K^+, and either serum aldosterone or captopril-suppressed aldosterone which they report has a superior diagnostic accuracy [38].

More than setting a strict cutoff value (conventional threshold ARR ≥ 20), it is essential that the clinician be aware of the variability of results based on the setting, laboratory variations, and the various effects of antihypertensive medications on the renin–aldosterone axis. Age, posture, time of day, medications, K^+, Na^+, and renal function can all lead to false results [4]. See Table 4 for various factors affecting the ARR. Alternatively, patients can be screened with a 24-h urinary aldosterone on a high-sodium diet.

Confirmatory suppression testing is recommended with either oral (5-g sodium diet for three days, 24-h urinary aldosterone level > 12 mcg confirms PA) or intravenous saline load (2-L saline infused over 4 h, serum aldosterone > 10 ng/dL confirms PA), captopril, or fludrocortisone as the specificity of screening tests are low; however, caution should be taken as testing can be potentially dangerous for patients (i.e., exacerbation of congestive heart failure (CHF)) and withdrawal of antihypertensive medication is needed [35, 39]. For the most accurate test, patients on MRA (spironolactone or eplerenone) should be discontinued for 6 weeks prior to confirmatory testing, hypokalemia should be corrected, and hypertension controlled. However, screening with ARR has been shown to still be useful without withdrawing antihypertensives or when changing the regimen to those that affect the ARR less and should be utilized in cases where withdrawal of medications may be deleterious [4, 7, 11].

Table 4 Factors that affect the aldosterone–renin ratio (ARR)

Factor	Effect on ARR
Increased age	FP
Hypokalemia	FN
Hypernatremia	FP
Pregnancy	FN
Renal failure	FP
Resistant hypertension	FN
Drugs	
Diuretics	FN
ACE inhibitors	FN
ARBs	FN
β-blockers	FP
CCB	FN

ACE angiotensin-converting enzyme, *ARBs* angiotensin II receptor blockers, *CCB* calcium channel blocker, *FP* false-positive, decreased specificity; *FN* false-negative, decreased sensitivity

Identifying Appropriate Patients for Surgery

Following serologic diagnosis of PA, differentiating APA and unilateral hyperplasia from BAH is essential to identify surgical candidates. While it has been shown that APA patients tend to be younger, and have higher systolic blood pressure, lower serum K^+, and higher serum aldosterone levels than BAH patients, no single serologic test is discriminating [40–42]. For instance, Rossi et al. found 48% of APA patients and 17% of BAH patients had spontaneous hypokalemia as did 7% of patients with primary hypertension [8]. Prior to proceeding, a discussion with the patient regarding the risks and benefits of surgery versus medical therapy as well as their desire for surgery is prudent prior to pursuing lateralization. Within this consent to proceed should be a discussion of the potential side effects of MRA.

Identifying appropriate patients for adrenalectomy remains a challenge. Traditional noninvasive imaging with abdominal CT detects many adrenal masses, but does not reflect functionality. Frequently, aldosteronomas are small, increasing false-negative imaging (sensitivity 75–80%). Rossi and colleagues found 17% of their cohort of PA patients had tumors <1 cm and 45% <2 cm [8]. Furthermore, nonfunctional adenomas increase with age, lending to a high false-positive rate and decreased specificity of CT in the older population. Magill and colleagues found an accuracy rate for CT of 37% in direct comparison to AVS [42]. Young and colleagues compared findings of 194 patients who underwent both AVS and CT for lateralization. In their cohort, 41% of patients that had negative CT scans had lateralizing AVS results and CT identified the wrong adrenal gland in 12/57 (21%), while AVS falsely diagnosed four patients with BAH [43]. Despite these limitations, however, most clinicians recommend structural imaging to assess for aldosterone-secreting ACC. Given that most aldosteronomas are small (<2 cm), suspicion for aldosterone-secreting

ACC should be high in patients with large tumors (>4 cm). Because of the deficiencies of CT, we recommend obtaining AVS in all patients wishing to pursue surgical treatment (Fig. 1). Due to the low incidence of incidental nonfunctional adrenal nodules in younger patients, the AACE/AAES and other guidelines state that one may proceed to surgery in patients younger than 40 with a unilateral microadenoma without AVS [12].

Adrenal venous sampling is recommended by many experts for lateralization, although indication, technique, and threshold values considered diagnostic vary significantly [40, 42–44]. Cost and access to centers performing AVS are also important considerations. The procedure entails cannulation and comparison of aldosterone and cortisol (to normalize dilution effects) levels in both adrenal veins and the inferior vena cava (IVC). Most centers use ACTH (cosyntropin) stimulation to augment potential laterality by minimizing stress-induced fluctuations during sequential sampling, aid in differentiating IVC versus right adrenal vein placement (adrenal to IVC cortisol ratio >5 indicates proper placement of right-sided catheter), and to maximize aldosterone secretion [17, 43]. Moreover, Rossi et al. report an adrenal cortisol-adjusted aldosterone ratio greater than two as 80% sensitive in classifying patients with PA that had poor localization with CT or MRI [40]. Most centers used a threshold cortisol-adjusted aldosterone lateralization ratio >4 to refer patients to surgery, with a sensitivity ranging from 78 to 98% [42, 43, 45].

Opponents of widespread use of AVS cite access to the procedure, technical difficulty, cost, lack of standardization, and potential complications such as hematoma, dissection, and adrenal infarction as arguments against using this modality regularly [46]. Ranges in the literature for successful determination of PA subtype (i.e., APA vs. BAH) are 63–97% [42, 47, 48]. Young and colleagues successfully cannulated both adrenal veins in 95% of their 194 catheterizations, with a 2.5% complication rate [43]. Rossi et al. cited successful AVS in 102/105 (97%) of procedures and one adrenal vein rupture. Successful bilateral adrenal vein cannulation is, however, related to volume of procedures with rates as low as 10% in low-volume centers [49]. Some experts recommend adrenalectomy following serologic diagnosis of PA and unilateral adrenal mass on CT [17]. Others, such as stated in the AACE/AAES guidelines, support AVS following CT only for patients >40 years old given the low prevalence of adrenal nodules in younger patients (Table 3, Fig. 1) [12].

Treatment

The treatment goal is to prevent the morbidity and mortality associated with hypertension and hypokalemia. The treatment is based upon whether the patient has unilateral (i.e.,

Fig. 1 Algorithm for diagnosis and treatment of surgically correctable primary aldosteronism

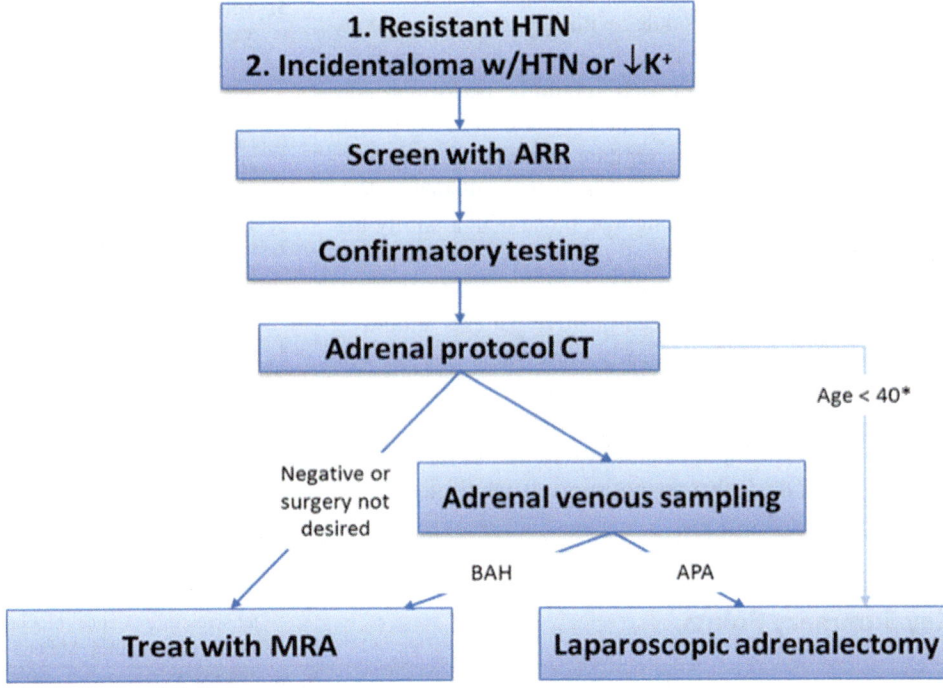

*with unilateral nodule >1 cm identified on CT

APA) or bilateral (i.e., BAH) aldosterone hypersecretion. Adrenalectomy for true APA or unilateral hyperplasia is effective and is shown to reverse not only the hypertension but also cardiovascular and renal complications [18, 50]. Lumachi et al. followed up patients for over 5 years subsequent to unilateral adrenalectomy for APA: mean blood pressure values improved in 97% of patients, and cure was achieved in 72% [51]. Persistent hypertension following adrenalectomy is significantly correlated with length of diagnosis and age [51, 52]. Rossi et al. documented improvement in blood pressure control, lessening of required antihypertensives in 57%, and complete cure in 30% of patients [53]. Similarly, Young and colleagues showed postoperative improvement in nearly all patients and cure in 36% and Letavernier's group found an improvement in HTN in 68–77% [43, 54]. Milliez and colleagues showed cure in 43% and improvement in an additional 29% [9]. Few studies report repeat ARR ratios following surgery in those patients that continue to require antihypertensives, likely indicating underlying primary hypertension.

Aldosterone hypersecretion in type I FH can be suppressed with exogenous administration of physiologic doses of glucocorticoids (e.g., dexamethasone 0.125–0.25 mg/day, prednisolone 2.5 or 5 mg/day) as the first-line therapy [21], while treatment with MRA (e.g., eplerenone) is considered an effective alternative or concomitant therapy if hypertension is uncontrolled on glucocorticoids alone [25]. Type II and type III FH should be treated the same way as sporadic forms of PA, with the exception of patients with severe forms of type III FH who may require bilateral laparoscopic adrenalectomy [34].

MRA, most commonly spironolactone or eplerenone, are also effective in treating all forms of PA, and should be considered in all patients with resistant hypertension, those with bilateral hyperplasia, or patients who refuse or are not candidates for surgery [55]. The appropriate dose for spironolactone has not been well defined for PA patients but it seems that a dose below 50 mg/day is considered both effective and safe [56, 57]. Spironolactone is also a progesterone agonist and androgen-receptor antagonist, and as a result is associated with side effects such as impotence, gynecomastia, and menstrual irregularities [57]. In the case of adverse effects with spironolactone, eplerenone which is a highly selective MRA with a low incidence of adverse effects could be used instead [58]. For patients who do not tolerate MRAs, a potassium-sparing diuretic (e.g., amiloride) could be used. Surgery appears to be more effective than MRAs in treating PA [59]. Additionally, the cost savings and quality of life improvement from coming off most if not all antihypertensive medications are substantial [60].

Summary

In conclusion, PA is a significant public health concern. Prevalence has increased with screening, with recent estimates over 10% in the hypertensive population. Given that approximately ½ of patients with PA have unilateral disease (i.e., 5% of the hypertensive population), the relative safety of laparoscopic adrenalectomy, and the potential for curing a great number of patients with surgically correctable (i.e., unilateral) disease, it is important to screen patients with both incidental adrenal nodules with hypertension or hypokalemia as well as patients with resistant hypertension for PA. Screening for PA with ARR should be performed after correcting K^+, in the morning after 15 min of being seated, and in consideration of concomitant antihypertensive medications altering the aldosterone–renin axis. Patients diagnosed with PA at a very young age, those with a family history of PA, or a personal or family history of cerebrovascular accidents at a young age should also be tested for familial PA. Type II familial PA screen-positive patients should be assessed for unilateral, surgically correctable disease with imaging (CT or MRI) and AVS where available. Laparoscopic adrenalectomy is a safe and highly effective treatment for patients with unilateral hyperplasia or APA. Those with BAH and those that are not surgical candidates should receive MRAs.

Key Summary Points

- PA is the most common form of secondary hypertension.
- Patients with PA have worse outcomes compared to matched patients with primary hypertension.
- PA is most commonly caused by an APA or BAH.
- Familial hyperaldosteronism is a group of autosomal dominant inherited diseases consisting of three subtypes.
- Treatment guidelines for PA vary; diagnosis should be focused on confirming hyperaldosteronism serologically followed by differentiation of unilateral versus bilateral disease with imaging (CT or MRI) and adrenal venous sampling.
- Laparoscopic adrenalectomy is a safe and highly effective treatment for patients with unilateral hyperplasia or APA.
- Patients with BAH and those that are not surgical candidates should receive an MRA.

References

1. James PA, Oparil S, Carter BL, Cushman WC, Dennison-Himmelfarb C, Handler J, et al. 2014 evidence-based guideline for the management of high blood pressure in adults: report from the panel members appointed to the Eighth Joint National Committee (JNC 8). JAMA. 2014;311(5):507–20. PubMed PMID: 24352797.
2. Green L. JNC 7 express: new thinking in hypertension treatment. Am Fam Physician. 2003;68(2):228, 30. PubMed PMID: 12892344.
3. Calhoun DA, Jones D, Textor S, Goff DC, Murphy TP, Toto RD, et al. Resistant hypertension: diagnosis, evaluation, and treatment: a scientific statement from the American Heart Association Professional Education Committee of the Council for High Blood Pressure Research. Circulation. 2008;117(25):e510–26. PubMed PMID: 18574054.
4. Funder JW, Carey RM, Fardella C, Gomez-Sanchez CE, Mantero F, Stowasser M, et al. Case detection, diagnosis, and treatment of patients with primary aldosteronism: an endocrine society clinical practice guideline. J Clin Endocrinol Metab. 2008;93(9):3266–81. PubMed PMID: 18552288.
5. Mulatero P, Stowasser M, Loh KC, Fardella CE, Gordon RD, Mosso L, et al. Increased diagnosis of primary aldosteronism, including surgically correctable forms, in centers from five continents. J Clin Endocrinol Metab. 2004;89(3):1045–50. PubMed PMID: 15001583.
6. Eide IK, Torjesen PA, Drolsum A, Babovic A, Lilledahl NP. Low-renin status in therapy-resistant hypertension: a clue to efficient treatment. J Hypertens. 2004;22(11):2217–26. PubMed PMID: 15480108.
7. Gallay BJ, Ahmad S, Xu L, Toivola B, Davidson RC. Screening for primary aldosteronism without discontinuing hypertensive medications: plasma aldosterone-renin ratio. Am J Kidney Dis. 2001;37(4):699–705. PubMed PMID: 11273868.
8. Rossi GP, Bernini G, Caliumi C, Desideri G, Fabris B, Ferri C, et al. A prospective study of the prevalence of primary aldosteronism in 1,125 hypertensive patients. J Am Coll Cardiol. 2006;48(11):2293–300. PubMed PMID: 17161262.
9. Milliez P, Girerd X, Plouin PF, Blacher J, Safar ME, Mourad JJ. Evidence for an increased rate of cardiovascular events in patients with primary aldosteronism. J Am Coll Cardiol. 2005;45(8):1243–8. PubMed PMID: 15837256.
10. Fardella CE, Mosso L, Gomez-Sanchez C, Cortes P, Soto J, Gomez L, et al. Primary hyperaldosteronism in essential hypertensives: prevalence, biochemical profile, and molecular biology. J Clin Endocrinol Metab. 2000;85(5):1863–7. PubMed PMID: 10843166.
11. Schwartz GL, Chapman AB, Boerwinkle E, Kisabeth RM, Turner ST. Screening for primary aldosteronism: implications of an increased plasma aldosterone/renin ratio. Clin Chem. 2002;48(11):1919–23. PubMed PMID: 12406976.
12. Zeiger MA, Thompson GB, Duh QY, Hamrahian AH, Angelos P, Elaraj D, et al. The American Association of Clinical Endocrinologists and American Association of Endocrine Surgeons medical guidelines for the management of adrenal incidentalomas. Endocr Pract. 2009;15(1):1–20. PubMed PMID: 19632967.
13. Fagugli RM, Taglioni C. Changes in the perceived epidemiology of primary hyperaldosteronism. Int J Hypertens. 2011;2011:162804. PubMed PMID: 21837271. Pubmed Central PMCID: 3151507.
14. Gordon RD, Stowasser M. Primary aldosteronism: the case for screening. Nat Clin Pract Nephrol. 2007;3(11):582–3. PubMed PMID: 17909546.
15. Lim PO, Rodgers P, Cardale K, Watson AD, MacDonald TM. Potentially high prevalence of primary aldosteronism in a primary-care population. Lancet. 1999;353(9146):40. PubMed PMID: 10023956.
16. Strauch B, Zelinka T, Hampf M, Bernhardt R, Widimsky J Jr. Prevalence of primary hyperaldosteronism in moderate to severe hypertension in the Central Europe region. J Hum Hypertens. 2003;17(5):349–52. PubMed PMID: 12756408.
17. Doppman JL, Gill JR Jr. Hyperaldosteronism: sampling the adrenal veins. Radiology. 1996;198(2):309–12. PubMed PMID: 8596821.
18. Lifton RP, Dluhy RG, Powers M, Rich GM, Gutkin M, Fallo F, et al. Hereditary hypertension caused by chimaeric gene duplications and ectopic expression of aldosterone synthase. Nat Genet. 1992;2(1):66–74. PubMed PMID: 1303253.
19. Kendrick ML, Curlee K, Lloyd R, Farley DR, Grant CS, Thompson GB, et al. Aldosterone-secreting ACCs are associated with unique operative risks and outcomes. Surgery. 2002;132(6):1008–11; discussion 12. PubMed PMID: 12490848.
20. Mulatero P, Tizzani D, Viola A, Bertello C, Monticone S, Mengozzi G, et al. Prevalence and characteristics of familial hyperaldosteronism: the PATOGEN study (Primary Aldosteronism in TOrino-GENetic forms). Hypertension. 2011;58(5):797–803. PubMed PMID: 21876069.
21. Ulick S, Chan CK, Gill JR Jr, Gutkin M, Letcher L, Mantero F, et al. Defective fasciculata zone function as the mechanism of GRA. J Clin Endocrinol Metab. 1990;71(5):1151–7. PubMed PMID: 2172271.

22. Lifton RP, Dluhy RG, Powers M, Rich GM, Cook S, Ulick S, et al. A chimaeric 11 beta-hydroxylase/aldosterone synthase gene causes glucocorticoid-remediable aldosteronism and human hypertension. Nature. 1992;355(6357):262–5. PubMed PMID: 1731223.

23. Rich GM, Ulick S, Cook S, Wang JZ, Lifton RP, Dluhy RG. Glucocorticoid-remediable aldosteronism in a large kindred: clinical spectrum and diagnosis using a characteristic biochemical phenotype. Ann Intern Med. 1992;116(10):813–20. PubMed PMID: 1567095.

24. Dluhy RG, Anderson B, Harlin B, Ingelfinger J, Lifton R. Glucocorticoid-remediable aldosteronism is associated with severe hypertension in early childhood. J Pediatr. 2001;138(5):715–20. PubMed PMID: 11343049.

25. McMahon GT, Dluhy RG. Glucocorticoid-remediable aldosteronism. Cardiol Rev. 2004;12(1):44–8. PubMed PMID: 14667264.

26. Sukor N, Mulatero P, Gordon RD, So A, Duffy D, Bertello C, et al. Further evidence for linkage of familial hyperaldosteronism type II at chromosome 7p22 in Italian as well as Australian and South American families. J Hypertens. 2008;26(8):1577–82. PubMed PMID: 18622235.

27. Carss KJ, Stowasser M, Gordon RD, O'Shaughnessy KM. Further study of chromosome 7p22 to identify the molecular basis of familial hyperaldosteronism type II. J Hum Hypertens. 2011;25(9):560–4. PubMed PMID: 20927129.

28. Young WF. Primary aldosteronism: renaissance of a syndrome. Clin Endocrinol (Oxf). 2007;66(5):607–18. PubMed PMID: 17492946.

29. Charmandari E, Sertedaki A, Kino T, Merakou C, Hoffman DA, Hatch MM, et al. A novel point mutation in the KCNJ5 gene causing primary hyperaldosteronism and early-onset autosomal dominant hypertension. J Clin Endocrinol Metab. 2012;97(8):E1532–9. PubMed PMID: 22628607. Pubmed Central PMCID: 3410272.

30. Choi M, Scholl UI, Yue P, Bjorklund P, Zhao B, Nelson-Williams C, et al. K+ channel mutations in adrenal aldosterone-producing adenomas and hereditary hypertension. Science. 2011;331(6018):768–72. PubMed PMID: 21311022. Pubmed Central PMCID: 3371087.

31. Mulatero P, Tauber P, Zennaro MC, Monticone S, Lang K, Beuschlein F, et al. KCNJ5 mutations in European families with nonglucocorticoid remediable familial hyperaldosteronism. Hypertension. 2012;59(2):235–40. PubMed PMID: 22203740.

32. Mussa A, Camilla R, Monticone S, Porta F, Tessaris D, Verna F, et al. Polyuric-polydipsic syndrome in a pediatric case of nonglucocorticoid remediable familial hyperaldosteronism. Endocr J. 2012;59(6):497–502. PubMed PMID: 22447138.

33. Scholl UI, Nelson-Williams C, Yue P, Grekin R, Wyatt RJ, Dillon MJ, et al. Hypertension with or without adrenal hyperplasia due to different inherited mutations in the potassium channel KCNJ5. Proc Natl Acad Sci U S A. 2012;109(7):2533–8. PubMed PMID: 22308486. Pubmed Central PMCID: 3289329.

34. Geller DS, Zhang J, Wisgerhof MV, Shackleton C, Kashgarian M, Lifton RP. A novel form of human mendelian hypertension featuring nonglucocorticoid-remediable aldosteronism. J Clin Endocrinol Metab. 2008;93(8):3117–23. PubMed PMID: 18505761. Pubmed Central PMCID: 2515083.

35. Mulatero P, Dluhy RG, Giacchetti G, Boscaro M, Veglio F, Stewart PM. Diagnosis of primary aldosteronism: from screening to subtype differentiation. Trends Endocrinol Metab. 2005;16(3):114–9. PubMed PMID: 15808809.

36. Mancia G, Fagard R, Narkiewicz K, Redon J, Zanchetti A, Bohm M, et al. 2013 ESH/ESC Guidelines for the management of arterial hypertension: the Task Force for the management of arterial hypertension of the European Society of Hypertension (ESH) and of the European Society of Cardiology (ESC). J Hypertens. 2013;31(7):1281–357. PubMed PMID: 23817082.

37. Weinberger MH, Fineberg NS. The diagnosis of primary aldosteronism and separation of two major subtypes. Arch Intern Med. 1993;153(18):2125–9. PubMed PMID: 8379804.

38. Rossi GP, Rossi E, Pavan E, Rosati N, Zecchel R, Semplicini A, et al. Screening for primary aldosteronism with a logistic multivariate discriminant analysis. Clin Endocrinol (Oxf). 1998;49(6):713–23. PubMed PMID: 10209558.

39. Mulatero P, Milan A, Fallo F, Regolisti G, Pizzolo F, Fardella C, et al. Comparison of confirmatory tests for the diagnosis of primary aldosteronism. J Clin Endocrinol Metab. 2006;91(7):2618–23. PubMed PMID: 16670162.

40. Rossi GP, Sacchetto A, Chiesura-Corona M, De Toni R, Gallina M, Feltrin GP, et al. Identification of the etiology of primary aldosteronism with adrenal vein sampling in patients with equivocal computed tomography and magnetic resonance findings: results in 104 consecutive cases. J Clin Endocrinol Metab. 2001;86(3):1083–90. PubMed PMID: 11238490.

41. Blumenfeld JD, Sealey JE, Schlussel Y, Vaughan ED Jr, Sos TA, Atlas SA, et al. Diagnosis and treatment of primary hyperaldosteronism. Ann Intern Med. 1994;121(11):877–85. PubMed PMID: 7978702.

42. Magill SB, Raff H, Shaker JL, Brickner RC, Knechtges TE, Kehoe ME, et al. Comparison of adrenal vein sampling and computed tomography in the differentiation of primary aldosteronism. J Clin Endocrinol Metab. 2001;86(3):1066–71. PubMed PMID: 11238487.

43. Young WF, Stanson AW, Thompson GB, Grant CS, Farley DR, van Heerden JA. Role for adrenal venous sampling in primary aldosteronism. Surgery. 2004;136(6):1227–35. PubMed PMID: 15657580.

44. Nishikawa T, Omura M. Clinical characteristics of primary aldosteronism: its prevalence and comparative studies on various causes of primary aldosteronism in Yokohama Rosai Hospital. Biomed Pharmacother. 2000;54(1):83–5. PubMed PMID: 10914999.

45. Satoh F, Abe T, Tanemoto M, Nakamura M, Abe M, Uruno A, et al. Localization of aldosterone-producing adrenocortical adenomas: significance of adrenal venous sampling. Hypertens Res. 2007;30(11):1083–95. PubMed PMID: 18250558.

46. Stewart PM, Allolio B. Adrenal vein sampling for Primary Aldosteronism: time for a reality check. Clin Endocrinol (Oxf). 2009. PubMed PMID: 19769616.

47. Young WF Jr, Stanson AW, Grant CS, Thompson GB, van Heerden JA. Primary aldosteronism: adrenal venous sampling. Surgery. 1996;120(6):913–9; discussion 9–20. PubMed PMID: 8957473.

48. Sheaves R, Goldin J, Reznek RH, Chew SL, Dacie JE, Lowe DG, et al. Relative value of computed tomography scanning and venous sampling in establishing the cause of primary hyperaldosteronism. Euro J endocrinol/Euro Fed Endocr Soc. 1996;134(3):308–13. PubMed PMID: 8616527.

49. Vonend O, Ockenfels N, Gao X, Allolio B, Lang K, Mai K, et al. Adrenal venous sampling: evaluation of the German Conn's registry. Hypertension. 2011;57(5):990–5. PubMed PMID: 21383311.

50. Sechi LA, Di Fabio A, Bazzocchi M, Uzzau A, Catena C. Intrarenal hemodynamics in primary aldosteronism before and after treatment. J Clin Endocrinol Metab. 2009;94(4):1191–7. PubMed PMID: 19141581.

51. Lumachi F, Ermani M, Basso SM, Armanini D, Iacobone M, Favia G. Long-term results of adrenalectomy in patients with aldosterone-producing adenomas: multivariate analysis of factors affecting unresolved hypertension and review of the literature. Am Surg. 2005;71(10):864–9. PubMed PMID: 16468537.

52. Celen O, O'Brien MJ, Melby JC, Beazley RM. Factors influencing outcome of surgery for primary aldosteronism. Arch Surg. 1996;131(6):646–50. PubMed PMID: 8645073.

53. Rossi GP, Bolognesi M, Rizzoni D, Seccia TM, Piva A, Porteri E, et al. Vascular remodeling and duration of hypertension predict outcome of adrenalectomy in primary aldosteronism patients. Hypertension. 2008;51(5):1366–71. PubMed PMID: 18347224.

54. Letavernier E, Peyrard S, Amar L, Zinzindohoue F, Fiquet B, Plouin PF. Blood pressure outcome of adrenalectomy in patients with primary hyperaldosteronism with or without unilateral adenoma. J Hypertens. 2008;26(9):1816–23. PubMed PMID: 18698217.

55. Vaclavik J, Sedlak R, Plachy M, Navratil K, Plasek J, Jarkovsky J, et al. Addition of spironolactone in patients with resistant arterial hypertension (ASPIRANT): a randomized, double-blind, placebo-controlled trial. Hypertension. 2011;57(6):1069–75. PubMed PMID: 21536989.

56. Batterink J, Stabler SN, Tejani AM, Fowkes CT. Spironolactone for hypertension. Cochrane Database Syst Rev. 2010;(8):CD008169. PubMed PMID: 20687095.

57. Ghose RP, Hall PM, Bravo EL. Medical management of aldosterone-producing adenomas. Ann Intern Med. 1999;131(2):105–8. PubMed PMID: 10419425.

58. Parthasarathy HK, Menard J, White WB, Young WF Jr, Williams GH, Williams B, et al. A double-blind, randomized study comparing the antihypertensive effect of eplerenone and spironolactone in patients with hypertension and evidence of primary aldosteronism. J Hypertens. 2011;29(5):980–90. PubMed PMID: 21451421.

59. Ahmed AH, Gordon RD, Sukor N, Pimenta E, Stowasser M. Quality of life in patients with bilateral primary aldosteronism before and during treatment with spironolactone and/or amiloride, including a comparison with our previously published results in those with unilateral disease treated surgically. J Clin Endocrinol Metab. 2011;96(9):2904–11. PubMed PMID: 21778218.

60. Lubitz CC, Sy S, Economopoulos KP, Gazelle GS, McMahon PM, Weinstein MC, et al. Cost-effectiveness of screening resistant hypertensive patients for primary aldosteronism: integrating lifetime cardiovascular risk and outcomes. 35th Annual Meeting of the American Association of Endocrine Surgeons. pp06.

Jerome W. Conn

1907–1994

Gregory A. Kline

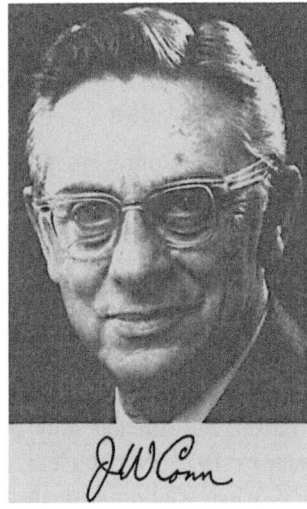

Jerome W. Conn, Professor Emeritus, University of Michigan. (From Office of the Home Secretary, National Academy of Sciences. *Biographical Memoirs V.71*; © 1997 The National Academies Press)

Dr. Jerome Conn belongs to the "golden age" of endocrinology, a time during the mid-twentieth century characterized by an explosion of interest in and discovery of classical endocrine hormones and the clinical syndromes produced by their dysregulation. It was a time when clinical biochemists worked side by side with inquisitive physician investigators, each one coming to the other for advice, even exchanging letters discussing the nuances and suggesting novel tests and solutions for individual patient cases. With scientific and clinical chemistry collaboration, a keen eye for clinical observation and the ability to admit patients to an investigation ward for months on end, Dr. Conn and others of his generation were able to unravel both rare and now common endocrinopathies that have since defined endocrinology practice around the world.

"Jerry" was born in New York City in 1907, the son of a lunch-shop owner. After graduating from Rutgers University in 1928, he received his M.D. from the University of Michigan in 1932 and remained at that institution for his entire career. His university expenses were paid by his two sisters who worked as secretaries to support him [1]. After a brief, 1-year flirtation with surgery, he switched to internal medicine and joined the Division of Clinical Investigation as assistant professor in 1938. At first, he worked under the supervision of Dr. Louis Newburgh who had clinical interests in the areas of diabetes and obesity. When Dr. Newburgh left to join the US Naval Research efforts, Dr. Conn became the director of the Division of Endocrinology and Metabolism in 1943, a position he held until his retirement 30 years later.

With World War II underway and the USA heavily involved in the South Pacific theatre, there was much interest in biomedical research of military importance. Dr. Conn became particularly interested in the science behind human acclimatization to heat and in 1950 published a complex paper in the *Journal of Clinical Endocrinology and Metabolism* demonstrating that the concentrations of sodium and chloride in human sweat were governed by steroids secreted by the adrenal cortex. In the same paper, he was able to demonstrate that the sweat electrolyte pattern could be used to evaluate the function of what he called "salt-active corticosteroids" [2]. In 1952, Simpson, Tait, and Bush isolated and identified a compound that eventually became known as "aldosterone" and thus opened the door to direct clinical measurement of Conn's "salt-active corticosteroid."

The clinical implications were not far behind these groundbreaking chemists' work. In June and November of 1954, Dr. M. D. Milne at Hammersmith Hospital in London and Dr. C. L. Cope (also in London) published separate reports of the same patient they had shared with an apparent diagnosis of "potassium-wasting nephritis" [3, 4]. The subject, a 41-year-old Nigerian woman had presented with severe hypertension and profound hypokalemic paralysis. Milne and Cope confirmed urinary potassium wasting and a high level of urinary "electrocortin" (aldosterone) but did not

G. A. Kline (✉)
Department of Medicine, Endocrinology, University of Calgary,
1820 Richmond Rd, SW, Calgary, AB T2T 5C7, Canada

J. L. Pasieka, J. A. Lee (eds.), *Surgical Endocrinopathies,* DOI 10.1007/978-3-319-13662-2_34,
© Springer International Publishing Switzerland 2015

appear to fully appreciate the connection and so a primary renal disease was postulated. Perhaps due to his established interest in adrenal steroids' effect upon electrolytes, it seems that Dr. Conn had begun similar investigations on a similar patient that same year but with a clearer understanding of the likely adrenal nature of his patient's problem. At the Central Society for Clinical Research meeting in October of 1954, Mader and Iseri from Detroit presented a paper detailing a case of hypertension and hypokalemia wherein an adrenal tumor had been found at surgical exploration in February of that year. But it was at the meeting's presidential address that Dr. Conn presented his own index case of what he called "primary aldosteronism". The patient was a 54-year-old woman with episodic weakness for several years. Over a 7-month inpatient investigation, Dr. Conn documented all the cardinal features of the syndrome: hypertension, hypokalemia not corrected with potassium salts, urinary potassium wasting, alkalosis, impaired urinary concentrating ability not corrected with vasopressin (hypokalemic nephrogenic diabetes insipidus). She had a low sodium to potassium ratio in her sweat and saliva, suggesting overproduction of a sodium-retaining substance. Conn postulated an aldosterone secreting adrenal tumor and indeed, an adrenal mass was discovered and surgically removed on December 10, 1954. The patient's potassium and blood pressure normalized within 12 days with disappearance of the polyuria and muscle weakness. This presentation appeared in print in January 1955 [5] and is considered the first published description of the disease with the appropriate linkage to primary aldosterone excess. A study of the literature of the time shows that within 4 years, this new disease was being called "Conn's syndrome" in the regular medical literature. Understanding of this newly described disease exploded and by 1962, Dr. Conn published a paper showing that his eponymous disease was not a rarity; in fact, within those 7 years, 145 similar cases were reported in the literature. Many clinicians also sought advice from Dr. Conn as he reported being aware of more than 50 other cases at the time that were as yet unpublished [6].

It is indeed a rare honor to have a novel and important disease named after its' discoverer, and especially so if such recognition occurs during their lifetime but for Dr. Conn, the discovery was just the beginning. Over the remaining years of his career, Dr. Conn described virtually all of what is known today regarding this illness, including:

a. Many patients have adrenal hyperplasia or multiple adenomas.
b. A high associated risk of heart disease, stroke, and death in those who do not get to surgery in time.
c. Not all patients are cured by adenoma removal (but most at least improved).
d. Many patients with confirmed disease do not have hypokalemia.
e. Salt loading appears to be an effective way to confirm the diagnosis.
f. Blood renin levels are an integral part of differentiating primary aldosteronism from other mineralocorticoid hypertension.
g. Black licorice ingestion may cause a similar clinical presentation.
h. "Failure to visualize (an adrenal mass) by various techniques now in vogue does not exclude their presence."
i. Functional adrenal masses may be detected by I131–19-iodocholesterol scanning.
j. Primary aldosteronism is far too common to be considered a rare disease.
k. Primary aldosteronism may overlap seamlessly with an essential hypertension population in clinical appearance.
l. Primary aldosteronism seems to be associated with impaired carbohydrate metabolism.

So comprehensive was Dr. Conn's research career that it is quite remarkable in the present day and age, many investigators in the field of primary aldosteronism are still publishing papers that, while appearing to be novel, are really just confirming or recapitulating an observation made earlier by Dr. Conn. One might even go so far as to state that aside from new studies of the genetics of aldosteronism, virtually everything of critical importance to the practice and knowledge base of aldosteronism was already fully described by Dr. Conn and his team by 1974. Nonetheless, it is particularly interesting to note, when reading through many of his 284 publications, Dr. Conn never referred to the syndrome by his own eponym, preferring to stick with the term "primary aldosteronism".

In addition to his contributions to primary aldosteronism, Dr. Conn also published in the fields of diabetes, obesity, **Cushing's** syndrome and even described what is likely the first case of "normocalcemic primary hyperparathyroidism" [7]. He served as the president of the American Diabetes Association, was elected to the National Academy of Sciences, and was a founding member of the Institute of Medicine.

It has been recorded that Dr. Conn had some sage advice for his younger brother Harold who followed him into a medical career: "(1) Stay in one place because every move will cost you at least one year, and (2) find a good umbrella [by this he meant a supportive chairman] and stay under it" to which he added, "do not be seduced into becoming an umbrella" [8]. Ironically, despite his recommendation to avoid becoming a chairman, Dr. Conn remained the figurehead of the Division of Endocrinology for almost 30 years, during which time innumerable young trainees matured into clinician-scientists under his tutelage and the University of Michigan gained and maintained a truly international reputation for excellence in endocrine research.

One of Conn's contemporaries recalled the following passage from an address given by Conn later in life:

> I am not old enough to have forgotten completely the perspective of younger colleagues. Their aspirations are pointed in your direction. They wish eventually to reach the standing and respect in clinical research which they believe you have achieved, and many of them will, and perhaps to a greater degree! Let us set for them a proper example of kindness, friendliness, and common decency. [8]

There is a general movement afoot today to remove the historical names from diseases and use more general pathologic terms. For Conn's keen insight, exemplary clinical investigation, comprehensive elucidation of an entire disease, and dedication to the furtherance of young researchers, perhaps "Conn's Syndrome" is an eponym that should be allowed to remain.

Dr. Jerome Conn died in 1994 in Naples, Florida.

References

1. Loriaux DL, Jerome W. Conn (1907–1994). Endocrinologist. 2008;18:159–60.
2. Conn JW, Louis LH. Production of endogenous "salt-active" corticoids as reflected in the concentrations of sodium and chloride of thermal sweat. J Clin Endocrinol Metab. 1950;10:12–23.
3. Cope CL, Garcia-LJ. The occurrence of electrocortin in human urine. Br Med J. 1954;1:1290–94.
4. Evans BM, Milne MD. Potassium losing nephritis presenting as a case of periodic paralysis. Br Med J. 1954;2:1067–71.
5. Conn JW. Presidential Address. II. Primary aldosteronism, a new clinical syndrome. J Lab Clin Med. 1955;45:3–17.
6. Conn JW, Knopf RF, Nesbit RM. Clinical characteristics of primary aldosteronism from an analysis of 145 cases. Am J Surg. 1964;107:159–72.
7. Johnson RD, Conn JW. Hyperparathyroidism with a prolonged period of normocalcemia. JAMA. 1969;210:2063–66.
8. Daughady WH. Jerome Conn. Biographical memoirs. Washington DC: National Academy of Sciences; 1997.

Cushing's Syndrome

Courtney J. Balentine and Rebecca S. Sippel

Overview

Cushing's syndrome (CS) refers to any state of excess cortisol and can be classified as from either exogenous or endogenous sources. Exogenous CS involves a medically induced hypercortisolism and is most commonly due to iatrogenic administration of steroids. By contrast, endogenous CS stems from overproduction of cortisol without any external stimulus, and this type of CS will be the focus of the current chapter. Endogenous CS is further divided into adrenocorticotropic hormone (ACTH)-independent and ACTH-dependent disease with the former involving autonomous cortisol secretion from the adrenal gland while the later stems from pituitary or extra-adrenal secretion of ACTH that drives cortisol excess.

Epidemiology and Classification

Precise estimates of the incidence of endogenous CS are somewhat variable due to difficulties with testing and confirming the diagnosis. Generally accepted figures for yearly incidence are up to 2.4 per million in an unselected population, and women are overall more likely than men to develop CS. Notably, the incidence of previously undiagnosed CS is higher among certain groups of patients including diabetics and those with obesity. Among individuals with incidentally discovered adrenal masses, cortisol may be elevated in 4–20% and 12.5% may develop overt CS within 1 year [1, 2].

CS is categorized according to the etiology as either ACTH-dependent or ACTH-independent with 80–85% of cases attributable to ACTH-dependent causes and the remaining 10–15% being ACTH independent (Table 1) [3].

ACTH-Dependent CS

Cushing's Disease: Pituitary Adenoma

The most common cause of ACTH-dependent CS is a pituitary adenoma or Cushing's disease (CD). Typically, the adenoma is relatively small in size (microadenoma) with an average diameter of <5 mm, though larger macroadenomas (>10 mm) do occur. It is important to note that autopsy studies suggest up to 27% of individuals will have incidental pituitary adenomas, so the mere presence of a mass seen on imaging does not necessarily mean that the patient has CD.

Ectopic ACTH Secretion

ACTH secretion can occur from sources other than the pituitary. Small-cell lung cancer frequently gives rise to paraneoplastic syndromes and can serve as a source of excess ACTH which stimulates adrenal cortisol secretion. Additionally, most neuroendocrine tumors including pheochromocytoma, gastrinoma, and carcinoids can secrete ACTH, as can medullary thyroid cancer and neuroblastoma [4].

ACTH-Independent CS

Unilateral Disease

Unilateral adrenal nodules causing CS can be due to either adenomas (60%) or carcinomas (40%) with the risk of cancer increasing with size. Nodules <4 cm carry a 2% cancer risk, while those >6 cm have a 25% risk of malignancy. Intermediate-sized nodules from 4 to 6 cm are found to be cancer in 6% of cases [5, 6].

R. S. Sippel (✉)
Chief of Endocrine Surgery, University of Wisconsin, K3/704 Clinical Sciences Center, 600 Highland Ave., Madison, WI 53792-7375, USA
e-mail: SIPPEL@surgery.wisc.edu

C. J. Balentine
Clinical Instructor in Surgery, University of Wisconsin, K3/704 Clinical Sciences Center, 600 Highland Ave., Madison, WI 53792-7375, USA

J. L. Pasieka, J. A. Lee (eds.), *Surgical Endocrinopathies,* DOI 10.1007/978-3-319-13662-2_35,
© Springer International Publishing Switzerland 2015

Table 1 Causes of Cushing's syndrome

ACTH dependent
Pituitary adenoma (Cushing's disease)
Ectopic ACTH secretion
ACTH independent
Adrenal adenoma
Adrenal carcinoma
ACTH-independent macronodular adrenal hyperplasia (AIMAH)
Primary pigmented nodular adrenal disease (PPNAD)
Other unilateral or bilateral adrenal disease

ACTH Adrenocorticotropic hormone

Bilateral Disease

ACTH-Independent Macronodular Adrenal Hyperplasia

ACTH-independent macronodular adrenal hyperplasia (AIMAH) is the underlying cause in <1 % of patients with CS and has also been referred to as massive macronodular adrenocortical disease, autonomous macronodular adrenal hyperplasia, ACTH-independent massive bilateral adrenal disease, and giant macronodular adrenal disease. Age of symptom onset is typically in the fifth or sixth decade, and men have a similar incidence as women [7, 8]. The classic imaging finding is multiple large adrenal nodules with pathology showing two distinct cell types: those containing clear cytoplasm or lipid-rich cells, and those with a compact cytoplasm or lipid-poor cells. It should be noted, however, that the disease may progress at a different rate in each adrenal gland so that what initially appears to be unilateral disease ultimately develops into bilateral nodules. Adrenal cortisol secretion is amplified due to an increased number of adrenocortical cells rather than greater production from individual cells.

Primary Pigmented Nodular Adrenocortical Disease

Unlike with AIMAH, the actual size of the adrenal gland may be normal but the structure is replaced with multiple nodules scattered throughout an atrophic cortex. On imaging, primary pigmented nodular adrenocortical disease (PPNAD) can have several different appearances ranging from a string of beads to several large nodules. On pathologic examination, most of the nodules are small (<4 mm) and clearly separate from the surrounding cortex. The nodules seen in PPNAD generally do not show a significant response to exogenous ACTH administration but demonstrate a paradoxical increase in cortisol secretion in response to dexamethasone.

The etiology of PPNAD is evenly split between sporadic and familial causes. The **Carney** complex is a multiple endocrine neoplasia syndrome involving myxomas (cutaneous and cardiac), spotty skin pigmentation, schwannomas, and several endocrine tumors. PPNAD is the most common endocrine tumor seen in the *Carney* complex (see Chap. 37 for more information on Carney) and can be found in one fourth of those patients. Additionally, PPNAD has been linked to mutations in the cyclic adenosine monophosphate (cAMP)-dependent protein kinase A (*PRKAR1A*) gene [9].

Presentation and Natural History

While the classic presentation of CS involves the characteristic physical changes such as a "buffalo hump" and purple striae, a wide array of other symptoms are associated with CS (Table 2), and the diversity of presentation frequently leads to delays in diagnosis. In particular, the manifestations of CS are quite similar to those of the metabolic syndrome and diabetes so a high index of suspicion is needed to make the diagnosis. Additional physical signs that can help distinguish CS from other disease processes include skin changes (easy bruising and fragile skin) and proximal muscle weakness.

CS significantly increases mortality primarily by increasing the risk of cardiovascular disease [10]. Compared to the normal population, the standardized mortality ratio for those with CS can be as high as 4.8 [11–13]. In addition to

Table 2 Signs and symptoms of Cushing's syndrome

Sign or symptom	Percentage of patients with symptom
Obesity	79–97
Plethora	78–94
Diabetes or impaired glucose tolerance	39–94
Moon facies	88–92
Hypertension	47–90
Muscle weakness	45–90
Menstrual changes	35–86
Hirsutism	58–84
Thin skin or easy bruising	17–84
Bone changes	48–83
Acne	21–82
Depression	25–67
Buffalo hump	34–67
Striae	50–64

ACTH Adrenocorticotropic hormone

Fig. 1 Diagnostic approach to Cushing's syndrome. *ACTH* adrenocorticotropic hormone, *CS* Cushing's syndrome, *MRI* magnetic resonance imaging

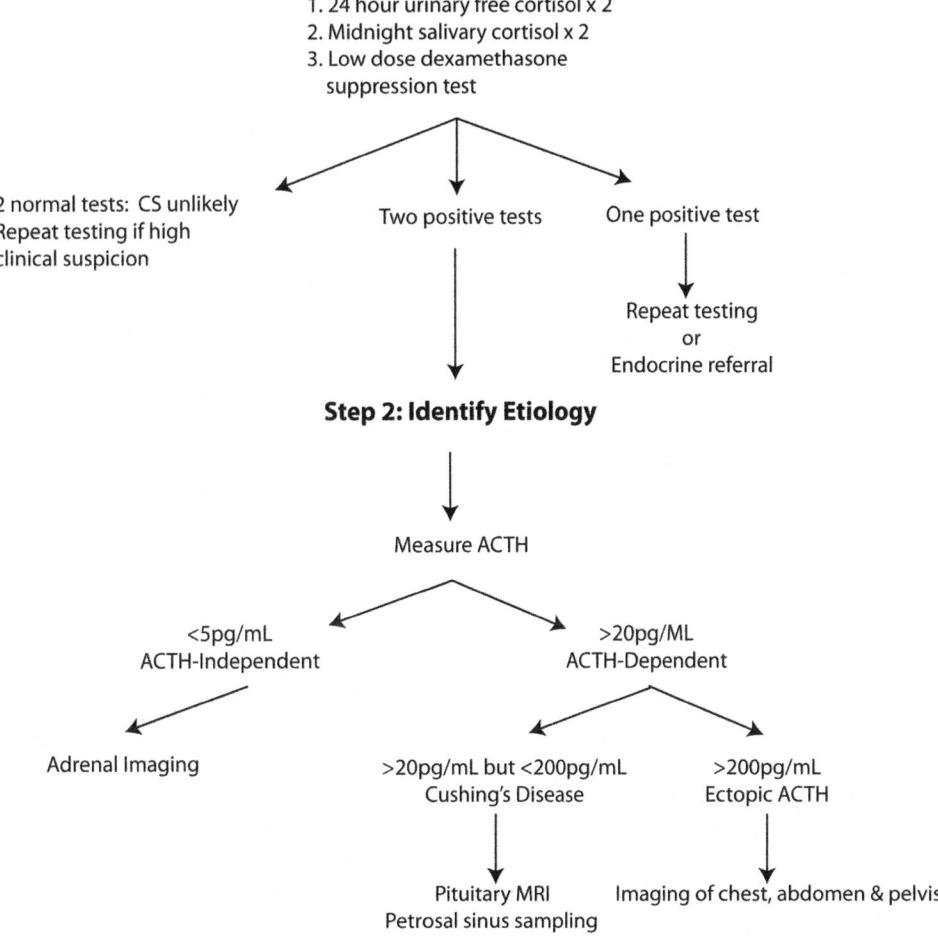

Step 1: Confirm Cortisol Excess

1. 24 hour urinary free cortisol x 2
2. Midnight salivary cortisol x 2
3. Low dose dexamethasone suppression test

2 normal tests: CS unlikely Repeat testing if high clinical suspicion

Two positive tests

One positive test

Repeat testing or Endocrine referral

Step 2: Identify Etiology

Measure ACTH

<5pg/mL ACTH-Independent

>20pg/ML ACTH-Dependent

Adrenal Imaging

>20pg/mL but <200pg/mL Cushing's Disease

>200pg/mL Ectopic ACTH

Pituitary MRI Petrosal sinus sampling

Imaging of chest, abdomen & pelvis

cardiovascular complications, CS is associated with hypercoagulability and an increased risk of deep vein thrombosis (DVT) and pulmonary embolus (PE) [14, 15]. This disease manifestation is particularly important when planning operative intervention. CS not only leads to physical changes and symptoms, there are also important psychological changes associated with the diagnosis. Depression and psychosis are commonly seen but more subtle abnormalities including fatigue and loss of concentration and memory also occur. Equally important is a sharp decline in measures of health-related quality of life (HRQL) covering multiple aspects of mental, social, and physical health [16–18]. In short, CS impacts multiple organ systems and the effects worsen the longer diagnosis and treatment are delayed.

Subclinical CS

A subset of patients with incidentally discovered adrenal masses will have elevated cortisol levels but lack the typical signs and symptoms associated with glucocorticoid excess. These patients are categorized as having "subclinical"

CS although they often present with hypertension, obesity, hyperlipidemia, and impaired glucose tolerance. The diagnostic tests which are discussed below are suboptimal when it comes to diagnosing subclinical CS as the biochemical changes are generally subtle and erratic. Consequently, no clear consensus has emerged regarding the best criteria or approach for diagnosing the condition. The same overall approach is used but a higher level of suspicion must be maintained in order to make the diagnosis.

Diagnostic Evaluation

The diagnosis of CS is complicated by the fact that there is no widely accepted gold standard test and each of the available tests has important limitations. In general, the diagnostic process can be broken down into discrete steps beginning with confirmation of excess cortisol (Fig. 1). Once a hypercortisol state is identified, the goal is to identify whether the underlying cause is autonomous secretion of cortisol due to adrenal disease or whether ACTH (or corticotropin-releasing hormone, CRH) secretion is driving adrenal oversecretion.

Table 3 Comparison of screening tests for Cushing's syndrome

	Low-dose dexamethasone suppression test	24 h urine-free cortisol	Midnight salivary cortisol
Performance advantages	Sensitivity up to 95%	Sensitivity >85%, specificity >90%	Sensitivity ≥92%
	1. Able to distinguish ACTH-independent from ACTH-dependent causes	1. Unaffected by changes in cortisol binding proteins	1. Easy administration
		2. Reflects 24 h total cortisol and not just a single time point	
Disadvantages	1. Interpretation complicated by medications altering dexamethasone metabolism	1. Difficult to collect	1. Need different measurement time if shift worker, or has sleep disorder
	2. False positives in pregnancy/ hormonal therapy	2. Sensitivity and specificity affected by renal function and volume of urine	2. Need to avoid licorice, tobacco
	3. Unreliable in renal failure		
Criteria for positive result	<1.8 µg/dL (higher specificity) <5 µg/dL (higher sensitivity)	Upper limit of normal for institutional assay	>145 ng/dL

Finally, if the diagnosis of ACTH-dependent disease is made, it is necessary to determine whether the source of ACTH comes from the pituitary or an ectopic source.

Screening for Hypercortisolism

Recent guidelines from the Endocrine Society recommend the use of any of three tests for confirmation of excess cortisol secretion: low-dose dexamethasone suppression (LDDST), 24 h urine cortisol, and midnight salivary cortisol [19]. Table 3 outlines the advantages, disadvantages, and what constitute a positive result for each test. These tests were selected based on their relatively high sensitivity since the consensus opinion was that the key to the initial diagnostic step is to avoid missing those who might actually have CS. The focus on sensitivity rather than specificity was based on the significant impact that untreated CS can have on mortality. The committee felt that, on balance, it would be better to have a few false positives which could be appropriately excluded by subsequent testing rather than missing those who might have CS and benefit from rapid evaluation and treatment. Since CS may be cyclic in nature or involve subtle derangements in the hypothalamic–pituitary–adrenal axis (HPA), it is frequently necessary to conduct multiple tests to confirm the diagnosis. Since there is no ideal or gold standard test for diagnosing CS, using two or more of these screening tests in combination may offer the best hope for accurate diagnosis. Collecting two separate samples for urine-free cortisol (UFC) or salivary cortisol is also useful as concordant results add support to the diagnosis of CS while discordant results should prompt additional testing.

Pseudo-Cushing's States

An important limitation of all tests for CS is the difficulty distinguishing true CS from conditions that lead to a temporary increase in cortisol (pseudo-Cushing states). Significant alcoholism, depression, panic attacks, obesity, stress, and intensive care unit (ICU) admission or critical illness can all transiently increase cortisol levels and lead to false-positive results. Additionally, the use of estrogens or oral contraceptives leads to increase in serum cortisol via higher levels of binding proteins (see section on UFC below). When attempting to diagnose CS, the presence of pseudo-Cushing states need to be considered and addressed when possible.

Low-Dose Dexamethasone Suppression Test

The rationale behind dexamethasone suppression testing is that the normal HPA responds to an increase in corticosteroids by suppressing ACTH secretion which leads to a drop in cortisol. In patients with ACTH-independent CS, the addition of dexamethasone should have minimal impact on serum cortisol because the feedback effect of excess cortisol has already suppressed ACTH secretion. Similarly, ectopic sources of ACTH secretion are generally not inhibited by receiving dexamethasone. Pituitary adenomas also tend not to be completely suppressed by low doses of dexamethasone, though there is often at least some decrease in serum cortisol after administration of dexamethasone. In practice, some patients with adrenal and even ectopic ACTH secretion (EAS) will have cortisol suppression in response to the LDDST. There are several methods for conducting the LDDST but one common approach involves oral administration of 1 mg dexamethasone between 2300 and 2400 h followed by plasma cortisol measurement between 0800 and 0900 h that morning. Overall sensitivity of LDDST may be as high as 95% with a cutoff point of 1.8 µg/dL, though there is some disagreement over where this threshold should be set. Using a higher cutoff of <5 µg/dL will decrease sensitivity but fewer false positives results in improved specificity [19–26].

The results of a LDDST can be affected by any of the pseudo-Cushing states mentioned above as well as by any process or medication that alters dexamethasone metabolism. These are discussed in more detail in a later section. Notably, women taking hormone supplementation may have up to a 50 % false-positive rate.

Twenty-Four-Hour UFC

Serum cortisol circulates in an inactive form bound to cortisol-binding protein. The active or free cortisol is a function of both total cortisol levels and concentration relative to binding proteins. Serum measurements are affected by medications and comorbidities that influence cortisol-binding globulin (CBG) levels. These include use of oral contraceptives by women as estrogen increases CBG production and this leads to elevated serum cortisol measurement. By contrast, UFC reflects the quantity of unbound cortisol that is filtered through the kidney and does not fluctuate with CBG concentration. Since UFC is collected over a 24-h period, it provides an overall assessment of free cortisol levels rather than relying on detecting elevated cortisol at a single time point. Sensitivity and specificity vary somewhat depending on the threshold set for an abnormal result but are typically >85 and 90 %, respectively [27, 28]. There are several limitations to measuring UFC. First, since the assay depends on renal filtration, alterations in kidney function can significantly alter cortisol levels. At a creatinine clearance of <60 cc/min, the rate of false negatives begins to increase substantially as less cortisol is filtered and collected in the specimen. At the opposite end of the spectrum, a substantial increase in fluid intake can lead to falsely elevated UFC as renal filtration increases. Additionally, performing the test can be something of a burden as patients need to provide a complete 24-h sample for the assay to be reliable.

Late-Night Salivary Cortisol

In otherwise healthy individuals, serum cortisol begins to rise prior to waking and peaks between 7 and 9 a.m. Cortisol then steadily declines throughout the day and reaches a nadir around midnight. This normal circadian rhythm is often interrupted in patients with CS so that midnight cortisol is substantially elevated. Plasma cortisol equilibrates with salivary levels and the concentration is not substantially affected by the amount of saliva produced. Equally important, increases in serum cortisol are rapidly reflected by increases in salivary cortisol. Since measurements of salivary levels do not require needle sticks and blood draws, this assay is a convenient way to measure cortisol in an outpatient setting. When a threshold value of >145 ng/dL is set, sensitivity and specificity are comparable to the previous assays and range from 92 to 100 % and 93 to 100 %, respectively [27–30].

Salivary glands express 11β-hydroxysteroid dehydrogenase type 2 which converts cortisol to cortisone; it is possible that medications or other substances which block the enzyme may have falsely elevated salivary cortisol. Substances such as licorice and tobacco fall into this category and should be avoided during testing. Since the assay functions based on assumptions of a normal circadian rhythm, patients who work in night shifts or have altered sleep–wake cycles should have the timing of the assay adjusted appropriately or the measurement will miss the actual nadir in cortisol.

Additional Confirmation of Elevated Cortisol

If one of the above high sensitivity tests are used to demonstrate elevated cortisol, it is important to confirm the diagnosis with additional testing. Two elevated tests are required to confirm the diagnosis. If the diagnosis is equivocal based on initial testing, additional advanced testing can help better identify patients who truly have CS. One option is use of the 48-h, 2 mg/day LDDST with or without addition of CRH stimulation. This test involves administering 0.5 mg doses of dexamethasone every 6 h for 48 h and then measuring serum cortisol 6 h later. The addition of 1 µg/kg intravenous (IV) ovine CRH 2 h after the last dose of dexamethasone may improve both sensitivity and specificity. The high-dose dexamethasone suppression test (HDDST) is another reasonable alternative though some studies suggest that this test adds little information compared to the LDDST [31]. Alternatively, the midnight serum cortisol test can help confirm the diagnosis of CS [32]. This test requires inpatient admission and can be performed in patients while sleeping or while awake with different thresholds set for each approach.

ACTH Dependent Versus Independent

After the presence of CS is confirmed, the next step in diagnosis is to determine whether cortisol excess is ACTH dependent (pituitary or ectopic ACTH) or ACTH independent (adrenal disease). This process involves a combination of biochemical and invasive testing to look for excess ACTH and imaging studies to localize the source.

ACTH-Independent CS

Low plasma ACTH (<5 pg/mL) and failure to suppress cortisol with the LDDST suggest an adrenal source for cortisol production and the diagnosis can generally be confirmed by either computed tomography (CT) or magnetic resonance imaging (MRI). Unilateral enlargement of an adrenal gland is generally due to adenoma or carcinoma while bilateral enlargement may be caused by AIMAH. Imaging features which may help distinguish benign adenoma from carcinoma include homogeneous appearance, CT attenuation ≤10 Hounsfield units, rapid washout, absence of necrosis, isointense relative to liver on T2 weighted MRI, and stable size over time [5]. If the adrenals do not appear grossly enlarged on imaging, then the CS may be due to PPNAD.

ACTH-Dependent CS

ACTH-dependent CS is suggested by an increase in ACTH over baseline. Once this finding is confirmed, the primary goal is to determine whether the excess ACTH is coming from the pituitary or from an ectopic source. Plasma ACTH >20 pg/mL is generally consistent with the diagnosis of CD, and even higher levels (>200 pg/mL) often suggest EAS. It should be noted, however, that in a large series from the National Institutes of Health (NIH) evaluating EAS, one third of patients actually had normal ACTH levels so a high level of suspicion must be maintained during diagnosis. Further distinguishing between CD and an ectopic source of ACTH relies on the observation that pituitary adenomas frequently retain some element of HPA regulation while ectopic tumors secreting ACTH are generally not responsive to cortisol or other elements of the axis. Classically, pituitary adenomas do not respond to low-dose dexamethasone but may decrease ACTH secretion in response to higher doses of dexamethasone. The HDDST involves administration of either 2 mg of dexamethasone every 6 h for 48 h or a single 8 mg dose with measurement of cortisol at the end of 48 h. A positive test consists of a drop in cortisol to <50 % of baseline level, and sensitivity is around 80 %. Recent studies have questioned the value of the HDDST as the LDDST appears to adequately predict response to higher doses of dexamethasone.

Another test used to identify the presence of CD is the CRH stimulation test using IV administration of either human or ovine CRH and measuring cortisol response. Depending on the cutoff value used for a positive result, sensitivity ranges from 86 to 93 %. Since neither of the above tests is ideal for discriminating between CD and EAS, the diagnosis often involves a combination of imaging and invasive testing.

Imaging the pituitary gland with MRI can be used to support the diagnosis of CD over EAS. Finding an adenoma >5 mm in the setting of cortisol suppression with dexamethasone or CRH strongly suggests that the primary disease is driven by the adenoma. Difficulty arises from the fact that pituitary adenomas are incidentally found in up to 10 % of patients who do not have CS and that 40–50 % of patients with CD will have apparently normal pituitary imaging.

When the diagnosis is unclear on the basis of imaging and noninvasive testing, the next step is bilateral inferior petrosal sinus sampling (BIPSS). This technique involves using catheters to measure ACTH concentration in both petrosal sinuses while simultaneously checking plasma ACTH. If ACTH is significantly higher in the petrosal sinuses compared to the periphery, then a pituitary source is likely. If there is no gradient, then efforts should focus on additional imaging studies to identify the source of ectopic ACTH. BIPSS is suggestive of a pituitary source when the petrosal sinus to peripheral ACTH ratio is >2:1 in an unstimulated patient or >3:1 following administration of CRH. Overall sensitiv-ity and specificity for BIPSS is >90 % when performed at centers with expertise in the technique, but both false negatives and false positives do occur [33–35]. One method to reduce false negatives is to record prolactin levels to serve as a control. Although sampling from both sinuses should, in theory, allow localization of the adenoma to either side of the pituitary gland this does not seem to be especially accurate in practice. Additionally, the technique does require the use of invasive catheters and complications such as bleeding and stroke can occur.

Special Cases

In addition to the standard evaluation for CS, the Endocrine Society recommendations also address difficult or unique situations that may complicate the diagnostic process.

Pregnancy

Cortisol levels increase significantly after the first trimester of pregnancy and can reach levels up to three times normal before delivery. Consequently, the threshold for diagnosing CS based on either urine or serum cortisol must also increase in pregnant women. At the same time, dexamethasone is less effective in suppressing the HPA during pregnancy so the LDDST is more likely to yield false positives in this population.

Seizure Medications

Several seizure medications can alter hepatic clearance of dexamethasone and complicate interpretation of the LDDST. Medications including phenytoin and carbamazepine both increase clearance via cytochrome P450 (CYP) enzymes and this effect tends to increase false positives when using the LDDST.

Renal Failure

Patients with poor renal function and glomerular filtration rate (GFR) <60 cc/min will have inadequate filtration and clearance of cortisol, so measurement of UFC becomes an unreliable reflection of serum concentrations. Moreover, at least one report suggests that serum cortisol levels are elevated in patients with renal disease who do not have CS. Finally, dexamethasone metabolism may be altered in the setting of significant renal disease so that LDDST is unreliable. Overall, having normal response to dexamethasone or a normal serum cortisol suggest that a diagnosis of CS is unlikely but abnormal values should be interpreted cautiously.

Cyclic CS

Some individuals with CS do not exhibit a consistently elevated cortisol level. Instead, oversecretion of cortisol is episodic or cyclic in nature so that multiple different tests will show normal cortisol levels. In this situation, it is probably best to repeat testing in several months if clinical suspicion remains high despite normal tests. Persistent or progressive signs and symptoms should especially prompt further investigation since patients without CS or other pathology should improve rather than worsening with time.

Treatment

ACTH-Dependent CS

Surgical

Definitive therapy for CD is surgical resection. The transsphenoidal approach is preferred for pituitary adenomas and is associated with initial remission rates of 60–80% when operating on a patient for the first time. Relapse rates following the initial surgery can be substantial, however, and appear to increase steadily with time to 20% or more depending on length of follow-up [36–39]. Risk factors for persistent disease after surgery include operating on macroadenomas rather than microadenomas, reoperation, and failure to identify an adenoma at the time of surgery. Transsphenoidal surgery is associated with low morbidity when performed by experts in the technique with a permanent hypopituitary state being the most significant complication.

Radiation

Pituitary radiotherapy is generally not a first-line therapy for CD but can be utilized after unsuccessful transsphenoidal resection or in patients who are not candidates for surgery due to other comorbidities. The biochemical response rate in the setting of failed pituitary surgery is >80%, but there is a considerable delay before remission actually begins. Most patients will show improvement within 2 years of radiation therapy but the timing ranges from 6 months to 5 years after treatment is complete [40].

Recurrent Disease

There are several options for patients with CD who fail to respond to transsphenoidal resection. One possibility is return to the operating room for additional resection. Most studies show that reoperation can successfully treat persistent or recurrent disease but is not as effective as the initial surgery. For those who do not desire additional surgery or are not candidates for another transsphenoidal resection, radiotherapy is a reasonable alternative. As mentioned above, radiotherapy is effective but there is a significant lag time between treatment and actual improvement. Any one or a combination of medical therapies can also be employed to help control symptoms from CS, though these are all associated with side effects and can become less effective over time.

Finally, bilateral adrenalectomy can be utilized as definitive therapy for both ACTH-independent and ACTH-dependent diseases by removing the final pathway for cortisol secretion. Bilateral adrenalectomy comes with a requirement for lifetime medical supplementation for adrenal insufficiency but does offer hope of cure for patients with otherwise refractory disease.

ACTH-Independent CS

Surgical

Laparoscopic adrenalectomy is the treatment of choice for CS due to adrenal glucocorticoid secretion from benign lesions. Both the transabdominal and retroperitoneal approaches are safe and produce similar outcomes with low complication rates [41, 42]. When adrenal cancer is suspected based on preoperative imaging characteristics (heterogeneity, elevated Hounsfield units, calcification, irregular borders, central necrosis), invasion into surrounding structures, or other factors, then the open approach is recommended. If it is entirely unclear whether a lesion is benign or malignant, it is reasonable to start with the laparoscopic approach with plans to convert upon any suspicious intraoperative findings. Larger lesions (>15 cm), coagulopathy, and previous abdominal operations or trauma are relative contraindications to the laparoscopic approach [43].

Postoperative adrenal insufficiency is common since glucocorticoid overproduction can lead to atrophy of the opposite gland. Unfortunately, there is no reliable method to determine who is most likely to develop adrenal insufficiency so all patients should be treated with perioperative steroids with plans for rapid taper to physiologic replacement levels. One approach to determining who will require longer-term steroid supplementation is to hold the evening steroid dose and check a morning cortisol level prior to the morning dose. If the value is low, then the patient is discharged with ongoing oral steroids and is evaluated later in clinic.

Since AIMAH can cause bilateral adrenal hyperplasia, the traditional approach has been to offer bilateral adrenalectomy. Recent papers have questioned whether this is truly necessary as unilateral adrenalectomy may offer significant reduction in symptoms without requiring medical management for adrenal insufficiency.

Medical

When patients are not surgical candidates or do not desire surgery, there are several medications which can be used to manage the symptoms of CS [44].

Dopamine receptors are expressed on most anterior pituitary cells and act to inhibit ACTH secretion. Dopamine agonists such as cabergoline were effective in treating recurrent or persistent CD in up to 40 % of patients after failed transsphenoidal surgery [45, 46].

Mitotane inhibits mitochondrial enzymes involved in adrenal cortisol production and can induce initial remission in > 80 % of patients, though most of these eventually relapse. Use of mitotane is generally limited to cases of adrenal cancer due to the considerable side-effect burden [47].

Etomidate is a drug commonly used for anesthesia induction but also has a rapid onset inhibition of cortisol production. Given the rapid onset and rapid decline in effect, etomidate is mostly used for the acute management of hypercortisolism and less for the long-term management of symptoms.

Metyrapone acts primarily by inhibiting the final step of cortisol synthesis by 11-β hydroxylase and leads to biochemical remission in up to 75 % of patients and clinical improvement in most [48]. Side effects stem mostly from loss of ACTH-mediated feedback inhibition with resultant increases in androgen and mineralocorticoids. Consequently, patients may develop hirsutism, acne, hypotension, and hypokalemia.

Ketoconazole leads to reduction in cortisol production via inhibiting several enzymes involved in steroid synthesis. Biochemical cure is obtained in greater than 50 % of patients and most individuals who respond to treatment will do so within 3 months. The most significant side effect is hepatotoxicity which necessitates measurement of liver function during therapy. Other notable side effects include gastrointestinal upset and hypogonadism in men. Plasma bioavailability is affected by proton pump inhibitors so these medications should not be used together.

Mifepristone, a glucocorticoid receptor antagonist, was recently evaluated for the treatment of CS in a multicenter trial which demonstrated that 87 % had at least some clinical improvement including improvement in diabetes, decrease in blood pressure, and weight loss.

Finally, since pituitary adenomas frequently express somatostatin receptors, that pathway has served as another target for controlling symptoms from CD. A recent phase III trial of the somatostatin analog pasireotide showed significant decrease in cortisol levels as well as symptomatic improvement in patients with CD who were not candidates for surgery [49].

Prognosis

Morbidity

Successful surgical intervention for CS results in considerable improvement both biochemically and from a symptom standpoint. The individual manifestations of CS have variable levels of improvement following successful treatment. Following successful surgical therapy, diabetes, obesity, blood pressure, and low-density lipoprotein (LDL)-cholesterol levels show significant improvement but may not ever return to levels seen in normal controls. Equally important, damage to the intima of major arteries and the increased presence of atherosclerotic plaques also persists even after remission which suggests that long-term damage to the vasculature occurs as a result of CS [50]. Similarly, although the neurologic and psychiatric manifestations of CS do tend to improve after treatment, overall HRQL remains persistently abnormal across nearly every dimension measured.

When treating patients with CS, it is important to counsel them that clinical improvement is gradual rather than immediate. Following adrenalectomy for CS, skin changes including striae and bruising may take 8–10 months to resolve [51]. Central obesity and moon facies tend to improve over a similar time frame while diabetes, depression, hirsutism, and the buffalo hump are more likely to resolve 10–12 months after surgery. Muscle weakness, skin hyperpigmentation, and acne all tend to persist for more than a year after surgery.

Mortality

Despite the delayed resolution of some symptoms and the lack of reversibility of all changes after treatment, mortality in patients with CD who undergo successful transsphenoidal surgery does not appear to differ from population controls. By contrast, those with persistent or recurrent disease continue to have persistently worse mortality.

Postoperative Steroids

Since CS represents a state of cortisol excess, the normal HPA axis is typically suppressed and may take considerable time to recover after surgical therapy. All patients undergoing unilateral adrenalectomy should be started on steroids postoperatively with plans to taper as the HPA axis normalizes. As with symptom improvement, however, it may take considerable time for the HPA axis to recover sufficiently to stop steroid supplementation. In fact, 65 % may require steroids for longer than 6 months with a median duration of 30 months following unilateral adrenalectomy [51].

Following bilateral adrenalectomy, patients need to understand that they will be on steroid medication for life and that they face the risk of **Addisonian** crisis as a result. The dosing will need to be monitored carefully in order to avoid an exogenous excess of cortisol and these patients will require stress dosing of steroids for any subsequent operations.

Key Summary Points

- CS can have significant impacts on morbidity, mortality and quality of life.
- Although early treatment can greatly reduce these problems, diagnosis is frequently difficult as the signs and symptoms are highly variable and often quite subtle.
- There is no ideal diagnostic test for CS and a high index of suspicion is often required to make the diagnosis.
- Treatment is surgical when possible. Second line therapies include medications and radiotherapy.

References

1. Barzon L, Fallo F, Sonino N, et al. Development of overt Cushing's syndrome in patients with adrenal incidentaloma. Eur J Endocrinol. 2002;146(1):61–6.
2. Terzolo M, Reimondo G, Bovio S, et al. Subclinical Cushing's syndrome. Pituitary. 2004;7(4):217–23.
3. Newell-Price J, Bertagna X, Grossman AB, et al. Cushing's syndrome. Lancet. 2006;367(9522):1605–17.
4. Ilias I, Torpy DJ, Pacak K, et al. Cushing's syndrome due to ectopic corticotropin secretion: twenty years' experience at the National Institutes of Health. J Clin Endocrinol Metab. 2005;90(8):4955–62.
5. Young WF, Jr. Clinical practice. The incidentally discovered adrenal mass. N Engl J Med. 2007;356(6):601–10.
6. Grumbach MM, Biller BM, Braunstein GD, et al. Management of the clinically inapparent adrenal mass ("incidentaloma"). Ann Intern Med. 2003;138(5):424–9.
7. Bourdeau I, Lampron A, Costa MH, et al. Adrenocorticotropic hormone-independent Cushing's syndrome. Curr Opin Endocrinol Diabetes Obes. 2007;14(3):219–25.
8. Lacroix A, Bourdeau I. Bilateral adrenal Cushing's syndrome: macronodular adrenal hyperplasia and primary pigmented nodular adrenocortical disease. Endocrinol Metab Clin North Am. 2005;34(2):441–58, x.
9. Stratakis CA, Kirschner LS, Carney JA. Clinical and molecular features of the Carney complex: diagnostic criteria and recommendations for patient evaluation. J Clin Endocrinol Metab. 2001;86(9):4041–6.
10. Dekkers OM, Biermasz NR, Pereira AM, et al. Mortality in patients treated for Cushing's disease is increased, compared with patients treated for nonfunctioning pituitary macroadenoma. J Clin Endocrinol Metab. 2007;92(3):976–81.
11. Etxabe J, Vazquez JA. Morbidity and mortality in Cushing's disease: an epidemiological approach. Clin Endocrinol (Oxf). 1994;40(4):479–84.
12. Clayton RN, Raskauskiene D, Reulen RC, et al. Mortality and morbidity in Cushing's disease over 50 years in Stoke-on-Trent, UK: audit and meta-analysis of literature. J Clin Endocrinol Metab. 2011;96(3):632–42.
13. Graversen D, Vestergaard P, Stochholm K, et al. Mortality in Cushing's syndrome: a systematic review and meta-analysis. Eur J Intern Med. 2012;23(3):278–82.
14. Trementino L, Arnaldi G, Appolloni G, et al. Coagulopathy in Cushing's syndrome. Neuroendocrinology. 2010;92(Suppl 1):55–9.
15. Manetti L, Bogazzi F, Giovannetti C, et al. Changes in coagulation indexes and occurrence of venous thromboembolism in patients with Cushing's syndrome: results from a prospective study before and after surgery. Eur J Endocrinol. 2010;163(5):783–91.
16. Wagenmakers MA, Netea-Maier RT, Prins JB, et al. Impaired quality of life in patients in long-term remission of Cushing's syndrome of both adrenal and pituitary origin: a remaining effect of long-standing hypercortisolism? Eur J Endocrinol. 2012;167(5):687–95.
17. Lindsay JR, Nansel T, Baid S, et al. Long-term impaired quality of life in Cushing's syndrome despite initial improvement after surgical remission. J Clin Endocrinol Metab. 2006;91(2):447–53.
18. Forget H, Lacroix A, Cohen H. Persistent cognitive impairment following surgical treatment of Cushing's syndrome. Psychoneuroendocrinology. 2002;27(3):367–83.
19. Nieman LK, Biller BM, Findling JW, et al. The diagnosis of Cushing's syndrome: an endocrine society clinical practice guideline. J Clin Endocrinol Metab. 2008;93(5):1526–40.
20. Arnaldi G, Angeli A, Atkinson AB, et al. Diagnosis and complications of Cushing's syndrome: a consensus statement. J Clin Endocrinol Metab. 2003;88(12):5593–602.
21. Boscaro M, Barzon L, Sonino N. The diagnosis of Cushing's syndrome: atypical presentations and laboratory shortcomings. Arch Intern Med. 2000;160(20):3045–53.
22. Elamin MB, Murad MH, Mullan R, et al. Accuracy of diagnostic tests for Cushing's syndrome: a systematic review and metaanalyses. J Clin Endocrinol Metab. 2008;93(5):1553–62.
23. Findling JW, Raff H, Aron DC. The low-dose dexamethasone suppression test: a reevaluation in patients with Cushing's syndrome. J Clin Endocrinol Metab. 2004;89(3):1222–6.
24. Isidori AM, Kaltsas GA, Mohammed S, et al. Discriminatory value of the low-dose dexamethasone suppression test in establishing the diagnosis and differential diagnosis of Cushing's syndrome. J Clin Endocrinol Metab. 2003;88(11):5299–306.
25. Newell-Price J. Diagnosis/differential diagnosis of Cushing's syndrome: a review of best practice. Best Pract Res Clin Endocrinol Metab. 2009;23(Suppl 1):S5–14.
26. Reimondo G, Allasino B, Bovio S, et al. Pros and cons of dexamethasone suppression test for screening of subclinical Cushing's syndrome in patients with adrenal incidentalomas. J Endocrinol Invest. 2011;34(1):e1–5.
27. Kidambi S, Raff H, Findling JW. Limitations of nocturnal salivary cortisol and urine free cortisol in the diagnosis of mild Cushing's syndrome. Eur J Endocrinol. 2007;157(6):725–31.
28. Putignano P, Toja P, Dubini A, et al. Midnight salivary cortisol versus urinary free and midnight serum cortisol as screening tests for Cushing's syndrome. J Clin Endocrinol Metab. 2003;88(9):4153–7.
29. Carroll T, Raff H, Findling JW. Late-night salivary cortisol measurement in the diagnosis of Cushing's syndrome. Nat Clin Pract Endocrinol Metab. 2008;4(6):344–50.
30. Papanicolaou DA, Mullen N, Kyrou I, et al. Nighttime salivary cortisol: a useful test for the diagnosis of Cushing's syndrome. J Clin Endocrinol Metab. 2002;87(10):4515–21.
31. Aron DC, Raff H, Findling JW. Effectiveness versus efficacy: the limited value in clinical practice of high dose dexamethasone suppression testing in the differential diagnosis of adrenocorticotropin-dependent Cushing's syndrome. J Clin Endocrinol Metab. 1997;82(6):1780–5.
32. Papanicolaou DA, Yanovski JA, Cutler GB, Jr., et al. A single midnight serum cortisol measurement distinguishes Cushing's syndrome from pseudo-Cushing states. J Clin Endocrinol Metab. 1998;83(4):1163–7.
33. Colao A, Faggiano A, Pivonello R, et al. Inferior petrosal sinus sampling in the differential diagnosis of Cushing's syndrome: results of an Italian multicenter study. Eur J Endocrinol. 2001;144(5):499–507.
34. Oldfield EH, Doppman JL, Nieman LK, et al. Petrosal sinus sampling with and without corticotropin-releasing hormone for the differential diagnosis of Cushing's syndrome. N Engl J Med. 1991;325(13):897–905.

35. Yanovski JA, Friedman TC, Nieman LK, et al. Inferior petrosal sinus AVP in patients with Cushing's syndrome. Clin Endocrinol (Oxf). 1997;47(2):199–206.

36. Atkinson AB, Kennedy A, Wiggam MI, et al. Long-term remission rates after pituitary surgery for Cushing's disease: the need for long-term surveillance. Clin Endocrinol (Oxf). 2005;63(5):549–59.

37. Hammer GD, Tyrrell JB, Lamborn KR, et al. Transsphenoidal microsurgery for Cushing's disease: initial outcome and long-term results. J Clin Endocrinol Metab. 2004;89(12):6348–57.

38. Porterfield JR, Thompson GB, Young WF, Jr., et al. Surgery for Cushing's syndrome: an historical review and recent ten-year experience. World J Surg. 2008;32(5):659–77.

39. Shimon I, Ram Z, Cohen ZR, et al. Transsphenoidal surgery for Cushing's disease: endocrinological follow-up monitoring of 82 patients. Neurosurgery. 2002;51(1):57–61; discussion 61–2.

40. Estrada J, Boronat M, Mielgo M, et al. The long-term outcome of pituitary irradiation after unsuccessful transsphenoidal surgery in Cushing's disease. N Engl J Med. 1997;336(3):172–7.

41. Poulose BK, Holzman MD, Lao OB, et al. Laparoscopic adrenalectomy: 100 resections with clinical long-term follow-up. Surg Endosc. 2005;19(3):379–85.

42. Meyer A, Behrend M. Cushing's syndrome: adrenalectomy and long-term results. Dig Surg. 2004;21(5–6):363–70.

43. Gagner M, Pomp A, Heniford BT, et al. Laparoscopic adrenalectomy: lessons learned from 100 consecutive procedures. Ann Surg. 1997;226(3):238–46; discussion 246–7.

44. Stewart PM and Petersenn S. Rationale for treatment and therapeutic options in Cushing's disease. Best Pract Res Clin Endocrinol Metab. 2009;23(Suppl 1):S15–22.

45. Feelders RA, Hofland LJ. Medical treatment of Cushing's disease. J Clin Endocrinol Metab. 2013;98(2):425–38.

46. Ferone D, Pivonello C, Vitale G, et al. Molecular basis of pharmacological therapy in Cushing's disease. Endocrine. 2014;46(2):181–98.

47. Morgan FH, Laufgraben MJ. Mifepristone for management of Cushing's syndrome. Pharmacotherapy. 2013;33(3):319–29.

48. Biller BM, Grossman AB, Stewart PM, et al. Treatment of adrenocorticotropin-dependent Cushing's syndrome: a consensus statement. J Clin Endocrinol Metab. 2008;93(7):2454–62.

49. Colao A, Petersenn S, Newell-Price J, et al. A 12-month phase 3 study of pasireotide in Cushing's disease. N Engl J Med. 2012;366(10):914–24.

50. Faggiano A, Pivonello R, Spiezia S, et al. Cardiovascular risk factors and common carotid artery caliber and stiffness in patients with Cushing's disease during active disease and 1 year after disease remission. J Clin Endocrinol Metab. 2003;88(6):2527–33.

51. Sippel RS, Elaraj DM, Kebebew E, et al. Waiting for change: symptom resolution after adrenalectomy for Cushing's syndrome. Surgery. 2008;144(6):1054–60; discussion 1060–1.

Harvey Cushing

1869–1939

Robert Udelsman

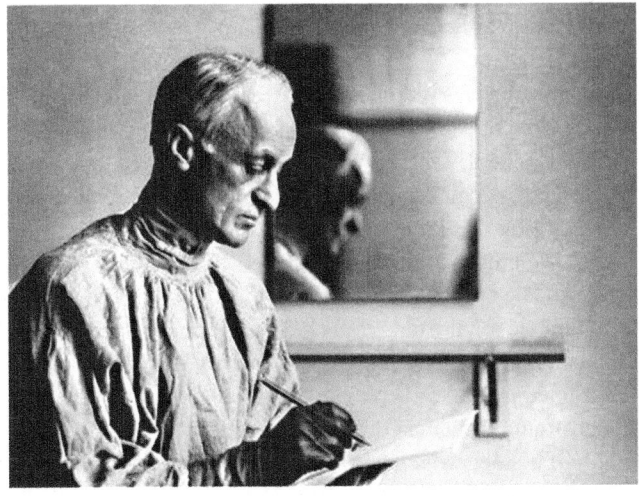

Photograph of Cushing in his dressing room. Immediately following surgery, Cushing would illustrate the operative findings. It was common for him to wear his operative gloves while drawing these illustrations. (Photograph by Walter Willard Boyd. Courtesy of the Cushing-Whitney Medical Historical Library, Yale University School of Medicine, New Haven, CT)

There are few individuals who have profoundly changed the course of medical history. Harvey Cushing (1869–1939) is one of them. His contribution to modern neurosurgery, critical care anesthesia, surgical education, research, medical illustration, and literature including a Pulitzer Prize for his biography of Sir William Osler demonstrate his enormous span of influence. Two excellent sources documenting Cushing's contributions and persona are the historical biography by John F. Fulton and the entertaining and insightful biography by Michael Bliss [1, 2].

Harvey William Cushing, the youngest of ten children, was born on April 8, 1869, in Cleveland, OH. His brother,

R. Udelsman (✉)
Surgery & Oncology, Yale-New Haven Hospital, Yale University School of Medicine, New Haven, CT, USA
e-mail: robert.udelsman@yale.edu

father, grandfather, and great-grandfather were all physicians who profoundly influenced his career. He benefited from a privileged lineage and a family that emphasized the importance of education. As a child he avidly collected and catalogued insects, minerals, and plants. He also demonstrated precocious talent as an illustrator, a skill he would subsequently refine and incorporate into his career [3]. He attended Yale University from 1887–1891, played for the Yale baseball team and was elected into the secret society "Scroll and Key".

He followed the lead of his brother Ned and attended Harvard Medical School from 1891 to 1895 where even as a medical student he made significant contributions including the creation and employment of the "ether chart" in 1894 and the implementation of X-rays that had been described 1 year earlier by Röntgen. Accordingly, he set the background for both critical care anesthesia and diagnostic radiology. He began his clinical training as a house pupil in Massachusetts General Hospital in 1895.

He left Boston to go to Baltimore in 1869, at the age of 27, to work as an assistant resident under the leadership of William S. Halsted of Johns Hopkins Hospital. At Hopkins, his clinical skills were enhanced and he also continued to refine his artistic talents under the tutelage of Max Brödel the founder of the Department of Art as Applied to Medicine and perhaps the greatest medical illustrator in the world [4]. Brödel's genius is demonstrated in his illustration of Cushing's approach to the pituitary gland (Fig. 1). Cushing took formal art lessons from Brödel and began a lifelong relationship with the master illustrator. Cushing became increasingly interested in intracranial surgery, but recognized that the inability to achieve hemostasis would limit the surgeon's ability to perform resectional therapy. In typical Cushing fashion, he attacked the problem with insight and experimental creativity and refined and incorporated the operative use of suction and coagulation devices while working with the engineer William Bovie; he would subsequently develop a vascular clip ("Cushing clip") to be applied to intracranial vessels. He developed the modern field of neurosurgery and

J. L. Pasieka, J. A. Lee (eds.), *Surgical Endocrinopathies,* DOI 10.1007/978-3-319-13662-2_36,

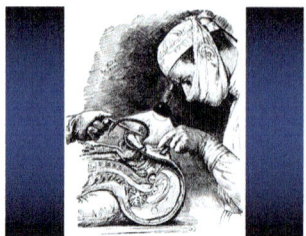

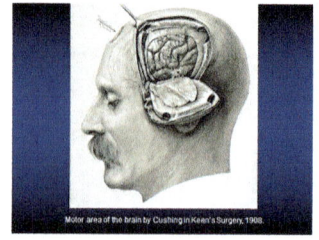

Fig. 1 Brödel illustration of Cushing performing surgery in 1912. Brödel used a real view of the surgeon and a sagittal view of the patient emphasizing the approach to the pituitary fossa. The operative light creates a powerful focus forcing the eye of both the surgeon and the observer through the patient's palate into the pituitary fossa. Black ink on Ross stippleboard; 1912. (Courtesy of the Max Brödel Archives, Department of Art as Applied to Medicine, Johns Hopkins University School of Medicine, Baltimore, MD)

Fig. 2 Cushing's illustration of a traumatic brain injury operation on the cerebral cortex. This sophisticated illustration employs techniques that can be attributed to the influence of Max Brödel. The face of the subject is remarkably similar to Cushing's mentor William Osler. It was more likely modeled after his older brother Ned, who bears a remarkable resemblance to Osler. Wolff's carbon pencil and dust on Ross stipple board. (Courtesy of the Cushing–Whitney Medical Historical Library, Yale University School of Medicine, New Haven, CT)

every subsequent neurosurgeon can trace their training based on a lineage to Harvey Cushing. At Hopkins, he worked with the founding fathers of Johns Hopkins Hospital: William Stewart Halsted (Surgery), William Osler (Medicine), William Henry Welch (Pathology), and Howard Atwood Kelly (Obstetrics). Osler was both his neighbor and mentor. They became lifelong colleagues sharing a profound interest in clinical medicine, scientific discovery, and collecting ancient medical books including the works of his historical hero Vesalius.

After training at Hopkins, Cushing, in the custom of the time, traveled to Europe to work with the greatest medical scientists. In Bern, he worked with **Theodore Kocher** and Hugo Kronecker exploring the relationship between intracranial hypertension and systolic blood pressure (Cushing's Reflex). In England, he worked with Victor Horsley and Sir Charles Scott Sherrington on the motor cortex. He also visited the surgical clinics and hospitals in Germany, Austria, France, and Italy.

He returned to Hopkins in 1902 and created the Hunterian Laboratory to both teach surgical technique and perform experiments. This laboratory would shape the scientific development of generations of medical students, house officers, and faculty members. His interest in neurosurgery became increasingly refined and he undertook evermore complex cases involving intracranial surgery. He developed a series of approaches to the pituitary gland for patients with acromegaly and he would subsequently recognize that pituitary basophil adenomas could cause the disease he discovered, Cushing's disease in the broader context of "Cushing's syndrome". He also developed approaches for acoustic neuroma, meningioma, and trigeminal neuralgia. He carefully documented his cases and immediately after surgery drew operative illustrations in exquisite and sophisticated detail as demonstrated in above Figure. He became not only the world's best known neurosurgeon but also the world's most distinguished and recognized physician.

In 1910, he was recruited to Boston to be surgeon-in-chief of the newly opened Peter Bent Brigham Hospital of Harvard Medical School. During World War I he served in France where he meticulously described the care of wounded soldiers. During this time, he cared for the only surviving child of his lifelong mentor and described the death of Edward Revere Osler. He served as chief of surgery of Peter Bent Brigham Hospital from 1910–1932 until he returned to New Haven as the Sterling professor of neurology (1933–1937). He trained a generation of neurosurgeons who would carry his profound influence throughout the world. He illustrated many of his operative approaches employing the techniques he had learned from Brödel (Fig. 2).

Harvey Cushing demonstrated enormous energy, creativity, and productivity. He published over 330 manuscripts and books and it was estimated that he wrote over 10,000 words a day. He was brilliant, driven, and intimidating. He was a man who according to Michael Bliss, "was respected by all, but loved by very few" [1].

In 1902, he married his childhood friend Katharine Stone Crowell and they had five children: William Harvey, Mary Benedict, Betsey, Henry Kirke, and Barbara. William Harvey would also go to Yale, but died in a tragic automobile accident in 1926. Cushing's influence extended well beyond surgery as he was well connected with the Roosevelt presidential family, and his daughters would assume prominent roles in high society in Manhattan and Washington, DC

During the latter part of life after he returned to Yale, he made plans to donate his extensive rare book collection of over 8000 items to Yale University and this would eventually form the core of the Cushing Historical Library. In addition, he documented and collected the clinical histories, operative procedures, and eventually the recovered brains from his patients and this extensive collection found a home in the newly opened Cushing Brain Tumor Registry in the Cushing Center at the Yale University School of Medicine which was organized under the guidance of Dennis Spencer, MD, the Cushing professor of neurosurgery at Yale.

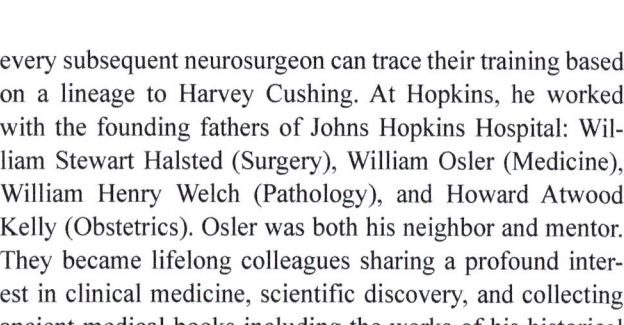

Cushing's honors are legendary: honorary degrees from nine American and thirteen European Universities, and innumerable awards and honorary memberships. His trainees founded the Harvey Cushing Society in 1932, and it would eventually become the American Association of Neurological Surgeons. Harvey Cushing was a driven individual who dominated and transformed medicine. He was an intellectual giant who employed his creative and technical skills to develop modern neurosurgery. He will be remembered as one of the most influential physicians of all times.

Acknowledgments Tracy Edwards is thanked for assisting with the preparation of this chapter.

References

1. Bliss M. Harvey Cushing, a life in surgery. Oxford: Oxford University Press; 2005.
2. Fulton JF. Harvey Cushing. A biography. Springfield: Charles Thomas; 1946.
3. Udelsman R. Presidential address: Harvey Cushing: the artist. Surgery. 2006;140(6):841–6.
4. Crosby RW, Cody J. Max Brödel, the man who put art into medicine. New York: Springer-Verlag; 1991.

J. Aidan Carney

1934–

Benzon M. Dy, Grace S. Lee and Melanie L. Richards

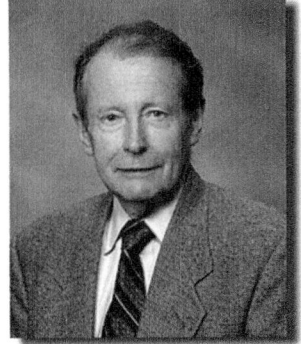

Aidan Carney. (Courtesy of Mayo Clinic)

Prior to genetic testing, the understanding of genetic endocrinopathies required the commitment and interest of astute clinicians treating patients with an interest in associating rare diseases. Conditions may have been described in only a single patient with a rare combination of diseases that required persistent and ongoing interest. Few have made contributions as important as J. Aidan Carney, M.D., Ph.D., in the field of endocrine surgery.

Dr. Carney's career at Mayo Clinic has spanned over five decades and continues today authoring more than 200 original articles including more than 90 articles after retirement. However, his interest in pathology and medicine began across the pond. Dr. Carney was born in Roscommon, Ireland on January 21, 1934. He was the son of Frances Howley Carney and Richard Gerard Carney. He attended Glongowes Wood College in Naas, Co. Kildare near Dublin from 1947 to 1952 and obtained his M.B.B. Ch in 1959 from the University College of Dublin. From 1959 to 1960, he was an intern in St. Vincent's Hospital in Dublin, Ireland, and

subsequently worked in the pathology department at both the University College and Richmond Hospital up to July 1962. He received his Ph.D. from the University of Minnesota in 1969, while working at Mayo Clinic, with his dissertation entitled "Morphology of Myosin and Thick Myofilament Diameter in Experimental Cardiac Hypertrophy." This special interest in the pathology of cardiac muscle was maintained throughout his career. At the time, he may not have realized that this interest would serve him well in understanding the complex pathologic relationship that would later bear his name.

He began his career at Mayo Clinic, Rochester, as a resident in the Department of Pathology from 1962 to 1966 and received an appointment as an assistant to the staff and associate consultant in 1966. Dr. Carney was married to Dr. Francoise Le Guen of Port Louis, Mauritius, on June 16, 1962. She was an accomplished anesthesiologist in her own right, appointed as a fellow in the Department of Anesthesiology in the Mayo Graduate School of Medicine from 1962 to 1965 as well as a member of the faculty of the Department of Anesthesiology in Mayo Clinic from October 1, 1965.

Dr. Carney's interest in endocrine disorders and syndromes began in 1966 after reading a paper by Dr. Dillwyn Williams which described the syndrome of multiple endocrine neoplasia 2B (MEN 2B). Dr. Carney's initial contribution included descriptions of medullary hyperplasia in bilateral pheochromocytomas in MEN 2B. Later, investigations led to reporting previously unrecognized syndromes—most notably Carney triad, Carney complex, and Carney Stratakis syndrome. Identification of these entities was accomplished through years of collecting unusual cases, establishing rapport with patients, exhaustive detective work with follow-up from around the world, and synthesis of seemingly unrelated findings into coherent clinical and pathological entities.

In understanding subtle connections between rare disease processes, Carney established several rules which he continues to abide by: (1) the concurrence of the tumors is statistically unlikely even in one patient because of their rarity; (2) the neoplasms are often multiple in the affected organs; (3)

B. M. Dy (✉)
Endocrine Surgery, Mayo Clinic, Rochester, MN, USA
e-mail: benzondymd@gmail.com

G. S. Lee · M. L. Richards
Department of Surgery, Mayo Clinic, Rochester 55905, MN, USA

J. L. Pasieka, J. A. Lee (eds.), *Surgical Endocrinopathies,* DOI 10.1007/978-3-319-13662-2_37,
© Springer International Publishing Switzerland 2015

Fig. 1 Characteristics of Carney complex. (Courtesy of Mayo Clinic)

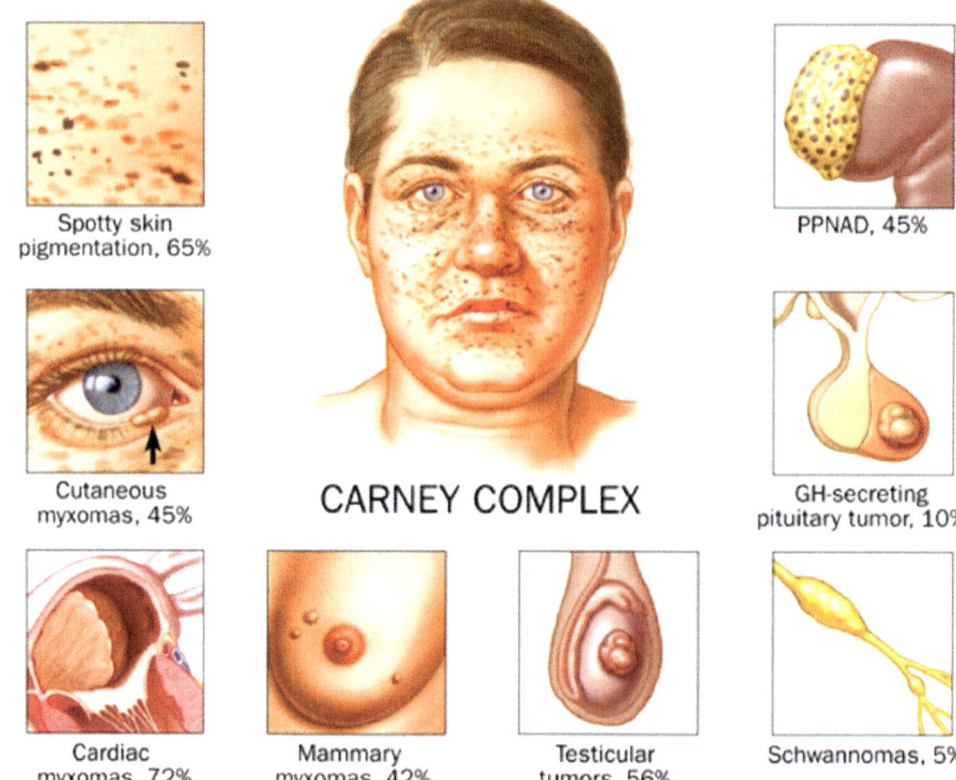

Spotty skin pigmentation, 65%

Cutaneous myxomas, 45%

Cardiac myxomas, 72%

CARNEY COMPLEX

Mammary myxomas, 42%

Testicular tumors, 56%

PPNAD, 45%

GH-secreting pituitary tumor, 10%

Schwannomas, 5%

the lesions appear at an age when tumors are not expected especially when compared to their sporadic counterpart; and (4) the association has a pronounced sex predilection—"then a case can be made for concluding that the concurrence of the tumors is likely not coincidental."

Based on the presence of these principles, the association involving gastric intestinal stromal tumors (GIST), pulmonary chondromas, and functional extra-adrenal paragangliomas became clearly evident. This constellation was one of Dr. Carney's first descriptions of syndromic associations and was described in *the New England Journal of Medicine* in 1977. This became to be known as Carney's triad [1].

His interest in this triad began after reviewing an article by Henry D. Appleman, M.D., from the University of Michigan in Ann Arbor. In line with his principles of understanding syndromic associations, he noted that out of 127 cases of GIST tumors, three occurred predominantly in women of young age, were multiple, and had an insidious development with slow-growing well-localized tumors compared to the other 124 cases which are most often presented in men in their fifth or sixth decade with malignant aggressive tumors.

In his initial report, he described the concurrent appearance of three unusual tumors in four young patients: pulmonary chondroma, epithelioid leiomyosarcomas, and functioning paragangliomas. In subsequent reports by himself and others who had developed an interest in the association,

the tumors of this triad occur at various times, often with long periods of time between their appearances in a given patient.

Over 30 years later, Carney continues to study his original triad and has found associations with two other entities, esophageal leiomyomas and adrenal adenomas, postulating that this may actually be a pentad in etiology [2]. With over 60 years of follow-up, Dr. Carney has published long-term results on patients he has diagnosed with Carney's triad with a disease-specific mortality rate of 80 % [3].

Another landmark association was achieved when Carney complex (Fig. 1) was described. This particular complex includes primary pigmented nodular adrenal disease (PPNAD), growth hormone secreting pituitary tumors, schwannomas, testicular tumors, mammary myxomas, cardiac myxomas cutaneous myomas, and spotted skin pigmentation in varying penetrances [4].

In 1984, PPNAD was described in four patients with **Cushing's** syndrome at the Mayo Clinic. At the time, a review of current literature had shown a clustering of this in two families with one patient dying of a cardiac myxoma. This led to further investigation by Dr. Carney. Due to his years of experience associated with endocrine pathology and special interest in cardiac pathology originating as early as his Ph.D. research, he "noted in a Swiss report two siblings with PPNAD and other disorders." In his review of these cases, he found two siblings with PPNAD but also a variety of other maladies. One suffered from eyelid fibromas and eventually developed hemiparesis. The other also had multiple fibromas. However, a third sibling without Cushing's syndrome or skin lesions, died of a cardiac myxoma at age 4 years. At the time, of the four patients diagnosed with PPNAD at Mayo Clinic and 19 in the literature, none had been diagnosed with a synchronous or metachronous cardiac myxoma which highlights the difficulty and persistence required to develop these associations.

This led Dr. Carney to pursue other routes for showing an association. None of the patients having undergone bilateral adrenalectomies up to 1982 had developed cardiac myxomas. Looking in reverse, no patients with cardiac myxomas in the literature or of the 51 diagnosed at Mayo Clinic had developed Cushing's syndrome. After searching through hundreds of records, he identified one case with "multiple cortical adrenal adenomas. The gross description of the glands was multiple cortical adrenal nodules in both adrenals. These are of a yellowish color but contain some brown and black dots." However, there were no cytologic features that were consistent with PPNAD described in the specimens.

It was not until he reviewed the slides that he diagnosed PPNAD in the specimen. He reported "It was surely not an accident that the cardiac myxoma was located in the left atrium." In addition, multiple fibromas and "nevi" throughout the body were described. Dr. Carney described that "it seemed almost impossible that all the patient's conditions, PPNAD, unusually situated or multiple cardiac myxomas, numerous pigmented moles, and a myxomatous fibroadenoma—could be encountered together in the particular circumstances in which they had been found and the events be unconnected." They must all be related. "They must constitute a syndrome."

Today, PPNAD occurs in approximately half of all patients with Carney complex. Genetic mutations in *PRKAR1A* and *PDE11A* have been identified in patients who manifest with the complex. However, not all patients with Carney complex have mutations in these gene sequences and additional mutations are being studied.

Although he is best known for his eponymous associations, his research interests spanned multiple areas including multiple endocrine neoplasia, testicular carcinoma, parathyroid disease, and adrenal disease. It is fitting that as mutational analysis and genetic correlation to phenotype abnormalities emerged, Dr. Carney was certainly at the forefront of these research endeavors. This is clearly evident in Carney–Stratakis syndrome in patients with paragangliomas and GIST tumors [5]. In 2001, Dr. Carney began working with Dr. Constantine Stratakis, a pediatric endocrinologist at the National Institutes of Health. Two notable findings were evident within this group of patients. First, they tended to occur in younger males as opposed to younger females as initially

described in the Carney triad in 1977. Second, despite long follow-up periods in these families, there appeared to be no emergence of pulmonary chondromas.

There was difficulty in distinguishing these syndromes given the long latency that can occur between the manifestations of the syndromes. There have been more than 20 families with this syndrome described. Although often clinically diagnosed, today, familial testing can be used to describe the syndrome in kindreds through mutations in subtypes of succinate dehydrogenase (SDH) mutations including *SDHB*, *SDHD*, and *SDHC*. With this understanding, future research into identifying targets for unresectable paragangliomas have emerged, including tyrosine kinase inhibitors and subsequent molecular targets.

In an editorial in *Mayo Clinic Proceedings,* Henry D. Appleman, M.D., reviewed the discovery of the Carney triad and raised the question, "has the Carney Triad had a clinical effect?" This can be extended to other rare associations including Carney Complex given the rarity of PPNAD, GIST tumors, and myxomas. In fact, even the most astute clinician may be unaware of these relationships and impact given that they have affected fewer than 500 patients in the literature. However, the road to describing these conditions was not straightforward. It required hundreds of hours of reviewing slide material, patient records and scouring the literature. There were countless approaches and creative and novel angles that had to be examined before a clear association could be established. At times, it may have been as few cases as a single patient that sparked a connection that would take over 20 years to be confirmed genetically. As Appleman so succinctly describes the Aidan Carneys of the world are insightful and creative, and they force us who are neither to keep our eyes open, observe things carefully, and question dogma frequently [6].

References

1. Carney JA, Sheps SG, Go VL, Gordon H. The triad of gastric leiomyosarcoma, functioning extra-adrenal paraganglioma and pulmonary chondroma. N Engl J Med. 1977 Jun 30;296(26):1517–8.
2. Carney JA, Stratakis CA, Young WF Jr. Adrenal cortical adenoma: the fourth component of the Carney triad and an association with subclinical Cushing syndrome. Am J Surg Pathol. 2013 Aug;37(8):1140–9.
3. Carney JA. Carney triad: a syndrome featuring paraganglionic, adrenocortical, and possibly other endocrine tumors. J Clin Endocrinol Metab. 2009;94:3656–62.
4. The discovery of the Carney Complex. Endocrinol Update. 2010;5(3).
5. Carney JA, Stratakis CA. Familial paraganglioma and gastric stromal sarcoma: a new syndrome distinct from the Carney triad. Am J Med Genet. 2002;108:132–9. doi:10.1002/ajmg.10235.
6. Appleman HD. The Carney Triad: a lesson in observation, creativity, and perseverance. Mayo Clin Proc. 1999;74(6):638–40.

Pheochromocytoma and Paraganglioma

Michael G. Johnston and James A. Lee

Introduction

Pheochromocytoma and paraganglioma are tumors of the chromaffin cells of the neuroendocrine system. These cells are called chromaffin cells due to their ability to turn dark brown when freshly incubated with potassium dichromate, which oxidizes the catecholamines stored therein to melanin [1, 2]. In 1912, Pick proposed the name "pheochromocytoma," creating it out of the Greek words *phaios* ("dusky"), *chroma* ("color"), and *cytoma* ("tumor") [3]. In 2004, the World Health Organization classified chromaffin tumors of the adrenal medulla, which make up approximately 85 % of chromaffin tumors, as *pheochromocytoma* [4, 5]. *Paraganglioma* refers to tumors of the extra-adrenal sympathetic and parasympathetic ganglia. In the case of pheochromocytomas and paragangliomas of the sympathetic ganglia, these tumors secrete excess catecholamines. Paragangliomas of the parasympathetic ganglia typically are nonfunctional. While the majority of pheochromocytomas and paragangliomas typically secrete excess catecholamines, they may also co-secrete adrenocorticotropic hormone (ACTH), parathyroid hormone-related protein (PTHrp), vasopressin, vasoactive intestinal polypeptide (VIP), and growth hormone-releasing hormone (GHrh) which may lead to clinically confusing presentations [2]. The details of pheochromocytoma are classically remembered by medical students and residents as the tumor that obeys the "rule of 10's," i.e. 10 % are inherited, 10 % are bilateral, 10 % are found in children, and 10 % are malignant. However, this mnemonic has largely been shown to be outdated as significantly higher proportions are shown to carry germ-line mutations [6]. The prevalence of pheo-chromocytoma and paraganglioma is estimated to be between 1 in 6500 and 1 in 2500, leading to an annual incidence in the USA of 500–1600 cases [7]. Autopsy studies in China, Australia, and New Zealand suggest a pheochromocytoma prevalence alone as high as 1 in 2000 [8, 9]. They can occur in any age group, although they usually present at a younger age if due to a germ-line mutation. They are generally considered to have an equal gender distribution, although there has been some suggestion of a 3:2 female predilection [10]. Pheochromocytomas and paragangliomas are rare causes of secondary hypertension, and account for approximately 0.1–0.6 % of screened secondary hypertensive cases [11].

Embryology/Cellular Biology

Since they can arise in either the adrenal medulla or anywhere along the sympathetic or parasympathetic ganglia, pheochromocytomas and paragangliomas have been reported in the head and neck (including the carotid and vagal bodies), the mediastinum, and the extra-adrenal abdomen and pelvis (including the celiac, superior, and inferior ganglia, organ of Zuckerkandl, and urinary bladder) [12] (Figs. 1 and 2).

In the chromaffin cell, tyrosine is first converted to 3,4-di-hydroxyphenylalanine (DOPA) by tyrosine hydroxylase. This is the rate-limiting step of catecholamine formation and serves as a point at which the physician can block catecholamine formation, either as part of the patient's preoperative preparation or as palliative treatment for unresectable disease with metyrosine. DOPA is then converted to dopamine by aromatic L-amino acid decarboxylase. Dopamine is then converted to norepinephrine by dopamine β-hydroxylase and norepinephrine is finally converted to epinephrine by phenylethanolamine N-methyltransferase (PMNT). PMNT is almost exclusively located in the adrenal medulla. Further, cortisol acts as a necessary cofactor in PMNT's mechanism of action. Thus, chromaffin tumors producing only norepinephrine as manifested by high normetanephrine levels are typically paraganglioma and not pheochromocytoma [2].

J. A. Lee (✉)

Associate Professor, Department of Surgery, Columbia University Medical Center, New York, NY 10032, USA
e-mail: jal74@cumc.columbia.edu

M. G. Johnston
General Surgery, Naval Medical Center Portsmouth, 620 John Paul Jones Circle, Portsmouth, VA 23708, USA

J. L. Pasieka, J. A. Lee (eds.), *Surgical Endocrinopathies*, DOI 10.1007/978-3-319-13662-2_38,
© Springer International Publishing Switzerland 2015

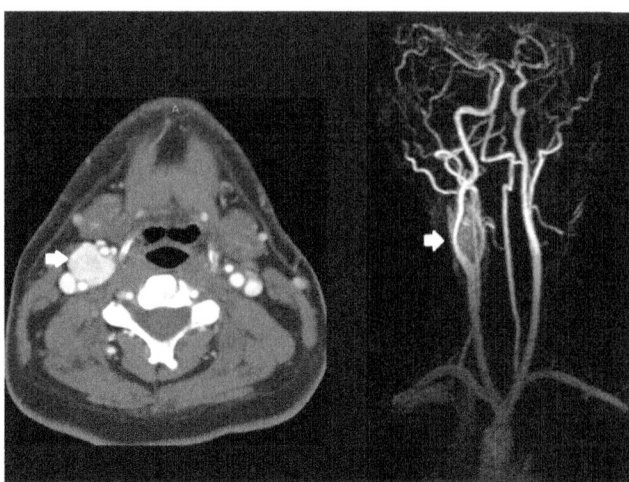

Fig. 1 A 31-year-old male noted to have a unilateral neck mass following an upper respiratory infection has a paraganglioma in the right carotid body (*white arrows*). (Images courtesy of John York, M.D., Department of Radiology, Naval Medical Center Portsmouth, Virginia)

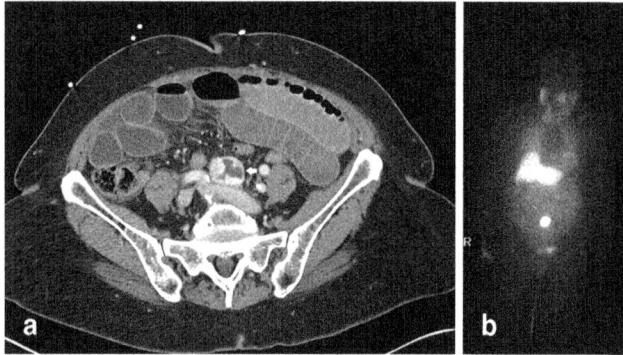

Fig. 2 An 83-year-old female, who presented with a small bowel obstruction, noted to have a mass at the aortic bifurcation found incidentally on CT. Subsequent planar and SPECT/ I-123-MIBG images demonstrated an organ of Zuckerkandl paraganglioma (*white arrows*). *CT* computed tomography, *SPECT* single photon emission computed tomography, *MIBG* metaiodobenzylguanidine. (Images courtesy of Thomas Nelson, M.D., Department of General Surgery, Naval Hospital Camp Pendleton and Robert Marks, M.D., Department of Radiology, Naval Medical Center San Diego)

The exception to this rule is the adrenal pheochromocytomas found in **von Hippel Lindau** disease [11].

Presentation

Given its rarity, pheochromocytoma and paraganglioma are generally not routinely sought out as a cause of secondary hypertension. Further complicating the issue, as many as 30 % of patients with pheochromocytoma or paraganglioma are either normotensive or experience only orthostatic hypotension [13]. However, in cases of heightened clinical suspicion, such as an early onset hypertension, or in a patient who presents with episodic, paroxysmal hypertension accompanied by the classic constellation of symptoms including headaches, palpitations and diaphoresis, the diagnosis of pheochromocytoma and paraganglioma should be considered. Only 10 % of patients will present with the classic constellation of symptoms and the key to making the diagnosis is first considering the possibility. Other symptoms of catecholamine excess may include pallor, hyperglycemia, anxiety, or a sense of foreboding, nausea, and/or vomiting. If these symptoms accompany micturition, a paraganglioma near the bladder should be considered. Further, a patient who demonstrates an unusually high blood pressure in response to an invasive procedure (such as general anesthesia, surgery, or interventional radiological interrogation) should undergo a workup for pheochromocytoma. The diagnosis of pheochromocytoma should also be entertained whenever an adrenal mass is uncovered on abdominal imaging either as an adrenal incidentaloma or as part of a metastatic workup for a known malignancy. Pheochromocytomas account for approximately 5–7 % of adrenal incidentalomas [14] and perhaps 20–30 % of current pheochromocytomas are discovered first as adrenal incidentalomas [15]. Left untreated, pheochromocytomas can cause catecholamine-induced cardiomyopathy, congestive heart failure, myocardial infarction, stroke, and death.

Workup

Epinephrine and norepinephrine are degraded by methylation through catechol-*O*-methyltransferase to metanephrine and normetanephrine, respectively, or by deamination through monoamine oxidase to vanillymandelic acid [16]. Measurements of plasma and urine catecholamines are unhelpful because the half-lives of the catecholamines are extremely short. In contrast, the metanephrine by-products have a longer half-life. Plasma-free metanephrines have a high sensitivity at 96–100 % but a lower specificity of 85–89 % [11]. Twenty-four-hour urine fractionated metanephrines have a sensitivity of 77–90 %, but a high specificity of 93–98 % [11]. In general, plasma metanephrines are the screening test of choice due to the ease of obtaining samples and the higher sensitivity [17, 18]. Metanephrine levels greater than two to three times the upper limit of normal carry a near 100 % positive predictive value for a pheochromocytoma and functional paraganglioma. Similarly, a metanephrine level that is less than one time the upper limit of normal has a very high negative predictive value [2]. When the metanephrine levels are between one and two times the upper limit of normal, there is a 30 % chance of having a pheochromocytoma or functional paraganglioma [19]. Unfortunately, no clinical factors have been shown to distinguish between patients with and without pheochromocytoma or functional paraganglioma in this latter group of patients. Of note, paraganglioma typically lack the *N*-methyl transferase necessary to convert norepinephrine to epinephrine, so a paraganglioma may have normal levels of metanephrine and only elevated normetanephrines while the total metanephrine should still be elevated. When testing metanephrine levels, it is important to eliminate confounding factors: the patient should ideally be in a stress-free state, lie supine for 20 min prior to phlebotomy and should refrain from intake of caffeine or other stimulants prior to testing. The list of medications that can potentially affect biochemical testing includes tricyclic antidepressants, levodopa, over-the-counter (OTC) decongestants, amphetamines, buspirone and other antipsychotic agents, prochlorperazine, reserpine, cocaine, nicotine, and ethanol. Withdrawal from clonidine and other stimulants can also affect biochemical testing [2]. In tumors that can secrete dopamine such as those caused by *SDHB* (see section "Genetic Syndromes") or *SDHD* mutations, consideration should be given to testing for dopamine and its metabolite methoxytyramine [20]. In general, testing for metanephrines should be done on two separate occasions to confirm the diagnosis.

After biochemical confirmation of the diagnosis, anatomic imaging (computed tomography (CT) scan or magnetic resonance imaging (MRI)) should be obtained followed by a functional imaging study (metaiodobenzylguanidine (MIBG) or positron emission tomography (PET) scan). Combining functional imaging in addition to anatomic imaging (especially in young patients and cases of paraganglioma) helps to identify multifocal lesions that may be missed with cross-sectional imaging alone and ensure that a nonfunctional anatomic abnormality is not removed instead of a "missed" functional lesion elsewhere. MRI and CT have sensitivity for pheochromocytoma of 98 and 89% respectively [11]. On CT, pheochromocytoma and paraganglioma can appear homogenous or heterogeneous and in addition to being solid, may be hemorrhagic, cystic, or necrotic compared to the usually homogenous and solid benign adenoma. Pheochromocytoma and paraganglioma have a higher density on CT than an adenoma and has a slower washout of contrast. Rarely, a pheochromocytoma can contain more lipid and be mistaken for an adenoma. On MRI, a pheochromocytoma is usually more signal intense, especially on T2-weighted imaging where approximately one third of the time it displays a "bright white light bulb" sign and has a slower washout phase [21]. An old adage is that a solid adrenal tumor that is bright on T2-weighted imaging is cancer or a pheochromocytoma until proven otherwise. Especially in younger patients or those with a higher suspicion for a genetic mutation, anatomic imaging from skull base to pelvis should be considered to look for paraganglioma.

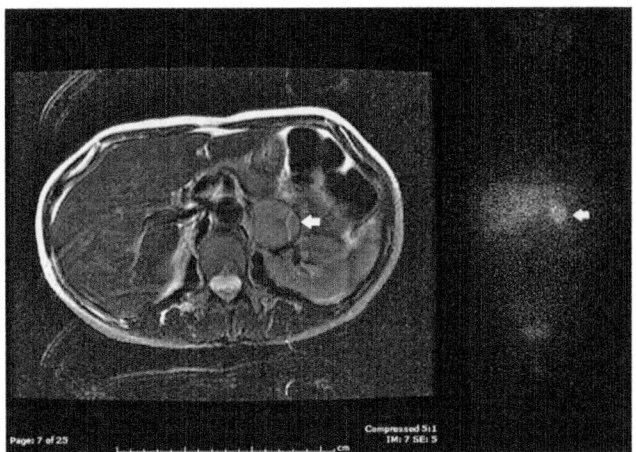

Fig. 3 T2 MRI and planar ^{131}I-MIBG of a left pheochromocytoma (*white arrows*). *MRI* magnetic resonance image, *MIBG* metaiodobenzylguanidine. (Images courtesy of Luisa Kropcho, M.D., and Ryan Restrepo, M.D., Department of General Surgery, Naval Medical Center Portsmouth, Virginia)

The two main functional studies for pheochromocytoma and paraganglioma are the MIBG scan either with 123-iodine or 131-iodine and the PET scan [22]. MIBG is an analog of norepinephrine and is readily taken up by the norepinephrine transporter. The overall sensitivity for ^{131}I-MIBG scanning is 77–90% and the specificity is even higher at 95–100%. Sensitivity improves with the use of ^{123}I-MIBG and single photon emission computed tomography (SPECT) imaging to 88–96% [23]. However, the sensitivity of MIBG imaging is lower in cases of familial disease, malignant disease, abdominal paraganglioma, and nonfunctional head and neck paraganglioma. The sensitivity is especially low in cases of small, multiple paraganglioma, thus rendering MIBG less helpful with succinate dehydrogenase (SDH)-related disease. Further drawbacks of the MIBG study include the need for thyroid blockade, the potential need for withdrawal of catecholamine-blocking medications, limited image resolution, and long study time. In contrast, PET scanning has emerged as an extremely valuable tool for all cases of pheochromocytoma and paraganglioma, but especially for cases of multiple paraganglioma. Several different tracers have been utilized, most notably ^{18}F-dopamine, ^{18}F-DOPA, and ^{18}F-flurodeoxyglucose (FDG). The sensitivity of ^{18}F-FDG PET has been reported between 92 and 100% and its specificity at 90% [23]. The sensitivity of ^{18}F-DOPA PET has been reported between 98 and 100% with a specificity of 100% [23]. [18]FDG is the only tracer currently in wide use, and most pheochromocytomas and paragangliomas accumulate [18]FDG (Fig. 3).

Adrenal tumors suspected of being a pheochromocytoma must not be biopsied as this may precipitate a "pheo crisis." In fact, there are very few situations in which biopsy of an adrenal tumor is indicated. Perhaps the only scenario in which

Table 1 Genetic mutations associated with common causes of familial pheochromocytomas and paragangliomas [15, 20]

Disease	Mutation	Predominant catecholamine	*Usual* location	Behavior	Associated findings
MEN 2a	RET	Epinephrine	Adrenal	Benign	MTC, HPT, cutaneous lichen amyloidosis
MEN 2b	RET	Epinephrine	Adrenal	Benign	MTC, mucosal neuromas, marfanoid habitus, Hirschprung's disease
Von Hippel-Lindau (type 2)	VHL	Norepinephrine	Adrenal (bilateral 40%)	Benign	Retinal angiomas, CNS hemangioblastomas, pancreatic cysts and NET's, renal cell carcinomas, epididymal cystadenomas
Von Recklinhausen (Neurofibromatosis)	NF1	Epinephrine	Adrenal	Benign (10% malignant)	Neurofibromas, Café-au-lait spots, axillary and groin freckling, iris hamartomas, macrocephaly, mental retardation
Familial paraganglioma syndrome (FPS)	SDHA	–	–	Benign (up to 14% malignant)	Leigh disease, GIST, renal cell carcinoma, pituitary adenoma
FPS type 4	SDHB	Norepinephrine but can produce dopamine	Extra-adrenal abdomen, mediastinum, pelvis	Malignant	Renal cell carcinoma, papillary thyroid cancer
FPS type 3	SDHC	Can be parasympathetic. Can produce norepinephrine, dopamine	Skull base/ neck	Benign	Renal cell carcinoma
FPS type 1	SDHD	Can be parasympathetic. Can produce norepinephrine, dopamine.	Skull base/ neck	Multiple. malignant	Renal cell carcinoma
FPS type 2	SDH AF2	–		Skull base/ neck	–	–

MEN multiple endocrine neoplasia, *RET* rearranged during transfection protooncogene, *MTC* medullary thyroid cancer, *HPT* hyperparathyroidism, *NET* neuroendocrine tumor, *NF1* neurofibromatosis, *SDHx* succinate dehydrogenase, *AF2* assembly factor 2, *CNS* central nervous system, *GIST* gastrointestinal stromal tumor

biopsy of an adrenal tumor is helpful is in the instance when a metastatic lesion is suspected and confirming the presence of an adrenal metastasis would change the management from surgical resection of the primary to systemic therapy.

Genetic Syndromes

Instead of the classic "10%" rate of germ-line mutation, it is now recognized that at least 30–35% of pheochromocytomas and paragangliomas demonstrate a germ-line mutation [15, 24, 25]. In children presenting with pheochromocytoma or paraganglioma, this rate of germ-line mutation has been cited to be as high as 40% [7]. There are at least 17 causative genes, including *RET, vHL, NF1, SDH* (*A, B, C, D,* and *AF2*), *MAX, PHD2, K1F1Bβ,* and *TMEM127* [14, 15, 26] (Table 1).

Genetic screening should be performed in patients with bilateral adrenal disease, paraganglioma, multifocal disease, and age younger than 50. However, given this higher rate of genetically linked disease, some groups advocate mandatory genetic testing for any patient with a pheochromocytoma or

paraganglioma. Using the patient's specific tumor characteristics combined with the information in Table 1, a directed, cost-effective testing strategy can be devised (Fig. 4).

In the evaluation of any suspected familial disease, particular attention should be paid to the dermatologic, head and neck, ophthalmologic, and neurologic evaluation [15].

Among the most common etiologies of heritable pheochromocytoma and paraganglioma are mutations in the *SDH* gene. The molecular basis for the SDHD mutation was first described in 2000 [15]. SDHB, the most common SDH mutation, and SDHC were subsequently identified followed by SDHA. Mutations in the SDH assembly factor 2 (SDHAF2) have also been described. These mutations cause a range of anatomic and clinical presentations, but usually lead to paragangliomas that secrete dopamine, the dopamine metabolite methoxytyramine, norepinephrine, or are clinically silent [14]. The mechanism of action for SDH-related tumor formation is thought to be increased degradation of the mutated enzyme followed by the loss of heterozygosity which combines to lead to decreased SDH action which in turn leads to an increase in succinate accumulation, increased DNA methylation, chronic hypoxia, and thus increased tumor formation

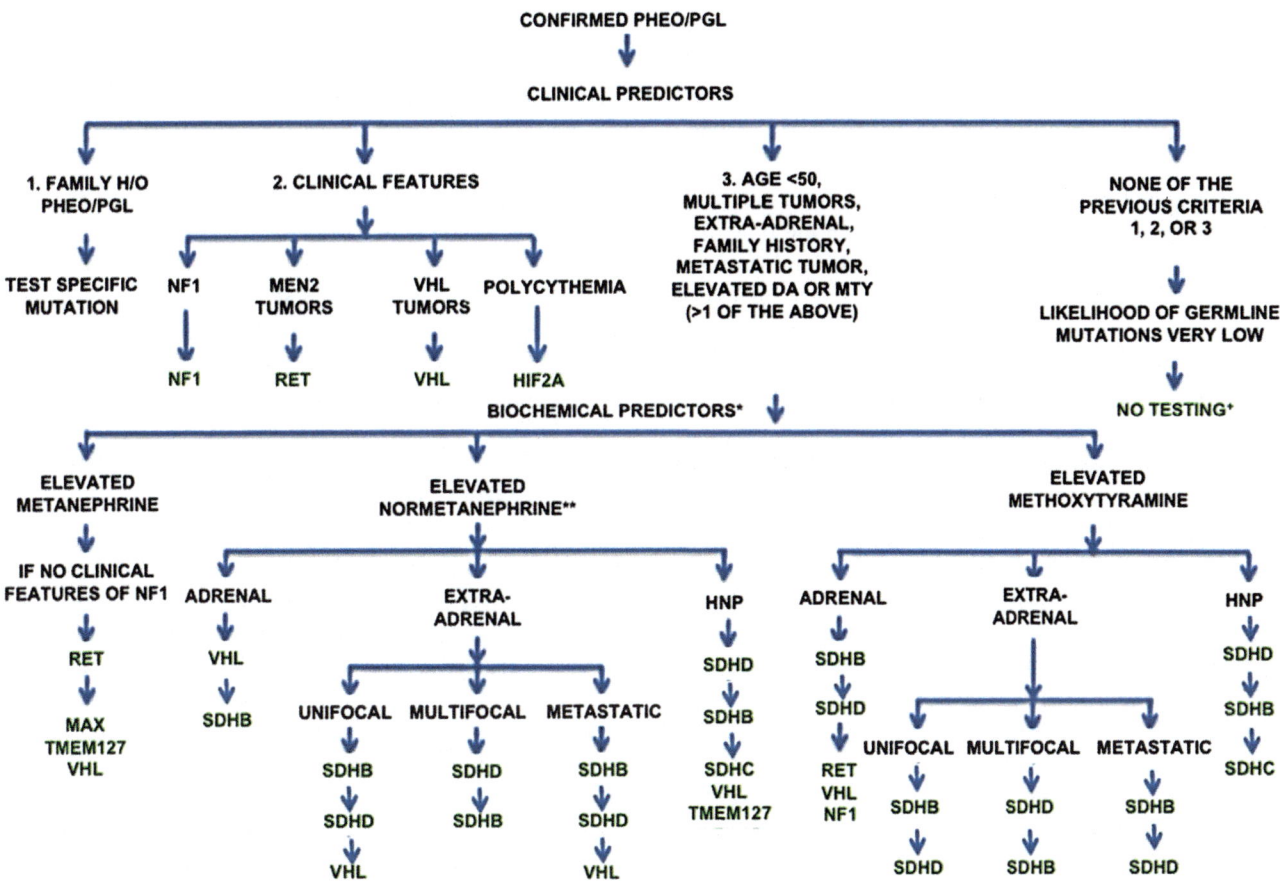

Fig. 4 Recommended genetic testing algorithm for patients with pheochromocytoma or paraganglioma. *If levels of both normetanephrine and methoxytyramine are elevated, follow the algorithm for methoxytyramine. If levels of both normetanephrine and metanephrine are elevated, follow the algorithm for metanephrine. **In patients with elevated levels of normetanephrine with clinical features that do not clearly indicated which gene to test, perform immunohistochemistry for SDHB and SDHA. + If tumor is adrenal, TMEM127 testing may be considered. *DA* dopamine, *HNP* head and neck paraganglioma, *h/o* history of, *MTY* methoxytyramine, *SDH* succinate dehydrogenase. (Reprinted from Martucci and Pacak [14] with permission from Elsevier, adapted from Karasek et al. [27] with permission from Nature Publishing Group)

[14, 24]. SDHB and SDHD mutations often cause thoracic and abdominal paragangliomas, such as in the organ of Zuckerkandl. SDHB mutations can present with metastases in up to 38 % of cases [24]. SDHD mutations also cause head and neck paragangliomas that can be clinically silent. Data on SDHC, SDHA, and SDHAF2 tumors are rare and not yet completely clear. Interestingly, the *SDHD* and *SDHAF2* genes undergo maternal imprinting and thus only patients with affected fathers develop the syndrome [14]. The overall penetrance of SDH mutations is low, which explains the apparent high rate of de novo mutations and the need for rigorous consideration of genetic testing in pheochromocytoma and paraganglioma patients [14].

Multiple endocrine neoplasia 2a and 2b (also called **Sipple**'s syndrome) are caused by a mutation in the rearranged during transfection (RET) proto-oncogene and occur in 10 % of germ-line mutations associated with pheochromocytoma. **Von Hippel Lindau** is a rarer cause of pheochromo-

cytoma accounting for only about 5 % of cases. Both Sipple syndrome and von Hippel Lindau syndrome are covered in detail in Chaps. 62 and 57, respectively. Carney–Stratakis dyad and **Carney** triad are also rare genetic causes of paraganglioma. The dyad consists of gastrointestinal stromal tumors in addition to paragangliomas whereas the triad also includes pulmonary chondromas. The specific genetic cause has yet to be isolated but is thought to be related to mutations in the SDH gene [14].

Treatment

Preoperative Preparation

Surgery is the mainstay of treatment for pheochromocytoma and paraganglioma and represents the only chance of curing the patient whether the disease is benign or malignant [2]. The first pheochromocytoma was resected without knowledge of the secretory effect this tumor had. **Charles Mayo** successfully removed this tumor via a flank approach in 1927. **Arthur Shipley** was the first surgeon to remove a pheochromocytoma knowingly, and as such was far better prepared to manage the consequences of manipulation and removal of such a tumor. Given the potentially life-threatening effects of increased catecholamine release, nowadays patients should undergo a preoperative cardiac evaluation, including at least an electrocardiogram with strong consideration given to obtaining an echocardiogram. In addition, patients should receive careful preoperative preparation.

The classic preoperative preparation for patients with pheochromocytoma and paraganglioma is alpha-blockade with an alpha-blocker such as phenoxybenzamine. Alpha-blockade is typically started at a low dose and is gradually increased until the patient experiences side effects such as a stuffy nose, mild orthostasis, and fatigue. As the alpha-blockade sets in, the chronic alpha-mediated vasoconstriction relaxes and the patient shows evidence of volume depletion. Therefore, it is critical to instruct the patient to drink extra fluid and take a little extra salt in the diet during this period of time. Adequate preoperative volume resuscitation will minimize the hypotension once the tumor is removed.

There are a number of alpha-blocking medications to choose from and generally fall into the categories of selective alpha-blockers such as doxazosin, terazosin, or prazosin and nonselective alpha-blockers such as phenoxybenzamine. Alpha-blockade with phenoxybenzamine results in less intraoperative hypertension but more postoperative hypotension due to its nonselective, noncompetitive, long-acting mechanism of action [28]. Selective, short-acting, competitive alpha-blockade results in more intraoperative hypertension and more use of intraoperative fluid resuscitation but less postoperative hypotension. However, there does not appear to be a difference in surgical outcome or hospital stay no matter which type is chosen [29].

Once the patient is alpha-blocked and volume resuscitated, he or she may demonstrate a reflex tachycardia. In that case, it is appropriate to add beta-blockade, whether selective or nonselective, in order to decrease the heart rate, diminish myocardial demand, and preserve coronary flow. It is critical to note that one must "not" begin beta-blockade until the patient is adequately alpha-blocked, or the patient will experience unopposed alpha stimulation, which can lead to potentially fatal cardiovascular events.

As an alternative or adjunct to traditional alpha-blockade, some surgeons prefer calcium channel blockers for their renal and cardiac protective effects. Some groups have shown that calcium channel blockers may minimize coronary vasospasm from a paroxysmal norepinephrine surge [20]. They

are also useful as a second-line agent if the patient continues to demonstrate hypertension even on maximal alpha blockade [16]. Calcium channel blockers reduce arterial hypertension by inhibiting norepinephrine-mediated transmembrane calcium influx in vascular smooth muscle [28].

In rare cases, metyrosine has been used for preoperative preparation. Metyrosine blocks the action of tyrosine hydroxylase, the enzyme responsible for the first step in catecholamine synthesis. Metyrosine, however, is quite expensive and carries with it a range of undesirable side effects including nightmares, galactorrhea, extrapyramidal symptoms, sedation, diarrhea, and anxiety [2].

Intraoperative Strategies

Anesthetic agents that increase sympathetic tone, such as succinylcholine, ketamine, ephedrine, pancuronium, and desflurane, should be avoided [28]. A smooth anesthetic induction is critical to avoid severe swings in blood pressure and heart rate; drugs such as propofol and dexmetatomadine are especially useful in this setting. An arterial line is highly recommended for close blood pressure monitoring as is central venous access for quick delivery of vasoactive drugs centrally. The anesthesiologist should prepare several drips of short-acting vasopressors and antihypertensives in advance, such as phentolamine, nitroprusside, and nicardipine, for acute lowering of blood pressure, lidocaine and esmolol for cardiac arrhythmias, and norepinephrine, phenylephrine, or vasopressin for blood pressure support if needed once the adrenal vein is ligated. Magnesium is also a useful anesthetic adjunct [30]. Many texts suggest early ligation of the adrenal vein to minimize systemic secretion of catecholamine, but this is often not necessary with good preoperative preparation and short-acting medications. While historical data suggest a perioperative mortality rate of 30–45%, modern series demonstrate a perioperative mortality rate of between 0 and 2.9% [16].

Pheochromocytomas and paragangliomas can be approached via open surgery, a transabdominal laparoscopic route, or through a posterior retroperitoneoscopic approach. Laparoscopic adrenalectomy has become the gold standard for resection of most pheochromocytomas and has been shown to have equivalent outcomes to laparoscopic adrenalectomy for other disease processes in the adrenal such as primary hyperaldosteronism and *Cushing*'s syndrome [31]. Indeed, there is a wealth of data to suggest that patients have better outcomes with a laparoscopic versus an open approach with regards to intraoperative blood loss, postoperative pain, length of stay, and return to work [20, 32, 33]. In the case of surgery for bilateral disease, consideration can be given to cortical-sparing adrenalectomy in order to save the patient from the lifelong sequelae of adrenal insufficiency [20, 33].

Postoperative Management

It is not uncommon, especially if the patient was prepared preoperatively with phenoxybenzamine, for patients to require vasopressor agents for a brief period postoperatively. Depending on the available resources, this can be monitored in either the recovery room or intensive care unit (ICU). While ICU care was once considered mandatory postoperatively, many modern series have demonstrated that many patients can be safely managed on the regular postsurgical floor [34]. In the case of laparoscopic adrenalectomy, patients can often be discharged on postoperative day 1 while patients who have had an open removal may require a longer hospitalization primarily for pain control.

Many groups will obtain a complete blood count 6 h postoperatively, given the hypervascular nature of these tumors. Repeat biochemical testing should be conducted at approximately 6 weeks postoperatively to demonstrate cure. Otherwise, there are no requisite postoperative laboratories until the time of subsequent surveillance for recurrence, which should occur annually. Some authors suggest close monitoring of the patient's blood sugar in the immediate postoperative period, due to the withdrawal of catecholamine stimulation on cellular glucose production.

Malignant and Recurrent Disease

Certain clinical factors are associated with an increased risk of malignancy including increased size, extra-adrenal location, SDHB mutation, and a high methoxytyramine level (a metabolite of dopamine) [19]. However, the only tried and true means of making the diagnosis of malignant pheochromocytoma or paraganglioma is if there is evidence of local invasion or metastatic disease or if there is a recurrence. Final pathology and scoring systems like the pheochromocytoma of the adrenal gland scaled score (PASS) are unable to reliably determine whether the tumor is malignant [35]. Therefore, it is imperative to treat every operation for pheochromocytoma or paraganglioma as a cancer operation and achieve adequate margins. Unfortunately, recurrent disease can present even following complete surgical removal [36]. Recurrence in sporadic cases has been reported at a rate of 14 % for pheochromocytoma and 30 % for paraganglioma [37]. The risk of recurrence in familial disease is 3.4 times that of sporadic disease [37]. Pheochromocytomas and paragangliomas metastasize most commonly to lung, liver, bone,

and lymph nodes [14]. All patients with a history of a pheochromocytoma or paraganglioma, especially those with a known mutation, should undergo yearly biochemical screening for recurrent disease. Given the different biochemical profiles of various familial pheochromocytomas and paragangliomas, the testing should be tailored to maximize the sensitivity and specificity of the screening process. For parasympathetic disease that does not secrete catecholamines, annual screening should be done with the appropriate imaging study.

In the case of metastatic disease, palliative debulking should be considered, given the tumor's biochemical activity. Chemotherapy options are limited but evolving. Results with traditional agents such as cyclophosphamide, vincristine, and dacarbazine have been disappointing, but future options may include LB1, a small molecule inhibitor of serine/threonine protein phosphatase 2A in combination with temzolamide or sunitinib [20]. When surgical palliation is not sufficient, chemical palliation may be achieved with metyrosine. Radiotherapy has been performed with ^{131}I-MIBG, yielding symptomatic improvement, decrease in tumor size, and improvement of the biochemical hormonal profile. Median survival has been reported at 4.7 years after treatment, with those patients who display a hormonal response more likely to experience a survival benefit [22]. Radiofrequency ablation and external beam radiation are also options for surgically inaccessible metastases [14].

Key Summary Points

- Pheochromocytomas and paragangliomas are tumors of the chromaffin cells of the neuroendocrine system involving the adrenal medulla and autonomic nervous system. They usually hypersecrete catecholamines and as such are a cause of secondary hypertension, cardiomyopathy, myocardial infarction, stroke, and death.
- Patients are best screened with plasma metanephrines and the diagnosis is confirmed with a 24-h urine study and subsequently localized with an anatomic study (such as CT or MRI) and a functional scan (such as MIBG or PET).
- Alpha-blockade and fluid resuscitation are the mainstays of preoperative preparation. A patient may be beta-blocked prior to surgery if he or she is tachycardic but beta-blockers must *never* begin until alpha-blockade has been established.
- Consider the diagnosis of pheochromocytoma in the case of any incidentally found adrenal mass and before any biopsy of an adrenal tumor. In general, adrenal biopsies should be avoided.

- Consider a directed genetic workup in the case of pheochromocytoma and especially with paraganglioma given the high rate (35%) of familial disease.
- All patients with pheochromocytoma or paraganglioma should under.go lifelong surveillance for recurrence and metastatic disease.

Disclaimer: The views expressed in this chapter are those of the authors and do not necessarily reflect the official policy or position of the Department of the Navy, Department of Defense, or the US Government.

Michael G. Johnston is a military service member (or employee of the US Government). This work was prepared as part of his official duties. Title 17, USC, § 105 provides that "Copyright protection under this title is not available for any work of the US Government." Title 17, USC, § 101 defines a US Government work as a "work prepared by a military service member or employee of the US Government as part of that person's official duties."

References

1. Maitra A. The endocrine system. In: Kumar V, Abbas AK, Fausto N, Aster JC, editors. Robbins and Cotran Pathologic basis of disease. professional edition, 8th ed. Philadelphia: Saunders Elsevier; 2009. p. 1159–61.
2. Young WF, Jr. Endocrine hypertension. In Melmed S, Polonksy KS, Larsen PR, Kronenberg HM, editors. Williams textbook of endocrinology, 12th ed. Philadelphia: Saunders Elsevier; 2011. p. 545–77.
3. Pick L. Das Ganglioma embryonale sympathicum (sympathoma embryonale), eine typische bösartige geschwuestform des sympathischen nervensystems. Berl Klin Wochenschr. 1912;49:16–22.
4. Eisenhofer G. Screening for pheochromocytomas and paragangliomas. Curr Hyptertens Rep. 2012;14(2):130–7.
5. World Health Organization. Pathology and genetics of tumours of endocrine organs. In: DeLellis RA, LLoyd RV, Heitz PU, Eng C, editors. Lyon: International Agency for Research on Cancer; 2004. ISBN 10: 9283224167/ISBN 13: 9789283224167.
6. Elder E. Pheochromocytoma and functional paraganglioma syndrome: no longer the 10% tumor. J Surg Oncol. 2005;89(3):193–201.
7. Chen H, Sippel RS, Pacak K. The NANETS consensus guideline for the diagnosis and management of neuroendocrine tumors: pheochromocytoma, paraganglioma & medullary thyroid cancer. Pancreas. 2010;39(6):775–83.
8. Lo CY, Lam KY, Wat MS, Lam KS. Adrenal pheochromocytoma remains a frequently overlooked diagnosis. Am J Surg. 2000;179(3):212–5.
9. McNeil AR, Blok BH, Koelmeyer TD, Burke MP, Hilton JM. Phaeochromocytomas discovered during coronial autopsies in Sydney, Melbourne, and Auckland. Aust N Z J Med. 2000;30(6):648–52.
10. Bajwa SS, Bajwa SK. Implications and considerations during pheochromocytoma resection: a challenge to the anesthesiologist. Indian J Endocrinol Metab. 2011;15(4):S337–44.
11. Tsirlin A, Oo Y, Sharma R, Kansara A, Gliwa A, Banerji MA. Pheochromocytoma: a review. Maturitas. 2014;77(3):229–38.
12. Gonzalez Lopez MT, Gonzalez SG, Garcia ES, Romero SG, de Loma JG. Surgical excision with left atrial reconstruction of a primary functioning retrocardiac paraganglioma. J Cardiothorac Surg. 2013;29(8):22.
13. Mazza A, Armigliato M, Marzola MC, Schiavon L, Montemurro D, Vescovo G, et al. Anti-hypertensive treatment in pheochromocytoma and paraganglioma: current management and therapeutic features. Endocrine. 2014;45(3):469–78.
14. Martucci VL, Pacak K. Pheochromocytoma and paraganglioma: diagnosis, genetics, management, and treatment. Curr Probl Cancer. 2014;38(1):7–41.
15. Shuch B, Ricketts CJ, Metwalli AR, Pacak K, Linehan WM. The genetic basis of pheochromocytoma and paraganglioma: implications for management. Urology. 2014;83(6):1225–32.
16. Fishbein L, Orlowski R, Cohen D. Pheochromocytoma/paraganglioma: review of perioperative management of blood pressure and update on genetic mutations associated with pheochromocytoma. J Clin Hypertens. 2013;15(6):428–34.
17. Kudva YC, Sawka AM, Young WF. Clinical review 164: the laboratory diagnosis of adrenal pheochromocytoma: the Mayo Clinic experience. J Clin Endocrinol Metab. 2003;88(10):4533–9.
18. NIH state-of-the-science statement on management of the clinically inapparent adrenal mass (incidentaloma). NIH Consens State Sci Statements. 2002 Feb 4–6;19(2):1–25. PMID: 14768652.
19. Lee JA, Zarnegar R, Shen WT, Kebebew E, Clark OH, Duh QY. Adrenal incidentaloma, borderline elevations of urine or plasma metanephrine levels, and the "subclinical" pheochromocytoma. Arch Surg. 2007;142(9):870–3.
20. Daerr R, Lenders JW, Hofbauer LC, Naumann B, Bornstein SR, Eisenhofer G. Pheochromocytoma—an update on disease management. Ther Adv Endocrinol Metab. 2012;3(1):11–26.
21. Raja A, Leung K, Stamn M, Girgis S, Low G. Multimodality imaging findings of pheochromocytoma with associated clinical and biochemical features in 53 patients with histologically confirmed tumors. Am J Roentgenol. 2013;201(4):825–33.
22. Castellani MR, Aktolun C, Buzzoni R, Seregni E, Chiesa C, Maccauro M, et al. Iodine-131 metaiodobenzylguanidine (I-131 MIBG) diagnosis and therapy of pheochromocytoma and paraganglioma: current problems, critical issues and presentation of a sample case. Q J Nucl Med Mol Imaging. 2013 ;57(2):146–52.
23. Rufini V, Treglia G, Castaldi P, Perotti G, Giordano A. Comparison of metaiodobenzylguanidine scintigraphy with positron emission tomography in the diagnostic work-up of pheochromocytoma and paraganglioma: a systematic review. Q J Nucl Med Mol Imaging. 2013;57(2):122–33.
24. Karasek D, Frysak Z, Pacak K. Genetic testing for pheochromocytoma. Curr Hypertens Rep. 2010;12(6):456–64.
25. Moraitis AG, Martucci VL, Pacak K. Genetics, diagnosis, and management of medullary thyroid carcinoma and pheochromocytoma/paraganglioma. Endocr Pract. 2014;20(2):176–87.
26 Tischler AS, Pacak K, Eisenhofer G. The adrenal medulla and extra-adrenal paraganglia: then and now. Endocr Pathol. 2014 Mar;25(1):49–58.
27. Karasek D, Shah U, Frysak Z, Stratakis C, Pacak K. An update on the genetics of pheochromocytoma. J Hum Hypertens. 2013;27(3):141–7.
28. Domi R, Laho H. Management of pheochromocytoma: old ideas and new drugs. Niger J Clin Pract. 2012;15(3):253–7.
29. Weingarten TN, Cata JP, O'Hara JF, Prybilla DJ, Pike TL et al. Comparison of two preoperative medical management strategies for laparoscopic resection of pheochromocytoma. Urology. 2010;76(2):508.e6–11.
30. Do S-H. Magnesium: a versatile drug for anesthesiologists. Korean J Anesthesiol. 2013;65(1):4–8.

31. Kalady MF, McKinlay R, Olson JA, Jr, Pinheiro J, Lagoo S, Park A, et al. Laparoscopic adrenalectomy for pheochromocytoma: a comparison to aldosteronoma and incidentaloma. Surg Endosc. 2004;18:621–25.

32. Sturgeon C, Kebebew E. Laparoscopic adrenalectomy for malignancy. Surg Clin N Am. 2004;84:755–74.

33. Brunt LM. Minimal access adrenal surgery. Surg Endosc. 2006;20:351–61.

34. Scholten A, Cisco RM, Vriens MR, Cohen JK, Mitmaker EJ, Liu C, et al. Pheochromocytoma crisis is not a surgical emergency. J Clin Endocrinol Metab. 2013;98(2):581–91.

35. Agarwal A, Mehrotra PK, Jain M, Gupta SK, Mishra A, Chand G, et al. Size of the tumor and pheochromocytoma of the adrenal gland scaled score (PASS): can they predict malignancy?. World J Surg. 2010;34(12):3022–8.

36. Lowery AJ, Walsh S, McDermott EW, Prichard RS. Molecular and therapeutic advances in the diagnosis and management of malignant pheochromocytomas and paragangliomas. Oncologist. 2013;18(4):391–407.

37. Amar L, Servais A, Gimenez-Roqueplo AP, Zinzindohoue F, Chatellier G, Plouin PF. Year of diagnosis, features at presentation, and risk of recurrence in patients with pheochromocytoma or secreting paraganglioma. J Clin Endocrinol Metab. 2005;90(4):2110–6.

38. Lin M, Wong V, Yap J, Jin R, Leong P, Campbell P. FDG PET in the evaluation of phaeochromocytoma: a correlative study with MIBG scintigraphy and Ki-67 proliferative index. Clin Imaging. 2013;37(6):1084–8.

Charles Horace Mayo

1855–1939

Jon A. van Heerden

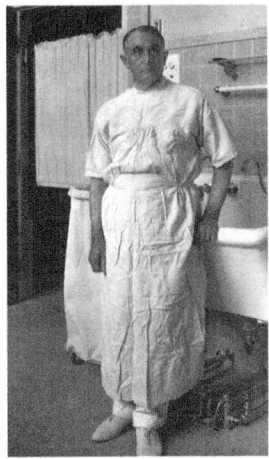

Dr. Charlie in scrubs

To have a continuing, tangible influence on the daily activities of a large medical institution, a century and a half after its origin, and 75 years after his own death, is a remarkable accomplishment.

Thus it was, and is, for C. H. (Charlie) Mayo. A perusal of his many wise aphorisms may give us some insight into the soul and spirit of this unique surgeon, affectionately known as Dr. Charlie [1–5].

> Carry out the two fundamental surgical requirements: see what you are doing and leave a dry field.

He was well renowned for his surgical dexterity and amazingly broad surgical practice which ranged from general, to urologic, to orthopedic, and even to neurosurgery. In 1937, his brother (**Dr William Mayo**) in an interview said, "Charlie had the widest scope of surgical ability of any man I have ever known. My field was restricted from the beginning to a few areas of the body, abdomen-pelvis-kidney, which I

developed one by one. Charlie seemed to have the ability to open up all fields." Indeed, Dr. Charlie's gift for excelling within all surgical disciplines lay in his tenacity for assuring that simplistic fundamental surgical principles were carried out: expose the diseased organ clearly, and maximize hemostasis with a meticulous technique. Although he considered himself a "simple surgeon," his adherence to these two surgical principles led him to a legendary career in surgery.

> Once you start studying medicine, you'll never get through with it.

Dr. Charlie had a lifelong passion for learning—both he and his brother assiduously set aside time each evening for scientific reading. If they were forced to miss their hour of reading for whatever reason, they made sure that they made up this "missed time" by doubling up on future sessions.

> More good would come to our country through tongue control than birth control.

In the operating room, hospital, and clinic, idle chatter was frowned upon by the Mayo brothers. They were the same at home; precise and concise use of the spoken language was deeply admired. This was their manner of speech, and especially so for Dr. Charlie.

> After all, the only thing a man can finally take with him is the love and respect of his fellow citizens. The more one forgets himself, the more the love, esteem and approbation of his fellow citizens.

Dr. Charlie loved his fellow man/woman. He was a loving husband, a gentle, but strict father, and a respected yet distant educator. All the while, he possessed a great sense of humor—what a unique combination of human traits.

What then was the pathway that led Dr. Charlie from humble beginnings to leaving an enduring legacy on what is today the largest, integrated, not-for-profit, private multispecialty medical practice in the world?

J. A. van Heerden (✉)
General Surgery, Medical University of South Carolina, 96 Jonathan Lucas Street, Charleston 29425-6730, SC, USA

J. L. Pasieka, J. A. Lee (eds.), *Surgical Endocrinopathies*, DOI 10.1007/978-3-319-13662-2_39,
© Springer International Publishing Switzerland 2015

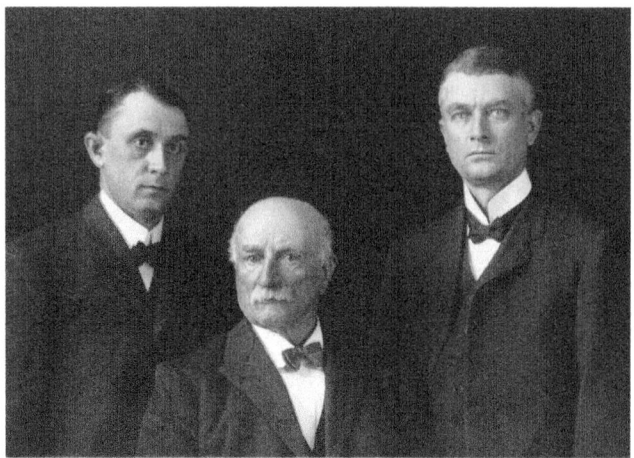

Fig. 1 Drs Will, WW, and Charlie

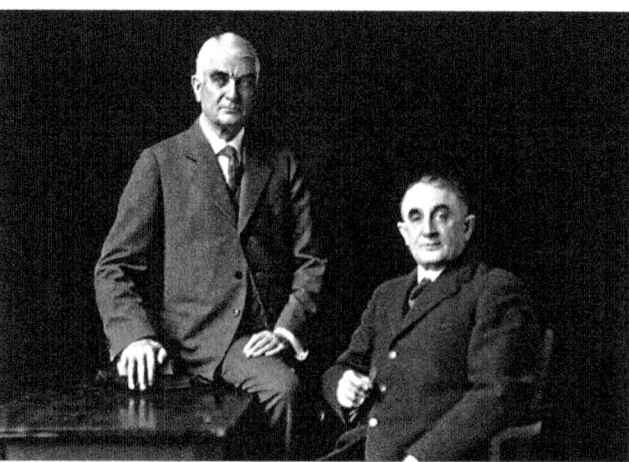

Fig. 2 Brothers Will (*left*) and Charlie

Charles Horace Mayo (CHM) was born in Rochester, Minnesota, in 1865 and died in Chicago, Illinois, in 1939. He was the younger son of Dr. William Worrall Mayo (Dr. WW) and Louise Abigail Wright Mayo. Dr. WW, who had emigrated from Manchester, England, in 1846, opened a solo medical practice in Rochester, Minnesota, in January of 1864. He was subsequently joined in practice by his eldest son William in 1883. The seed of Mayo Clinic was germinating.

CHM graduated with his medical degree from the Chicago Medical College in 1888 after 3 years of study before joining his father and brother in practice (Fig. 1).

An act of nature and the love of brothers are both noteworthy and significant. In 1883, a tornado devastated the town of Rochester. The Franciscan nuns and the Mayos came together in response to this tragedy with the Sisters funding construction of a hospital (Saint Mary's) and the Mayos providing medical and surgical care for its patients. The hospital was finished as Charlie graduated medical school. What an alignment of the cosmos!

The lifelong relationship between Charlie and Will was unique. Each brother, without exception, spoke of their accomplishments in terms of "my brother and I"—a phrase which was frequently the opening salvo of a scientific presentation or a public address. When called into consultation on a complex patient, each would independently request that the medical team have the other brother see the patient as well. They practiced the philosophy that "no man is big enough to be independent of others" and, in doing so, in a collegial fashion led to the inner core of the Mayo Clinic, then and now, which is: "the needs of the patient come first" and that "the best interest of the patient is the only interest to be considered." It is not a surprise that both brothers died within months of each other in 1939. Dr. Charlie succumbed to pneumonia—he was 73 years young (Fig. 2). In 1937,

Dr. Will reflected on this unique brotherly bond. "When our opportunity came, we were prepared. We had travelled, observed, and applied. And because of this we were able to do all sorts of surgery, and do it better than many of the older surgeons of wider operative experience. We were successful because we were two men who loved each other and had absolute confidence in each other, who lived out of the same purse, who were anxious to do what we could, who came into activity at just the right time in the development of medicine and surgery. My brother was quiet, studious, and friendly, interested in people and was the most loveable man I have ever known. He never gave me a cross word and I needed it often, because when I got my eye on the ball, I went ahead, regardless. The whole point was that I was the cavalry leader, Charlie brought up the infantry and when he got there, the big guns began to roar. If I did not already have the enemy on the retreat, he soon did. Charlie is truly a gentle man, salt and pepper, but never mustard. He has never desired to develop what would rebound especially to his own credit. He had, I think, the least self-glorification of any man I know who had accomplished great things."

It is worthy of reflection to consider just what it was that led from such a minute, embryonic beginning, to an institution that has today an annual budget of US$ 8.8 billion dollars, sees more than a million patients annually, does 500 + operations daily, and employs 4100 physicians-scientists as well as 53,600 allied personnel. And amazingly, each of these health-care professionals know about Dr. Charlie and Dr. Will and continue to carry out their original ideals to the betterment of mankind.

Drs. Pasieka and Lee have been insightful in suggesting "a couple of words" about Charles Mayo following this chapter. They felt that this commentary would be incomplete if the brief story of Dr. Charlie and Sister Mary Joachim was not told. It is the story of the first successful resection of a pheochromocytoma which was not diagnosed prior to resection, in North America.

Sister Joachim was a 30-year-old nun from Chatham in Ontario, Canada, who was referred to the Mayo Clinic in June of 1926 by Dr. J. H. Duncan because of "spells" that he felt were due to an "incompetent liver." She was hospitalized in Saint Mary's Hospital "for observation of spells" for a full 5 months! During observation of her many spells, she was tremulous, perspired profusely, and had blood pressures that ranged from 100/70 to 280/190 mmHg. An excretory urogram suggested the presence of a left juxta-renal mass. Dr. Charlie was called in consultation. He felt that she was most likely functional but there was a possibility that the mass might be "secreting toxins" which were "affecting the sympathetic." He recommended resection.

Resection was performed on October 11, 1926, under open-drop mask ether and ethylene. No intravenous or central lines were placed, and she had no urinary catheter. The operation, skin to skin, lasted 56 min. The tumor was enucleated with no vascular ligation taking place. Blood loss was severe with a large pack being left in place in an attempt to control the bleeding. Dr. Charlie thought that the mass was an "enormous enlargement of the ganglion which rested on the renal vessels." When he bisected the enucleated mass, he commented that "it resembled brain tissue."

Mary Joachim's only "stimulants" during her precarious recovery were coffee enemas which sustained her blood pressure at 90 mmHg systolic! She miraculously rallied and left for Chatham on December 13—almost 6 months after her admission.

Dr. Charlie had a long-standing friendship with Dr. **Harvey Cushing** at the Peter Bent Brigham Hospital in Boston, Massachusetts. They exchanged correspondence about Mary Joachim with Dr. Cushing being intrigued by her paroxysmal hypertension. He pondered to Dr. Charlie: "Should the growth have recurred, one would naturally expect a recurrence of her former symptoms of hypertension. I am puzzling my mind over some hypertensions now under observation here."

After her return to Canada, she led a productive life as a nun who loved to teach music. She died of a myocardial infarct in 1944, 18 years after her operation by Dr. Charlie.

Medicine gives only to those who give, but her reward for those who serve is finer than much fine gold. 1926–CHM

Dr. Charlie was a shining example of just such a man.

References

1. Olsen KD, Dacy MD. Mayo Clinic—150 years of serving humanity through hope and healing. Mayo Clin Proc. 2014:89(1):8–15.
2. Berry LL, Seltman KD. Management lessons from Mayo Clinic: inside one of the world's most admired service organizations. New York: McGraw Hill; 2008.
3. Mayo CH. Tomorrow's education seen by Dr. Mayo. In: Northwestern University Alumni News vol. 10. Evanston: Northwestern University; 1931.
4. Clapsattle H. The doctors Mayo. 1st ed. Minneapolis: University of Minnesota Press; 1941.
5. Mayo CH. When does disease begin? Can this be determined by health examination? Minn Med. 1932;15(1):40–42.

Arthur M. Shipley

1878–1955

Minerva Angélica Romero Arenas, Jon A. van Heerden and Nancy Dugal Perrier

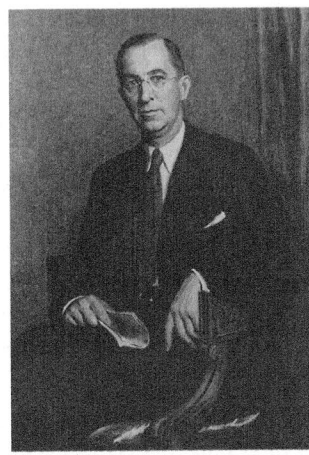

Portrait of Dr. Arthur M. Shipley. (Reproduction by Mark Teske, professional photographer at University of Maryland School of Medicine)

Introduction

Dr. Arthur M. Shipley was a renowned American surgeon and native Marylander. In 1911, Dr. Shipley was appointed chairman of surgery at the University of Maryland in Baltimore. He was a wartime surgeon and published 80 diverse manuscripts ranging from femoral fractures to dehisced abdominal incisions. Of historical significance is the fact that Dr. Shipley resected the first preoperatively diagnosed pheochromocytoma on June 27, 1928. He was well known by his contemporaries as a clinician with compulsive attention to detail and in-depth knowledge of the medical and surgical literature. Dr. Shipley was elected to membership in the Southern Surgical Association in 1927, and in 1943 served as vice president of the American Surgical Association. He remained at the University of Maryland School of Medicine until his retirement in 1948 (Fig. 1).

Background

Dr. Shipley was a fifth-generation member of the Shipley family and was born in Maryland in 1878 to Roderick O. and Wilhelmina Clark Shipley. As a student at the University of Maryland School of Medicine, Dr. Shipley maintained a brilliant scholastic record and was recognized as a man of great potential. He graduated in 1902 serving important administrative hospital duties as a senior resident. During the First World War (1917–1919), Dr. Shipley was chief of surgical services at the 8th American Evacuation Hospital in Juilly, France [1]. This position afforded him the opportunity to see many soldiers with infected and nonhealing wounds. In this regard, he wrote, "These wounds were all heavily infected. The streptococci exist in various strains, some are more vicious than others and have an uncanny ability to break down the local defenses of the body. The time (for aggressive early treatment) factor was most important" [2].

In 1911, at the early age of 33 years, he became professor of surgery and chief of the surgical service at the University of Maryland (1911). This position provided an opportunity for the exercise and development of his gifts as a teacher and organizer. He was widely recognized as one of the outstanding teachers of clinical surgery in the USA, with a broad base of knowledge, expert organization, and a forceful and stimulating method of presentation.

Endocrine Surgery

Dr. **Charles Mayo** is credited with resecting the first pheochromocytoma in the USA. This resection was performed in 1926 on the now famous patient, Sister Joachim. That it was a pheochromocytoma was, however, determined only by the final postoperative pathologic determination of the specimen [3]. The honor of resecting the first preoperatively

N. Dugal Perrier (✉)
Surgical Oncology, MD Anderson Cancer Center, The University of Texas, 1400 Pressler Dr., Unit 1484, Houston, TX 77030, USA
e-mail: NPerrier@mdanderson.org

M. A. Romero Arenas
Surgery, Sinai Hospital of Baltimore, Baltimore, MD, USA

J. A. van Heerden
General Surgery, Medical University of South Carolina, Charleston, SC, USA

J. L. Pasieka, J. A. Lee (eds.), *Surgical Endocrinopathies*, DOI 10.1007/978-3-319-13662-2_40,
© Springer International Publishing Switzerland 2015

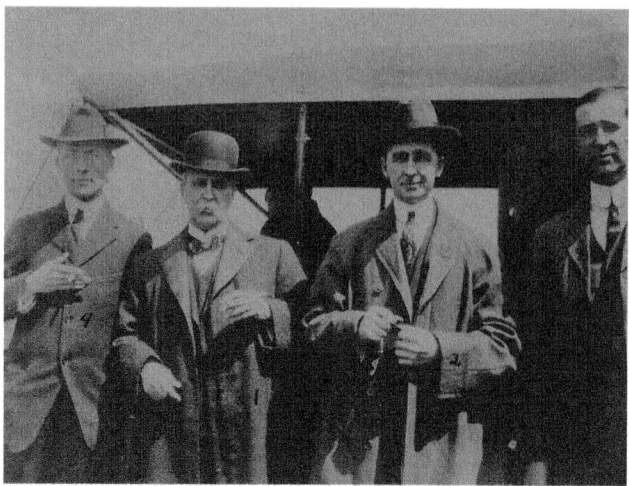

Fig. 1 Dr. Arthur M. Shipley and other prominent surgeons at the old Baltimore City Hospital (now Johns Hopkins Bayview), 1913—from *left to right*, Thomas Boggs, William Osler, Thomas B. Futcher, and Shipley

diagnosed pheochromocytoma belongs clearly to Dr. Shipley. In 1928, Dr. Shipley was called in consultation on a patient by the chairman of medicine in Baltimore, Dr. Maurice C. Pincoffs. The patient was a 26-year-old woman with worsening "attacks with palpitation of the heart" over a 10-year period. In addition to what would now be considered classical, paroxysmal hypertensive attacks, the patient had a positive family history. Interestingly, her sister had a superior mediastinal mass "which interfered with breathing and caused distention of the neck vessels." Physical examination of the patient revealed nothing remarkable at rest; however, during the attacks, her blood pressure rose from 120/90 to 219/110 mmHg and she was observed to have facial flushing, tremulous hands, tachycardia, and hyperpnoea. A preoperative diagnosis of a medullary tumor of the adrenal gland was made by Doctor Pincoffs. Because cross-sectional imaging and biochemical profiles were not available until the next decade, Shipley had no information about the characteristics of the suspected mass, or of its laterality. Dr. Shipley pondered: "The thing that immediately concerned us was to determine which gland was involved." Undaunted, Dr. Shipley planned an elective exploratory operation on June 14, 1928.

The peritoneal cavity was entered via a high left rectus incision and the retroperitoneum and perirenal area were carefully explored and it was determined that no tumor was present on the left side. The right side of the abdomen was then palpated and a large mass was felt above the kidney. "It could not be reached through the left rectus incision and so it was decided to close the abdomen and wait until healing had taken place and then to approach the tumor through a different incision." Thirteen days later, the patient underwent the planned reoperation.

After mobilizing the right colon, the tumor was visualized. "It was smooth, almost as large as the patient's kidney and lay immediately above and in contact with the kidney and was tucked up close to the undersurface of the liver; laterally it lay against the posterior abdominal wall and medially it was abutting the inferior vena cava for several inches." Shipley described the tumor as being firm, smooth, and surrounded by areolar tissue containing numerous vessels (Fig. 2). Multiple clamps were "applied wherever veins were visible" and hemorrhage was noted below the tumor and between the tumor and kidney. Shipley noted the direct return of venous blood to the inferior vena cava, and that "considerable difficulty was encountered in finding room enough between the tumor and the vena cava to apply clamps." Once removed, "some bleeding in this area and a good deal of anxiety was felt in controlling it, as it was feared that the vena cava would be torn". Altogether, the patient lost about 8 oz. of blood.

During the operation, Dr. Pincoffs maintained a careful record of the patient's blood pressure. Shipley wrote, "The patient's blood pressure varied sharply during the operation and she was infused on the table with normal salt solution." "The patient left the table badly shocked and her blood pressure remained very low for hours after the operation. Her condition during this time was critical," he writes. By the first postoperative day, the patient's condition markedly improved and she was reported to be free from attacks at 10 months following the operation. Her only complication was a thrombophlebitis of a leg that responded to treatment within a few days. Pathology found an encapsulated tumor of the adrenal medulla weighing 115 g and measuring $9 \times 7 \times 3.5$ cm. Gross examination revealed hemorrhage. On microscopic evaluation, the tumor tissue was positive on chromaffin staining and was diagnosed as a paraganglioma.

This event generated a publication in the *Annals of Surgery* in November 1929 entitled, "Paroxysmal Hypertension Associated with Tumor of the Suprarenal" (Fig. 3) [4]. Only 30 cases of medullary tumors had been reported in the literature at that time. Dr. Shipley noted, "No one has proven, up to the present that an increase of epinephrine is found in the blood of patients with hypertension." "The clinical aspects

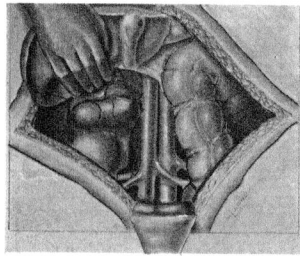

Fig. 2 Illustration of the resected specimen (from Dr. Shipley's 1929 manuscript). (Courtesy of UAB Archives, University of Alabama at Birmingham)

of the patient's case were described as those not resembling any type of paroxysmal hypertension previously seen." It is noteworthy that Dr. **George Crile**, of Cleveland, Ohio, was in the audience and urged caution in proclaiming an effect of the tumor on the patient's blood pressure. Describing his own experience of 12 cases, Crile was noted to be "unconvinced that he produced any results" since the patients' blood pressures would run an irregular course postoperatively.

PAROXYSMAL HYPERTENSION ASSOCIATED WITH TUMOR OF THE SUPRARENAL

BY ARTHUR M. SHIPLEY, M.D.
OF BALTIMORE, MD.

THIS report has to do *with paroxysmal hypertension* associated with *tumors of the medulla of the suprarenal body*. The patient whose case is reported was referred to me by Dr. Maurice C. Pincoffs, who reported the point of view of diagnosis and clinical aspects before the Association of American Physicians on May 8. Portions of the tumor after removal were used for experimental work by Dr. William H. Shultz, and the three of us will publish a full report of all phases of the case later.

We are not concerned in this report with tumors of the suprarenal cortex. The medulla of the suprarenals is a part of the chromaffin system which is not confined to the suprarenal body. The two portions of the suprarenal, cortex and medulla develop from entirely different tissues; the cortex develops from the mesoderm. "The immediate anlage of the suprarenal medulla and the anlages of the remainder of the chromaffin organs lie in the sympathetic ganglions, which, in turn, are derived from the cells of the neural crest." These primitive cells of the ganglions are called sympathogonia or the sympathetic formative cells. In early fœtal life these cells migrate laterally toward the suprarenals. "During the migration, portions of the embryonic tissue may become split off; these develop as separate organs at varying distances from the aorta in the region of the renal arteries or the inferior mesenteric artery to form the organs of Zuckerkandl."

The first report of a tumor of the medulla of the suprarenal body was by Berdez,[1] in 1892. That these tumors may be associated with hypertension was pointed out by Neusser,[2] in 1898, who reported two tumors of the adrenals described by him as carcinoma. Vaquez,[3] in 1904, associated hypertension with increase of epinephrin in the blood. No one has proven, up to the present, that an increase of epinephrin is found in the blood in patients with hypertension. Many clinical observations in patients with chromaffin cell tumors of the suprarenal glands indicate that this is true, but the proof is not forthcoming.

Oppenheimer and Fishberg[4] give three varieties of tumors derived from the medulla of the suprarenal.

1. Sympathoblastomas, made up of immature sympathoblasts.

2. Ganglioneuromas, consisting of relatively mature sympathetic ganglion cells.

3. Paragangliomas, which is the type of tumor with which we are concerned in this paper. These are rare tumors and Rabin[5] was able to find only thirty cases in the literature, and in an excellent article in the *Archives of Pathology* for February, 1929, he discusses these cases and reports one of his own.

742

Fig. 3 Manuscript published in *Annals of Surgery*, 1929. (Courtesy of UAB Archives, University of Alabama at Birmingham)

Legacy

The inaugural publication of *Reflexions* by the senior class of the School of Medicine and Nursing was dedicated to Dr. Shipley in 1946. The dedication text reads: To Arthur Marriott Shipley, surgeon, student, teacher and gentleman this first edition of *Reflexions* is dedicated as an expression of the admiration and esteem held for him by those of us who have come under his influence. May we in the days ahead pause to remember the sincerity of the efforts and wisdom of the teachings of the man known affectionately as "King Arthur."

Dr. Arthur M. Shipley retired from the University of Maryland in 1948 and died 7 years later in 1955 at the age of 77 years. In paying tribute, Dr. Stone wrote, "To the medical world and to younger men in the profession, his death meant the passing of a prominent figure. To those close to him, it meant the loss of a desired example and of a beloved friend." To the current endocrine surgeon, his death meant the passing of a giant who epitomized the most sound of clinical and surgical judgment. Today, an accurate preoperative endocrine diagnosis and tumor localization is a daily given. The courage and surgical fortitude to blindly explore a patient with a pheochromocytoma is worthy of wondrous contemplation and admiration.

References

1. Roderick E, Arthur Shipley papers, Special Collections, University of Maryland Libraries. http://hdl.handle.net/1903.1/1288. Accessed 19 Feb 2015.
2. Shipley AM, Considine AT. The officers and nurses of evacuation eight, with a complete roster of all those who served with the unit. New Haven: Yale University Press; 1929. http://Hdl.Handle.Net/2027/Mdp.39015027342719. Accessed 19 Feb 2015.
3. Mayo C.H. Paroxysmal hypertension with tumor of the retroperitoneal nerve. JAMA. Sept 1927;89(13):1047–50. doi:10.1001/jama.1927.02690130035013.
4. Shipley AM. Paroxysmal hypertension associated with tumor of the suprarenal. Ann Surg. 1929; 90: 742–9.

Emil Zuckerkandl

1849–1910

Leigh W. Delbridge

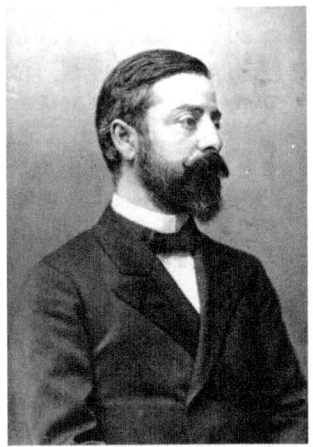

Emil Zuckerkandl. (Circa 1890, author unknown, public domain)

Emil Zuckerkandl was born on September 1, 1849, in Györ, Hungary, and died on May 28, 1910, in Vienna. He was a professor and anatomist whose name is well known to endocrine surgeons for his description of two important anatomical entities: the "tubercle of Zuckerkandl" in the neck and the "organ of Zuckerkandl" in the abdomen.

Zuckerkandl studied medicine at the University of Vienna in 1867, completing his degree in 1874. His younger brother, Otto, also studied medicine and went on to become a professor and urologist in Vienna. Emil was an exceptionally able student who so impressed his anatomy teacher, Joseph Hyrtl, at the Vienna School of Anatomy, that he was appointed as a demonstrator in anatomy, and later sent to the University of Utrecht in Amsterdam as a prosector. In 1873, he returned to Vienna to work with Langer at the Vienna School of Anatomy, the world's leading anatomy center for over half a century [1]. Following the death of Langer in 1888, he assumed

the chair of descriptive and topographic anatomy in Vienna. In 1905, Zuckerkandl edited Heitzmann's *Atlas of Descriptive Anatomy of Man,* with over 600 illustrations. As professor, he was noted for his observational powers and critical appraisal. He made significant contributions to normal and pathological anatomy and was known to anatomists and surgeons from around the world as the most indefatigable worker. He published over 160 papers, although the writer of his obituary, published in *The Lancet* in 1910, did note that he was "a patient and diligent worker, too ready to publish perhaps, and somewhat urgent and short-sighted in his claims for priority" [2].

The organ of Zuckerkandl (Fig. 1) was described by Zuckerkandl in 1901 [3] and comprises a collection of chromaffin cells located between the origin of the inferior mesenteric artery and the aortic bifurcation. It is thought to have a physiologic function in early gestation in relation to blood pressure control; however, it regresses late in the third trimester. Its importance to endocrine surgeons arises from its propensity to be a site in which extra-adrenal pheochromocytoma may develop.

The subsequent year, in 1902, he published his description of the tubercle of Zuckerkandl [4]. Prior to this, he had in fact described aspects of thyroid anatomy during his dissections of the oral cavity, noting in 1878 the presence of "glandular masses with the structure of thyroid, embedded in the tongue above the hyoid" (presumably a lingual thyroid). In his drawings of the tubercle of Zuckerkandl (Fig. 2), a clear appreciation of the relationship between a posterolateral projection of thyroid tissue immediately lying adjacent to the normal position of the superior parathyroid gland can be seen. Although its clinical significance was almost certainly appreciated by Zuckerkandl at the time, knowledge of the structure was lost to endocrine surgeons until "rediscovered" decades later [5]. The tubercle of Zuckerkandl is now considered to be the key to understanding the surgical anatomy of the thyroid and parathyroid glands [6]. The vascular relationship of the tubercle of Zuckerkandl to the superior parathyroid gland and the terminal part of the recurrent laryngeal

L. W. Delbridge (✉)
Surgery, University of Sydney, PO Box 3, St. Leonards, Sydney, NSW 2065, Australia
e-mail: leighd@med.usyd.edu.au

J. L. Pasieka, J. A. Lee (eds.), *Surgical Endocrinopathies,* DOI 10.1007/978-3-319-13662-2_41,
© Springer International Publishing Switzerland 2015

is critical to safe thyroid lobectomy, [7] while failure to appreciate nodular change within the tubercle of Zuckerkandl (Fig. 3) is a common cause of recurrent disease after total thyroidectomy [8].

In fact, Zuckerkandl's name is associated with considerably more eponymous anatomical structures than just those two structures hitherto described which are of primary interest to endocrine surgeons. There are at least seven anatomical structures that bear his name. In addition to the organ of Zuckerkandl and the tubercle of Zuckerkandl, Emil also described: the concha of Zuckerkandl—a rarely found small nasal concha situated above the supreme nasal concha; Zuckerkandl's dehiscence—small gaps occasionally seen in the layers of the ethmoid bone; Zuckerkandl's gyrus (Zuckerkandl's convolution)—the thin sheet of gray/white

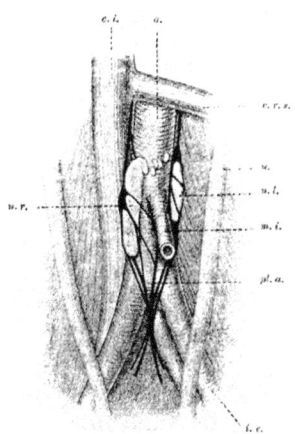

Fig. 1 Zuckerkandl's drawing of the "organ of Zuckerkandl." (Public domain, [3])

substance in front of, and ventral to, the genu of the corpus callosum; Zuckerkandl's fascia—the posterior layer of the renal fascia; and the suprapleural membrane of Zuckerkandl and Sebileau—a thickening of connective tissue covering the lung apex [1].

While this list of structures is at first sight seemingly random, there was a clear link throughout his research career leading him to uncover and describe each in turn. That lifetime link was carefully outlined by the anonymous author of his obituary in *The Lancet* [2] in which is described how the many different lines of research all began from his very first observation, made at the age of 26 when he was an acting prosector at the School of Anatomy in Vienna. At that point in time, very early in his career, Zuckerkandl obtained a collection of human cranial specimens brought home from an expedition of the Austrian ship *Novara*. He compared these skulls to the collection of over 300 crania already held in the department and published a monograph entitled *Morphology of the Facial Skeleton* in 1877. In this, he determined that the shape and structure of the nasal cavities were the determining factor of cranial shape, leading to further extensive research into the structure and function of the nasal cavity and respiratory tract. In subsequent publications, including *Comparative Anatomy of the Nasal Cavities* and *Anatomy and Diseases of the Nose,* he described the concha of Zuckerkandl (one of the nasal conchae) and Zuckerkandl's dehiscence in the ethmoid bone. When he was appointed to the chair of anatomy in Vienna, his research on the nose led him to investigate adjacent regions of the body, with the aim of understanding the incidence and pathogenesis of diseases of the nasopharynx, laryngopharynx, and neck. Over ensuing years, he undertook further research on adjacent anatomical structures including the thyroid, thymus, trachea, and airways

Fig. 2 Zuckerkandl's drawing of the tubercle demonstrating the clear relationship with the superior parathyroid glands. ([4])

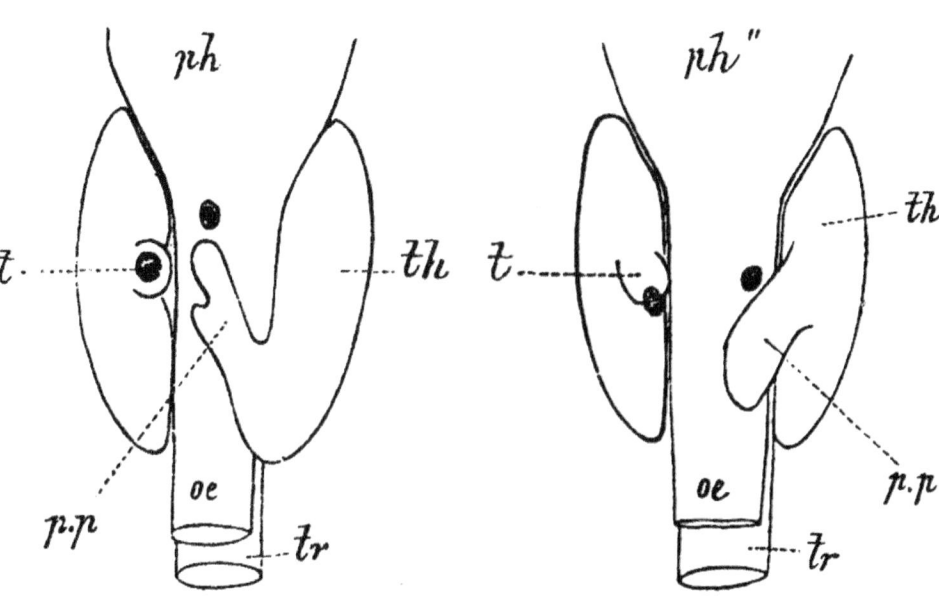

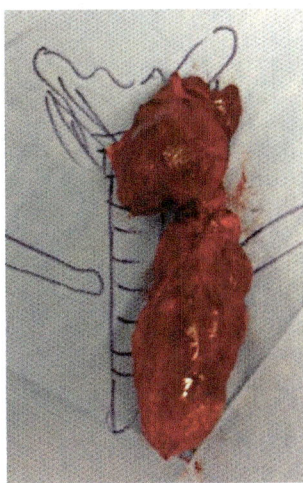

Fig. 3 Very large retrosternal nodule arising from the tubercle of Zuckerkandl on the posterolateral border of the left thyroid lobe, then passing down alongside the esophagus to enter the posterior superior mediastinum

(during which he described the suprapleural membrane of Zuckerkandl and Sebileau). Following on from his research interest in the nasal cavities, Zuckerkandl also began investigating the anatomy of the brain, with a view to locating the center for smell and in 1900 he published a paper on the olfactory center. His study of the brain led to the description of Zuckerkandl's gyrus, also known as Zuckerkandl's convolution, ventral to the corpus callosum. His study of the brain and the intricacy of its arterial supply was also responsible for his other principal research interest, namely the arterial system. He published further monographs on the anatomy and development of the arteries of the forearm before turning his attention to the pelvis and lower limb with the publication of *Morphology of the Arteries of the Extremities* in 1907. It was this research that led him to observe and separately describe the organ of Zuckerkandl, extraadrenal chromaffin tissue at the aortic bifurcation, and Zuckerkandl's fascia, posterior to the kidney.

Zuckerkandl was also one of those famous men of science who is remembered as much for his wife, Berta Zuckerkandl-Szeps, as for his own scientific contributions. Berta was one of the most remarkable personalities of the intellectual Jewish society in Vienna during the last decades of the Austro-Hungarian Empire. She was the daughter of the editor of Vienna's leading morning newspaper *Morgenpost* and

the sister-in-law of the French Prime Minister Clemenceau, and after her marriage to Emil, she went on to become a renowned journalist in her own right. Their house became the meeting point for the avant-garde in arts and science, including Auguste Rodin (sculptor), Gustav Mahler (composer), Gustav Klimt (painter), Otto Wagner (architect), Hermann Bahr (writer), and Arthur Schnitzler (playwright) [1].

Emil Zuckerkandl was clearly a great man of science in the tradition of his time. Shoja [1] comments that Emil Zuckerkandl left a tremendous legacy regarding anatomical knowledge and was credited with the statement that "anatomy is the war map for the operations of the physician." Despite having as his major interest the study of human anatomy and morphology rather than being engaged in clinical practice, he never lost sight of the fundamental principle underlying medical research. The final paragraph of his obituary [2] commends the deceased Zuckerkandl for "keeping steadfastly in mind that the medical man studies the human body with the object of understanding and curing disease." As such, he endeavored to make the study of anatomy "subservient" to clinical practice and is credited with being the father of clinical anatomy [1].

References

1 Shoja MM, Tubbs RS, Loukas M, Shokouhif W, Oakes J. Emil Zuckerkandl (1849–1910): anatomist and pathologist. Ann Anat. 2008;190:33–6.

2 Anonymous. Obituary—Professor Emil Zuckerkandl. The Lancet. 1910 (June 4); 175(4527): 1564–65.

3 Zuckerkandl, E. Ueber Nebenorgane des Sympathicus im Retroperitonealraum des Menschen. Verhandl Anat Ges. 1901;15:85–107.

4 Zuckerkandl, E. Die Epithelkorperchen von Didelphys Azara (Epithelkorperchen des Menchen). Vienna, 1902;19(1):59–84.

5 Pelizzo MR, Toniato A, Gemo G. Zuckerkandl's tuberculum: an arrow pointing to the recurrent laryngeal nerve (constant anatomical landmark). J Am Coll Surg. 1998;187:333–36.

6 Gauger PG, Delbridge LW, Thompson NW, Crummer P, Reeve TS. Incidence and importance of the tubercle of Zuckerkandl in thyroid surgery. Eur J Surg. 2001;167:249–54.

7 Serpell JW. New operative surgical concept of two fascial layers enveloping the recurrent laryngeal nerve. Ann Surg Oncol. 2010 17:1628–36.

8 Snook KL, Stalberg PL, Sidhu SB, Sywak MS, Edhouse P, Delbridge L. Recurrence after total thyroidectomy for benign multinodular goiter. World J Surg. 2007 31:593–8.

Insulinomas

Jane S. Lee and William B. Inabnet III

Historical Background

Paul Langerhans discovered and described pancreatic islet cells while he was still a medical student in 1869 [1]. It was not until 1922 that insulin was successfully extracted from canine pancreatic tissue by the works of **Banting** and **Best** [1]. A year later, Banting et al. described symptoms of hypoglycemia from insulin excess [3]. That same year, Harris discussed the possibility of hyperinsulinism as a disease process [4]. In 1927, **Charles Mayo** described a case of hyperinsulinism from a pancreatic tumor [4]. Graham performed the first successful surgical resection of an insulinoma, which was reported in 1929 [4]. In 1935, **Whipple** and Frantz described the diagnostic triad that defines insulinoma [4].

Epidemiology

Insulinomas are the most common functioning neuroendocrine tumors of the pancreas. However, they are rare tumors with an incidence of approximately one to four per million population. There have been some autopsy studies showing a higher incidence, consisting of 0.8–10% of the population [5].

Insulinomas can occur at any age with a mean around 50 years and are slightly more predominant in females [6]. The majority of these tumors are benign, solitary, and relatively small in size (<2 cm). Most are located in the pancreas with an even distribution throughout the pancreatic head, body, and tail. Extrapancretic occurrences are rare, reported to be less than 2%, and these are mainly found in the duodenal wall [7].

The majority of insulinomas are sporadic; however, 5–10% are associated with multiple endocrine neoplasia type 1 (MEN-1) syndrome. Also known as *Wermer's* syndrome, MEN-1 is an autosomal dominant disorder with a mutation in the *menin* gene on chromosome 11q13 [8, 9]. The syndrome consists of parathyroid hyperplasia, anterior pituitary adenomas, and tumors of the endocrine pancreas and duodenum. Insulinomas associated with MEN-1 develop earlier in life and are frequently multicentric, with higher risk of recurrence (21% at 10 and 20 years) compared to patients without MEN-1 (5% at 10 years, 7% at 20 years) [6]. Malignant insulinomas are characterized by local invasion into surrounding soft tissue or metastasis to liver, lymph nodes, bone, and peritoneum, occurring in 5–15% of cases [10, 11].

Anatomy and Physiology

Normal blood glucose levels are closely regulated between 60 and 100 mg/dL in a negative feedback system [12]. The consumption of food increases blood glucose levels, which, in turn, stimulates insulin production. The reverse is true when blood glucose levels are low. Insulin production decreases in response to low blood glucose levels. Insulinomas are characterized by intermittent insulin secretion by tumor cells even during times of low glucose, leading to episodes of symptomatic fasting hypoglycemia [7]. In patients with insulinoma, insulin production by normal beta cells is suppressed.

At the cellular level, rodent models have allowed the discovery of the mechanisms of insulin secretion and its regulation. Elevated levels of glucose induce glycolysis and the citrate cycle, increasing the ratio of intracellular adenosine triphosphate (ATP) to adenosine diphosphate (ADP), leading to closure of ATP-sensitive potassium channels [13, 14]. Plasma membrane depolarization opens voltage-dependent calcium channels, resulting in action potentials and calcium influx into the cell, triggering calcium-dependent exocytosis of insulin granules [13, 14]. There are important variations in humans, including involvement of voltage-gated sodium channels in the process [13, 14].

W. B. Inabnet III (✉)
Chairman, Department of Surgery, Mount Sinai Beth Israel, First Ave at 16th St., Baird Hall, 16th Floor, Suite 20, New York, NY 10003, USA
e-mail: william.inabnet@mountsinai.org

J. S. Lee
Surgery, Mount Sinai Hospital, New York, NY 10029, USA

J. L. Pasieka, J. A. Lee (eds.), *Surgical Endocrinopathies*, DOI 10.1007/978-3-319-13662-2_42,
© Springer International Publishing Switzerland 2015

Clinical Presentation

Patients present with episodes of hypoglycemia with associated symptoms. The diagnosis of insulinoma, although rare, should be considered in the differential for fasting hypoglycemia in an otherwise healthy patient. Patients can present with an array of symptoms categorized into adrenergic and neuroglycopenic symptoms. Adrenergic symptoms caused by catecholamine secretion consist of anxiety, diaphoresis, tremors, palpitations, and hunger [15, 16]. Many of these patients gain weight resulting in obesity due to the frequent meals and snacks they consume to relieve hypoglycemic symptoms. Neuroglycopenic symptoms are caused by the low glucose supply to the nervous system and may consist of headache, dizziness, confusion, behavioral changes, personality changes, visual disturbances, amnesia, and in rare cases seizures and coma (Table 1) [15, 16].

These symptoms present in the fasting state and can become evident following physical exertion. They normally occur at plasma glucose levels less than 50 mg/dL, and central nervous system (CNS) symptoms mainly present at plasma glucose levels less than 45 mg/dL [5]. Some patients may not manifest significant symptoms even with significant hypoglycemia, which is termed hypoglycemic unawareness, when the CNS adapts to frequent episodes of hypoglycemia [17].

Diagnosis

Patients often present with bizarre symptoms not unique to hypoglycemia. These patients are often falsely diagnosed with psychiatric or neurologic disorders, resulting in a delay in diagnosis of insulinoma. The mean duration to diagnosis has been reported to range from several months to even more than several decades. One study reported a median of 18 months (range 1–240 months) to diagnosis [18]. In another study, the mean duration was noted to be 3.8 years ranging from 1 h (in a newborn) to 34 years [19].

The classic diagnosis is achieved by the presence of Whipple's triad:

1. Fasting hypoglycemia (plasma glucose <50 mg/dL)
2. Neuroglycopenic symptoms
3. Relief of symptoms after administration of glucose

The normal negative feedback mechanism is altered in patients with insulinoma. Insulin production is not dependent on the blood glucose level and continues during periods of low blood glucose levels. The biochemical diagnosis is obtained by measuring elevated insulin in the presence of hypoglycemia. The gold standard biochemical diagnosis consists of the 72-h fast requiring hospitalization with measurement of plasma glucose, insulin, C-peptide, and proinsulin. It is able to detect 99% of insulinomas [20].

The patient is admitted for a monitored fast. During the fasting period, the patient is allowed to drink calorie-free fluids and is encouraged to ambulate. Blood glucose is initially measured every 6 h [21, 22]. Once the plasma glucose level reaches less than 60 mg/dL, measurements are taken every 1–2 h [21, 22]. When the glucose level reaches 40–45 mg/dL with the presence of symptoms, blood is drawn to measure glucose, insulin, C-peptide, β-hydroxybutyrate, and sulfonylurea [21, 22]. The fast is then terminated. The presence of low glucose ($\leq$40 mg/dL), high insulin ($\geq$6 μU/L), elevated C-peptide ($\geq$200 pmol/L), and absence of sulfonylurea in toxicology exam are all defining features of insulinoma [23]. Level of proinsulin $\geq$5 pmol/L and β-hydroxybutyrate levels $\leq$2.7 mmol/L are also measurements that can guide diagnosis [23].

Proinsulin is a precursor to endogenous insulin, which undergoes enzymatic cleavage into insulin and C-peptide [22]. With surreptitious insulin use or oral hypoglycemia, the proinsulin level would be normal or decreased, allowing the test to distinguish other conditions causing fasting hypoglycemia [24]. Factitious hypoglycemia due to exogenous insulin would also result in low C-peptide levels [24].

After completion of the test, some centers administer 1 mg of intravenous glucagon and take measurements of plasma glucose levels after 10, 20, and 30 min to measure the response of beta-hydroxybutyrate and glucose, which increases the sensitivity of the test [25]. Insulin is an antiketogenic and glycogenic agent; therefore, low levels of beta-hydroxybutyrate $\leq$2.7 mmol/L at time of hypoglycemia or increase in plasma glucose >25 mg/dL within 30 min of the glucagon bolus can be used as surrogate markers of hyperinsulinemia [22].

Table 1 Characteristic symptoms of insulinoma and frequencies. (Data from [18])

Adrenergic symptoms	Palpitations (5%)
	Diaphoresis (30%)
	Anxiety (12%)
	Tremors (12%)
	Hyperphagia/obesity (44%)
Neuroglycopenic symptoms	Visual changes/diplopia (42%)
	Confusion/altered mental status (67%)
	Amnesia (8%)
	Abnormal behavior (16%)
	Lethargy/weakness/fatigue (28%)
	Headache (7%)
	Seizures (16%)
	Coma

In more recent years, a 48-h fast has been suggested to replace the traditional 72-h fast with the diagnosis of insulinoma achieved in 90–97 % of patients [26].

Outpatient fast protocols have also been developed [25]. Patients are instructed to start the fast at home overnight, and the office visit is timed for when the usual hypoglycemic symptoms occur. If the glucose level does not drop during the visit, the patient is admitted for continued fast as an inpatient.

Differential Diagnosis

Hypoglycemia can be caused by diabetes mellitus, sepsis, drugs, critical illness, renal/hepatic failure, and hypocortisolism. Hypoglycemia in healthy-appearing patients can also be caused by noninsulinoma pancreatogenous hypoglycemia syndrome (NIPHS), factitious hypoglycemia, strenuous exercise, and ketotic hypoglycemia. NIPHS is an endogenous hyperinsulinism not caused by a functional tumor [25]. Diffuse islet cell hyperplasia/nesidioblastosis can also cause exaggerated insulin response to glucose ingestion. These conditions present with postprandial hypoglycemia 1–4 h after meals, with similar symptoms as insulinomas, but with different timing and pathology [12]. Autoimmune hypoglycemia which consists of elevated insulin due to anti-insulin antibodies or anti-insulin receptor antibodies can also be part of the differential diagnosis [27].

Localization

Preoperative localization of insulinomas is important in determining the surgical approach and the amount of resection needed as well as in decreasing the operation time. The failure rate of preoperative localization is reported to be around 10–27 % [28]. Some suggest that preoperative localization is not necessary because they are successfully localized intraoperatively, but the need for imaging still exists to rule out metastatic disease and to decide on the extent and type operation [29, 30].

Several methods of noninvasive imaging are utilized with varying sensitivities and advantages. Transabdominal ultrasound is an easily accessible, cost-efficient modality without exposure to radiation, but it is highly operator dependent and limited by the patient's body habitus. Obesity, which is a common characteristic of insulinoma patients, decreases its effectiveness. Resolution is also often limited by the presence of bowel gas overlying the pancreas [25]. However, when used appropriately, it can be useful in identifying the size, location, and relationship of the tumor to surrounding structures. Sensitivity ranges from 9 to 67 % and therefore can be used as a preliminary study, but most patients undergo other imaging modalities [8].

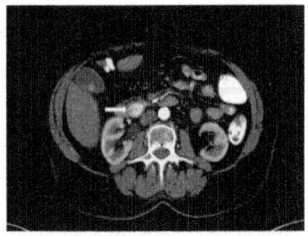

Fig. 1 CT of the abdomen. A 74-year-old female patient with a 1.8-cm insulinoma in the head of the pancreas inferior to ampulla of Vater

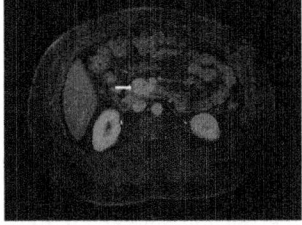

Fig. 2 MRI of the abdomen. A 49-year-old male patient with a 3.6-cm insulinoma in the uncinate process

On dual-phase computed tomography (CT), insulinomas often appear as a hypervascular, well-defined, round, homogenous mass with enhancement during the arterial phase. Atypical appearances can occur with hypoattenuation, cystic mass, and calcification, which is discrete, nodular, and more common in malignant tumors [31, 32]. Dynamic CT is especially useful due to the small size of most insulinomas. The location of the tumor, its relationship to surrounding structures, as well as lymphadenopathy and presence of metastasis can all be evaluated. CTs have the advantage of being easily interpreted by the operating surgeon. With the recent advances in CT technology, sensitivities have increased [33]. The latest multiphase helical CTs can localize 50–80 % of insulinomas [24]. Multidetector CTs can visualize 94.4 % of insulinomas (Fig. 1) [34].

Magnetic resonance imagings (MRIs) have become a superior modality for small insulinomas. They are safe and noninvasive, and have the ability to detect metastasis. Insulinomas have low signal intensity on T1-weighted images and high signal intensity on T2-weighted images.

Sensitivity is reported to be 40–95 % [33]. Diffusion-weighted MRI offers even better imaging. MRIs also have the advantage of being more sensitive than CT for liver metastasis (Fig. 2) [24].

Despite the common use of CT and MRI for insulinoma localization, there is a significant number of insulinomas that are undetectable by these noninvasive means. The subsequent use of some invasive techniques may allow localization of these tumors.

Endoscopic ultrasonography (EUS) is an invasive procedure that requires sedation and is operator dependent but has high detection rates of 86.6–92.3 % [35]. Sensitivity varies from 37 to 94 % depending on the location of the lesion [8, 36–39]. Sensitivity is higher in the head of the pancreas and lower for the tail and splenic hilum area. Using a high-frequency transducer (7.5–10 MHz), EUS is able to detect

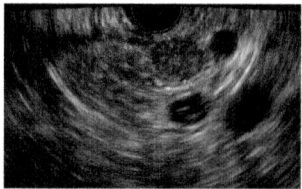

Fig. 3 EUS showing 11-mm insulinoma in the body of pancreas appearing as a round, hypoechoic lesion with well-defined borders. FNA confirmed pancreatic endocrine tumor and patient underwent a laparoscopic enucleation of the tumor

lesions as small as 5 mm. Insulinomas have a characteristic appearance on EUS: They are homogeneously hypoechoic, round and have distinct margins. In young, female patients with low body mass index (BMI), tumors can be isoechoic and easily missed by EUS [40]. EUS-guided fine-needle aspiration (FNA) can also be performed when the appearance of the tumor is unusual to confirm the diagnosis, raising the sensitivity of the technique. Fritscher-Ravens et al. used a 22-gauge needle to obtain adequate tissue in two to three passes to diagnose and differentiate neuroendocrine tumors from each other as well as from other malignancies (Fig. 3) [41].

Angiography and arterial stimulation venous sampling was previously one of the major localization methods with sensitivity of 87.5–100 %. However, due to its invasive and technically demanding nature, and the development of other imaging modalities, it is no longer the first-line modality [42, 43].

Transhepatic portal-venous sampling (THPVS) requires percutaneous and transhepatic catheterization of a branch of portal vein. The catheter is then advanced into small veins that drain the pancreas. It requires intra-arterial and intra-venous catheterization. This technique had a localization rate of 64–100 % [8]. However, it has now been replaced by intra-arterial calcium stimulation with hepatic venous sampling [44, 45].

Intra-arterial calcium stimulation with hepatic venous sampling provides additional information. The tumor can be localized by its hormonal function allowing development of an accurate surgical approach and avoidance of reoperation [46]. The accuracy of this technique is around 94–100 % (17431724) and sensitivity of 77–100 % [8, 42, 43, 47–49].

The tumor appears as a well-defined, round/oval vascular blush, with increased vascularity [25]. It is visualized in the early arterial phase and continues through the venous phase. The mechanism involves increased calcium in vessels causing degranulation of cells, releasing insulin into the portal venous system, leading to a detectable increase in insulin in venous samples obtained from the hepatic vein [50]. Selective catheterization of splenic (body/tail), gastroduodenal (anterosuperior head), superior mesenteric (posteroinferior

head), and proper hepatic (hepatic mets) arteries is performed with simultaneous venous catheterization of the right hepatic vein for obtaining blood samples [25]. Sequentially 0.025 mEq/kg of calcium gluconate are injected, and blood samples are obtained to measure insulin levels from right and left hepatic veins prior to and 30, 60, and 120 s after calcium infusion [51]. A twofold increase in insulin concentration from baseline localizes the insulinoma to its respective region. It is important to account for aberrant anatomy because localization depends on normal anatomy of the pancreatic vasculature.

Unlike other pancreatic neuroendocrine tumors, somatostatin receptor scintigraphy is not helpful for insulinomas. The test is positive in only 46 % of benign insulinomas. Not all insulinoma cells express somatostatin receptor type 2, which explains the low yield of this test. Malignant insulinomas can have a higher rate of positive yield [23].

Management

Surgical resection is the primary treatment modality for all localized tumors. Surgery has a high success rate with cure obtained in more than 90 % of patients [19, 44].

Patients are generally admitted 1 day prior to surgery for monitoring of blood glucose. After midnight, the patient is maintained on a 10 % dextrose infusion. Some centers promote the use of diazoxide preoperatively for glucose control. Precise intraoperative glucose monitoring is highly important. The level of blood glucose is kept above 40–50 mg/dL using dextrose boluses if necessary [25]. The open approach involves a bilateral subcostal incision and the abdomen is first examined for any signs of metastases [25]. An extended **Kocher** maneuver is performed to access the head, and uncinate or medial mobilization of the spleen and distal pancreas is performed if tumor location is distal. Manual palpation has a sensitivity of 75–95 % in locating the tumor [52]. Intraoperative ultrasound (IOUS) is also used with sensitivity of 80–100 % (Fig. 4) [53, 54].

The combination of palpation and IOUS allows 83–98 % of tumors to be detected [24]. IOUS is useful for defining the anatomy—the relationship of the tumor to pancreatic and bile ducts as well as the vasculature. Benign, solitary lesions are amenable to enucleation, with complete excision of the capsule to prevent local recurrence [22]. Usually, a clear dissection plane exists between the tumor and the pancreatic parenchyma. Even when the tumor is located close to the common bile duct (CBD) or pancreatic duct, enucleation can be performed in most cases because the tumor usually does not invade or constrict the ducts [25]. Enucleation and partial pancreatectomy preserve the pancreatic parenchyma and reduce the risk of exocrine/endocrine insufficiency [55]. Distal pancreatectomy may be required, if the tumor is located deep

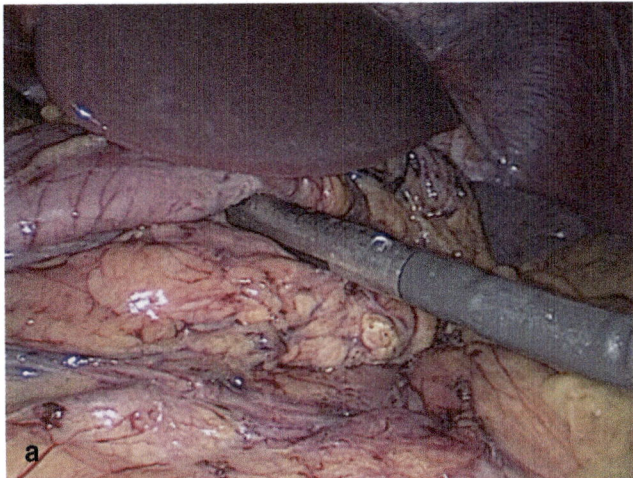

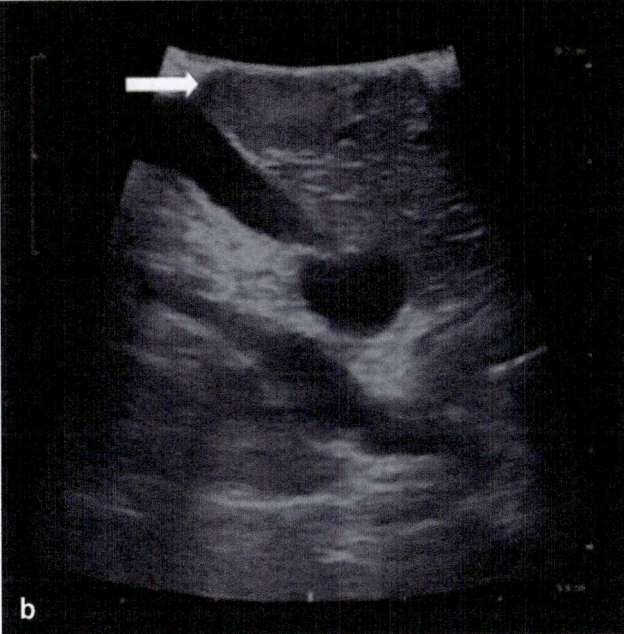

Fig. 4 a Intraoperative ultrasound can be performed to localize insulinoma. **b** Ultrasound showing 1.5-cm tumor located in body of pancreas

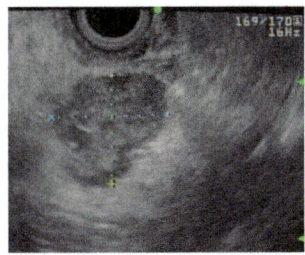

Fig. 5 Patient with MEN-1 and multifocal insulinoma. EUS showing well-defined 2.1-cm irregular mass in the pancreatic body, numerous subcentimeter lesions throughout the rest of the body of the pancreas, and single subcentimeter lesion in the tail of the pancreas. Patient underwent a laparoscopic spleen-preserving distal pancreatectomy and pathology confirmed multifocal insulinoma

in the tail, and in some rare cases, pancreatoduodenectomy may be necessary, if the tumor is located deep in the head [18]. Also extended resections may be necessary for multiple tumors, large tumors > 4 cm, tumors that are not well encapsulated, or those suspicious for malignancy—tumors that are hard, infiltrating, or puckering, or have evidence of pancreatic duct dilatation, indicating duct involvement and probable malignancy. In cases of suspected or proven malignancy, peripancreatic lymphadenectomy should be performed to verify the extent of disease [25]. The open approach may be indicated for MEN-1-associated insulinomas, because multifocal disease and presence of other tumors must be considered. These tumors may require subtotal pancreatectomy in addition to enucleation (Fig. 5) [56, 57].

Once the tumor is removed, blood glucose levels may rapidly rise to 120–140 mg/dL. Glucose is administered intravenously for an additional 24 h postoperatively. High glucose levels may persist for several days to weeks, and the patient may require doses of insulin administration. Blood glucose is measured frequently during this period. Normalization of glucose levels is observed usually within 2–3 weeks after surgery [25].

In cases where the tumor could not be localized intraoperatively, blind distal pancreatectomy was performed historically. However, this approach has been abandoned due to a low success rate. Since there is equal distribution of insulinomas throughout the pancreas, a blind distal pancreatectomy would only resolve half of the tumors, those located in the body and tail. With the current multimodality preoperative imaging options as well as improved intraoperative ultrasound, blind resections are no longer recommended [58].

Laparoscopic resection of insulinomas was started in 1996 by Gagner et al. [59]. Others soon followed and there are multiple publications regarding the technique, which is becoming more and more popular for benign, small insulinomas located in the body or tail of the pancreas. Distal pancreatectomy can be performed with electrocautery or other endoscopic sealing device [25]. Preoperative localization is even more important in these cases because intraoperative palpation is not performed. Laparoscopic IOUS can now identify > 85 % of tumors. Laparoscopic resection has a success rate of 70–100 % and is valued for its shorter duration of stay and faster recovery of patients [24, 60, 61].

Postoperative complications include pancreatic leaks that can present as fistulas or intra-abdominal collections, which are self-limited and most can be treated conservatively. Fistula rates have been reported to be around 15–43 % [24, 62–64].

Abscesses requiring percutaneous drainage consist about 4–6 % [24]. Delayed gastric emptying occurs in 4–8 % of patients and is mainly managed with medical treatment. Other possible complications are hemorrhage, pseudocyst, diabetes, and pancreatitis [25]. Up to 40–50 % can present with these various complications [25].

Overall morbidity and mortality rates have been reported at 10–43 % and 0–4 %, respectively, and laparoscopic rates are comparable [8, 60, 61, 65, 66]. More extensive resections such as distal pancreatectomy and pancreatoduodenectomy indicated for malignant tumors or failed enucleation of multiple insulinomas have higher complication rates. For distal pancreatectomy, pancreatic fistula rates are around 15–40 % [5]. The morbidity and mortality rates for pancreatoduodenectomy are < 5 and 50 %, respectively [5].

Medical Management

Medical management of insulinoma may be necessary during the preoperative period to normalize blood glucose, or for patients unable or unwilling to undergo surgery. It can be necessary in cases where surgery is contraindicated, for example, in patients with diffuse beta-cell disease, multiple insulinomas, or unresectable malignant insulinoma. It involves dietary modification to prevent prolonged periods of fasting by eating small frequent meals during the day and even at night as well as pharmacologic interventions of which diazoxide is the most commonly used. Diazoxide is a nondiuretic benzothiadiazine derivative, which was initially developed for the treatment of hypertension, but also has the ability to induce hyperglycemia [8]. It can be prescribed 50–300 mg/day and titrated up to 600 mg/day to maintain levels of plasma glucose in insulinoma patients [67]. The mechanism of diazoxide involves suppression of insulin secretion by directly acting on beta cells via stimulation of alpha-adrenergic receptors and enhancing glycogenolysis via cyclic adenosine monophosphate phosphodiesterase inhibition [8, 24]. Diazoxide is effective in approximately 50 % patients, with its main side effect being fluid retention and hirsutism [68]. All these side effects tend to be mild and well tolerated [68].

Octreotide, a somatostatin analog that inhibits insulin secretion, is another pharmacologic agent that has been used in the treatment of insulinoma. It has been found to lower plasma insulin and alleviate symptoms in approximately 50 % patients [69]. The half-life of this medication is 100 min, and a dose of 50 or 100 µg can be administered every 12 h [8].

The most common side effects are pain at the injection site and gastrointestinal (GI) disturbance including nausea/vomiting, heartburn, abdominal pain, constipation, or diarrhea [70, 71].

Another alternative way of administration is 50 µg subcutaneous injection two or three times daily, increased to 1500 µg daily [24]. Octreotide suppresses the release of glucagon and growth hormone, and it can therefore occasionally worsen hypoglycemia in some patients [8]. The mean duration of treatment tolerated is 1 year until patients develop tachyphylaxis [24]. Long-term use may also lead to side effects such as mild diabetes, cholelithiasis, malabsorption, and weight loss [8].

Other medications, such as verapamil, glucocorticoids, and phenytoin, have also been used in the treatment of surgically unresectable insulinomas. However, their effects have not been well studied due to the small number of these patients. Phenytoin can be administered as a maintenance dose of 300–600 mg daily and works by inhibiting the release of insulin from beta cells [24]. Only one third of patients who take this medication benefit from its effects [24]. Glucocorticoids and glucagon can be administered alone or simultaneously with diazoxide [24].

Malignant Insulinoma

The treatment of malignant insulinoma varies. The World Health Organization classification of malignant insulinomas involves the presence of metastases, gross invasion into surrounding tissue, tumor size, percentage of mitoses, proliferative index, and vascular invasion. Chemotherapy can be administered for malignant insulinoma [8]. Studies have been performed using streptozocin, doxorubicin, 5-fluorouracil (5-FU), and chlorozotocin. Palliation via primary tumor resection, radical debulking surgery, hepatic embolization, hepatic arterial chemoperfusion, radiofrequency ablation, cryoablation, and ethanol ablation are also treatment modalities that have been used in malignant insulinoma patients [10, 23, 72].

Antitumor agents, such as everolimus, a mammalian target of rapamycin (mTOR) inhibitor, have also been recently studied as an effective treatment for metastatic malignant insulinoma and refractory hypoglycemia (Figs. 6 and 7) [73, 74].

Prognosis and Follow-Up

Insulinomas are considered cured after complete surgical removal of the tumor. Most benign, solitary lesions have a cure rate of 89–96 %, and patients with benign disease have a normal life span after resection of the tumor. Therefore, no special follow-up is required beyond the basic postoperative visit [25]. However, when there is a return of hypoglycemic signs or symptoms, recurrence, MEN-1, or malignant disease should be considered and followed up promptly [25].

For patients with malignant insulinomas and MEN-1, follow-up is highly important. The need for reoperation is more common with metastatic disease, multiple tumors, and MEN-1 patients [8]. Danforth et al. have shown that primary malignant tumors are often single, large with a mean

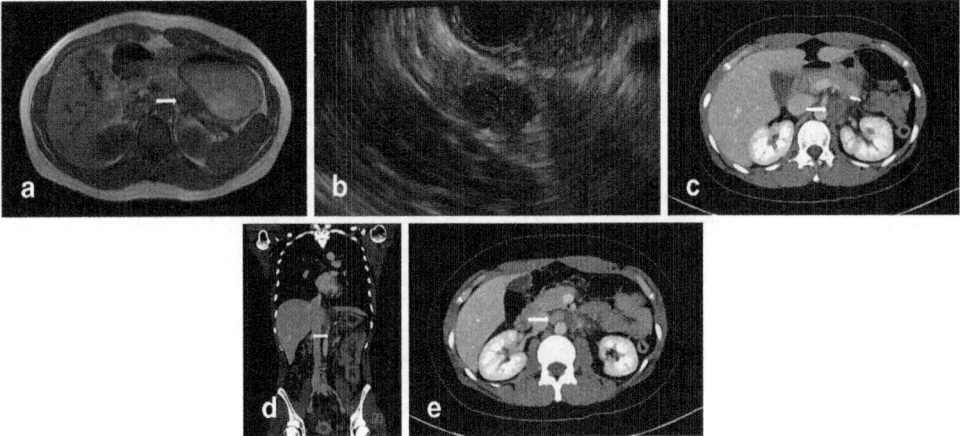

Fig. 6 Thirty-three-year-old female with metastatic insulinoma. **a** MRI identified a 3.2 × 1.4-cm lesion in the body of the pancreas. Laparoscopic distal pancreatectomy and splenectomy were performed. She continued to have persistent episodes of hypoglycemia. Pathology revealed well-differentiated insulinoma with two positive peripancreatic lymph nodes. **b** Post surgery, EUS–FNA identified periportal lymph nodes with malignant cells. **c, d, e** Follow-up CT of the abdomen showing enlarged retroperitoneal and left para-aortic lymph nodes. *CT* computed tomography, *EUS* endoscopic ultrasonography, *FNA* fine-needle aspiration, *MRI* magnetic resonance imaging

Fig. 7 Forty-four-year-old female with multifocal insulinoma. Preoperative imaging revealed three lesions. Distal lesions were removed by distal pancreatectomy. EUS-guided ethanol ablation performed for lesion in the head of pancreas

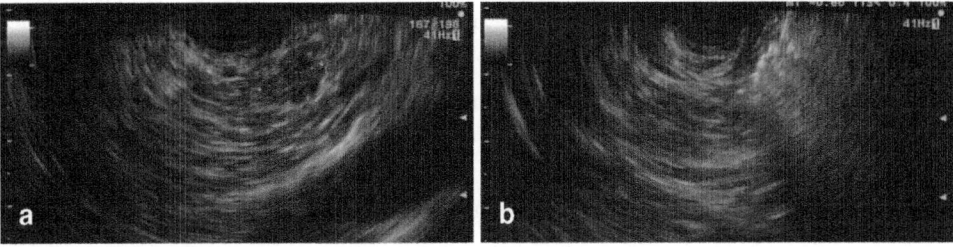

diameter of 6 cm, median disease-free survival of 5 years, and recurrence of 63 % at median 2.8 years after curative resection [75]. They have a varied course with up to 35 % of patients surviving longer than 5 years. The biology of tumor determines survival after resection. Malignant insulinomas, which are often slow-growing and symptomatic, have a better prognosis than adenocarcinomas. The 10-year survival of patients with malignant insulinoma is reported to be 29 % [10, 72, 73].

Future Studies

Although insulinomas are the most common neuroendocrine tumors of the pancreas, there is still much to be discovered, most likely due to the rare incidence of the disease. Further studies need to be conducted to define the molecular etiology of the disease. Localization techniques, which have become essential in planning the surgical resection, are being developed and enhanced to raise their sensitivities. The laparoscopic approach is becoming more and more common in the treatment of insulinomas and has promising results thus far. The management of malignant disease is also an area to be further studied with the use of continuous glucose infusion pumps and molecular-targeted therapies against the glucagon-like peptide-1 (GLP-1) receptor.

References

1. Sakula A. Paul Langerhans (1847–1888): a centenary tribute. J R Soc Med. 1988;81(7):414–5.
2. Frederick Grant Banting (1891–1941), codiscoverer of insulin. JAMA. 1966 Nov 7;198(6):660–1. PMID: 5332306.
3. Banting FG, Campbell WR, Fletcher AA. Further clinical experience with insulin (pancreatic extracts) in the treatment of diabetes mellitus. Br Med J. 1923;1(3236):8–12.
4. Whipple AO, Frantz VK. Adenoma of islet cells with hyperinsulinism: a review. Ann Surg. 1935;101(6):1299–335.
5. Vaidakis D, Karoubalis J, Pappa T, Piaditis G, Zografos GN. Pancreatic insulinoma: current issues and trends. Hepatobiliary Pancreat Dis Int. 2010;9(3):234–41.
6. Service FJ, McMahon MM, O'Brien PC, Ballard DJ. Functioning insulinoma–incidence, recurrence, and long-term survival of patients: a 60-year study. Mayo Clin Proc. 1991;66(7):711–9.
7. Oberg K, Eriksson B. Endocrine tumours of the pancreas. Best Pract Res Clin Gastroenterol. 2005;19(5):753–81.
8. Shin JJ, Gorden P, Libutti SK. Insulinoma: pathophysiology, localization and management. Future Oncol. 2010;6(2):229–37.
9. Larsson C, Skogseid B, Oberg K, Nakamura Y, Nordenskjold M. Multiple endocrine neoplasia type 1 gene maps to chromosome 11 and is lost in insulinoma. Nature. 1988;332(6159):85–7.

10. Hirshberg B, Cochran C, Skarulis MC, Libutti SK, Alexander HR, Wood BJ, et al. Malignant insulinoma: spectrum of unusual clinical features. Cancer. 2005;104(2):264–72.

11. Starke A, Saddig C, Mansfeld L, Koester R, Tschahargane C, Czygan P, et al. Malignant metastatic insulinoma-postoperative treatment and follow-up. World J Surg. 2005;29(6):789–93.

12. Service GJ, Thompson GB, Service FJ, Andrews JC, Collazo-Clavell ML, Lloyd RV. Hyperinsulinemic hypoglycemia with nesidioblastosis after gastric-bypass surgery. N Engl J Med. 2005;353(3):249–54.

13. Rutter GA, Hodson DJ. Minireview: intraislet regulation of insulin secretion in humans. Mol Endocrinol. 2013;27(12):1984–95.

14. Rutter GA. Nutrient-secretion coupling in the pancreatic islet beta-cell: recent advances. Mol Aspects Med. 2001;22(6):247–84.

15. Cryer PE. Mechanisms of hypoglycemia-associated autonomic failure and its component syndromes in diabetes. Diabetes. 2005;54(12):3592–601.

16. Suzuki K, Miyamoto M, Miyamoto T, Hirata K. Insulinoma with early-morning abnormal behavior. Intern Med. 2007;46(7):405–8.

17. Gerich JE, Mokan M, Veneman T, Korytkowski M, Mitrakou A. Hypoglycemia unawareness. Endocr Rev. 1991;12(4):356–71.

18. Nikfarjam M, Warshaw AL, Axelrod L, Deshpande V, Thayer SP, Ferrone CR, et al. Improved contemporary surgical management of insulinomas: a 25-year experience at the Massachusetts General Hospital. Ann Surg. 2008;247(1):165–72.

19. Boukhman MP, Karam JH, Shaver J, Siperstein AE, Duh QY, Clark OH. Insulinoma–experience from 1950 to 1995. West J Med. 1998;169(2):98–104.

20. Service FJ, Natt N. The prolonged fast. J Clin Endocrinol Metab. 2000;85(11):3973–4.

21. Service FJ. Hypoglycemic disorders. N Engl J Med. 1995;332 (17):1144–52.

22. Grant CS. Insulinoma. Best Pract Res Clin Gastroenterol. 2005;19 (5):783–98.

23. de Herder WW, Niederle B, Scoazec JY, Pauwels S, Kloppel G, Falconi M, et al. Well-differentiated pancreatic tumor/carcinoma: insulinoma. Neuroendocrinology. 2006;84(3):183–8.

24. Mathur A, Gorden P, Libutti SK. Insulinoma. Surg Clin North Am. 2009;89(5):1105–21.

25. Vanderveen K, Grant C. Insulinoma. Cancer Treat Res. 2010;153: 235–52.

26. Hirshberg B, Livi A, Bartlett DL, Libutti SK, Alexander HR, Doppman JL, et al. Forty-eight-hour fast: the diagnostic test for insulinoma. J Clin Endocrinol Metab. 2000;85(9):3222–6.

27. Iglesias P, Diez JJ. Management of endocrine disease: a clinical update on tumor-induced hypoglycemia. Eur J Endocrinol. 2014;170(4):R147–57.

28. Grant CS. Gastrointestinal endocrine tumours. Insulinoma. Baillieres Clin Gastroenterol. 1996;10(4):645–71.

29. Hashimoto LA, Walsh RM. Preoperative localization of insulinomas is not necessary. J Am Coll Surg. 1999;189(4):368–73.

30. Daggett PR, Goodburn EA, Kurtz AB, Le Quesne LP, Morris DV, Nabarro JD, et al. Is preoperative localisation of insulinomas necessary? Lancet. 1981;1(8218):483–6.

31. Balci NC, Semelka RC. Radiologic features of cystic, endocrine and other pancreatic neoplasms. Eur J Radiol. 2001;38(2):113–9.

32. Kurosaki Y, Kuramoto K, Itai Y. Hyperattenuating insulinoma at unenhanced CT. Abdom Imaging. 1996;21(4):334–6.

33. McAuley G, Delaney H, Colville J, Lyburn I, Worsley D, Govender P, et al. Multimodality preoperative imaging of pancreatic insulinomas. Clin Radiol. 2005;60(10):1039–50.

34. Gouya H, Vignaux O, Augui J, Dousset B, Palazzo L, Louvel A, et al. CT, endoscopic sonography, and a combined protocol for preoperative evaluation of pancreatic insulinomas. AJR Am J Roentgenol. 2003;181(4):987–92.

35. Goh BK, Ooi LL, Cheow PC, Tan YM, Ong HS, Chung YF, et al. Accurate preoperative localization of insulinomas avoids the need for blind resection and reoperation: analysis of a single institution experience with 17 surgically treated tumors over 19 years. J Gastrointest Surg. 2009;13(6):1071–7.

36. Sotoudehmanesh R, Hedayat A, Shirazian N, Shahraeeni S, Ainechi S, Zeinali F, et al. Endoscopic ultrasonography (EUS) in the localization of insulinoma. Endocrine. 2007;31(3):238–41.

37. Glover JR, Shorvon PJ, Lees WR. Endoscopic ultrasound for localisation of islet cell tumours. Gut. 1992;33(1):108–10.

38. Schumacher B, Lubke HJ, Frieling T, Strohmeyer G, Starke AA. Prospective study on the detection of insulinomas by endoscopic ultrasonography. Endoscopy. 1996;28(3):273–6.

39. Rösch T, Lightdale CJ, Botet JF, Boyce GA, Sivak MV, Jr, Yasuda K, et al. Localization of pancreatic endocrine tumors by endoscopic ultrasonography. N Engl J Med. 1992;326(26):1721–6.

40. Kann PH, Ivan D, Pfutzner A, Forst T, Langer P, Schaefer S. Preoperative diagnosis of insulinoma: low body mass index, young age, and female gender are associated with negative imaging by endoscopic ultrasound. Eur J Endocrinol. 2007;157(2):209–13.

41. Fritscher-Ravens A, Izbicki JR, Sriram PV, Krause C, Knoefel WT, Topalidis T, et al. Endosonography-guided, fine-needle aspiration cytology extending the indication for organ-preserving pancreatic surgery. Am J Gastroenterol. 2000;95(9):2255–60.

42. Doppman JL, Chang R, Fraker DL, Norton JA, Alexander HR, Miller DL, et al. Localization of insulinomas to regions of the pancreas by intra-arterial stimulation with calcium. Ann Intern Med. 1995;123(4):269–73.

43. Brown CK, Bartlett DL, Doppman JL, Gorden P, Libutti SK, Fraker DL, et al. Intraarterial calcium stimulation and intraoperative ultrasonography in the localization and resection of insulinomas. Surgery. 1997;122(6):1189–93; discussion 93–4.

44. Doherty GM, Doppman JL, Shawker TH, Miller DL, Eastman RC, Gorden P, et al. Results of a prospective strategy to diagnose, localize, and resect insulinomas. Surgery. 1991;110(6):989–96; discussion 96–7.

45. Finlayson E, Clark OH. Surgical treatment of insulinomas. Surg Clin North Am. 2004;84(3):775–85.

46. Morita S, Machida H, Kuwatsuru R, Saito N, Suzuki K, Iihara M, et al. Preoperative localization of pancreatic insulinoma by super selective arterial stimulation with venous sampling. Abdom Imaging. 2007;32(1):126–8.

47. Tseng LM, Chen JY, Won JG, Tseng HS, Yang AH, Wang SE, et al. The role of intra-arterial calcium stimulation test with hepatic venous sampling (IACS) in the management of occult insulinomas. Ann Surg Oncol. 2007;14(7):2121–7.

48. Doppman JL, Miller DL, Chang R, Shawker TH, Gorden P, Norton JA. Insulinomas: localization with selective intraarterial injection of calcium. Radiology. 1991;178(1):237–41.

49. Kaplan EL, Rubenstein AH, Evans R, Lee CH, Klementschitsch P. Calcium infusion: a new provocative test for insulinomas. Ann Surg. 1979;190(4):501–7.

50. Jackson JE. Angiography and arterial stimulation venous sampling in the localization of pancreatic neuroendocrine tumours. Best Pract Res Clin Endocrinol Metab. 2005;19(2):229–39.

51. Brandle M, Pfammatter T, Spinas GA, Lehmann R, Schmid C. Assessment of selective arterial calcium stimulation and hepatic venous sampling to localize insulin-secreting tumours. Clin Endocrinol (Oxf). 2001;55(3):357–62.

52. Wong M, Isa SH, Zahiah M, Azmi KN. Intraoperative ultrasound with palpation is still superior to intra-arterial calcium stimulation test in localising insulinoma. World J Surg. 2007;31(3):586–92.

53. Shin LK, Brant-Zawadzki G, Kamaya A, Jeffrey RB. Intraoperative ultrasound of the pancreas. Ultrasound Q. 2009;25(1):39–48; quiz

54. Grover AC, Skarulis M, Alexander HR, Pingpank JF, Javor ED, Chang R, et al. A prospective evaluation of laparoscopic exploration with intraoperative ultrasound as a technique for localizing sporadic insulinomas. Surgery. 2005;138(6):1003–8; discussion 8.

55. Falconi M, Bettini R, Boninsegna L, Crippa S, Butturini G, Pederzoli P. Surgical strategy in the treatment of pancreatic neuroendocrine tumors. JOP. 2006;7(1):150–6.

56. Norton JA, Fang TD, Jensen RT. Surgery for gastrinoma and insulinoma in multiple endocrine neoplasia type 1. J Natl Compr Canc Netw. 2006;4(2):148–53.

57. Demeure MJ, Klonoff DC, Karam JH, Duh QY, Clark OH. Insulinomas associated with multiple endocrine neoplasia type I: the need for a different surgical approach. Surgery. 1991;110(6):998–1004; discussion -5.

58. Hirshberg B, Libutti SK, Alexander HR, Bartlett DL, Cochran C, Livi A, et al. Blind distal pancreatectomy for occult insulinoma, an inadvisable procedure. J Am Coll Surg. 2002;194(6):761–4.

59. Gagner M, Pomp A, Herrera MF. Early experience with laparoscopic resections of islet cell tumors. Surgery. 1996;120(6):1051–4.

60. Berends FJ, Cuesta MA, Kazemier G, van Eijck CH, de Herder WW, van Muiswinkel JM, et al. Laparoscopic detection and resection of insulinomas. Surgery. 2000;128(3):386–91.

61. Sweet MP, Izumisato Y, Way LW, Clark OH, Masharani U, Duh QY. Laparoscopic enucleation of insulinomas. Arch Surg. 2007;142(12):1202–4; discussion 5.

62. Park BJ, Alexander HR, Libutti SK, Huang J, Royalty D, Skarulis MC, et al. Operative management of islet-cell tumors arising in the head of the pancreas. Surgery. 1998;124(6):1056–61; discussion 61–2.

63. Fernandez-Cruz L, Blanco L, Cosa R, Rendon H. Is laparoscopic resection adequate in patients with neuroendocrine pancreatic tumors? World J Surg. 2008;32(5):904–17.

64. Menegaux F, Schmitt G, Mercadier M, Chigot JP. Pancreatic insulinomas. Am J Surg. 1993;165(2):243–8.

65. Isla A, Arbuckle JD, Kekis PB, Lim A, Jackson JE, Todd JF, et al. Laparoscopic management of insulinomas. Br J Surg. 2009;96(2):185–90.

66. Lo CY, Chan WF, Lo CM, Fan ST, Tam PK. Surgical treatment of pancreatic insulinomas in the era of laparoscopy. Surg Endosc. 2004;18(2):297–302.

67. Fajans SS, Floyd JC, Jr., Thiffault CA, Knopf RF, Harrison TS, Conn JW. Further studies on diazoxide suppression of insulin release from abnormal and normal islet tissue in man. Ann N Y Acad Sci. 1968;150(2):261–80.

68. Gill GV, Rauf O, MacFarlane IA. Diazoxide treatment for insulinoma: a national UK survey. Postgrad Med J. 1997;73(864):640–1.

69. Vezzosi D, Bennet A, Rochaix P, Courbon F, Selves J, Pradere B, et al. Octreotide in insulinoma patients: efficacy on hypoglycemia, relationships with Octreoscan scintigraphy and immunostaining with anti-sst2A and anti-sst5 antibodies. Eur J Endocrinol. 2005;152(5):757–67.

70. Lamberts SW, van der Lely AJ, de Herder WW, Hofland LJ. Octreotide. New Engl J Med. 1996;334(4):246–54.

71. Maton PN, Gardner JD, Jensen RT. Use of long-acting somatostatin analog SMS 201–995 in patients with pancreatic islet cell tumors. Dig Dis Sci. 1989;34(3 Suppl):28S–39S.

72. Ferrer-Garcia JC, Iranzo Gonzalez-Cruz V, Navas-DeSolis S, Civera-Andres M, Morillas-Arino C, Merchante-Alfaro A, et al. Management of malignant insulinoma. Clin Transl Oncol. 2013;15(9):725–31.

73. de Herder WW, van Schaik E, Kwekkeboom D, Feelders RA. New therapeutic options for metastatic malignant insulinomas. Clinic Endocrinol (Oxf). 2011;75(3):277–84.

74. Bernard V, Lombard-Bohas C, Taquet MC, Caroli-Bosc FX, Ruszniewski P, Niccoli P, et al. Efficacy of everolimus in patients with metastatic insulinoma and refractory hypoglycemia. Eur J Endocrinol. 2013;168(5):665–74.

75. Danforth DN Jr, Gorden P, Brennan MF. Metastatic insulin-secreting carcinoma of the pancreas: clinical course and the role of surgery. Surgery. 1984;96(6):1027–37.

Sir Fredrick Grant Banting

1891–1941

Janice L. Pasieka

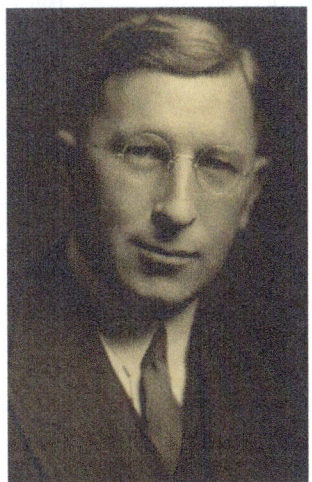

Fredrick Grant Banting. (Courtesy of Banting House National Historic Site of Canada)

On August 27, 1923, the cover of *Time* magazine featured Dr. Fredrick Grant Banting, the man responsible for the discovery of insulin (Fig. 1). He and J. J. R. MacLeod were later that year awarded the Nobel Prize in Physiology or Medicine. The story of the discovery of insulin is filled with controversy, drama, academic bickering, and the excitement and reward that come with making an impact in the lives of millions of patients suffering from the then fatal disease, diabetes. For most, the discovery of insulin is credited to this bright young surgeon and the medical student assigned to assist him in the laboratory in the summer of 1921, **Charles Best**. Yet the discovery and purification of an insulin extract involved a team effort, one shared with J. J. R. McLeod, C. H. Best, and **J. B. Collip**.

FIFTEEN CENTS

TIME

The Weekly News-Magazine

VOL. I. NO. 26   DR. FREDRICK GRANT BANTING   AUGUST 27, 1923
"*From the Islands of the Langerhans—*"
See Page 19

Fig. 1 Cover of *Time* magazine of Fredrick G. Banting, the man responsible for the discovery of insulin. August 1923. (Courtesy of Banting House National Historic Site of Canada)

Fredrick Grant Banting was born on November 14, 1891, at the family farmhouse in Alliston, ON, Canada. Banting was the son of a rural farmer, William Thompson Banting, and his wife Margaret Grant. Fred or Freddie as he was called was the youngest of six children. William Banting was a hardworking and progressive farmer in the community. He diversified the 100-acre farm to raise livestock, fruits, grains, and vegetables. The Bantings were considered well-off, and

J. L. Pasieka (✉)
Divisions of General Surgery and Surgical Oncology, Faculty of Medicine, University of Calgary, 1403 29th Street, NW, Calgary, AB T2N T29, Canada
e-mail: Janice.pasieka@albertahealthservices.ca

J. L. Pasieka, J. A. Lee (eds.), *Surgical Endocrinopathies*, DOI 10.1007/978-3-319-13662-2_43,
© Springer International Publishing Switzerland 2015

Fred enjoyed a comfortable boyhood on the farm [1, 2]. He was a shy and unsocial boy, who struggled to make passing grades in the early years of grammar school. As Fred developed into a young man, his aspirations beyond middle school were set high compared to most rural farm boys. His father offered each of his sons a gift when they turned 21 that they could use any way they saw fit. The gift consisted of $ 1500, a horse, harness, and buggy [1]. Although his older brothers all spent their gift helping to establish themselves as farmers, Fred spent his on university education.

In 1910, Banting enrolled in general arts at Victoria College at the University of Toronto. He failed to successfully complete all of his first-year courses (failing French) and was denied entrance into the second year. He returned to Victoria College to repeat his first year in 1911 having at some point decided on becoming a doctor. Admission into medical school required successful completion of first-year university. Banting petitioned the university's senate to be allowed to enter medicine in February 1912. His petition was granted on the condition he completed his missing arts course during his medical school training. Although he struggled to complete the last art course to meet the first year's requirements, his marks in medicine were significantly better. He was considered slightly above average in his medical school class.

On August 4, 1914, Canada entered the Great War. It was the following day that Banting tried to enlist in the army, but was refused due to poor eyesight. Following his third year in medicine, he tried again and was now accepted in the Canadian Army Medical Service. He was soon promoted to sergeant, spending the summer of 1915 in a military training camp in Niagara Falls, ON. After completion of his fourth year, the University of Toronto condensed the fifth year of medical school into a special summer session in order to speed up the training of the much-needed army doctors. Sometime during this period, Banting decided on surgery as his specialty. He was fortunate to have trained as a fifth-year medical student under C. L. Starr, an orthopedic surgeon at Toronto Hospital for Sick Children. Banting's medical class of 1917 finished their final exams in October 1916, graduated on December 9, and on December 10, 1916, all able-bodied members of his class reported for military duty [1]. He was promoted to lieutenant and left for Britain in March 1917. Starr, who by then was posted abroad at the Granville Canadian Special Hospital in Britain, requested young Banting be assigned to assist him. Banting worked with Starr for the next 18 months before being transferred to France in June 1918 [1, 2]. Captain Banting was injured near the front lines by a piece of shrapnel to his forearm for which he was awarded the Military Cross. Banting was discharged from the army in July 1919, returning to Toronto Hospital for Sick Children to complete his surgical training [1–3].

Much to Banting's disappointment upon completing his surgical training, he was not given a consulting position in Toronto. So in June 1920, he headed for London, ON, to start up his own surgical practice [4]. The house on Adelaide Street that served as his home and office now houses the Banting Museum. Banting became a lecturer at the University of Western while he struggled to establish his surgical practice. In November 1920, he was scheduled to give a lecture to the medical students on the function of the pancreas. Little was known at that time about the pancreas except that it made digestive juices, and when experimentally removed from dogs, the symptoms of the metabolic disorder, called diabetes, developed.

In preparation for this talk, Banting read the recently published article by M. Barron entitled "The Relation of the Islets of Langerhans to Diabetes with Special Reference to Cases of Pancreatic Lithiasis" [1, 6]. Barron observed that blockage of the pancreatic duct resulted in atrophy of the acinar cells with preservation of the islets. This observation along with others supported the hypothesis, put forth by many, that some internal secretion from the islets was responsible for the prevention of diabetes. In his notebook from that night, Banting conceived the idea for his landmark experiments writing:

> Ligate pancreatic ducts of dogs. Keep dogs alive till acini degenerate leaving Islets. Try to isolate the internal secretion of these to relieve glycosuria. [1]

Banting was encouraged by several faculty members at Western to consult with a leading expert in carbohydrate metabolism J. J. R. MacLeod, the professor of physiology at the University of Toronto, about his idea. Records indicate that their first meeting did not go well. Banting was poorly prepared, knowing very little about diabetes or experimental design. MacLeod soon realized that Banting was very much a novice when it came to research yet recognized that his idea had some merit. MacLeod cautioned Banting that success was unlikely, as many far more experienced researchers had failed thus far, yet negative results would still be of value. MacLeod also told him that a substantial commitment from Banting himself would be required for MacLeod to provide the laboratory facilities required for this project [1, 2, 5, 6]. Banting returned to London to reflect upon the offer by MacLeod.

Banting's mentor C. L. Starr advised him to stay in London and build his practice. Although his professional life in London continued to improve, his personal life suffered. His long-standing engagement to his childhood sweetheart ended, and by the spring of 1921, Banting decided to leave London. He initially decided to commit himself to a summer research project, allowing him the possibility to return to London in September. MacLeod provided Banting with two research students, **Charles Best** and Clark Noble, who would divide their time in his laboratory over the summer. Best won the toss and was assigned to assist Banting for the first half of the summer [5].

Starting in May 1921, Banting and Best started working on dogs, some of which were obtained from the streets of

Toronto, paying up to three dollars for the unwanted animals. In June, MacLeod left the team for a 3-month sabbatical to Scotland while the team worked on developing an extract from ligated pancreases. By August, Banting reported to MacLeod that he and Best had an extract that reduced the blood and urinary sugar and improved the clinical condition of diabetic dogs [1]. In November, the team set out to demonstrate how long a diabetic dog could be kept alive with their extract. The labor-intensive process of making the extract from ligated pancreatic ducts forced Banting to come up with another method. Banting knew that the islet developed early in the fetus, and that cattle were often impregnated to help fatten them up before slaughter. So he and Best went to the local abattoir and retrieved fetal pancreases. The extract from these worked and allowed the team to start a longevity experiment [7]. They soon encountered difficulty with standardization of the extract called "isletin." In December 1921, **J. B. Collip**, a biochemist visiting from the University of Alberta, helped the team purify the extract and developed a method of standardizing the potency.

Keen to move from the laboratory to clinical trials, the team administered the first injection of insulin to a 14-year-old boy named Leonard Thompson. The insulin injections on young Thompson improved his clinical condition and normalized his blood sugar. Further clinical testing proved that insulin had great promise in the treatment of this fatal disease. Unfortunately, by this time the group was no longer functioning as a team. Banting, always mistrusting of MacLeod, started to tell people the he suspected MacLeod was taking credit for his work. On top of that, Collip, who was able to improve upon Banting and Best's extract, refused to tell Banting how he had done it. The bickering and accusations of breach of academic integrity disrupted the team's ability to work together, resulting in numerous setbacks. In an attempt to broker a truce, MacLeod proposed the names on the research paper would be listed alphabetically, giving Banting and Best the lead authorship. However, it was MacLeod who presented this paper to the Association of American Physicians, in effect, announcing the discovery of insulin in May 1922 [8]. Unfortunately, neither Banting nor Best attended the conference.

The clinical testing of insulin took on a unique course in Toronto in the months that followed. The university had denied Banting an academic appointment to the Faculty of Medicine and as such he could not be involved in the clinical trials at the Toronto General Hospital. In the spring of 1922, Banting opened a private office and a specialized diabetes clinic at the Christie Military Hospital in Toronto. The university soon realized that it was not in their best interest to continue to have insulin testing occurring outside the Toronto General. Banting wrote: "Things were stalemated. Best and I had control of the production of insulin and I had the clinic at Christie Street Hospital and had more private patients than I knew what to do with. So I decided that the Department of Medicine and the Toronto General Hospital could not have insulin for use on its wards until I had an appointment on staff" [1, 3]. Also, at this time, Banting was being heavily recruited to the USA and as such pressure was put on the university to ensure that Banting stay in Canada. The university soon reversed their decision and gave Banting an appointment to the hospital staff, and the Toronto General Hospital became the sole site for insulin testing.

In October 1923, the announcement came that Banting and MacLeod were awarded the Nobel Prize for Physiology or Medicine for their discovery of insulin. Banting was outraged at having to share this award with MacLeod and upset that Best was not included. His initial reaction was to refuse the prize. Fortunately, he was convinced that as the first Canadian to receive the award, it would be best for the country and the advancement of science for him to accept. Banting in his telegram to Best publicly shared his prize with Charles (see Fig. 1 in the chapter 44). Not to be upstaged, in the days that followed, MacLeod announced that he was sharing his half of the prize with Collip. At the time, this controversy continued to create a rift among faculty and friends between those in Banting's camp versus those backing MacLeod. The two gentlemen rarely spoke and were never seen in public together again. Sadly, Banting, not wanting to share the stage with MacLeod, did not attend the Nobel Prize Ceremony in Stockholm that year. It was a few years later that he finally went to Stockholm to receive his award [9, 10].

It is a sad piece of Canadian history to discover that the first Canadian to receive the Nobel Prize did not attend the grand ceremony that celebrates such a wonderful accomplishment. Upon reflection, biographers such as Michael Bliss have clearly documented that Banting did not have the capability or scientific knowledge to discover insulin on his own [1, 5]. This discovery was clearly a group effort. MacLeod's research skills and knowledge likely did play a significant role in helping the team isolate the hormone. Without the expertise of Collip, needed to purify the crude extract created by Banting and Best, insulin would never have gone on so quickly to the human trials that confirmed its usefulness in the treatment of diabetes.

Following the Nobel Prize, Banting was catapulted into the spotlight, a place he rarely felt comfortable. Numerous awards and honorary degrees from universities and medical societies, including Knight Commander of the Civil Division of the Order of the British Empire, were bestowed upon him. The Canadian government in 1923 provided Banting a life annuity of $7500 per year. His discomfort with his newfound fame is best revealed in a poem he wrote:

> But mark you who are young and ambitious,
> Who strive to rise above the world,
> The thing that made you famous,
> Will be a curse in the end [11]

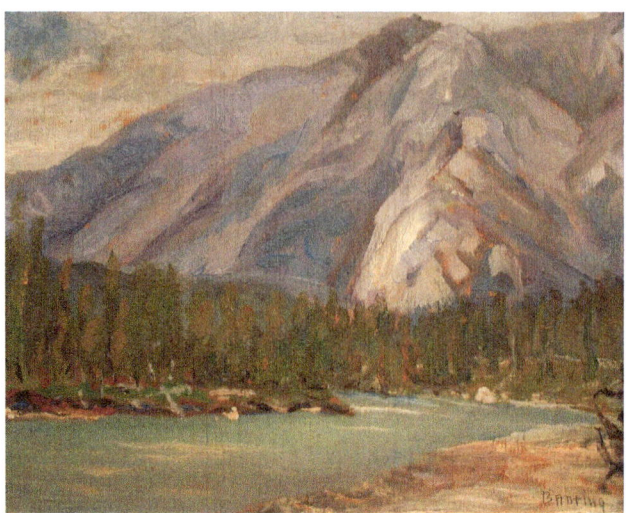

Fig. 2 Banting's early artistic work. This, a painting from Jasper, AB, was painted in 1926. (Courtesy of Banting House National Historic Site of Canada)

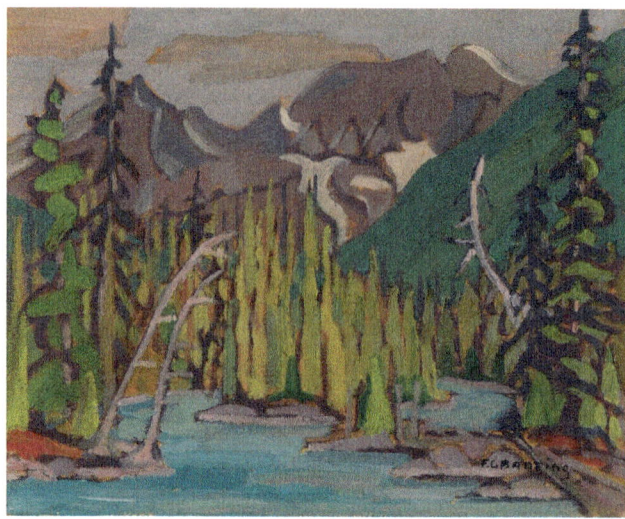

Fig. 3 Rockies Mountains close to Calgary painted in 1933 clearly demonstrates the influence his dear friend A. Y. Jackson had on his work. (Courtesy of Banting House National Historic Site of Canada)

Like the celebrities of today, Banting's personal life was the subject of many tabloid-like stories in the national newspapers. His much-publicized divorce from Marion Robertson was featured as a scandalous affair in the Toronto papers for all to see. Banting's public humiliation took a personal toll on him. He retreated into a quiet life as the director of Medical Research at the newly created Banting Institute for Medical Research. He took up painting as a hobby and soon befriended several members of the newly formed Group of Seven Painters. In 1925, Lawren Harris nominated Banting for membership in the Arts and Letter Club of Toronto, a private men-only club for artisans in the Toronto area. It was here that Banting forged a lifelong friendship with A. Y. Jackson. Banting accompanied Jackson on several sketching expeditions, including one to the Canadian Arctic in 1927. By the 1930s, Banting was one of Canada's best-known amateur artists. His work was clearly influenced by his mentor and friend A. Y. Jackson (Figs. 2 and 3).

Banting spent the next several years maintaining and enlarging the research activities at the University of Toronto. He evolved into an ambassador for medical science both in Canada and abroad [1]. In 1937, Banting agreed to serve on Canada's National Research Council (NRC). When war broke out in 1939, the NRC shifted its focus to wartime research efforts, including aviation research. Banting's involvement in this wartime effort resulted in traveling to Britain on numerous occasions. It was on one such trip, departing from Gander, NF, that Banting's plane crashed not long after takeoff. The two crew members were killed on impact; however, the pilot survived and was able to pull an unconscious Banting from the wreck. Rescue efforts were impeded by bad weather, and by the time the plane wreckage

was discovered, Sir Fredrick Banting had succumbed to his injuries on February 21, 1941. Rumors of sabotage surrounded his death well into the 1980s [12]. Fueled by both the statement the pilot's widow made to biographer Michael Bliss, that two members of the ground crew at Gander had put sand in the fuel tank and later confessed to the crime and had been executed and failure to uncover any official reports of the inquiry into the crash made this story plausible [1, 5]. However, as Bliss pointed out later, sabotage was likely not the case [1]. The class of plane involved in the crash was later discovered to have a faulty oil cooling system that had a tendency to rupture in the extreme cold upon takeoff.

Sir Fredrick Grant Banting was a decorated soldier, an artist, and a young surgeon who had an idea. His dedication and perseverance brought about the discovery of insulin and ultimately changed the lives for millions of people. Fredrick Banting was Canada's first Nobel laureate. And to date remains the youngest recipient of the award at the age of 32. This remarkable discovery was by no means an individual effort. Although he clearly did not agree, his team, including Best, MacLeod, and Collip, all deserve credit for the discovery of one of the first hormones discovered in the early days of modern-day endocrinology.

Acknowledgment I am grateful for the help and insight provided to me by Grant Maltman, curator of the Banting House National Historical Site of Canada, London, ON. Michael Bliss's books on both Banting [1] and the discovery of insulin [5] provided much of the background for this chapter.

References

1. Bliss M. Banting a biography. Toronto: McClelland and Stewart; 1984.
2. Stevenson L. Sir Fredrick Banting. Springfield: Ryerson; 1947.
3. Banting Papers. Fisher Rare Books Library, University of Toronto.
4. Bliss M. Dr Fredrick Banting: getting out of town. CMAJ. 1984;130:1215–23.
5. Bliss M. The discovery of insulin. Toronto: McClelland and Stewart; 1982.
6. Barron M. The relation of the islets of Langerhans to diabetes with special reference to cases of pancreatic lithiasis. Surgery Gyne Ob. 1920:31(5):437.
7. Banting FG, Best CH. The internal secretion of the pancreas. J Lab Clinic Med. 1922;7:256–71.
8. Banting FG, Best CH, Collip JB, Campbell WR, Fletcher AA, Macleod JJR, Noble EC. The effect produced on diabetes by extracts of the pancreas. Trans Assoc Am Phys. 1922;37:337–47.
9. Nobel Lectures in physiology or medicine 1922–1941. Amsterdam: Elsevier; 1965.
10. www.nobelprize.org.
11. Katz S. A new informal glimpse at Dr Fredrick Banting. CMAJ. 1983;129:1229–32.
12. Callahan William R. The Banting enigma: the assassination of Sir Fredrick Banting. St. John's Newfoundland: Flanker Press; 2005.

Charles Herbert Best

1899–1978

Philip I. Haigh, MD, MSc

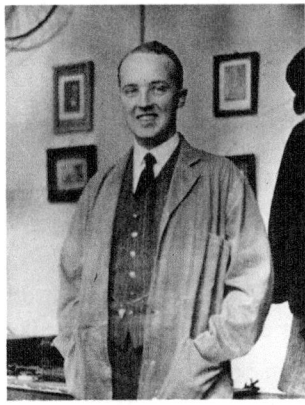

Photograph of Charles Best taken by Professor A.V. Hill, University College, London, 1928. (Courtesy of the University of Toronto Fisher Library, The Discovery and Early Development of Insulin online collection, digital ID, L10070. http://link.library.utoronto.ca/insulin/digobject.cfm?idno=P10070)

Charles Herbert Best was born on February 27, 1899, in Maine, USA, the second child of Dr. Herbert and Luella Best, both parents originally from Nova Scotia, Canada. His father was a "country doctor," and Charles spent much of his boyhood years in and around the towns of Pembroke, Easton, and Eastport [1]. After high school in Pembroke, at the urging of his parents, he moved to Toronto and studied at Harbord Collegiate to synchronize into the Canadian education system, and then enrolled in 1916 at the University of Toronto in general arts. He transferred into physiology and biochemistry after the first year, which was interrupted by a short stint with the Canadian military with duties in Great Britain during World War I, and then he resumed his studies back at the University of Toronto and graduated with a bachelor of arts degree in 1921 [1].

In the summer of 1921, in a few short months, Charles Best was the codiscoverer of insulin. At the time, he and his friend Edward Clark Noble were honors master's students working under the supervision of John James Rickard Macleod, professor and head of physiology and biochemistry at the University of Toronto. **Frederick Banting** required assistance to work on his idea of investigating the "internal secretion of the pancreas" and Macleod introduced him to the two graduate students. They were to take turns over the summer working with Banting, and according to many reports, Best won a coin toss to start his month first [1]. Work began in mid-May 1921, and quickly escalated at a feverish pace. Working into the early morning hours and most nights in hot, humid conditions, Banting and Best conducted experiments on dogs to isolate the pancreatic extract, initially by ligating the pancreatic duct, which resulted in atrophy of the acini, leaving viable islet cells allowing easier capture of the extract, which was then administered to dogs that had undergone total pancreatectomy. During the hot summer months and with conditions in the animal laboratory suboptimal, many dogs died from sepsis, with Best complaining to Macleod that it was "next to impossible to keep a wound clean" [2].

In August, a few months after starting the experiments, Best wrote to Macleod: "We made an extract from a pancreas, the ducts of which had been tied for 5 weeks. We followed your directions in preparing the extract—chilled mortar, cold Ringer's solution, etc. Our first trial was on a dog (410) whose pedicle had been removed on July 18th. …The extract seemed to have a marked effect" [2]. At the injection of extract, the blood sugar dropped dramatically. The letter continued: "Our most convincing experiment is the record of Dog 408. The whole of the large chart is devoted to this dog. We are also inclosing a copy of our notes as entered during the experiment. We hope that the curves and rough notes will make all the points sufficiently clear…. Until we hear from you sir we intend to conduct experiments on two dogs as follows—we will remove the whole pancreas from each and place the dogs in metabolism cages—we will treat

P. I. Haigh (✉)
Department of Surgery, Kaiser Permanente Los Angeles Medical Center, Los Angeles, CA 90027, USA
e-mail: philip.i.haigh@kp.org

J. L. Pasieka, J. A. Lee (eds.), *Surgical Endocrinopathies*, DOI 10.1007/978-3-319-13662-2_44,
© Springer International Publishing Switzerland 2015

one dog with the extract and have the other as a control. ... Sincerely yours. F. G. Banting C. H. Best" [2]. Banting also wrote to Macleod on the same day, with more details of the research findings. He also requested to continue with Best, rather than to switch assistants to Clark Noble as agreed on the initial introduction: "Mr Best has expressed the desire to work with me and I should be more than pleased to have him. His work has been excellent and he is absolutely honest, careful and impartial, and has taken a great interest in the work. He has assisted me in all the operations and taught me the chemistry so that we work together all the time and check up each others readings. I hope that you will be able to make out our report" [3].

By November of 1921, Banting and Best had collected enough data to present their initial findings intramurally in Toronto at a Physiological Journal Club, and then publicly at a meeting of the American Physiological Society in New Haven, CT, on December 30, 1921. Soon afterwards, the "Internal Secretion of the Pancreas" was published in the *Journal of Laboratory and Clinical Medicine* in February 22, 1922, which concluded primarily that

> Intravenous injections of extract from dog's pancreas, removed from seven to ten weeks after ligation of the ducts, invariably exercises a reducing influence upon the percentage sugar of the blood and the amount of sugar excreted in the urine. [4]

The work continued, and after several modifications such as changing substrate to fetal calf pancreas, the pancreatic extract became more potent, which led to greater success at more durable reductions in blood sugar levels. The most dependable results, and more readily feasible for larger-scale production, came after switching to adult beef whole pancreas and using alcohol to extract the hormone instead of saline, and also with the refinements to the purification by **James Bertram Collip**, a visiting biochemist on sabbatical from the University of Alberta in Edmonton. Collip took Best's product and increased the alcohol percentage, and when the extract itself precipitated, he used the reconstituted powder as the injectable. The advancements culminated in a preliminary paper published in the *Canadian Medical Association Journal* in March 1922 as Banting, Best, Collip, Campbell, and Fletcher (the latter two authors were clinicians at Toronto General Hospital), mentioning that the extract was used in seven patients and markedly reduced blood sugar and abolished glycosuria, as shown in detail in the first patient, a young diabetic boy [5]. The next major publication, authored by Banting, Best, Collip, Campbell, Fletcher, Macleod, and Noble, which was presented in May 1922 by Macleod at the annual meeting of the Association of American Physicians in Washington, DC, introduced to the world the term "insulin" for the extract [6]. Later, Macleod regretted not insisting that Banting and Best accompany him to Washington for this seminal paper [7].

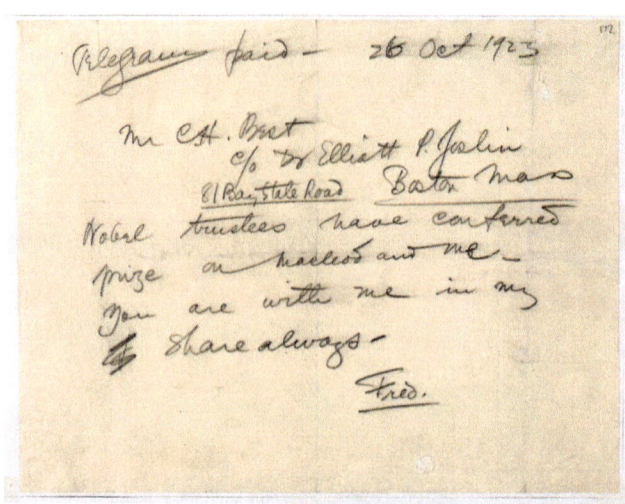

Fig. 1 Draft of telegram sent by Frederick Banting to Charles H. Best on October 26, 2014. (Courtesy of the University of Toronto Fisher Library, The Discovery and Early Development of Insulin online collection, digital ID, L10058. http://link.library.utoronto.ca/insulin/digobject.cfm?idno=L10058)

After the initial clinical testing of insulin, Charles Best changed direction and oversaw large-scale insulin production, and he became director of the Insulin Division at Connaught Laboratories at the University of Toronto and at the same time was a medical student at the University of Toronto. For about 2 months, insulin production at a larger scale sputtered as Collip was unable to produce the insulin as before, and none was produced. Best worked diligently with the team to get production back on track, and he succeeded in May 1922. He and Collip then collaborated with Eli Lilly and Company to try and improve larger-scale production.

The year after, Banting and Macleod were nominated by August Krogh, the prior Nobel laureate who visited Macleod in Toronto, and by several others for consideration by the Nobel Committee, and the Nobel Prize for Physiology was awarded to them on October 25, 1923, for the discovery of insulin. Banting, after learning Macleod was corecipient, immediately shared the prize with Charles Best. Best was in Boston, MA, as a visiting professor, and Banting drafted a personal telegram for him on October 26, 1923 (Fig. 1), which was then made more formal for public audience and read by Dr. Elliott Joslin, his host: "At any meeting or dinner please read following. I ascribe to Best equal share in discovery. Hurt that he is not so acknowledged by Nobel trustees. Will share with him. Banting" [8]. In a personal letter to Dr. Henry Geyelin, Banting stated that he thought that the "whole thing was an injustice to Best" [9]. A few days later, Best wrote to his wife Margaret: "It seems that the Boston papers speaking editorially and otherwise had heralded the coming of 'The Most Famous Medical Student in the World.' It has to be the most something. I went to the Peter Bent Brigham

Hospital at 2.30 and stayed there until nearly four. Went then to the Harvard Medical School where the students had congregated. The largest Hall available was filled to overflowing. President Elliot or Eliott or otherwise who is over ninety introduced me. He said that Dr. Banting a surgeon had come to Toronto to investigate a problem but that I had supplied the necessary knowledge to enable the problem to be investigated therefore that I was the real discoverer of insulin. Hurrah: cried the students. They really gave me a great reception both before and after my little talk. At the end of my talk Dr. Joslin read a telegram he had just received from Banting saying—'I assign to Best equal share discovery insulin. Hurt that Nobel trustees did not so acknowledge him. Will share with him. Please read this telegram at any dinner or meeting—Banting.' Dr. Joslin read it at the students meeting and at the dinner at night. I am going down to get a bite now, dear. I have thought about you continually during this trip, sweetheart. I love you more and more. Charley" [10].

The prize in 1923 certainly generated controversy, and according to Henry Best, Charles' son, "the process of awarding the prize failed to operate properly in 1923 and is most responsible for the unfortunate result that has embarrassed the Nobel Committee ever since" [1]. Almost five decades later, it was stated in 1972 in an official history of the Nobel Prize that Best should also have won the prize: "Although it would have been right to include Best among the prizewinners, this was not formally possible, since no one had nominated him—a circumstance which probably gave the Committee a wrong impression of the importance of Best's share in the discovery" [7]. Almost another decade after the official history, Rolf Luft, a former chairman of the Nobel selection committee for the physiology or medicine award, told the National Institutes of Health (NIH) that in his opinion, the 1923 award to Banting and Macleod was the worst error of commission, and he thought the prize should have gone to Banting, Best, and Paulescu (Nicolae Paulescu was a Romanian physiologist who also contributed to the discovery of insulin) [7].

Best married Margaret Mahon in September 1924. He completed his medical studies as class president and graduated with a bachelor of medicine degree (MB was conferred in those years, modeled after the British medical system) in June 1925 [1]. He won the Ellen Mickle Fellowship of the Faculty of Medicine for the highest rank in the medical class, and another award for highest grade in pathology. After medical school, he completed his doctor of science degree at the University of London working with renowned physiologists Henry Hallett Dale and Archibald Vivian Hill. He then accepted a position back at the University of Toronto in 1928 as the professor and head of the Department of Physiological Hygiene, and 1 year later became professor and head of the Department of Physiology, succeeding perhaps with some irony, John J. R. Macleod, who left Toronto for the Univer-

sity of Aberdeen. Best had a long and successful career as a medical research scientist and was also known for his work in the nutritional effects of choline in preventing fatty liver, the discovery of histaminase, and in the purification and clinical use of heparin.

After Banting's death in 1941, Best became the professor and head of the Banting and Best Department of Medical Research, and retired in 1967. He was awarded several research awards and prizes, and was also given many international honorary degrees. He was a member of a pantheon of societies, including an honorary member of the American Diabetes Association since its founding in 1940, and he was its president in 1948–1949 [1]. Best was coauthor of a textbook of physiology with Norman Taylor—"Best and Taylor's Physiological Basis of Medical Practice," for near ten editions, and the title is still in circulation today. Additional honors were plenty, including the annual Charles H. Best Lecture of the Toronto Diabetes Association that was established in 1970, and the Charles H. Best Postdoctoral Fellowship in the Banting and Best Department of Medical Research established in 1971. The University of Toronto Charles H. Best Lectureship and Award was later established in 1995 by an endowment to recognize outstanding contributions in the field of diabetes research [1].

Charles Herbert Best collapsed from a ruptured aorta on March 26, 1978, the day after the sudden death of his eldest son Charles Alexander Best, and then died several days later on March 31, 1978.

References

1. Best HBM. Margaret and Charley: the personal story of Dr. Charles Best, the co-discoverer of insulin. Toronto: The Dundurn Group; 2003.
2. C.H. Best's draft of letter to J.J.R. Macleod. http://link.library.utoronto.ca/insulin/digobject.cfm?idno=L10027. August 9, 1921.
3. F. G. Banting's draft of letter to J.J.R. Macleod. http://link.library.utoronto.ca/insulin/digobject.cfm?idno=L10026. August 9, 1921.
4. Banting FG, Best CH. The internal secretion of the pancreas. J Lab Clin Med. 1922;7:256–71.
5. Banting FG, Best CH, Collip JB, Campbell WR, Fletcher AA. Pancreatic extracts in the treatment of diabetes mellitus. CMAJ. 1922;12:141–6.
6. Banting FG, Best CH, Collip JB, Campbell WR, Fletcher AA, JJR Macleod, Noble EC. The effect produced on diabetes by extracts of the pancreas. Trans Assoc Am Phys 1922;37:337–47.
7. Rosenfeld L. Insulin: discovery and controversy. Clin Chem. 2002;48:2270–88.
8. Telegram from Frederick Banting to Elliott Joslin. http://link.library.utoronto.ca/insulin/digobject.cfm?idno=L10036.
9. Letter to Dr. Geyelin from Frederick G Banting. http://link.library.utoronto.ca/insulin/digobject.cfm?idno=L10336.
10. Letter to Margaret Mahon from Charles H Best. http://link.library.utoronto.ca/insulin/digobject.cfm?idno=L10478.

Allen Oldfather Whipple

1881–1963

Jean M. Butte and Elijah Dixon

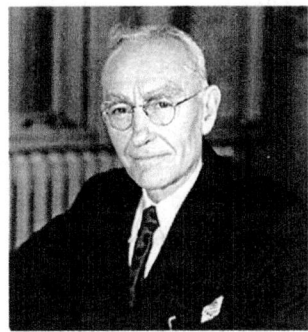

Dr. Allen Oldfather Whipple. (Courtesy of Samir Johna, MD)

Introduction

Allen Oldfather Whipple, called Oldfather by his closer friends, was born on September 2, 1881, in Oroomisha, Persia (currently Iran), where his parents were working as missionaries. He was always considered the eldest child because his three older siblings died at the ages of 1, 2, and 3 in Persia. The family moved back to the USA in 1896 with the aim of obtaining a better education for their children [1].

Whipple graduated from Princeton in 1904, and then attended Columbia University's College of Physicians and Surgeons, becoming a physician in 1908. He then completed a 2-year internship at Roosevelt Hospital in New York [1].

Whipple was appointed chairman of the Department of Surgery at Columbia-Presbyterian with the rank of professor of surgery in 1921, when he was only 39 years old [2]. Over the course of his career, he introduced the concepts of multi-

disciplinary teams, prospective collection of data for analysis, and critical assessment of postoperative morbidity and mortality. In addition, he made important contributions to the field including a better understanding of neuroendocrine tumors of the pancreas, the development of the *Whipple procedure*, and insights into portal hypertension [3–6]. He became president of a number of important surgical organizations including the American Board of Surgery and the American Surgical Association. After his retirement in 1946, he completed his career at Princeton where he was a professor of biology and a counselor of students. He died on April 16, 1963, in Princeton, New Jersey. Dr. Allen O. Whipple should be recognized for his tremendous influence in multiple aspects of surgery and for his impact on generations of surgeons.

Living in Persia and His First Years in the USA

Allen Whipple's parents, William and Mary Louise, graduated from seminary school in Ohio and went to Persia to work as missionaries. They went on a *Christian mission* and had nine children, four of whom died in Iran. Whipple was born when his parents had been overseas for 9 years, and his family always considered him the eldest child [1].

The Whipples' stayed in Persia for 25 years in total (1872–1896), with intermittent visits to the USA (1877–1880 and 1889–1890). The young Whipple had several run-ins with medicine including a bout of typhoid fever lasting 2 months and surviving a cholera epidemic in Tabriz that sparked his interest in medicine. However, he first became interested in surgery when his sister had surgery to relieve a small bowel obstruction [1, 2].

Whipple moved back to Oroomiah without his family to attend school in 1894. He lived with the Coans' family and attended the *College Hospital Compound*. In 1895, the wife of one of the local physicians died from pneumonia and the Coans (including Whipple) moved into his house to help him. Whipple was greatly impressed with the doctor, not only for his work but also for the compassion and interest he

E. Dixon (✉)
Division of General Surgery, Faculty of Medicine, University of Calgary, EG - 26, Foothills Medical Centre, 1403 - 29 Street NW, Calgary, AB, Canada
e-mail: Elijah.Dixon@albertahealthservices.ca

J. M. Butte
Hepato-Pancreato-Biliary, Foothills Medical Centre, University of Calgary, Calgary, AB, Canada

J. L. Pasieka, J. A. Lee (eds.), *Surgical Endocrinopathies,* DOI 10.1007/978-3-319-13662-2_45,
© Springer International Publishing Switzerland 2015

had in his patients. Whipple helped him in his clinical practice and clearly, these activities helped influence his decision to study medicine [1].

The Whipple family returned to the USA to prepare their children for college in 1896. Before leaving Tabriz, they donated all their belongings including their house to create the "Whipple Hospital for Women." Thus, they traveled with minimal goods, without a lot of money, and were supported by their families and friends after arriving. They settled in Duluth, Minnesota, where they rented half of the house where William's brother lived [1]. Allen initially attended the *Duluth Central High School,* where he was seen as a different person because he spoke four languages. The head of his school knew the dean of Princeton and helped Allen to obtain a scholarship to study there.

The Princeton Years (1900–1904)

While at Princeton, Whipple received a full scholarship with a US$ 150 annual stipend. He supplemented the scholarship by tutoring Latin and working at the *Princetonian,* the college newspaper. Years later, he said that this work gave him the ability to express his ideas adequately [1, 2]. He performed well and was in the upper 20–30 % of his class. Throughout his time at Princeton, he continued to work hard and eventually went on to manage the Robador dinning club, participated in the Colonial Club, and worked at the Blakeley Laundry. He spent the summer in Evanston teaching a classmate and attended the surgical clinic of Dr. Graham, in the afternoons.

He met many important people in his life while at Princeton. In particular, Charles McClure, a professor of biology, became one of his lifelong mentors. Whipple had planned to attend Johns Hopkins Medical School, but Professor McClure arranged for him to attend Columbia University's College of Physicians and Surgeons with a full scholarship.

Columbia University, College of Physicians and Surgeons (1904–1908)

Whipple continued to excel at Columbia. Of the 160 students in his class, only 79 graduated and Whipple was the third in his class [1]. After graduating medical school, Whipple wanted to continue his training at Roosevelt Hospital, which was the primary teaching hospital of Columbia. He started his residency training on January 1, 1909. However, important changes in the organization of the hospitals occurred during his residency. Abraham Fleuxner conducted studies into the organization of the medical schools of the USA, Canada, and

Newfoundland. One of the primary findings was that medical schools should incorporate a teaching hospital when feasible. Roosevelt Hospital was given the option to become the teaching hospital of Columbia University. However, they declined and Columbia subsequently partnered with the Presbyterian Hospital. This decision had an important effect on Whipple, since his surgical mentor, Professor Blake, was transferred to the Presbyterian Hospital. Blake was a senior surgeon, with important experience in and out of the operating room. Despite this setback, Whipple completed 2 years of internship at Roosevelt Hospital even though the standard training included only 1 year of internship. During the first year, he administered anesthetics during the morning, worked in the laboratory, and evaluated patients during the afternoon. He worked as the medical house officer over the next 6 months. During this time, there was a severe epidemic of typhoid fever in New York, and Whipple performed a cholecystectomy on 32 typhoid carriers, interrupting the life cycle of the typhoid *Bacillus* that harbors in the gallbladder and helping to stop the epidemic [7]. During his second year, he functioned as a surgical intern. However, he never completed a formal training program in general surgery.

Whipple was reunited with his mentor when Professor Blake offered him an academic appointment at his outpatient department as the second assistant attending surgeon. Whipple started on January 1, 1911, and was in charge of the fourth-year clerks. During this time, he worked with Dr. Bill Clarke, who was a surgical pathologist, and participated in research into angiogenesis. He also maintained an outpatient practice in the hospital clinic, worked as a part-time surgical pathologist at Englewood Hospital in New Jersey, and maintained his practice in anesthesia and some practice in obstetrics. However, during this time, he was not performing major surgery.

Notwithstanding, the dean considered him an important part of the academic team and appointed him as a junior attending at the Presbyterian Hospital in 1914. This marked his return to the operating room. He was primarily interested in the surgery of the biliary tract as well as postoperative care, specifically in pneumonia, and published at least one manuscript every year.

His Family

In the spring of 1911, Whipple was invited by a friend to meet two young ladies. Miss Mary Neales was coming to New York to be with her sister. After this initial meeting, the two maintained the relationship, and Dr. Whipple visited her in Boston, when she underwent an appendectomy. They were married on September 26, 1912, at Woods Hall,

Massachusetts. They were married for 47 years until her death in February 1959 from a possible myocardial infarction.

They had three children—Mary Allen Whipple (1913–1990) who married Dr. Richard Being, a famous cardiologist; Allen Oldfather Whipple Jr., (1915–1963) who studied history at Princeton; and William Neales Whipple (1917–1933), who was involved in a severe accident near New York. Dr. Whipple was called in to evaluate his son and traveled with him in the ambulance back to Presbyterian Hospital. Unfortunately, he succumbed to his wounds and passed away after emergency surgery.

Contributions to Surgery

Dr. Whipple contributed to the surgical field in many different ways [8–10]. However, he was specifically interested in the spleen (especially the after effects of removal) and portal hypertension, determining that the latter was a consequence of a liver disease. In 1945, he published their experience of 1189 patients treated in 17 years in *Annals of Surgery* [4].

Much of his research focused on postoperative complications. Indeed, he noticed that many patients developed a particular form of pneumonia after surgery. He studied this finding and wrote a paper called "A study of postoperative pneumonitis." In this series, 97 of 3719 (2.3%) patients developed this condition [8]. This was the first study to define postoperative atelectasis and its clinical implications.

Whipple created the first system to record the inpatient and outpatient records into a single document in 1916 and emphasized this comprehensive collection of data in his first paper about pancreatic disease published in 1918. That year he presented a protocol for the collection of information on

Table 1 A summary of Dr. Whipple's experience treating neuroendocrine tumors of the pancreas

Characteristics	N
Patients explored	39
Tumor found (patients)	34 (87%)
Operations	N=44
Simple excision	21
Partial pancreatectomy	10
Reoperation and resection	7
Whipple procedure	1
Exploration and failure to find the tumor	5
Diagnosis	N=43
Adenoma	27
Carcinoma (functional)	3
Carcinoma (nonfunctional)	1
Probably malignant	9
Adenomatosis	3

patients with diseases of the biliary tract and pancreas, which was one of the first prospective protocols.

Dr. Whipple became interested in pancreatic tumors, especially in *islet cell tumors of the pancreas*, while he was studying the spleen and portal hypertension. He initially studied the insulinoma, which was the first hormone-secreting tumor of the islets of Langerhans to be recognized. The concept of "spontaneous hyperinsulinism" was first reported in 1924 within a year of the discovery of insulin by **Banting** and **Best**. Patients presented with symptoms similar to those of an insulin overdose. After **William Mayo** first described hyperinsulinemia from a malignant islet cell tumor in 1927, and Rosco Graham in 1929 successfully removed the first benign insulinoma, many patients were operated on for symptoms of hypoglycemia, yet the success of finding an insulinoma was only 32%. It was Whipple who put together a series of 62 patients from the world literature operated on for hypoglycemia and developed a clinical tool to help establish the diagnosis of an insulinoma from other causes of hypoglycemia [5]. In this landmarked article, Whipple introduced his Whipple's triad, which consisted of (1) clinical symptoms of hypoglycemia following fasting, (2) low blood glucose levels at the moment of symptoms, and (3) temporary relief of symptoms with the administration of glucose [3, 5, 11]. By the time he retired, Whipple had operated on 39 cases of insulinoma, the largest published series at that time (Table 1). Whipple's triad is still utilized today in the diagnosis of insulinoma.

The Whipple Procedure

Until Whipple's innovations in pancreatic surgery, the formal resection of the pancreas was a highly morbid procedure. Between 1882 and 1905, 21 surgeons removed part of the head/body/uncinate process of the pancreas in 24 patients, with a mortality rate of 53% in 19 [1]. Codivilla performed the first pancreatoduodenectomy in 1898, but the patient died 24 days after surgery. That same year, Dr. Halsted performed the first local resection of a carcinoma of the ampulla de Vater [1].

Whipple observed that the main problem associated with the resection of the head of the pancreas was bleeding due to the hypocoaguable state caused by jaundice. It was not yet known that the underlying issue was a lack of vitamin K (a fat-soluble vitamin) absorption due to the disruption of the biliary system [12, 13]. However, the discovery of insulin in 1921, the description of human blood groups in 1930, and the discovery of vitamin K in 1929 helped improve the outcome of pancreatic surgery significantly. Whipple performed the first two-stage Whipple procedure in 1934 [6]

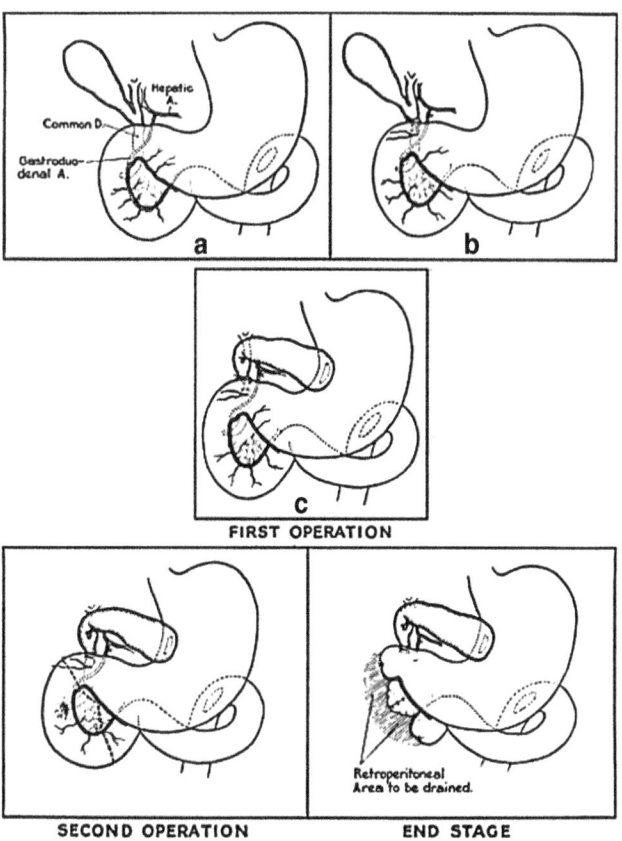

Fig. 1 The two-stage Whipple operation. (From Whipple et al. [6]. Reprinted with permission from Wolters Kluwer Health)

(Fig. 1), while the first one-stage procedure was not performed until 1940 [3]. On March 6, 1940, Whipple operated on a 33-year-old woman who was thought to have a possible gastric cancer. During the operation, he felt a mass in the pylorus and transected the stomach in the middle part. He examined the posterior wall and did not find a tumor in the pylorus, but instead found a small tumor located in the head of the pancreas. He performed a one-stage pancreaticoduodenectomy, removing the distal part of the stomach, the head of the pancreas, the duodenum, and the distal bile duct. He then closed the pancreatic stump and duct and anastomosed the bile duct to the stomach (Fig. 2). The patient had made an excellent recovery. The final pathology was a glucagonoma, which was the first reported glucagonoma resected. The patient died 9 years later from liver metastases. Whipple presented the case at the New York Academy of Medicine after 5 years of follow up and published the operation in *Annals of Surgery* that year [3]. Whipple would later publish a series comparing the mortality rate of 38 % in eight patients treated with two-stage surgery and 31 % in 19 patients treated with one-stage surgery lending support to the superiority of a one-stage procedure.

Involvement in Surgical Societies

Whipple was active in many surgical societies at the time. He served as president of the American Board of Surgery (ABS), the American Surgical Association (ASA), and the Society of Clinical Surgeons (SCS) among others. One of his great passions was surgical training. In 1935, he presented a paper "Opportunities for graduate teaching of surgery in larger qualified hospitals" [14]. The president of the ASA subsequently recommended creating an American Board of Surgery to help distinguish surgeons practicing surgery at a higher level and Whipple was vice-chairman of the initial task force. Whipple served as vice-president of the ABS for 4 years and president for another 2 years. Whipple served as the chairman of the commission that selected the questions for the first certifying examination. Whipple was also a governor of the ACS between 1938 and 1948 and received the gold medal from the American Medical Association for his distinguished service in 1951 [15, 16]. He served as president of the American Surgical Association in 1939 and his presidential address expounded on the subject of wound healing. Whipple was elected president of the Society of Clinical Surgeons in 1935 and traveled to Europe with the Society in 1937. The night before his departure, his mother developed a bowel obstruction from an inoperable tumor. He traveled to Wisconsin to see her, and she died 2 days later. He then joined his colleagues in Europe.

Time at Memorial Hospital (1947–1951)

In January 1961, Whipple received the Judd award from Memorial Hospital in recognition of his contribution to the field of cancer. He was subsequently approached by the director of the Memorial Hospital to serve as the clinical director. Although Whipple had planned to go to Beirut after retiring from Presbyterian Hospital, he ended up taking the position. His main objectives were to develop an academic residency, increase the standards, and create an autonomous surgical service. He created the most modern and well-equipped experimental laboratory of the country 1 year before retirement. Whipple did not like administration, finding the job very uninteresting, and happily left for retirement [1].

Retirement

Whipple moved to Princeton where he was appointed as an advisor to the students and continued with his studies on the splenic circulation in the laboratory of Professor Parpart, publishing these results in 1954 [17]. Whipple was honored

Fig. 2 The one-stage Whipple operation. (From Whipple [3]. Reprinted with permission from Wolters Kluwer Health)

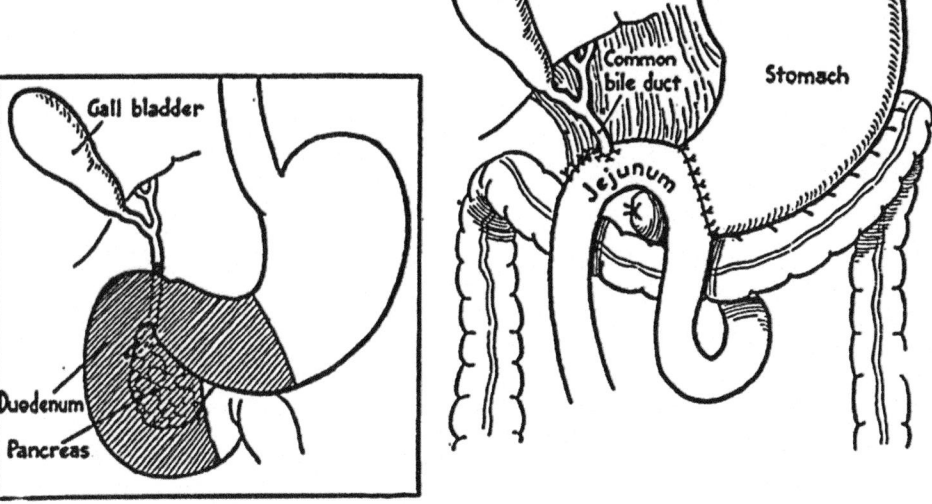

with a dinner in the Grand Ballroom of the Plaza Hotel in New York City on September 22, 1952. The *Whipple Surgical Society* was created that day and consisted of 217 surgeons who had been trained by Whipple. The Whipple Society closed in 1978 but reopened in 2003 [18].

Whipple continued on at Princeton as a visiting lecturer and professor of biology. He also became a trustee of Princeton University from 1943–1952 and was granted a doctor of science in September 1956 followed by the Woodrow Wilson Award in February 1958 for his lifetime of achievements. During this time, he was also the chairman of the advisory committee that guided in the building of a hospital in Shiraz, Iran.

Dr. Whipple attended the annual meeting of the ASA in 1961, but had two episodes of chest pain and returned immediately to Princeton. He was transferred to Presbyterian Hospital and was admitted for 6 weeks. He was found dead possibly of a myocardial infarction in his house, in Princeton, on April 16, 1963. His son had died just 8 days before. Allen O. Whipple will always be recognized as a pioneer in surgery and his work in the treatment of pancreatic disease. Surely, many generations of health care professionals will continue to refer to Whipple's triad and the Whipple procedure.

Acknowledgments The authors would like to highlight that relevant information in this chapter was obtained from two important sources:

1. The life and times of Allen Oldfather Whipple. *The Missionary and the Surgeon*, by John M Howard.
2. *The Memoirs of Allen Oldfather Whipple: The Man Behind the Whipple Operation* by Allen Oldfather Whipple, Samir Johna, M.D. (editor), Moshe Schein, M.D. (editor)

References

1. Howard JM. The life and times of Allen Oldfather Whipple: the missionary and the surgeon. 2007;1&2:1–1242.
2. Johna S, Schein M, editors. The memoirs of Allen Oldfather Whipple. The man behind the Whipple operation. First edition, 2003;1–222.
3. Whipple AO. Pancreaticoduodenectomy for islet carcinoma: a five-year follow-up. Ann Surg. 1945;121(6):847–52.
4. Whipple AO. The problem of portal hypertension in relation to the hepatosplenopathies. Ann Surg. 1945;122(4):449–75.
5. Whipple AO, Frantz VK. Adenoma of islet cells with hyperinsulinism: a review. Ann Surg. 1935;101(6):1299–335.
6. Whipple AO, Parsons WB, Mullins CR. Treatment of carcinoma of the ampulla of Vater. Ann Surg. 1935;102(4):763–79.
7. Whipple AO. The surgical treatment of bile typhoid carriers. Ann Surg. 1929;90(4):631–42.
8. Whipple AO. A study of postoperative pneumonitis. Surg Gynecol Obstet. 1918;26:29.
9. Whipple AO. The organization of a surgical department in a university clinic. Tufts Med J. 1947;15(1):3–8.
10. Whipple AO. The training of the surgeon. J Natl Med Assoc. 1957;49(5):295–304.
11. Whipple AO. Islet cell tumors of the pancreas. Can Med Assoc J. 1952;66(4):334–42.
12. Whipple AO. Observations on radical surgery for lesions of the pancreas. Surg Gynecol Obstet. 1946;82:623–31.
13. Whipple AO. The use of the duodenal tube in the pre-operative study of the bacteriology and pathology of the biliary tract and pancreas. Ann Surg. 1921;73(5):556–67.
14. Whipple AO. Opportunities for graduate teaching of surgery in larger qualified hospitals. Ann Surg. 1935;102(4):516–30.
15. Whipple AO. The continuing history of the society of clinical surgery. Ann Surg. 1959;150:783–9.
16. In Memoriam Allen O. Whipple, Md. 1881–1963. Ann Surg. 1963;158:148.
17. Whipple AO, Parpart AK, Chang JJ. A study of the circulation of the blood in the spleen of the living mouse. Ann Surg. 1954;140(3):266–9.
18. Longmire WP, Allen O Jr. Whipple surgical society. Summary of the meeting. Surgery. 1972;72(4):495–7.

William J. Mayo

1861–1939

Clive S. Grant

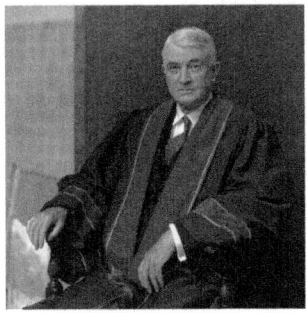

Dr. William Mayo.

The story of the first operation for insulinoma is fascinating but tragic. After struggling with recurrent bouts of abdominal pain and a perineal rash that seemed to defy diagnosis for 5 years, Dr. Dickinson Wheelock, an orthopedic surgeon from South Dakota, was referred to the Mayo Clinic by his local physician, Dr. D. A. Gregory, for abdominal pain accompanied by a constellation of additional symptoms. Excerpts of his referral letter are poignant and enlightening.

> I think someone picked him for a 'nut'…about a year ago he noticed that he would develop a tremor, sweating, and nervousness after going without food or after severe exertion. He discovered taking sugar would prevent the recurrence of these attacks…. About three weeks ago I saw him in one of his typical attacks caused by his going without breakfast and not having enough candy. He resembled an acute alcoholic, great motor activity, dancing and talking, squinting and frowning, apparently having hallucination of sight and hearing, negativistic and difficult to control. I had great difficulty in getting him to take a coca cola full of syrup, but after taking it, he recovered in about five minutes…. Several times he has become comatose…. This man is not a nut but has become rather soured on his professional confreres because he has not got to first base on a diagnosis… [He] is an exceptional case and I can find nothing about hypo-

glycemia. Try and get someone interested in him and don't let him die because he sure will if he goes too long without carbohydrate. (Referral letter to Dr. Davis at Mayo Clinic, 1926 [1])

Dr. Wheelock remained in hospital for months under the care of Dr. Russell M. Wilder, a noted endocrinologist. True to the story, the patient's hypoglycemia was so severe as to require an estimated 25 g of glucose per hour to ameliorate his symptoms. But no medical therapy could resolve his problem, and Dr. Will Mayo was consulted, principally because his surgical expertise was abdominal and pelvic surgery (Fig. 1). On Saturday, December 4, 1926, surgical exploration was undertaken. Portions of Dr. Mayo's operative note follow:

> The pancreas was normal from the head to the top of the spine and from then on it curved like a shrimp and seemed to grasp the spine. The consistency of this portion was hard, irregular. Secondarily there is a tumor the size of an orange in the middle of the right lobe of the liver…. A specimen about five cm wedge-shaped by about 4 cm at the point of the wedge was removed for diagnosis.

Extracts of the tumor and the normal liver were subsequently prepared which were injected intravenously into rabbits—and behaved exactly like an insulin preparation. Sadly, Dr. Wheelock continued to suffer symptoms when not receiving his glucose infusion, and remained hospitalized until he died on January 3, 1927. Autopsy confirmed carcinoma of the pancreas with metastases to the liver, intestine, and regional lymph nodes.

Pertinent to Dr. William Mayo's involvement in endocrine surgery is his first and only experience with thyroid surgery. In his own words, "Dr. Will" recounts this story as part of his touching eulogy for **Dr. Henry S. Plummer** in 1938 [2]:

> Away back in 1889, when St. Mary's Hospital was first opened, one of the earliest operative cases we had was one of goiter, the largest thyroid tumor I have ever seen, in J.S., a Scotchman aged about sixty-two years…. The huge tumor was a degenerating thyroid, and the man had great difficulty in breathing and was in a very serious condition. I had heard something about the use of iodine to cause shrinkage of large thyroid tumors, and I injected this tumor with iodine in a number of situations…. The patient's condition was precarious, and I knew, that whatever happened,

C. S. Grant (✉)
Department of Surgery, Mayo Clinic, 200 1st St SW, Rochester, MN 55905, USA
e-mail: cgrant@mayo.edu

J. L. Pasieka, J. A. Lee (eds.), *Surgical Endocrinopathies,* DOI 10.1007/978-3-319-13662-2_46,
© Springer International Publishing Switzerland 2015

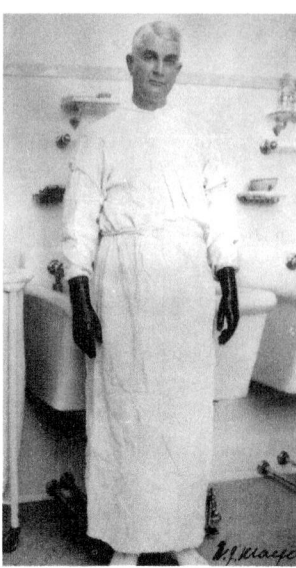

Fig. 1 Dr. William Mayo at the scrub sink. (By permission of the Mayo Foundation for Medical Education and Research. All rights reserved)

the tumor must come out. We put him on the table, using a small amount of the old ACE anesthetic mixture (alcohol one part, chloroform two parts, and ether three parts), incised the skin and superficial tissues…and rapidly enucleated the tumor with our hands. The bleeding was profuse…and knowing the efficacy of turpentine to stop this type of bleeding…the sponge soaked with turpentine was placed in the cavity from which the goiter had been removed, and the wound was sutured tightly over it…a large dressing was bandaged in place as tightly as the patient's breathing capacity would permit. After some days the incision was opened and the sponge removed. The wound healed perfectly and the patient made a fine recovery…. My brother, who recently had graduated from Northwestern University, in 1888, assisted me in the operation. This was the beginning and end of my work in the goiter field. The problem passed entirely over to my brother.

While the stories of the first insulinoma ever operated, and the collaboration of the Mayo brothers faced with resecting a huge goiter as their first thyroid operation are amazing and remarkable, the sustained prominence of William and Charlie Mayo goes far beyond. Their incredible, single-minded, lifelong dedication to serving mankind laid the foundation for what evolved into the most prestigious medical center worldwide. This account focuses on "Dr. Will", as "**Dr. Charlie's**" career is summarized elsewhere. But their success, fame, and respect were earned and shared equally. Their story can hardly be more eloquently recounted than to rely largely on their own words.

Will and Charlie were fortunate to have exemplary parents as role models—their father, William Worall Mayo, was a highly respected doctor. They recognized and appreciated their heritage. Charlie once stated, "the biggest thing Will and I ever did was to pick the father and mother we had" [3]. Will said, "It never occurred to us that we could be anything but doctors…. From the beginning Charlie and

I always went together. We were known as the Mayo boys" [3]. They learned the principle of *noblesse oblige* from their father. Will set lofty goals for himself—at the age of 22, after working in his father's medical office for 1–2 years, Will told a friend of his father's that "I expect to remain in Rochester and become the greatest surgeon in the world" [3]. Will eventually graduated from medical training at the University of Michigan on June 28, 1883, the same year that a devastating tornado ravaged through Rochester which prompted the building of St. Mary's Hospital (SMH), currently supporting 1400 beds. Charlie earned his medical degree from Chicago Medical College (subsequently Northwestern University) on March 27, 1888.

For the first decade of practice, Will and Charlie assisted each other in the operating room (Fig. 2). Only 5 years after finishing his training, at the age of 27, Will presented his operative experience with appendectomy to the Minnesota State Medical Society which was impressive enough for him to be elected chairman of the surgical section for the following year. Adopting the principles of antisepsis, they entered what for them was a golden era of surgery from 1890 to 1910. Their surgical experience grew exponentially. Following the opening of SMH in 1889, over 1000 patients had been treated by 1893. Abdominal operations escalated from 54 in the first 3 years, to 612 in 1900, to 2157 in 1905 [3]. That same year, nearly 4000 operations were performed at SMH, largely by Dr. Will and Dr. Charlie. After a while, the brothers developed different surgical interests and expertise; Dr. Will, pelvic and abdominal surgery; Charlie, eye, ear, nose, throat, bones and joints, brain, nerves, and neck. Tongue-in-cheek, Dr. Will commented that "I was driven to cover by a better surgeon. Charlie drove me down and down until I reached the belly" [3]. In December 2004, Dr. Charlie read to the Southern Surgical Association his and his brother's joint report of 1000 operations for gall bladder disease.

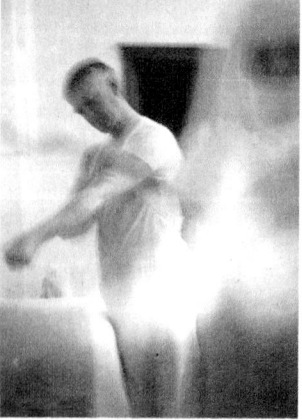

Fig. 2 Dr. "Will" scrubbing for an operation. (By permission of the Mayo Foundation for Medical Education and Research. All rights reserved)

In 1905, Dr. Will was considered the foremost American authority on stomach surgery. He read "A review of 500 cases of gastroenterostomy" at the American Surgical Association that year. In response, a Dr. Moore of Minneapolis pointed out that "the evolution of an operation...generally comes to us through the experience of a large number of men. Today we have had something which is almost anomalous in the history of surgery. We have been given the whole evolution of surgery within the experience of one man" [3]. A Dr. Haggard described a comparison of the two brothers as surgeons, "Dr. Will is a wonderful surgeon; Dr. Charlie is a surgical wonder."

Dr. Will expressed his views regarding education, especially as it related to patient care. His June 15, 1910 address at the Rush Medical College commencement, was one of the most important principles he ever emphasized, one that remains at the very core of Mayo Clinic philosophy. "Errors of judgment in student days were made harmless by the care and attention of your teachers. From now on you will have no such check upon your actions, and your mistakes will be costly because they concern the health and happiness, if not the life of individuals.... As we grow in learning, we more justly appreciate our dependence upon each other.... **The best interest of the patient is the only interest to be considered....** Write papers; they will do you much good, although at first they may not benefit anyone else. In order to write papers, you will institute a wider range of reading and investigation, you will learn to crystallize your thoughts and expressions, and, finally, to produce work worthy of your efforts" [4]. Even nearly a century ago, Will recognized the value of critical thinking over mere memorization: "Today we are suffering from too much knowledge too widely diffused.... Without intending to criticize unkindly, I believe that we devote too much effort to driving home detailed information and too little to the development of perspective" [5]. "We must bear in mind the difference between thoroughness and efficiency. Thoroughness gathers all the facts, but efficiency distinguishes the two-cent pieces of non-essential data from the twenty dollar gold pieces of fundamental fact" [6]. And beyond the education of just the individual, he stated, "What a man may do with his own hands is small compared with what he may do to implant ideals and scientific spirit in many men who in endless chains will carry on the same endeavor" [3].

The Mayo brothers were taught early by their father that "No man is big enough to be independent of others" [3]. Evolving from that principle, they recognized the value and power of collaboration. "In an endeavor to give the patient the very best in the way of medical treatment, a system of interrelation has been devised in which cooperation adds to the success of special practice" [7]. In contrast to the potential corruption of financially motivated physician group practice, Dr. Will described his model in a personal letter to Dr. W.L. Wallace, dated 1922, "Those clinics which are operated for the best interest of the patient and on the ethical principles of the American Medical Association will live, and will deserve to live, and that those which are essentially commercial...will die." Specifically, regarding Mayo Clinic: "...All its properties and funds, and all its earnings over a reasonable compensation to the physicians and surgeons of its staff go to create endowments. Everyone associated with the institution is on a fixed salary." Further, in a letter to Dr. J. Panteleone in 1930, "Properly considered, group medicine is not a financial arrangement, except for minor details, but a scientific cooperation for the welfare of the sick. Medicine's place is fixed by its services to mankind; if we fail to measure up to our opportunity it means state medicine, political control, mediocrity, and loss of professional ideals." "One can trace through the development of specialization, like the theme of a melody, the consistent purpose of carrying the benefits of modern medicine to the sick.... A sound understanding of diseases of the thyroid has been almost entirely a development of the last decade. The chemist, the research worker, the internist, and the surgeon have organized and combined to bring about the safety with which patients with exophthalmic and toxic goiters are now restored to health by surgical means" [8].

Will summarized the three keys he considered of vital importance to Mayo Clinic: an active ideal of service instead of personal profit, a primary and sincere concern for the care of the sick and for the individual patient, and an unselfish interest of every member of the group in the professional progress of every other member [3]. A different perspective was offered by an English fellow in training many years ago, "The most amazing thing of all about the Mayo Clinic is the fact that five hundred members of the most highly individualistic profession in the world could be induced to live and work together in a small town on the edge of nowhere and like it!" [3]. Reflecting on his professional life, Will stated, "What are the rewards of so laborious a life? They cannot be measured, because there is no standard of comparison. To realize that one has devoted himself to the most holy of all callings, that without thought of reward he has alleviated the sufferings of the sick and added to the length and usefulness of human life, is a source of satisfaction money cannot buy.... The medical profession can be the greatest factor for good in America" [9].

Addressing the American Surgical Association on the occasion of his 70th birthday, Will made the following comments—once again paying tribute to his brother, and addressing the new generation of surgeons to follow. "... Your chairman, in his kind remarks, has forgotten the most important factor in what I may have accomplished: that is, my association with my brother...Charlie (Fig. 3) has stimulated me by precept and example, and our association has been unique not only in the love and confidence we have for

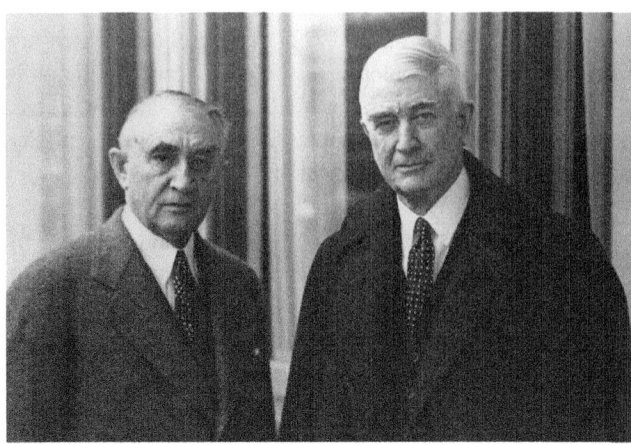

Fig. 3 Drs. William and Charles Mayo. (By permission of the Mayo Foundation for Medical Education and Research. All rights reserved)

each other, but in having made an opportunity for two men to work as one and to share equally such rewards as have come. Even to this day, not only have our fraternal contacts been maintained, but also our habit of having a common pocketbook, in which each has wanted the other to have the greater share. And with due regard to the statement of a truth, my brother, Charles H. Mayo, is not only the best clinical surgeon from the standpoint of the patient that I have ever known, but he has that essential attribute of the true gentleman, consideration for others." "Each day as I go through the hospitals surrounded by younger men, they give me of their dreams and I give them of my experience, and I get the better of the exchange…. I look through a half-opened door into the future, full of interest, intriguing beyond my power to describe, but with a full understanding that it is for each generation to solve its own problems and that no man has the wisdom to guide or control the next generation. It is a comfortable feeling, to be interested in what is to happen, but in bringing it about to be in no way responsible" [10].

On February 8, 1915, the Mayo Foundation for Medical Education and Research was incorporated, with funding amounting to US$ 1.5 million from the Mayos'. Four years later, the Mayos' transferred the ownership of all the properties of the Mayo Clinic from the building itself down to the last test tube, case record, and pathological specimen in it, along with all accumulated cash and securities. By 1925, the properties were valued at US$ 5 million and securities at US$ 5.5 million [3].

May 26, 1939, newspapers reported "Dr. Charlie is dead" from pneumonia. Almost 2 months later to the day, on July 28, Dr. Will died of stomach cancer. Their colleagues commented, "We are too close to this grief to describe it…. True sorrow makes a silence in the heart" [3].

References

1. Van Heerden J, Churchward M. Dr Dickinson Ober wheelock–a case of sporadic insulinoma or multiple endocrine neoplasia type 1? Mayo Clin Proc. 1999;74:735–8.
2. Mayo W. The work of Dr. Henry S. Plummer (eulogy). Proc Staff Meetings Mayo Clinic. 1938;13(27):417–22.
3. Clapesattle H. The doctors mayo. Minneapolis: The University of Minnesota Press; 1941.
4. Mayo W. The necessity of cooperation in the practice of medicine. Collected Papers St Mary's Hospital Proceedings Staff Meetings Mayo Clinic. 1910:557–66.
5. Mayo W. Medical education for the general practitioner. JAMA. 1927;88:1377–9.
6. Mayo W. Looking backward and forward in medical education. J Iowa State Med Soc. 1929;19:41–6.
7. Mayo W. The future of the clinic. Trans Assoc Resident Ex Resident Phys Mayo Clinic. 1924;5:21–4.
8. Mayo W. Progress of surgery in the last two decades. Surg Gynecol Obstet. 1925 June:737–9.
9. Mayo W. The medical profession and the issues which confront it. JAMA. 1906;46:1737–40.
10. Mayo W. Seventieth birthday anniversary of William J. Mayo. Ann Surg. 1931;94:799–800.

Gastrinoma

Naris Nilubol

In 1955, **Robert M. Zollinger** and **Edwin H. Ellison** described two patients with primary nonspecific jejunal ulcers associated with marked gastric hypersecretion and hyperacidity despite complete vagal resection and radical gastric resection [1]. The first patient suffered from complications of gastric hypersecretion, including recurrent marginal jejunal ulcers, gastrointestinal (GI) obstruction, and recurrent bleeding that eventually required total gastrectomy; the patient eventually succumbed to severe protein-calorie malnutrition and postoperative complications. A postmortem examination revealed 1-cm pancreatic islet-cell tumor at the tail of the pancreas. The second patient suffered from multiple recurrent esophageal, gastroduodenal, and jejunal ulcers and underwent a subtotal, followed by a total gastrectomy, to control gastric hypersecretion. One small pancreatic-tail islet-cell tumor with capsular invasion was identified, and a lymph node with metastatic islet-cell tumor was removed. The authors described a diagnostic triad of "ulcerogenic potential" of these pancreatic islet-cell tumors that included (1) the presence of peptic ulcers in unusual locations or recurrent stomal ulcers following gastric surgery, (2) gastric hypersecretion despite adequate conventional and surgical therapy (at that time), and (3) the identification of nonspecific pancreatic islet-cell tumors. The eponym Zollinger–Ellison syndrome (ZES) was proposed by Dr. Ben Eiseman at the Society of University Surgeons meeting in February 1956 to credit their discovery [2].

Since then, the understanding of gastrinoma and the management of this rare disease have improved significantly because of the scientific contribution from a number of well-known physicians and scientists [2]. These distinguished individuals (and their discoveries) include, but are not limited to: R. A. Gregory and H. J. Tracy (identification of gastrin, 1960), L. O. Underdahl, **Paul Werner**, and S. Wells (multiple endocrine neoplasia type I, 1953–1954), H. Oberhelman (duodenal gastrinoma, 1964), R. S. Yalow and S. A. Berson (immunoassay, 1960), J. McGuigan and W. L. Trudeau (detection of gastrin by immunoassay, 1966), J. I. Isenberg (paradoxical effect of secretin on serum gastrin in patients with ZES, 1972), E. Passaro and B. Stabile (gastrinoma triangle, 1984), **Norman Thompson** and J. Norton (importance of duodenotomy, 1989), R. T. Jensen (pharmacologic control of gastric acid hypersecretion), T. M. O'Dorisio and L. Kvols (role of somatostatin in neuroendocrine tumors; NETs).

Epidemiology

ZES is a rare disease caused by gastrinoma, the second most common functional pancreatic neuroendocrine tumor (PNET) following insulinoma [3]. The incidence of gastrinoma in the USA is one to three cases per million individuals per year [4]. ZES accounts for 0.1–1 % of patients with peptic ulcer disease [4]. For all patients, there is a slight male predominance (1.3:1) with a mean age at onset of ZES of 41 years. The onset of ZES in patients with multiple endocrine neoplasia type 1 (MEN1) occurs at an earlier age compared to that of sporadic ZES (mean age of 33.7 vs. 43.2 years) [5]. While most gastrinomas occur sporadically, approximately 20–25 % of patients with ZES have underlying MEN1 [6, 7, 8]. Gastrinoma is the most common functional NET in patients with MEN1, as half of patients with MEN1 have ZES. Thus, phenotypes of MEN1 must always be evaluated in patients with ZES [3].

Clinical Manifestation

Patients with gastrinoma typically present with symptoms of ZES as a result of acid hypersecretion. Historically, most patients presented with chronic diarrhea, refractory peptic

N. Nilubol (✉)
Endocrine Oncology Branch, National Cancer Institute, The National Institutes of Health, 10 Center Drive, Building 10, Room 4-5932, Bethesda, MD 20817, USA
e-mail: naris.nilubol@nih.gov

J. L. Pasieka, J. A. Lee (eds.), *Surgical Endocrinopathies,* DOI 10.1007/978-3-319-13662-2_47,
© Springer International Publishing Switzerland 2015

ulcer disease, or complications of hyperacidity, such as GI hemorrhage, esophagitis and stricture, and peptic ulcer perforation [2, 5]. Since effective treatments for acid hypersecretion, such as histamine H2 receptor antagonists (H2Rs) and proton pump inhibitors (PPIs), have become widely available, "classic" presentation has been substantially reduced. At present, in most patients treated at the National Institutes of Health (NIH), ZES manifests with symptoms of abdominal pain from peptic ulcer disease and diarrhea (70%), gastroesophageal reflux disease (44%), nausea (33%), vomiting (25%), and weight loss (17%) [5]. Chronic diarrhea is the only manifestation in 3–10% of patients [5, 9]. Because the clinical presentation often overlaps with common GI symptoms in other diseases, misdiagnosis and delay in diagnosis are common. Thus, a high index of suspicion is required for early diagnosis of ZES.

Although widespread use of effective antisecretory agents (e.g., PPIs) decreases the complications from acid hypersecretion, this type of treatment may increase delayed diagnosis. Ellison and Sparks reported an increased rate of patients presenting with metastatic gastrinoma during times when PPIs were widely used (55%) as compared to the prior decade (29%) [10].

Patients with MEN1 syndrome and gastrinoma can present with synchronous or metachronous endocrinopathy such as primary hyperparathyroidism (90–99%), pituitary tumors (30–40%), GI NETs and PNETs (30–70%), adrenocortical tumor (40%), bronchopulmonary NETs (2%), thymic NETs (2%), and gastric NETs (10%) [11].

Despite increased awareness of ZES, diagnosis is still often delayed. Several features should lead the physician to suspect ZES and reduce the delay in diagnosis: (1) the combination of abdominal pain, diarrhea, and weight loss, (2) recurrent or refractory ulcers, (3) hypertrophic gastric rugal folds as the result of chronic gastrin stimulation documented on endoscopy, and (4) GI symptoms with or without ulcers occurring in a MEN1 patient. Patients with any of these symptoms should have a fasting serum gastrin evaluation, while off PPIs, for a minimum of 72 h and possibly up to 7 days [2].

Diagnosis

Gastrinoma is a neuroendocrine neoplasm arising in the duodenum and pancreas and is composed of epithelial cells with neuroendocrine differentiation. Histologically, these tumor cells typically have round to oval nuclei with "salt and pepper" chromatin. Most gastrinomas are well differentiated and have a trabecular and pseudoglandular or nesting pattern. All gastrinomas have positive gastrin staining by immunohistochemistry (Fig. 1) [7]. Well-differentiated NETs are commonly characterized by expression of Chromogranin A and

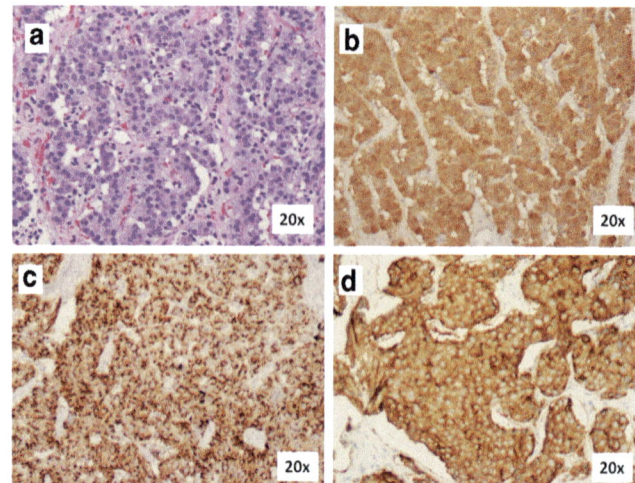

Fig. 1 Histology of grade 1, well-differentiated, duodenal neuroendocrine tumor (gastrinoma) from a patient with MEN1-associated ZES. **a** Hematoxylin and eosin stain. **b** Immunohistochemistry for gastrin. **c** Chromogranin A. **d** Synaptophysin. *MEN1* multiple endocrine neoplasia type 1, *ZES* Zollinger–Ellison syndrome

synaptophysin as seen by immunohistochemistry (Fig. 1) [12].

Once a diagnosis of ZES is suspected, the initial workup should include an evaluation of gastric acid hypersecretion and fasting serum gastrin levels. Because PPIs inhibit acid secretion, serum gastrin is commonly elevated as physiologic response to lowered intraluminal acidity. Therefore, PPIs and H2Rs should be held for 1 week and 2 days, respectively, if tolerated by the patient [2]. However, ZES patients can develop complications from acid hypersecretion and peptic ulcer disease during withdrawal from PPIs or H2-blockers; therefore, caution should be used when discontinuing these agents [13]. It is prudent to wait until peptic ulcer disease is significantly improved before holding PPIs or H2Rs for evaluation of serum gastrin. Patients with no active peptic ulcer disease can be treated with a high-dose H2-blocker while PPI is withdrawn for 3–7 days, then H2Rs should be stopped for 24 h to assess gastric acidity and fasting serum gastrin [14–17].

Criteria to diagnose ZES include (1) a fasting gastrin more than ten-fold higher than normal with a gastric pH less than 2 (40% of patients) or (2) a fasting gastrin less than ten-fold, of upper limit of normal, gastric pH less than 2, and a positive secretin-stimulation test or gastric hypersecretion (60% of patients). A positive secretin-provocative test (> 120 pg/ml increase) is frequently used to establish the diagnosis of ZES in questionable cases and has a sensitivity of 94% and specificity of 100% [18]. The later studies are needed in patients with less than a tenfold elevation of ZES, because a number of other diseases can also result in hyperchlorhydria/hypergastrinemia in this range, including *Helicobacter pylori* infections, renal failure, antral hyperplasia/

hyperfunction, retained antrum syndrome, and extensive small bowel resections.

A negative secretin stimulation test is extremely rare in patients with ZES. If the secretin test is negative, but there is still a suspicion of ZES, either a repeated secretin stimulation test or a calcium stimulation test can be performed. The calcium stimulation test is used less commonly, as it is less sensitive (63 vs. 94%) and has the potential for serious side effects from the intravenous infusion of calcium [18].

Because of the challenges in diagnosing patients with ZES and the potential complications from PPI withdrawal, the best approach may be to refer the patient to an institution with experience in ZES diagnosis [15, 16, 19].

Tumor Localization

The location of the gastrinoma and the extent of the disease are crucial for the management of ZES. Approximately, 80% of gastrinomas are located within the "gastrinoma triangle," which is defined by (1) the junction of the cystic and common bile ducts superiorly, (2) the junction of the second and third part of the duodenum inferiorly, and (3) the junction of neck and body of pancreas medially (Fig. 2) [20, 21]. Gastrinomas are frequently located in the duodenum (60%), especially in patients with negative imaging studies. However, hepatic metastasis is more common when tumors are located to the left of the superior mesenteric artery, compared to those in the triangle [22].

Although thin-sectioned computed tomography (CT) and magnetic resonance imaging with contrast enhancement are the most commonly used preoperative localization studies because of widespread availability, the sensitivity of these

modalities depends on the size of the lesions. Tumors less than 1 cm can be missed by cross-sectional imaging studies [16, 23]. Most authors recommend a biphasic or triphasic imaging protocol or pancreatic protocol [24]. Somatostatin receptor scintigraphy (SRS) in the USA is commonly performed using 111 indium-labeled somatostatin analogues with single-photon emission computed tomography (SPECT). Cross-sectional imaging studies detect 30–50% of small primary gastrinomas (less than 1–2 cm) and 60–70% of liver metastasis, whereas SRS with 111 indium-labeled somatostatin analogues has slightly higher sensitivity, at 60–70% and 85–95%, respectively [25–27]. The sensitivity of SRS using 111 indium is dependent on tumor size; 96% of tumors larger than 2 cm could be detected, but, in one study, SRS missed a third of gastrinomas identified at surgery [28]. Recently, 68 gallium-labeled somatostatin analogues with positron emission tomography have been shown to be more sensitive than traditional 111 indium-labeled somatostatin analogues in detecting small NETs, including gastrinoma (Fig. 3) [29, 30]. Thus, this technique is likely to gain wide acceptance as the imaging procedure of choice for identifying NETs. This imaging is currently available in several centers in Europe and a few centers in the USA, including the NIH.

Endoscopic ultrasound (EUS) has a high sensitivity for detection of pancreatic gastrinoma, ranging from 75 to 93%, and enlarged peripancreatic lymph nodes [31]. However, the sensitivity of EUS for detection of duodenal gastrinomas is lower, ranging from 11 to 50% [31]. The procedure allows cytologic evaluation of primary tumors as well as lymph nodes. Selective arterial secretagogue injection (SASI) test (with either secretin or calcium) and portal venous sampling was first described by Imamura et al. in 1987 to localize gastrinoma [32]. This test regionalizes the location of gastrinomas by selectively injecting secretagogue into arterial branches supplying the pancreas and duodenum and measuring the gastrin level by collecting venous samples from portal veins. A blush of contrast from angiography can reveal the location of NET as it is often very well vascularized. A step up in gastrin level helps localize the gastrinoma within the area supplied by the corresponding artery [33]. Although SASI has high sensitivity in localizing sporadic gastrinomas (86%) and MEN1-associated gastrinomas (81%) [34], it is used infrequently at present as other less invasive tests have improved diagnostic accuracy, and intraoperative maneuvers, such as intraoperative ultrasound, intraluminal illumination, and bimanual palpation, can successfully identify localized gastrinomas that preoperative localizing studies miss [34].

Ectopic gastrinomas have been reported in the stomach [35], heart [36], ovary [37], liver [38], kidney [39], and bile duct [40]. Excision of such lesions may cure ZES and is associated with long-term survival.

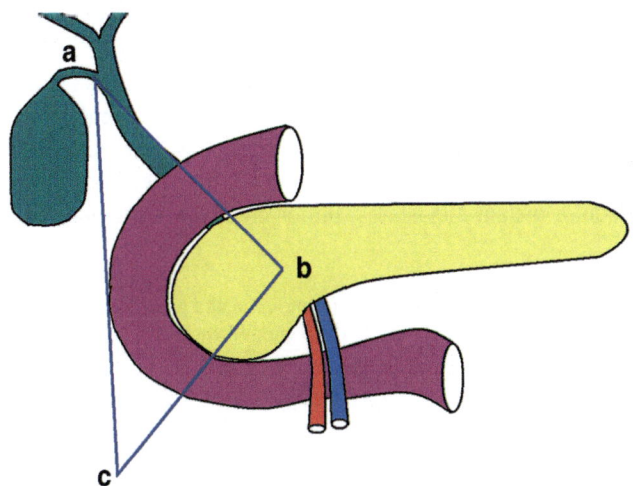

Fig. 2 Gastrinoma triangle. **a** The junction of cystic and common bile duct. **b** The junction of pancreatic neck and body. **c** The junction of second and third part of duodenum

Fig. 3 Preoperative imaging
studies in a patient with MEN1-
associated ZES and metastatic
neuroendocrine tumor. **a** 111 In
somatostatin analogue scintigraphy demonstrated an avid left
lung nodule with no other sites
of disease. **b** 68-Ga DOTATATE
scintigraphy demonstrates
multiple abdominal-avid nodules,
in addition to left lung nodule.
c 68-Ga DOTATATE positron
emission test/computed tomography revealed multiple, avid,
paraduodenal lymph nodes and
duodenal lesions. **d** Corresponding arterial phase of contrast-
enhanced computed tomography.
MEN1 multiple endocrine neoplasia type 1, *ZES* Zollinger–Ellison
syndrome

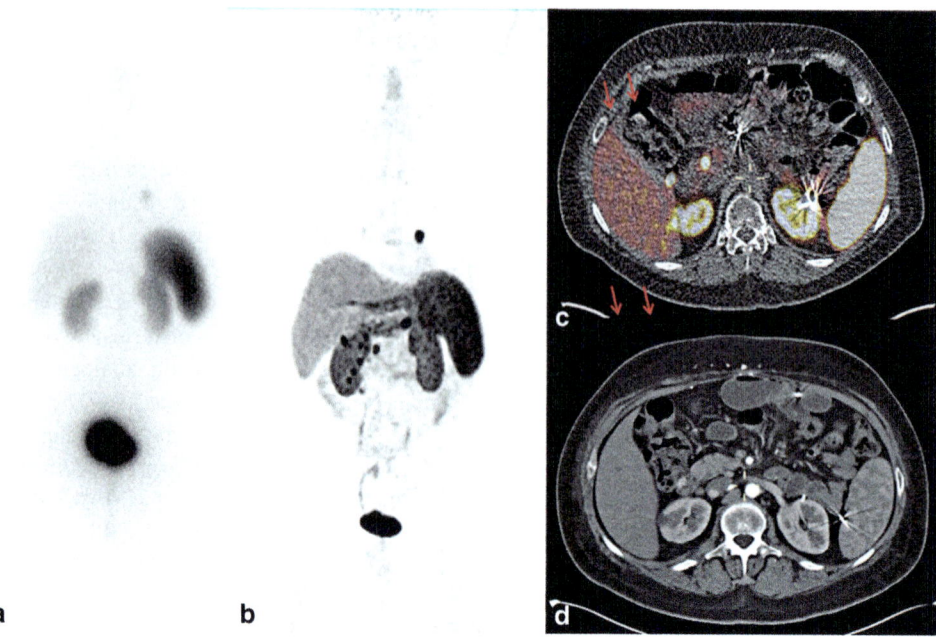

Classification

Prior to recent standardized nomenclature, NETs comprised
various entities based on organ of origin, mechanism of development, function, histologic pattern, and biological behavior. These entities include carcinoid tumor, pancreatic
islet-cell tumor, NET, and carcinoma. Recently, a number
of organizations such as the World Health Organization
(WHO), the European Neuroendocrine Tumor Society
(ENETS), and the American Joint Committee on Cancer
(AJCC)/Union for international Cancer Control (UICC) have
developed standardized guidelines to classify NETs [41–47].
While differences in parameters exist among the classification systems, there is considerable overlap in the essential
information used in each system; proliferative index is a
fundamental characteristic used in grading system. While in
concept, tumor grade and level of differentiation are related,
subtle differences exist [45]. Tumor grade refers to inherent
biological aggressiveness, whereas differentiation refers to
the extent to which tumor cells retain or recapitulate nonneoplastic cellular features. For example, well-differentiated
neuroendocrine neoplasms (grade 1 or grade 2 NETs) retain
morphology similar to nonneoplastic neuroendocrine cells,
including the presence of nesting, trabecular or organoid
pattern, and strong expression of neuroendocrine differentiation makers such as Chromogranin A and synaptophysin.
Ki-67-positive cells in grade 1 and grade 2 NETs are usually less than 20%. In contrast, poorly differentiated NETs
have less resemblance and are less organized than normal
neuroendocrine cells. Proliferative index (Ki-67) in poorly
differentiated NETs is frequently greater than 20%, while
immunostaining for neuroendocrine markers are often not
avid and may only have focal staining [48].

Proliferative rate is typically assessed by performing mitotic count or by calculating the percentage of tumor cells
that stain positive for Ki-67 expression. In 2010, the WHO
incorporated proliferative indices such as mitotic count and
Ki-67 expression as criteria to classify and consolidated all
NETs into three groups: (1) well-differentiated NET grade
1 (mitotic count per 10 HPF < 2, Ki-67 < 2%), (2) well-differentiated NET grade 2 (mitotic count per 10 HPF = 2–20,
Ki-67 = 3–20%), and (3) poorly differentiated neuroendocrine carcinoma grade 3 of small and large cell type (mitotic
count per 10HPF > 20, Ki-67 > 20%; Table 1).

To further improve prognostic stratification of WHO classification for NETs, ENETS includes site-specific tumor,
node, metastasis (TNM)-classifications, in addition to a
three-tiered tumor grading system based on mitotic count
and Ki-67 activity for GI and PNETs (see below) [42, 43].

An informative pathological report that aids in risk stratification should include diagnosis, tumor size, extent of primary tumor invasion, including lymphovascular, perineural
invasion, resection margins, presence of necrosis, lymph
node or distant metastases, tumor grade and differentiation,

Table 1 Grading criteria for gastrointestinal and pancreatic neuroendocrine tumors by WHO and ENETS classifications

Tumor grade	Proliferative indices	
	Mitotic count (per 10 HPF)	Ki-67 activity (%)
Grade 1 (low grade)	<2	<3
Grade 2 (intermediate grade)	2–20	3–20
Grade 3 (high grade)	>20	>20

HPF high-power field, *WHO* World Health Organization, *ENETS*
European Neuroendocrine Tumor Society

immunohistochemical staining for NETs, and proliferative rate (Ki-67 or mitotic count), as well as TNM staging [48].

Molecular Biology of Gastrinoma

The exact origin of the cells that give rise to pancreatic gastrinomas remains controversial. Some suggest that pancreatic gastrinomas may originate from islet and/or ductal cells [49, 50]. Duodenal gastrinomas originate from duodenal G cells. In patients with MEN1 or Werner's syndrome, an increase in duodenal G-cell proliferation was observed concomitantly with loss of heterozygosity at the MEN1 locus (11q13) [50, 51]. The most common inherited syndrome associated with gastrinoma is MEN1, an autosomal-dominant syndrome caused by inactivating mutations in *MEN1* gene that result in an alteration of menin protein. Germ-line mutation of this tumor suppressor gene is identified in 70–90 % of affected members of MEN1 families [52]. Because MEN1 syndrome can be diagnosed clinically in patients with two or more clinical features of MEN1 (pituitary tumor, pancreatic and/ or duodenal NET, hyperparathyroidism), negative germ-line mutation does not exclude the diagnosis of MEN1 syndrome as the affected individual may have large intronic mutations that are not recognized by polymerase chain reaction [53, 54]. The importance of *MEN1* tumor suppressor gene is further highlighted by the observation that 33–44 % of sporadic GI-PNETs harbor somatic inactivating mutations of *MEN1* [55–57], that result in a loss of menin protein expression or an expression of truncated menin protein.

Menin is a 610-amino acid protein that is typically located in the nucleus but is also detected in cytoplasm and around telomerases [58, 59]. Menin binds to double-stranded DNA in a sequence-independent manner via its C-terminal region. Menin normally regulates transcription by stabilizing or modifying histone proteins ultimately resulting in inhibition of cell division [60]. The loss of a direct DNA binding by menin results in a failure to repress cell proliferation and cell-cycle progression [61] Menin interacts with numerous proteins, such as transcription factors, DNA repair factors, and cytoskeletal proteins. The first menin-interacting protein partner identified was JunD; interaction of menin with JunD forms a growth-suppressor complex [62]. Deacetylation of histones is an essential mechanism of repression. Molecularly, MEN1 syndrome can be visualized by the role of menin in direct regulation of cyclin-dependent kinase (CDK) inhibitors p27 and p18 expression. Menin activates transcription by a mechanism involving recruitment of mixed-lineage leukemia (MLL) protein, a histone methyltransferase, to the p27 and p18 promoters and coding regions. Loss of menin function from inactivating mutations in *MEN1* results in downregulation of p27 and p18 expression, and thereby cell-cycle dysregulation resulting in abnormal cell growth and tumorigenesis in neuroendocrine cells [62]. There are over 25 proteins that interact with menin; however, the significance of all of these interactions for the development of NETs is largely unclear [63]. Functions of menin and interactions with JunD and MLL are shown in Fig. 4.

Multiple genetic alterations have been described in sporadic NETs. In addition to *MEN1* gene mutations, which commonly occur in sporadic NETs (up to 44 %), two other common mutations are death-domain associated protein (*DAXX*; 25 %) and alpha thalassemia/mental retardation

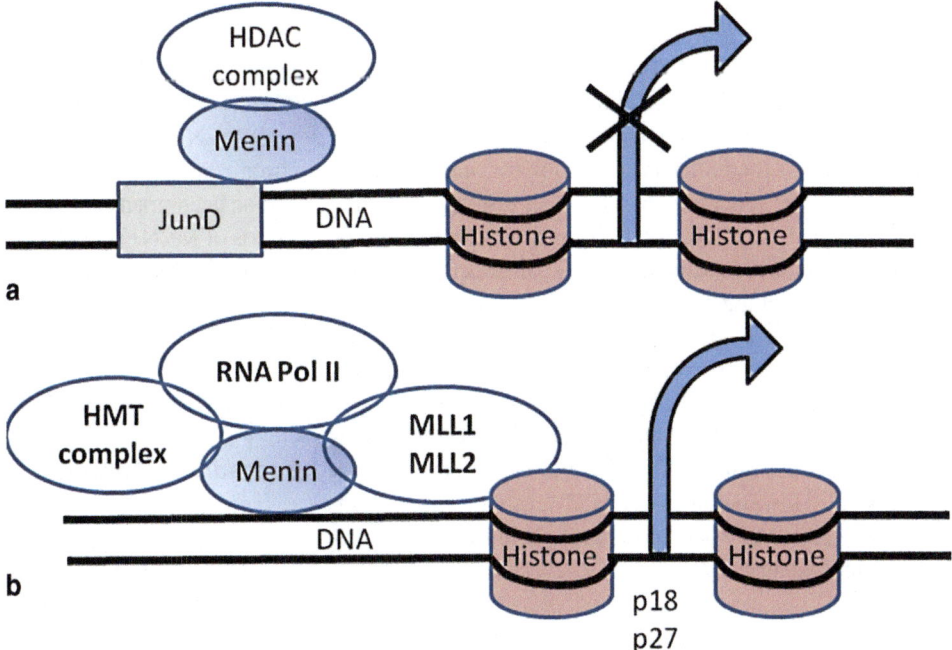

Fig. 4 The function of menin in transcription regulation by stabilizing or modifying histone proteins. **a** Menin interacts with JunD which binds to DNA and represses JunD-mediated transcription by recruiting histone-deacetylating protein complex. **b** Menin is a component of histone methyltransferase complex and interacts with MLL1 and MLL2. MLL and menin regulate expression of CDK inhibitors (p18 and p27). *MLL* mixed lineage leukemia, *CDK* cyclin-dependent kinase, *HDAC* histone deacetylase, *HMT* histone methyltransferase, *RNA Pol II* RNA polymerase II

syndrome X-linked (*ATRX*; 18%) encode two subunits of a transcription and chromatin remodeling complex [55]. DAXX and ATRX proteins interact and both associate with histone H3 machinery to deposit the histones on the DNA. Both proteins are required for histone H3 incorporation at telomeres, a function that might be important for maintaining genome stability [55, 63].

Clinically, mutations in *MEN1* and *DAXX/ATRX* genes are associated with a better prognosis. Patients with mutations in both *MEN1* and *DAXX/ATRX* survived at least 10 years, whereas patients lacking these mutations died within 5 years of diagnosis [55]. However, a recent study described the association of loss of DAXX or ATRX protein and alternative lengthening of telomeres with chromosomal instability, tumor stage, metastasis, reduced recurrent-free survival, and tumor-associated survival [64].

Approximately, 15% of sporadic NETs have mutation in the genes involved in phosphoinositide 3-kinase/Akt/mammalian target of rapamycin (PI3K/Akt/mTOR) signaling pathway such as *PTEN* (7%), *TSC2* (9%), and *PI3KCA* (1.4%) [55]. Both Akt and mTOR play important role in multiple cellular processes including cellular proliferation, survival, and migration as well as glucose metabolism. Microarray expression profiling of PNETs showed downregulation of PTEN and TSC2, tumor suppressors involved in PI3K/Akt/mTOR signaling pathways, in the majority of primary PNETs [65]. In addition, lower expression was associated with shorter disease-free and overall survival [65]. These findings suggest that activation of PI3K/Akt/mTOR signaling pathway contributes to the development and behavior of NETs. Jiao et al. demonstrated that all *PTEN*-mutated tumors have secondary mutation of *MEN1* and/or *DAXX,* suggesting that dysregulation of multiple pathways may be involved in the development of sporadic PNETs [55].

Most GI-NETs and PNETs exhibit a high degree of vascularization. Pancreatic islet cells express high levels of proangiogenic proteins, such as vascular endothelial growth factor (VGEF), a factor that is critical for islet microvasculature and islet-cell function [66–68]. Other proteins including platelet-derived growth factor, c-kit, and those in the mTOR and hypoxic-induced factor 1 (HIF-1) pathways have a significant role in angiogenesis of NETs [69].

A unique feature specific to NETs is that low-grade benign-appearing PNETs exhibit higher microvascular density than high-grade tumors. In addition, unlike most epithelial tumors and carcinomas, higher microvascular density is associated with a survival benefit and better prognosis in PNETs [70]. However, high-grade PNETs still have activation of key regulatory pathways involved in hypoxic signaling and angiogenesis [69].

Treatment

Medical Control of Gastric Acid Hypersecretion

The most important initial treatment for a patient with ZES is to adequately control gastric hypersecretion with antisecretory drugs. PPIs, such as omeprazole, esomeprazole, rabeprazole, pantoprazole, and lansoprazole, are the medications of choice because of their potency and effectiveness as well as their long half-life that allows daily or twice-daily dosing [15, 23]. For treatment of ZES, the recommended dose for omeprazole, lansoprazole, and rabeprazole is 60 mg daily. The maximum dose varies based on response to treatment but can be as high as 240 mg per day in a divided dose. A divided dose is recommended once the required dosage to control the acid hypersecretion exceeds 120 mg per day. The recommended dose of pantoprazole and omeprazole is 40 mg twice daily with a maximum dose of 240 mg per day in a divided dose [2]. Intravenous PPIs are the treatment of choice in patients who cannot tolerate oral PPIs because of GI obstruction, ileus, vomiting, or postoperative restriction; PPIs, such as intravenous (IV) pantoprazole, can be administered twice daily, whereas a high-dose of IV H2Rs must be given continuously [71].

Long-term PPI treatment in patients with ZES is well tolerated with minimal side effects and has great compliance. The long-term complications include malabsorption of vitamin B12, iron, and calcium due to hypo or achlorhydria [71–73]. Patients who are on long-term PPI treatment should have their vitamin B12 checked periodically. Although not specific to patients with ZES, long-term use of PPIs is associated with increased risk of bone fractures [73, 74]. Unlike animal studies, prolonged exposure to hypergastrinemia in humans does not increase the incidence of gastric NETs (previously known as gastric carcinoids), as patients with sporadic ZES rarely develop gastric NETs [71, 75]. In contrast, gastric NETs develop in 23% of patients with MEN1-associated ZES [76] and are not uncommon in chronic atrophic gastritis/pernicious anemia [77], suggesting that an accompanying defect may be needed in humans, such as loss of MEN1 or the presence of chronic atrophic gastritis, at least for the short-term development of gastric carcinoids (<10 years).

Surgical Treatment for Localized Gastrinoma

Sporadic Gastrinoma

The goal of surgery is to provide biochemical cure (normalized fasting serum gastrin and negative secretin stimulation test), prevent disease progression, and prolong survival.

The impact of surgery depends on the stage of the tumor. Preoperative imaging studies localize primary gastrinoma in 60–70 % of patients. Surgical exploration should be offered to patients with sporadic gastrinoma even in those with negative preoperative localizing studies; however, primary gastrinoma may not be found in 15 % of these patients [2]. A recent study suggests that an experienced surgeon will find a gastrinoma in 98 % of patients, and 46 % will be cured in patients with negative preoperative imaging studies [78]. In this study, patients with negative imaging had a significantly longer delay from the onset of ZES to surgery compared with those with positive localizing studies (mean delay of 7.9 years), and 7 % of patients had liver metastases at the time of surgery [78]. In addition, patients with negative imaging studies had higher rates of duodenal gastrinoma and longer survival [78]. Surgical exploration should include (1) a wide **Kocher** maneuver to facilitate thorough examination of the head of the pancreas, uncinated process, and duodenum; (2) mobilization of the body and tail of the pancreas for bimanual palpation; (3) intraoperative ultrasound; (4) duodenal transillumination and duodenotomy for exploration of duodenal mucosa; and (5) removal of lymph nodes in the gastrinoma triangle.

Duodenotomy is indicated in all patients undergoing surgery for ZES and was first highlighted by **N. W. Thompson**. Duodenotomy is the most effective method of identifying duodenal gastrinomas, which represent 60 % of gastrinomas [79]. Biochemical cure increased from 30 to 60 % with duodenotomy and removal of duodenal gastrinoma [80, 81]. The choice of operation (enucleation versus anatomical resection) for pancreatic gastrinoma depends on the location of tumor and the proximity to pancreatic duct. Enucleation is the procedure of choice for superficial tumors or tumors that are not close to pancreatic duct. Systematic lymphadenectomy with retrieval of ≥ 10 lymph nodes during initial surgery may reduce the risk of persistent disease and improve survival [82].

MEN1-Associated Gastrinoma

It has been well accepted that patients with MEN1-associated ZES who have primary hyperparathyroidism should undergo parathyroidectomy first to reduce gastrin stimulation from hypercalcemia [2]. On the other hand, the role of surgery in MEN1-associated gastrinoma continues to be controversial. Several studies have revealed that > 85 % of patients with MEN1-associated ZES have multiple duodenal gastrinomas that often are small (< 0.5 cm.) and are associated with lymph node metastasis in 40–60 % of patients [7, 34, 83]. Because biochemical cure in these patients is unlikely [34], and medical control of gastric acid hypersecretion is very effective, timing of surgical intervention and the extent of surgery are the subjects of ongoing debate because of the lack

of prospective, controlled data. Some authors suggest that a cure can only be achieved by performing a pancreaticoduodenectomy; however, many of these studies lack long-term follow-up and inconsistent utilization of secretin stimulation testing [2, 7, 84]. Although pancreaticoduodenectomy provides a good chance for biochemical cure for gastrinoma in patients with MEN1 syndrome, recent guidelines by Thakker et al. do not recommend this procedure because of associated morbidities and because lesser operations in these patients are associated with excellent long-term survival [11]. Thompson et al. reported eugastrinemia in 68 % of patients with MEN1-associated ZES undergoing aggressive targeted resection, which included a distal pancreatectomy, enucleation of any head, uncinate, and duodenal tumors as well as peripancreatic lymphadenectomy (the Thompson procedure) [85]. Less extensive surgery that focuses on identified lesions (enucleation or segmental resection of involved pancreas, with peripancreatic and periduodenal lymphadenectomy) has been currently used by groups at the NIH and the Ohio State University [86]. The rationale supporting this approach includes the indolent course of ZES in patients with MEN1, and the observation that most patients have longevity without undergoing radical resection that can decrease quality of life because of short- and long-term complications. Furthermore, a survival benefit can be achieved when no residual tumor is grossly visualized without normalization of postoperative gastrin [86]. The role of surgery for patients with MEN1-associated gastrinoma is largely determined by preoperative imaging studies. Surgery should be considered if lymph node metastasis is suspected, even in the absence of distant metastasis. While previous reports from the NIH recommended surgery in patients with tumors > 2–2.5 cm [87, 88], others do not use size to determine the time of intervention and consider surgery if localizing studies identify suspicious lesion(s) [2].

Treatment of Advanced, Metastatic Gastrinoma

Despite indolent clinical course, most gastrinomas are malignant, and the disease recurrence or progression occurs in 40–60 % of patients with sporadic disease, while most MEN1-associated ZES will not be cured surgically [2, 23]. Because effective treatments are available to control symptoms from hormonal overproduction, the treatment strategy for patients with advanced or metastatic gastrinoma (and other NETs) should target tumor progression both locoregionally and systemically. Because of the rarity of ZES, most studies that have patients with advanced gastrinoma include all other different kinds of PNETs since the treatments for advanced PNETs are similar. The presence of liver metastasis is one of the most important prognostic factors in patients with ZES. The 10-year survival for patients with diffuse metastatic gastrinoma in the liver ranges from 15 to 35% [86, 89, 90].

Fasting serum gastrin levels greater than 700 pg/ml are associated with poor survival; only 20% of patients survive 10 years compared with 100% of patients with a fasting gastrin levels less than 700 pg/ml [91]. Other factors associated with a poor survival for PNETs are extensive liver metastasis (>70–75% of liver volume involved), polyhormonal secretion (particularly adrenocorticotropic hormone; ACTH), extrahepatic metastases (in particular, bone metastases), and an unresected primary tumor.

There are several treatment modalities available for patients with advanced PNETs, including gastrinoma, such as cytoreductive surgery, liver-directed therapy (radiofrequency ablation (RFA), embolization, chemoembolization, or radioembolization), liver transplantation, biotherapy (somatostatin analogues, interferon alpha), targeted-molecular therapy (everolimus and sunitinib), and peptide receptor radionuclide therapy (PRRT).

Cytoreductive Surgery

The benefit of cytoreductive surgery in patients with metastatic gastrinoma is difficult to assess because most series combine PNETs, including gastrinoma and carcinoid tumors. In addition, there have been no case–control studies, and selection bias in retrospective studies can be a contributing factor for survival benefit. It is important to confirm that surgical candidates have (1) well-differentiated NETs (G1 or G2), (2) no extra-abdominal metastasis, and (3) no diffuse or unresectable peritoneal carcinomatosis. It is generally accepted and recommended by ENETS that cytoreductive surgery can result in long-term survival in selected cases, and a survival benefit has been reported when at least 90% of visible metastatic tumors are removed or ablated [2, 92–94]. Resection of the primary tumor, in the presence of unresectable liver metastasis, may be considered to avoid local complications such as intestinal obstruction, mesenteric retraction, and hemorrhage. If surgery is indicated, a cholecystectomy may be considered to prevent ischemic complications of the gallbladder following (chemo)embolization. Gallstones are less frequently observed with somatostatin analogue SSA therapy than previously expected, thus preventive cholecystectomy may not necessarily be required [92].

Liver-Directed Therapy

The indication for liver-directed therapy in patients with metastatic gastrinoma is usually progressive liver involvement, since ZES and gastric acid hypersecretion can be well managed medically. There are several modalities of liver-directed therapy for patients with advanced NETs. Percutaneous RFA or intraoperative RFA uses the thermal energy to ablate the tumor. Despite a high response rate of ablated

tumor (80–95%), it remains unclear if patient survival is comparable to medical therapy or palliative liver resection due to lack of randomized clinical trials. Because most hepatic metastasis from NETs have abundant blood supply from the hepatic artery, a selective hepatic artery embolization using a coil or beads coated with a chemotherapeutic agent or radioactive material is a good option for patient with bi-lobar liver metastasis and/or large tumors (>5 cm), situations which are considered unsuitable for RFA. Post-embolization complications are not uncommon. These include tumor necrosis and abscess, gallbladder necrosis, pancreatitis, and hepatic transaminitis.

The choice of an ablative procedure (RFA, chemoembolization, radioembolization, etc.) depends on the experience of the operator, location(s), number, and size of the tumors. Recurrence and progression after RFA for metastatic NET are common (60% in 10-month follow-up) [95].

Biotherapy

This includes somatostatin analogues and/or interferon. These agents have a tumoristatic effect and result in disease stabilization in 40–80% of patients, while less than 15% of tumor response rate [92, 96]. The clinical benefit of the antiproliferative effect of somatostatin analogues in patients with advanced gastrinoma or PNETs is unknown. A prospective, randomized, double-blind study in GI midgut carcinoid tumors (PROMID trial) using long-acting octreotide demonstrated a significantly longer time to tumor progression in the treatment group (14.3 vs. 6 months) [97]. The ENETS 2012 guidelines conclude that somatostatin analogues may provide some benefit in patients with advanced well-differentiated PNETs and that interferon should be considered in those patients if the PNET is somatostatin-receptor negative [92]. The Controlled Study of Lanreotide Antiproliferative Response in Neuroendocrine Tumors (CLARINET) trial has been designed to assess the benefit of somatostatin analogue in patients with advanced nonfunctioning GI-NETs and PNETs. Lanreotide was associated with significantly prolonged progression-free survival (median progression-free survival, not reached vs. 18.0 months, $p<0.001$), compared to placebo. The estimated rates of progression-free survival at 24 months were 65% in the lanreotide group and 33% in the placebo group [98].

Molecular-Targeted Therapy

Everolimus and sunitinib are currently approved treatment options for progressive, locally advanced, or metastatic well-differentiated PNETs, including gastrinoma. Although tumor remission is rare, 60–80% of patients experience disease stabilization [92]. The use of everolimus for PNETs has been approved by Food and Drug Administration (FDA) based on a large ($n=410$) prospective, randomized, placebo-controlled phase III trial that demonstrated significantly longer progression-free survival in the treatment group (11.0 vs. 4.6 months) [99]. However, no difference in overall survival was observed, likely because of the crossover. Everolimus has an acceptable safety profile and may be considered as the first-line therapy in select patients with advanced well-differentiated (low or intermediate grade) PNETs. The most frequent side effects included stomatitis (64%), rash (49%), and diarrhea (34%), and the most frequent grade 3/4 side effects were stomatitis (7%), anemia (6%), and hyperglycemia (5%) [99].

Sunitinib is an FDA-approved, multiple tyrosine kinas inhibitor for patients with progressive, well-differentiated PNETs. Raymond et al. conducted a prospective, randomized, placebo-controlled phase III trial that evaluated progression-free survival, objective response rate, and overall survival in patients receiving sunitinib [100]. The study was discontinued early after 171 patients were accrued (target accrual: $n=340$), because the primary endpoint of the study, progression-free survival, was superior in the sunitinib arm with 11.1 months compared to 5.5 months in the placebo. In addition, overall survival was significantly better in patients receiving sunitinib. The objective remission rate was less than 10%. The most frequent side effects included diarrhea (59%), nausea (45%), vomiting (33%), asthenia (33%), and fatigue (32%). Adverse events were rarely grade 3 or 4 and included hypertension (10%) and neutropenia (12%) as the most frequent serious side effects [100]. Similar to everolimus, sunitinib may be considered as a first-line therapy in selected cases.

Systemic Chemotherapy

Systemic cytotoxic agents are indicated in patients with progressive, metastatic, well-differentiated PNETs, especially with inoperable liver metastasis. Chemotherapy is the first-line treatment for poorly differentiated neuroendocrine carcinoma (G3) [92]. Streptozotocin in combination with 5-fluorouracil and/or doxorubicin remains an important treatment in patients with metastatic gastrinomas [101]. While this regimen produces a response rate of 20–45%, and there is no durable, long-term remission, side-effects, especially nephrotoxicity, are not uncommon. A recent study in 30 patients with metastatic PNETs demonstrated that 70% of patients receiving a combination of temozolomide and capecitabine had partial response with a median progression-free survival of 18 months and 2-year overall survival of 92% [102]. Additional studies are required to confirm the effectiveness of this regimen, and the efficacy in patients with metastatic gastrinoma remains to be proven.

Peptide Receptor Radionuclide Therapy (PRRT)

PRRT is a promising treatment that targets NETs that express somatostatin receptor in patients with advanced disease using Yttrium 90 or 177 Lutetium-labeled DOTATOC,

or DOTATATE. Based on several small, retrospective phase II trials, PRRT resulted in a partial response rate that ranged from 0 to 37%. The response rate is higher for PNETs than midgut NETs [103–106]. Bushnell et al. conducted a prospective, multicenter, phase II trial of 90 Y-DOTATOC and found that 4% of patients had a partial response, and the disease stabilization rate was 70% [106]. A prospective, randomized clinical trial to assess the benefit of PRRT in patients with advanced NETs is currently in progress. The use of PRRT should be considered in patients with advanced NETs after failing first-line medical therapy. The presence of somatostatin receptor as demonstrated by somatostatin receptor imaging is a prerequisite for the use of PRRT. Most patients tolerate the treatment well. Serious side effects include severe bone marrow disease (acute myelogenous leukemia, myelodysplastic syndrome; both in patients with and without prior chemotherapy). Kidney failure and liver failure occur in 3–5% of patients [103, 104].

Staging and Prognosis

The seventh edition of the AJCC cancer staging manual and ENETS staging both use TNM system and have included staging parameters for NETs of all sites. Because most gastrinomas are in either the duodenum or the head of the pancreas, the staging system discussed here will be for duodenal and PNETs. Although the TNM staging of duodenal NET is similar between the AJCC/UICC system and ENETS system (Table 2), there is a notable difference between the two staging systems for PNET in the extent of tumor (T2 and T3; Table 3).

In general, gastrinomas have indolent clinical course with a combined 5-year survival rate of 65% and a 10-year survival rate of 51% [108]. Even with metastatic disease, a 10-year survival of 46% (lymph node metastases) and 40% (liver metastases) has been reported with complete tumor resection have 5- and 10-year survivals of 90–100% [108].

In contrast to a very-low-cure rate in MEN1-associated gastrinoma, postoperative cure can be achieved in 60% of patients with sporadic gastrinoma. Disease recurs in 23% of patients, thus the 5-year cure rate is 40%, and the 10-year cure rate is 34%. Ten-year overall survival was 94% in a large surgical series [34].

Surgical resection of gastrinoma improves disease-specific survival in patients with sporadic disease. Norton et al. compared the outcome in 160 patients with ZES (21% had MEN1) who underwent surgery for gastrinoma with curative intent to that in 35 comparable controlled patients who did not undergo surgery (26% had MEN1). There was a significantly higher rate of liver metastasis in the nonsurgical group (29% vs. 5%, $p<0.01$). Overall and disease-specific mortality were significantly higher in nonsurgical group (54%

Table 2 The American Joint Committee on Cancer Staging for Neuroendocrine tumor of the small intestine. (Used with permission of the American Joint Committee on Cancer (*AJCC*), Chicago, Illinois. The original and primary source for this information is the AJCC Cancer Staging Manual, Seventh Edition (2010) published by Springer Science+Business Media)

Stage	Tumor staging	Extent or size of tumor	Regional lymph node metastasis	Distant metastasis
I	T1	Tumor invades lamina propria or submucosa and size 1 cm or less	N0	M0
IIA	T2	Tumor invades muscularis propria or size greater than 1 cm		
IIB	T3	Tumor invades muscularis propria into subserosal tissue without penetration of overlying serosa (jejuna or ileal tumors) or invades pancreas or retroperitoneum (ampullary or duodenal tumors) or into non-peritonealized tissues		
IIIA	T4	Tumor invades visceral peritoneum (serosa) or other organs or adjacent structures		
IIIB	Any T		N1	
IV	Any T		Any N	M1

Table 3 A comparison of the American Joint Committee on Cancer and the European Neuroendocrine Tumor Society TNM staging systems on pancreatic neuroendocrine tumors [107]

AJCC/UICC[a]				ENETS[b]				
Stage	Tumor staging	Extent or size of tumor	Regional lymph node metastasis	Stage	Tumor staging	Extent or size of tumor	Regional lymph node metastasis	Distant metastasis
IA	T1	Limited to pancreas, <2 cm	N0	I	T1	Limited to pancreas, <2 cm	N0	M0
IB	T2	Limited to pancreas, >2 cm		IIA	T2	Limited to pancreas, 2–4 cm		
IIA	T3	Beyond the pancreas but not involving celiac or SMA[c]		IIB	T3	Limited to pancreas, >4 cm. or invading duodenum or CBD		
IIB	T1-T3	See above	N1	IIIA	T4	Invading adjacent structures		
III	T4	Involving celiac axis or SMA	Any N	IIIB	Any T		N1	
IV	Any T		Any N	IV	Any T		Any N	M1

[a] *AJCC/UICC* the American Joint Committee on Cancer/Union for International Cancer Control
[b] *ENETS* the European Neuroendocrine Tumor Society
[c] *SMA* superior mesenteric artery
TNM tumor, node, metastasis, *CBD* common bile duct

vs. 21%, $p<0.01$ and 23% vs. 1%, $p<0.01$, respectively). Fifteen-year disease-specific survival was higher in the surgical group (98% vs. 74%, $p<0.01$) [80]. Ellison et al. reported that patients with sporadic gastrinoma who underwent R0 (normal postoperative gastrin) and R1 (postoperative hypergastrinemia but no measurable residual disease) had significantly higher disease-specific survival rate, compared with nonsurgical patients and patients with gross residual tumors postoperatively (R2; 60% vs. 20%, $p<0.01$) [86].

The prognosis of patients with MEN1-associated gastrinoma is difficult to assess because (1) metastatic NETs in patients with MEN1 syndrome can be from multiple origins such as nonfunctioning PNET, gastrointestinal NET (carcinoid tumors), or gastrinoma; (2) there is no consensus in treatment strategy because of a lack of controlled studies for this rare syndrome to determine the appropriate timing and role of surgery. An earlier study suggested that patients with MEN1-associated gastrinoma generally have excellent long-term survival, with or without surgery. Fifteen-year survival of patients with metastatic disease was over 50% [87]. However, the progression of gastrinoma and/or other NETs is probably the most important factor affecting long-term survival in patients with MEN1 syndrome [109].

Summary

There have been several advances in understanding the molecular pathogenesis of NETs including gastrinoma and in the molecular imaging modalities that provide superior diagnostic accuracy. As a result of insights into the molecular biology of NETs, new treatment options such as targeted-molecular therapy and PRRT are available for patients with advance disease. Despite recent advances in diagnosis and treatment, early diagnosis probably has the greatest impact on patient survival; however, delay in diagnosis is still common. Because effective medical control of gastric acid hypersecretion is widely available, the goal of surgery is to intervene before distant metastasis occurs. All patients with sporadic gastrinoma should undergo surgery as it can provide a cure and improve survival. The timing and the extent of surgery in MEN1-associated ZES continues to be a subject of controversy. While radical surgery may provide a cure in some patients, patients who receive a lesser operation have excellent long-term survival with medical treatment to control acid output.

Key Summary Points

- ZES is a rare disease caused by gastrinoma, the second most common functioning NET. Approximately, 20–25 % of patients with ZES have underlying MEN1.
- Because effective medical treatments for acid hypersecretion are widely available, classic presentation of ZES (chronic diarrhea, refractory peptic ulcer disease, or complication of acid hypersecretion) has been reduced. Abdominal pain, diarrhea, and gastroesophageal reflux disease are common presenting symptoms. High index of suspicion for ZES can reduce delayed diagnosis.
- Initial workup of ZES includes an evaluation of gastric acid hypersecretion and fasting serum gastrin levels. Diagnostic criteria of ZES include (1) a fasting serum gastrin more than tenfold higher than normal with gastric pH < 2 or (2) a fasting serum gastrin less than tenfold of upper normal limit, while gastric pH < 2 *and* a positive secretin-stimulation test.
- Eighty percent of gastrinomas are located within "gastrinoma triangle." Preoperative imaging studies such as CT scan, MRI, somatostatin analogue scintigraphy, and endoscopic ultrasound can help identify primary and metastatic gastrinoma. Recent studies suggest that 68-Gallium-labeled somatostatin analogues scintigraphy with positron emission tomography provides higher accuracy and sensitivity in identifying gastrinoma.
- NETs, including gastrinoma, are classified by tumor grade and level of differentiation. The WHO and the ENETS use proliferative indices (mitotic count and Ki-67 activity) to categorize NETs into three grades. NETs can be classified by a level of differentiation (well-, or poorly differentiated NETs). ENETS and the AJCC have recently published site-specific TNM staging systems for NETs.
- Advances in molecular pathogenesis of NETs show several dysregulated molecular pathways and gene mutations involved in tumor initiation and progression. Dysregulated pathways include PI3K/AKT/mTOR pathways, VGEF, hypoxic-induced factor (HIF-1) and other factors associated with angiogenesis. Mutation in *MEN1, DAXX,* and *ATRX* genes in sporadic tumors have recently been described.
- Because the effective treatment of gastric acid hypersecretion in patients with ZES using PPIs is widely available, the indication for surgery has shifted to prevent disease progression and offer a chance of biochemical cure in patients with sporadic gastrinoma. Enucleation or anatomical resection of pancreas may be performed in patients with sporadic gastrinoma. Surgical treatment for patients with MEN1-associated ZES remains controversial. Periduodenal and peripancreatic lymph node dissection should be performed in all patients with ZES undergoing surgery, as lymph node metastasis is not uncommon in patients with gastrinoma.
- Several treatment options for patients with metastatic gastrinoma are available. These include cytoreductive surgery, liver-directed therapy, biotherapy (somatostatin analogue), molecular-targeted therapy (sunitinib, everolimus), systemic chemotherapy, and PRRT

References

1. Zollinger RM, Ellison EH. Primary peptic ulcerations of the jejunum associated with islet cell tumors of the pancreas. Ann Surg. 1955;142(4):709–23 (discussion 24–8).
2. Ellison EC, Johnson JA. The Zollinger–Ellison syndrome: a comprehensive review of historical, scientific, and clinical considerations. Curr Probl Surg. 2009;46(1):13–106.
3. Krampitz GW, Norton JA. Pancreatic neuroendocrine tumors. Curr Probl Surg. 2013;50(11):509–45.
4. Gibril F, Jensen RT. Zollinger–Ellison syndrome revisited: diagnosis, biologic markers, associated inherited disorders, and acid hypersecretion. Curr Gastroenterol Rep. 2004;6(6):454–63.
5. Roy PK, Venzon DJ, Shojamanesh H, Abou-Saif A, Peghini P, Doppman JL, et al. Zollinger–Ellison syndrome. Clinical presentation in 261 patients. Medicine (Baltimore). 2000;79(6):379–411.
6. Ito T, Igarashi H, Uehara H, Berna MJ, Jensen RT. Causes of death and prognostic factors in multiple endocrine neoplasia type 1: a prospective study: comparison of 106 MEN1/Zollinger-Ellison syndrome patients with 1613 literature MEN1 patients with or without pancreatic endocrine tumors. Medicine (Baltimore). 2013;92(3):135–81.
7. Jensen RT, Niederle B, Mitry E, Ramage JK, Steinmuller T, Lewington V, et al. Gastrinoma (duodenal and pancreatic). Neuroendocrinology. 2006;84(3):173–82.
8. Benya RV, Metz DC, Venzon DJ, Fishbeyn VA, Strader DB, Orbuch M, et al. Zollinger–Ellison syndrome can be the initial endocrine manifestation in patients with multiple endocrine neoplasia-type I. Am J Med. 1994;97(5):436–44.
9. Simmons LH, Guimaraes AR, Zukerberg LR. Case records of the Massachusetts General Hospital. Case 6-2013. A 54-year-old man with recurrent diarrhea. N Engl J Med. 2013;368(8):757–65.
10. Ellison EC, Sparks J. Zollinger-Ellison syndrome in the era of effective acid suppression: are we unknowingly growing tumors? Am J Surg. 2003;186(3):245–8.
11. Thakker RV, Newey PJ, Walls GV, Bilezikian J, Dralle H, Ebeling PR, et al. Clinical practice guidelines for multiple endocrine neoplasia type 1 (MEN1). J Clin Endocrinol Metab. 2012;97(9):2990–3011.

12. Kloppel G, Couvelard A, Perren A, Komminoth P, McNicol AM, Nilsson O, et al. ENETS consensus guidelines for the standards of care in neuroendocrine tumors: towards a standardized approach to the diagnosis of gastroenteropancreatic neuroendocrine tumors and their prognostic stratification. Neuroendocrinology. 2009;90(2):162–6.

13. Poitras P, Gingras MH, Rehfeld JF. The Zollinger–Ellison syndrome: dangers and consequences of interrupting antisecretory treatment. Clin Gastroenterol Hepatol. 2012;10(2):199–202.

14. Ito T, Igarashi H, Jensen RT. Pancreatic neuroendocrine tumors: clinical features, diagnosis and medical treatment: advances. Best Pract Res Clin Gastroenterol. 2012;26(6):737–53.

15. Jensen RT, Cadiot G, Brandi ML, de Herder WW, Kaltsas G, Komminoth P, et al. ENETS consensus guidelines for the management of patients with digestive neuroendocrine neoplasms: functional pancreatic endocrine tumor syndromes. Neuroendocrinology. 2012;95(2):98–119.

16. Kulke MH, Anthony LB, Bushnell DL, de Herder WW, Goldsmith SJ, Klimstra DS, et al. NANETS treatment guidelines: well-differentiated neuroendocrine tumors of the stomach and pancreas. Pancreas. 2010;39(6):735–52.

17. Ito T, Cadiot G, Jensen RT. Diagnosis of Zollinger-Ellison syndrome: increasingly difficult. World J Gastroenterol. 2012;18(39):5495–503.

18. Berna MJ, Hoffmann KM, Long SH, Serrano J, Gibril F, Jensen RT. Serum gastrin in Zollinger-Ellison syndrome: II. Prospective study of gastrin provocative testing in 293 patients from the National Institutes of Health and comparison with 537 cases from the literature. evaluation of diagnostic criteria, proposal of new criteria, and correlations with clinical and tumoral features. Medicine (Baltimore). 2006;85(6):331–64.

19. Metz DC, Jensen RT. Gastrointestinal neuroendocrine tumors: pancreatic endocrine tumors. Gastroenterology. 2008;135(5):1469–92.

20. Stabile BE, Morrow DJ, Passaro E Jr. The gastrinoma triangle: operative implications. Am J Surg. 1984;147(1):25–31.

21. Howard TJ, Zinner MJ, Stabile BE, Passaro E Jr. Gastrinoma excision for cure. A prospective analysis. Ann Surg. 1990;211(1):9–14.

22. Howard TJ, Sawicki MP, Stabile BE, Watt PC, Passaro E Jr. Biologic behavior of sporadic gastrinoma located to the right and left of the superior mesenteric artery. Am J Surg. 1993;165(1):101–5 (discussion 5–6).

23. Ito T, Igarashi H, Jensen RT. Zollinger–Ellison syndrome: recent advances and controversies. Curr Opin Gastroenterol. 2013;29(6):650–61.

24. Noone TC, Hosey J, Firat Z, Semelka RC. Imaging and localization of islet-cell tumours of the pancreas on CT and MRI. Best Pract Res Clin Endocrinol Metab. 2005;19(2):195–211.

25. Gibril F, Jensen RT. Diagnostic uses of radiolabelled somatostatin receptor analogues in gastroenteropancreatic endocrine tumours. Dig Liver Dis. 2004;36(Suppl. 1):S106–20.

26. Gibril F, Reynolds JC, Doppman JL, Chen CC, Venzon DJ, Termanini B, et al. Somatostatin receptor scintigraphy: its sensitivity compared with that of other imaging methods in detecting primary and metastatic gastrinomas. A prospective study. Ann Intern Med. 1996;125(1):26–34.

27. Termanini B, Gibril F, Reynolds JC, Doppman JL, Chen CC, Stewart CA, et al. Value of somatostatin receptor scintigraphy: a prospective study in gastrinoma of its effect on clinical management. Gastroenterology. 1997;112(2):335–47.

28. Alexander HR, Fraker DL, Norton JA, Bartlett DL, Tio L, Benjamin SB, et al. Prospective study of somatostatin receptor scintigraphy and its effect on operative outcome in patients with Zollinger–Ellison syndrome. Ann Surg. 1998;228(2):228–38.

29. Naswa N, Sharma P, Soundararajan R, Karunanithi S, Nazar AH, Kumar R, et al. Diagnostic performance of somatostatin receptor PET/CT using 68 Ga-DOTANOC in gastrinoma patients with negative or equivocal CT findings. Abdom Imaging. 2013;38(3):552–60.

30. Srirajaskanthan R, Kayani I, Quigley AM, Soh J, Caplin ME, Bomanji J. The role of 68 Ga-DOTATATE PET in patients with neuroendocrine tumors and negative or equivocal findings on 111In-DTPA-octreotide scintigraphy. J Nucl Med. 2010;51(6):875–82.

31. McLean AM, Fairclough PD. Endoscopic ultrasound in the localisation of pancreatic islet cell tumours. Best Pract Res Clin Endocrinol Metab. 2005;19(2):177–93.

32. Imamura M, Takahashi K, Adachi H, Minematsu S, Shimada Y, Naito M, et al. Usefulness of selective arterial secretin injection test for localization of gastrinoma in the Zollinger–Ellison syndrome. Ann Surg. 1987;205(3):230–9.

33. Imamura M, Komoto I, Ota S. Changing treatment strategy for gastrinoma in patients with Zollinger–Ellison syndrome. World J Surg. 2006;30(1):1–11.

34. Norton JA, Fraker DL, Alexander HR, Venzon DJ, Doppman JL, Serrano J, et al. Surgery to cure the Zollinger–Ellison syndrome. N Engl J Med. 1999;341(9):635–44.

35. Liu TH, Zhong SX, Chen YF, Lin Y, Chen J, Li DC, et al. Gastric gastrinoma. Chin Med J (Engl). 1989;102(10):774–82.

36. Noda S, Norton JA, Jensen RT, Gay WA Jr. Surgical resection of intracardiac gastrinoma. Ann Thorac Surg. 1999;67(2):532–3.

37. Primrose JN, Maloney M, Wells M, Bulgim O, Johnston D. Gastrin-producing ovarian mucinous cystadenomas: a cause of the Zollinger–Ellison syndrome. Surgery. 1988;104(5):830–3.

38. Smith AL, Auldist AW. Successful surgical resection of an hepatic gastrinoma in a child. J Pediatr Gastroenterol Nutr. 1984;3(5):801–4.

39. Nord KS, Joshi V, Hanna M, Khademi M, Saad S, Marquis J, et al. Zollinger–Ellison syndrome associated with a renal gastrinoma in a child. J Pediatr Gastroenterol Nutr. 1986;5(6):980–6.

40. Martignoni ME, Friess H, Lubke D, Uhl W, Maurer C, Muller M, et al. Study of a primary gastrinoma in the common hepatic duct—a case report. Digestion. 1999;60(2):187–90.

41. Hochwald SN, Zee S, Conlon KC, Colleoni R, Louie O, Brennan MF, et al. Prognostic factors in pancreatic endocrine neoplasms: an analysis of 136 cases with a proposal for low-grade and intermediate-grade groups. J Clin Oncol. 2002;20(11):2633–42.

42. Rindi G, Kloppel G, Alhman H, Caplin M, Couvelard A, de Herder WW, et al. TNM staging of foregut (neuro)endocrine tumors: a consensus proposal including a grading system. Virchows Arch. 2006;449(4):395–401.

43. Rindi G, Kloppel G, Couvelard A, Komminoth P, Korner M, Lopes JM, et al. TNM staging of midgut and hindgut (neuro) endocrine tumors: a consensus proposal including a grading system. Virchows Arch. 2007;451(4):757–62.

44. Kloppel G, Perren A, Heitz PU. The gastroenteropancreatic neuroendocrine cell system and its tumors: the WHO classification. Ann N Y Acad Sci. 2004;1014:13–27.

45. Klimstra DS, Modlin IR, Coppola D, Lloyd RV, Suster S. The pathologic classification of neuroendocrine tumors: a review of nomenclature, grading, and staging systems. Pancreas. 2010;39(6):707–12.

46. Edge S, Byrd DR, Compton CC, Fritz AG, Greene FL, Trotti A, editors. AJCC cancer staging manual. 7th ed. New York: Springer; 2010.

47. Rindi G, Arnold R, Bosman FT. Nomenclature and classification of neuroendocrine neoplasms of the digestive system. In: Bosman FT, Carneiro F, Hruban RH, Theise ND, editors. WHO classification of tumours of the digestive system. 4th ed. Lyon: IARC Press; 2010. p. 13–4.

48. Klimstra DS. Pathology reporting of neuroendocrine tumors: essential elements for accurate diagnosis, classification, and staging. Semin Oncol. 2013;40(1):23–36.

49. Vortmeyer AO, Huang S, Lubensky I, Zhuang Z. Non-islet origin of pancreatic islet cell tumors. J Clin Endocrinol Metab. 2004;89(4):1934–8.

50. Kloppel G, Anlauf M, Perren A. Endocrine precursor lesions of gastroenteropancreatic neuroendocrine tumors. Endocr Pathol. 2007;18(3):150–5.

51. Anlauf M, Perren A, Henopp T, Rudolf T, Garbrecht N, Schmitt A, et al. Allelic deletion of the MEN1 gene in duodenal gastrin and somatostatin cell neoplasms and their precursor lesions. Gut. 2007;56(5):637–44.

52. Larsson C, Skogseid B, Oberg K, Nakamura Y, Nordenskjold M. Multiple endocrine neoplasia type 1 gene maps to chromosome 11 and is lost in insulinoma. Nature. 1988;332(6159):85–7.

53. Chandrasekharappa SC, Guru SC, Manickam P, Olufemi SE, Collins FS, Emmert-Buck MR, et al. Positional cloning of the gene for multiple endocrine neoplasia-type 1. Science (New York, NY). 1997;276(5311):404–7.

54. Emmert-Buck MR, Lubensky IA, Dong Q, Manickam P, Guru SC, Kester MB, et al. Localization of the multiple endocrine neoplasia type I (MEN1) gene based on tumor loss of heterozygosity analysis. Cancer Res. 1997;57(10):1855–8.

55. Jiao Y, Shi C, Edil BH, de Wilde RF, Klimstra DS, Maitra A, et al. DAXX/ATRX, MEN1, and mTOR pathway genes are frequently altered in pancreatic neuroendocrine tumors. Science (New York, NY). 2011;331(6021):1199–203.

56. Zhuang Z, Vortmeyer AO, Pack S, Huang S, Pham TA, Wang C, et al. Somatic mutations of the MEN1 tumor suppressor gene in sporadic gastrinomas and insulinomas. Cancer Res. 1997;57(21):4682–6.

57. Wang EH, Ebrahimi SA, Wu AY, Kashefi C, Passaro E Jr, Sawicki MP. Mutation of the MENIN gene in sporadic pancreatic endocrine tumors. Cancer Res. 1998;58(19):4417–20.

58. Guru SC, Olufemi SE, Manickam P, Cummings C, Gieser LM, Pike BL, et al. A 2.8-Mb clone contig of the multiple endocrine neoplasia type 1 (MEN1) region at 11q13. Genomics. 1997;42(3):436–45.

59. Guru SC, Goldsmith PK, Burns AL, Marx SJ, Spiegel AM, Collins FS, et al. Menin, the product of the MEN1 gene, is a nuclear protein. Proc Natl Acad Sci U S A. 1998;95(4):1630–4.

60. Dreijerink KM, Hoppener JW, Timmers HM, Lips CJ. Mechanisms of disease: multiple endocrine neoplasia type 1-relation to chromatin modifications and transcription regulation. Nat Clin Pract Endocrinol Metab. 2006;2(10):562–70.

61. La P, Silva AC, Hou Z, Wang H, Schnepp RW, Yan N, et al. Direct binding of DNA by tumor suppressor menin. J Biol Chem. 2004;279(47):49045–54.

62. Balogh K, Racz K, Patocs A, Hunyady L. Menin and its interacting proteins: elucidation of menin function. Trends Endocrinol Metab. 2006;17(9):357–64.

63. Oberg K. The genetics of neuroendocrine tumors. Semin Oncol. 2013;40(1):37–44.

64. Marinoni I, Kurrer AS, Vassella E, Dettmer M, Rudolph T, Banz V, et al. Loss of DAXX and ATRX are associated with chromosome instability and reduced survival of patients with pancreatic neuroendocrine tumors. Gastroenterology. 2014;146(2):453–60.

65. Corbo V, Dalai I, Scardoni M, Barbi S, Beghelli S, Bersani S, et al. MEN1 in pancreatic endocrine tumors: analysis of gene and protein status in 169 sporadic neoplasms reveals alterations in the vast majority of cases. Endocr-Relat Cancer. 2010;17(3):771–83.

66. Inoue M, Hager JH, Ferrara N, Gerber HP, Hanahan D. VEGF-A has a critical, nonredundant role in angiogenic switching and pancreatic beta cell carcinogenesis. Cancer Cell. 2002;1(2):193–202.

67. Lammert E, Gu G, McLaughlin M, Brown D, Brekken R, Murtaugh LC, et al. Role of VEGF-A in vascularization of pancreatic islets. Curr Biol. 2003;13(12):1070–4.

68. Lammert E, Cleaver O, Melton D. Induction of pancreatic differentiation by signals from blood vessels. Science (New York, NY). 2001;294(5542):564–7.

69. Zhang J, Francois R, Iyer R, Seshadri M, Zajac-Kaye M, Hochwald SN. Current understanding of the molecular biology of pancreatic neuroendocrine tumors. J Natl Cancer Inst. 2013;105(14):1005–17.

70. Marion-Audibert AM, Barel C, Gouysse G, Dumortier J, Pilleul F, Pourreyron C, et al. Low microvessel density is an unfavorable histoprognostic factor in pancreatic endocrine tumors. Gastroenterology. 2003;125(4):1094–104.

71. Ito T, Igarashi H, Uehara H, Jensen RT. Pharmacotherapy of Zollinger–Ellison syndrome. Expert Opin Pharmacother. 2013;14(3):307–21.

72. Termanini B, Gibril F, Sutliff VE, Yu F, Venzon DJ, Jensen RT. Effect of long-term gastric acid suppressive therapy on serum vitamin B12 levels in patients with Zollinger–Ellison syndrome. Am J Med. 1998;104(5):422–30.

73. Ito T, Jensen RT. Association of long-term proton pump inhibitor therapy with bone fractures and effects on absorption of calcium, vitamin B12, iron, and magnesium. Curr Gastroenterol Rep. 2010;12(6):448–57.

74. Yang YX, Lewis JD, Epstein S, Metz DC. Long-term proton pump inhibitor therapy and risk of hip fracture. JAMA. 2006;296(24):2947–53.

75. Peghini PL, Annibale B, Azzoni C, Milione M, Corleto VD, Gibril F, et al. Effect of chronic hypergastrinemia on human enterochromaffin-like cells: insights from patients with sporadic gastrinomas. Gastroenterology. 2002;123(1):68–85.

76. Berna MJ, Annibale B, Marignani M, Luong TV, Corleto V, Pace A, et al. A prospective study of gastric carcinoids and enterochromaffin-like cell changes in multiple endocrine neoplasia type 1 and Zollinger–Ellison syndrome: identification of risk factors. J Clin Endocrinol Metab. 2008;93(5):1582–91.

77. O'Toole D, Delle Fave G, Jensen RT. Gastric and duodenal neuroendocrine tumours. Best Pract Res Clin Gastroenterol. 2012;26(6):719–35.

78. Norton JA, Fraker DL, Alexander HR, Jensen RT. Value of surgery in patients with negative imaging and sporadic Zollinger–Ellison syndrome. Ann Surg. 2012;256(3):509–17.

79. Norton JA. Intraoperative methods to stage and localize pancreatic and duodenal tumors. Ann Oncol. 1999;10(Suppl 4):182–4.

80. Norton JA, Fraker DL, Alexander HR, Gibril F, Liewehr DJ, Venzon DJ, et al. Surgery increases survival in patients with gastrinoma. Ann Surg. 2006;244(3):410–9.

81. Doherty GM, Thompson NW. Multiple endocrine neoplasia type 1: duodenopancreatic tumours. J Intern Med. 2003;253(6):590–8.

82. Bartsch DK, Waldmann J, Fendrich V, Boninsegna L, Lopez CL, Partelli S, et al. Impact of lymphadenectomy on survival after surgery for sporadic gastrinoma. Br J Surg. 2012;99(9):1234–40.

83. MacFarlane MP, Fraker DL, Alexander HR, Norton JA, Lubensky I, Jensen RT. Prospective study of surgical resection of duodenal and pancreatic gastrinomas in multiple endocrine neoplasia type 1. Surgery. 1995;118(6):973–9 (discussion 9–80).

84. Jensen RT, Berna MJ, Bingham DB, Norton JA. Inherited pancreatic endocrine tumor syndromes: advances in molecular pathogenesis, diagnosis, management, and controversies. Cancer. 2008;113(7 Suppl):1807–43.

85. Thompson NW. Current concepts in the surgical management of multiple endocrine neoplasia type 1 pancreatic-duodenal disease. Results in the treatment of 40 patients with Zollinger–Ellison syndrome, hypoglycaemia or both. J Intern Med. 1998;243(6):495–500.

86. Ellison EC, Sparks J, Verducci JS, Johnson JA, Muscarella P, Bloomston M, et al. 50-year appraisal of gastrinoma: recommendations for staging and treatment. J Am Coll Surg. 2006;202(6):897–905.

87. Norton JA, Alexander HR, Fraker DL, Venzon DJ, Gibril F, Jensen RT. Comparison of surgical results in patients with advanced and limited disease with multiple endocrine neoplasia type 1 and Zollinger–Ellison syndrome. Ann Surg. 2001;234(4):495–505 (discussion 6).

88. Gibril F, Venzon DJ, Ojeaburu JV, Bashir S, Jensen RT. Prospective study of the natural history of gastrinoma in patients with MEN1: definition of an aggressive and a nonaggressive form. J Clin Endocrinol Metab. 2001;86(11):5282–93.

89. Yu F, Venzon DJ, Serrano J, Goebel SU, Doppman JL, Gibril F, et al. Prospective study of the clinical course, prognostic factors, causes of death, and survival in patients with long-standing Zollinger–Ellison syndrome. J Clin Oncol. 1999;17(2):615–30.

90. Weber HC, Venzon DJ, Lin JT, Fishbein VA, Orbuch M, Strader DB, et al. Determinants of metastatic rate and survival in patients with Zollinger–Ellison syndrome: a prospective long-term study. Gastroenterology. 1995;108(6):1637–49.

91. Miller CA, Ellison EC. Therapeutic alternatives in metastatic neuroendocrine tumors. Surg Oncol Clin N Am. 1998;7(4):863–79.

92. Pavel M, Baudin E, Couvelard A, Krenning E, Oberg K, Steinmuller T, et al. ENETS Consensus Guidelines for the management of patients with liver and other distant metastases from neuroendocrine neoplasms of foregut, midgut, hindgut, and unknown primary. Neuroendocrinology. 2012;95(2):157–76.

93. Kunz PL, Reidy-Lagunes D, Anthony LB, Bertino EM, Brendtro K, Chan JA, et al. Consensus guidelines for the management and treatment of neuroendocrine tumors. Pancreas. 2013;42(4):557–77.

94. Ito T, Igarashi H, Jensen RT. Therapy of metastatic pancreatic neuroendocrine tumors (pNETs): recent insights and advances. J Gastroenterol. 2012;47(9):941–60.

95. Berber E, Flesher N, Siperstein AE. Laparoscopic radiofrequency ablation of neuroendocrine liver metastases. World J Surg. 2002;26(8):985–90.

96. Krampitz GW, Norton JA, Poultsides GA, Visser BC, Sun L, Jensen RT. Lymph nodes and survival in pancreatic neuroendocrine tumors. Arch Surg. 2012;147(9):820–7.

97. Rinke A, Muller HH, Schade-Brittinger C, Klose KJ, Barth P, Wied M, et al. Placebo-controlled, double-blind, prospective, randomized study on the effect of octreotide LAR in the control of tumor growth in patients with metastatic neuroendocrine midgut tumors: a report from the PROMID study group. J Clin Oncol. 2009;27(28):4656–63.

98. Caplin ME, Pavel M, Ćwikła JB, Phan AT, Raderer M, Sedláčková E, Cadiot G, Wolin EM, Capdevila J, Wall L, Rindi G, Langley A, Martinez S, Blumberg J, Ruszniewski P, CLARINET Investigators. Lanreotide in metastatic enteropancreatic neuroendocrine tumors. N Engl J Med. 2014;371(3):224–33.

99. Yao JC, Shah MH, Ito T, Bohas CL, Wolin EM, Van Cutsem E, et al. Everolimus for advanced pancreatic neuroendocrine tumors. N Engl J Med. 2011;364(6):514–23.

100. Raymond E, Dahan L, Raoul JL, Bang YJ, Borbath I, Lombard-Bohas C, et al. Sunitinib malate for the treatment of pancreatic neuroendocrine tumors. N Engl J Med. 2011;364(6):501–13.

101. von Schrenck T, Howard JM, Doppman JL, Norton JA, Maton PN, Smith FP, et al. Prospective study of chemotherapy in patients with metastatic gastrinoma. Gastroenterology. 1988;94(6):1326–34.

102. Strosberg JR, Fine RL, Choi J, Nasir A, Coppola D, Chen DT, et al. First-line chemotherapy with capecitabine and temozolomide in patients with metastatic pancreatic endocrine carcinomas. Cancer. 2011;117(2):268–75.

103. Kwekkeboom DJ, de Herder WW, Kam BL, van Eijck CH, van Essen M, Kooij PP, et al. Treatment with the radiolabeled somatostatin analog [177 Lu-DOTA 0,Tyr3]octreotate: toxicity, efficacy, and survival. J Clin Oncol. 2008;26(13):2124–30.

104. Kwekkeboom DJ, de Herder WW, van Eijck CH, Kam BL, van Essen M, Teunissen JJ, et al. Peptide receptor radionuclide therapy in patients with gastroenteropancreatic neuroendocrine tumors. Semin Nucl Med. 2010;40(2):78–88.

105. Kwekkeboom DJ, Krenning EP, Lebtahi R, Komminoth P, Kos-Kudla B, de Herder WW, et al. ENETS consensus guidelines for the standards of care in neuroendocrine tumors: peptide receptor radionuclide therapy with radiolabeled somatostatin analogs. Neuroendocrinology. 2009;90(2):220–6.

106. Bushnell DL Jr, O'Dorisio TM, O'Dorisio MS, Menda Y, Hicks RJ, Van Cutsem E, et al. 90Y-edotreotide for metastatic carcinoid refractory to octreotide. J Clin Oncol. 2010;28(10):1652–9.

107. Strosberg JR, Cheema A, Weber J, Han G, Coppola D, Kvols LK. Prognostic validity of a novel American Joint Committee on Cancer Staging Classification for pancreatic neuroendocrine tumors. J Clin Oncol. 2011;29(22):3044–9.

108. Kloppel G. Classification and pathology of gastroenteropancreatic neuroendocrine neoplasms. Endocr-Relat Cancer. 2011;18(Suppl 1): S1–16.

109. Doherty GM, Olson JA, Frisella MM, Lairmore TC, Wells SA Jr, Norton JA. Lethality of multiple endocrine neoplasia type I. World J Surg. 1998;22(6):581–6 (discussion 6–7).

Robert Milton Zollinger

1903–1992

Quan-Yang Duh

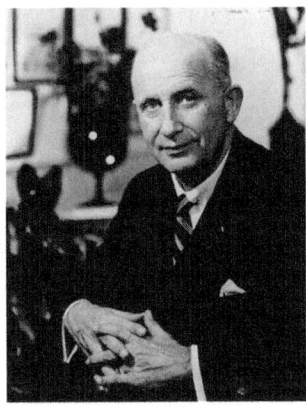

Robert M. Zollinger. Photograph taken for cover of Modern Medicine, May 25, 1964

Surgeons and physicians will always associate Dr. Zollinger with gastrinoma, the "Zollinger–Ellison syndrome," which he and Dr. Ellison described in 1955 [1]. He is also remembered as one of the giants of twentieth-century American surgery.

Robert Milton Zollinger was born on September 4, 1903, in Millersport, OH, USA [2]. He grew up on his family's farm. As a boy, he had a business delivering milk and vegetables from his family farm to the neighbors. He was athletic and lettered in basketball during high school. He initially wanted to attend West Point, but when he decided to become a doctor, he went to Ohio State University, where he received a BA in 1925 and MD in 1927. He was a competitive young medical student: "I got a C in surgery and I said then I was coming back as a professor of surgery" [3].

Q.-Y. Duh (✉)
Surgical Service, VA Medical Center, 4150 Clement St.,
San Francisco, CA 94121, USA
e-mail: Quan-Yang.Duh@ucsfmedctr.org

Department of Surgery, Section of Endocrine Surgery,
University of California, San Francisco CA, USA

Dr. Zollinger was offered an internship at Peter Bent Brigham Hospital by **Harvey Cushing**. Dr. Cushing sent him to Western Reserve in Cleveland to work with Cushing's pupil Elliot Carr Cutler (1888–1947) for 6 months before starting the internship at the Brigham in 1928.

After his internship, Zollinger returned to work with Cutler in 1929, as a surgery resident at Lakeside Hospital and Western Reserve University in Cleveland. When Cutler took over from Cushing as the Mosley Professor at the Brigham in 1932, Zollinger went with him as his chief resident. Cutler and Zollinger subsequently published the first of nine editions of the *Atlas of Surgical Operations*. In 1939, Zollinger was appointed assistant professor at Harvard at Peter Bent Brigham Hospital.

Dr. Zollinger joined the army before the start of World War II (WWII) in 1941 and served until 1945. He joined the Harvard Unit as a major in the Medical Corp of the US Army in Ireland and was the assistant chief of the Surgical Service. Because of his farm experience and love of roses, he planted a garden and cultivated roses and was appointed the post, beautification officer. Dr. Zollinger was promoted to colonel and was senior consultant in surgery to the European Theater of Operation, and commander of the 5th General Hospital in France. He was awarded the Legion of Merit by the US Army for the development of mobile surgical teams (with Colonel Dr. Michael DeBakey and others). He earned Battle Stars for Normandy, Northern France, and Rhineland, and the European–African–Middle Eastern Service Medal.

Dr. Zollinger returned to Harvard after WWII. However, soon after in 1946, he returned to his alma mater Ohio State University as professor of surgery. Within a year, he became chairman of the Department of Surgery. He built and grew the Department of Surgery at Ohio State University until he retired as professor emeritus in 1974. Dr. Zollinger continued his surgical practice until January of 1983, retiring at age 79 [3, 4]. He died from pancreatic cancer, on June 12, 1992, in Columbus, OH, USA [5].

J. L. Pasieka, J. A. Lee (eds.), *Surgical Endocrinopathies*, DOI 10.1007/978-3-319-13662-2_48,
© Springer International Publishing Switzerland 2015

The Paper

Dr. Zollinger recruited Dr. **Edwin Homer Ellison** as soon as he arrived at Ohio State in 1946. Dr. Ellison was a medical student at Ohio State, studied biochemistry, and had just finished his surgical residency at Ohio State in 1946 [6]. They became close friends and collaborators over the next decades. In 1967, Dr. Ellison became professor and chairman of surgery at the Marquette School of Medicine in Milwaukee.

Zollinger and Ellison presented the paper "Primary peptic ulceration of the jejunum associated with islet cell tumors of the pancreas" before the American Surgical Association in Philadelphia on April 29, 1955 [1]. They described two patients in detail. One was a 36-year-old woman, a patient of Ellison, who had recurrent jejunal ulceration that required several resections and finally had a total gastrectomy, esophago-duodenotomy for bleeding, and eventually died of anastomotic perforation (Fig. 1). Autopsy showed a well-encapsulated 1-cm nodule in the tail of the pancreas with other smaller surrounding nodules. The other patient was a 19-year-old woman, a patient of Zollinger. She had two

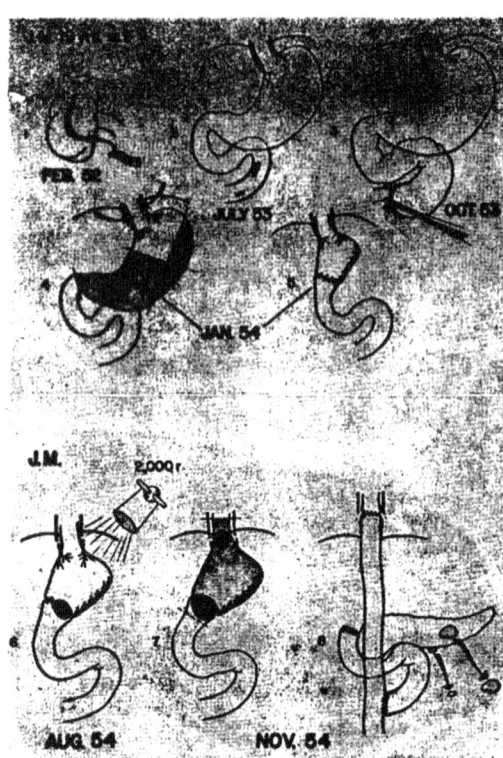

Fig. 2 Schematic representation of clinical course of case 2 [1]

episodes of jejunal perforation and uncontrollable ulcers with hypersecretion of gastric acid. She had already undergone a truncal vagotomy, proximal gastrectomy, and irradiation of gastric remnant. Dr. Zollinger performed a total gastrectomy, pancreas resection, and node dissection (Fig. 2). Following the suggestion of Dr. Hilger Jenkins of Chicago to look for an insulinoma, Dr. Zollinger was initially disappointed after not finding any obvious tumor in the pancreas during the operation. However, subsequent final pathology exam showed a small pancreatic tumor with metastatic lymph nodes.

In addition to these two patients, they reviewed the literature for possibly four more patients with a similar condition. They postulated "an ulcerogenic humoral factor of pancreatic islet origin" and suggested "a clinical entity consisting of hypersecretion, hyperacidity, and atypical peptic ulceration associated with non-insulin-producing islet cell tumors of the pancreas." The postulated gastrin was finally identified by RA Gregory and Hilda Tracy of the University of Liverpool in 1960.

The discussants of Zollinger and Ellison's paper were in sequence: Dr. Higer Perry Jenkins of Chicago, IL (who suggested to Zollinger the possibility of an insulinoma), Dr. **Allen Oldfather Whipple** (1981–1963, of the "Whipple procedure") of Princeton, NJ, Dr. Lester R. Dragstedt (1893–1975, who developed vagotomy for the treatment of peptic ulcer) of Chicago, IL, Dr. Edgar J. Poth (1899–1989) of Galveston,

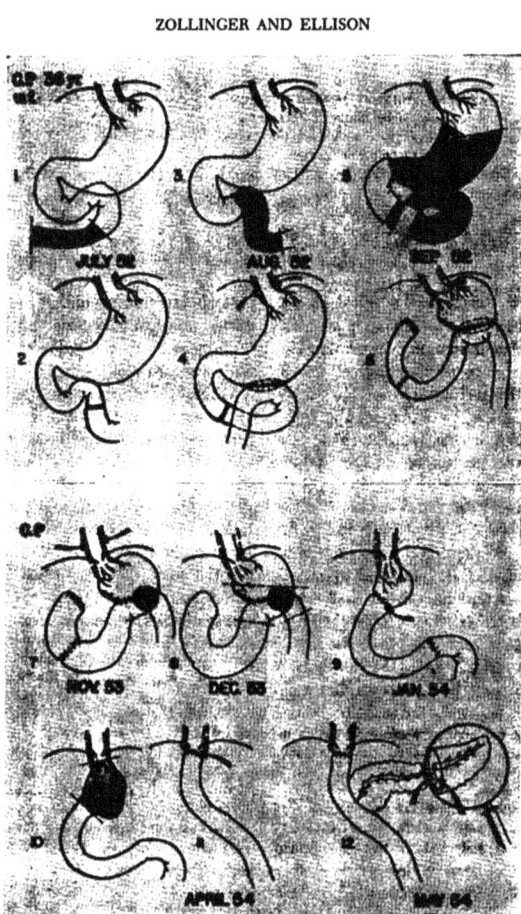

Fig. 1 Schematic representation of clinical course of case 1 [1]

TX, and Dr. Carl A. Moyer (1908–1970, head of surgery at Washington University, 1951–1965) of St. Louis, MO. Each congratulated Ellison and Zollinger for the presentation and presented their own similar cases of possible gastrinoma.

Although most of us continue to use the eponym Zollinger–Ellison syndrome to refer to the syndrome of gastrinoma, as initially suggested by Dr. Ben Eiseman of University of Colorado [6], Dr. Zollinger "would never refer to the eponym, preferring the term gastrinoma" [7].

As Zollinger's successor to the editor-in-chief of the *American Journal of Surgery,* Dr. Hiram Polk remarked: "Long after the unique personality, the special skills, and the scientific insights have been dimmed, Dr. Zollinger will be remembered as the individual who moved surgical endocrinology into the 21th century! His discovery with his esteemed colleague Edwin Ellison of the gastrin-secreting tumor of the pancreas set the stage for the clinical discovery of the endocrine nature of the alimentary tract and its appendages, has revolutionized not only surgery but the entire practice of medicine, and redefined the forefront of clinically relevant research" [5].

Academic Achievements

During his tenure at Ohio State, Dr. Zollinger grew the training program at the Department of Surgery from 8 residents and 3 professors to 65 residents and 42 full-time faculty [8]. The R. M. Zollinger Club was conceived by Edwin H. Ellison and founded by Zollinger's surgical residents in his honor in 1955 [7, 8]. The Robert M. Zollinger Chair of Surgery was established in Dr. Zollinger's honor, and it has been held by Dr. Stuart S. Roberts (1930–2001), Dr. Larry C. Carey, Dr. Olga Jonasson (1934–2006), and Dr. E. Christopher Ellison [9].

Over his lifetime, Dr. Zollinger published more than 350 papers [3]. He edited *Atlas of Surgical Operations* with Dr. Cutler, and also coedited the *Textbook of Surgery* with Dr. Warren H. Cole (1898–1990).

Dr. Zollinger was one of the giants of twentieth-century American medicine and surgery. He was one of only a handful of surgeons who had been the president of the American College of Surgeons (1961–1962), the chairman of the American Board of Surgery (1963), and the president of the American Surgical Association (1965). He was also a founding member and president of the Society of University Surgeons (1947). Dr. Zollinger served for 28 years as the editor-in-chief of the *American Journal of Surgery* from 1958 to 1986.

Dr. Zollinger received an honorary degree from the University of Lyons, France (1965) and held honorary fellowships at the Royal College of Surgeons of England (1965) and the Royal College of Surgeons of Edinburgh (1966) [8].

In 1977, he received the American Medical Association's highest honor, the Sheen Award, recognizing him as the Outstanding Doctor of Medical Sciences in the USA.

"Respected By His Peers, Feared By His Students and Loved By His Patients" [3]

Dr. Zollinger was known as "The Big Z" or "Zolly" to his friends and peers [3]. He was "one of the most honored of the world's surgeons." "Dr. Zollinger's cutting wit and repartee made him the perpetual star of the College's Clinical Congress and the most feared of examiners of the American Board of Surgery" [5]. "He was a great entertainer, but he practiced every line, including the jokes" [7]. Zollinger was a stickler for details and insisted on carefully prepared slides for presentation. In 1961, Dr. Zollinger, Dr. William Pace, and George Kuenzle, chief of School of Journalism at Ohio State, developed a paperback guide on making medical presentation slides [6].

Dr. Zollinger was described by those who have operated with him as "a master technical surgeon, very quick and very gentle, but not tolerant of assistants, especially residents"[4]. Dr. Zollinger was "notorious for being a stern taskmaster who used to bully his students towards excellence" [3]. Caring for his patients was of utmost importance to Dr. Zollinger. "We saw his silver Thunderbird parked at the hospital before most of us arrived in the mornings and it was often still there when we left at night. He demanded a call at 9:00 p.m. every night from the resident covering his personal patients" [4]. Although he was a member of the Columbus Country Club for 40 years, he never set foot on the golf course [3]. He was offered, but turned down the job as the president of Ohio State University because he would not have been able to continue his surgical practice [3].

"Teacher, Surgeon, Soldier and Farmer" [2]

Dr. Zollinger married Louise Kiewit in 1929 after returning to Cleveland (at that time Brigham interns could not be married). Since Zollinger was being paid only US$ 50 a week as a resident, Mrs. Zollinger supported the family during his residency by teaching. They had two children, Myra Louis Waud (Chapel Hill, NC, USA) and Robert M. Zollinger Jr (who became professor of surgery at Case Western Reserve University, Cleveland, OH, USA). In addition to roses, Dr. Zollinger had a passion for photography and enjoyed his winters on Sanibel Island. "He never lost the Ohio farm in the boy who was pulled from the school each spring for planting until his grade fell to a C. This fueled a determined competitiveness, which resulted in his becoming President of the American Rose Society (1966) while tending over 400 roses plus gourds in all available yard spaces at Club 83 (his Bexley home for 45 years)" [7]. Dr. Zollinger was a friend of the famous Ohio State University football coach Woody Hayes, who once told him "I am sure glad I never coached against you" [3].

When asked how he would like to be remembered, he replied "They should write on my tombstone: 'teacher, surgeon, soldier and farmer'. And my wife may remember that she says I'm an amusing fellow to live with" [2].

References

1. Zollinger RM, Ellison EH. Primary peptic ulceration of the jejunum associated with islet cell tumors of the pancreas. Ann Surg. 1955;142:709–23 (Discussion pages 724–6).
2. Zollinger RM. The Ohio State University Library Blogs. Posted April 11, 2011 by Rodgers.102@osu.edu. http://library.osu.edu/blogs/mhcb/2011/04/11/robert-m-zollinger-md/.
3. Fiely D, Ellison EC. The wit and wisdom of master surgeon Robert Zollinger. Am J Surg. 2003;186:242–4 (Originally published in September 4, 1985 issue of the Columbus Dispatch on his 82nd birthday).
4. Carey LC, Elliot DW, Ellison EC, Fabian TC, Roberts L. Recollection of Robert M Zollinger, MD. Am J Surg. 2003;186:226–33.
5. Polk HC Jr. In Memoriam: Robert M. Zollinger, MD. Am J Surg. 1992;164A:14.
6. Zollinger RM Sr, Ellison EC. A history of the Ohio State University Department of Surgery. Am J Surg. 2003;186:208–10 (Zollinger wrote it before he died in 1992).
7. Zollinger RM Jr, Ellison EC. Robert M Zollinger, Sr., as a father, teacher and mentor. Am Surg. 2011;11:1428–9.
8. Pace WG. Robert Milton Zollinger. Am J Surg. 1974;128: 585–7.
9. Pontious B, Daly J. A history of the Robert M Zollinger chair of surgery. Am J Surg. 2003;186:224–5.

Edwin H. Ellison

1918–1970

Stuart D. Wilson

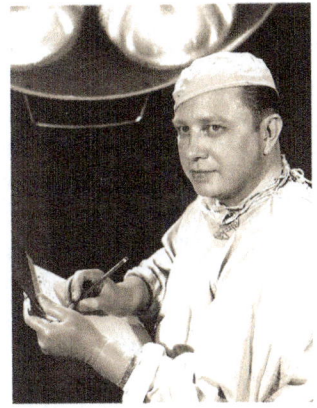

Edwin H Ellison. Ellison Library Archives, Department of Surgery, Medical College of Wisconsin

Edwin H. Ellison was born in Dayton, OH, September 4, 1918. His father was a chemist and his mother was a school teacher. His father died during the influenza epidemics when "Eddie," as he was known by his friends, was only a youngster. He and his mother moved to Columbus, OH, where he resided for the next 25 years attending public schools, Ohio State University (BA 1939) and Ohio State College of Medicine (MD Cum Laude 1943). During the ensuing busy, sometimes chaotic years of World War II (WWII) and residency training, Dr. Ellison managed to complete all the requirements for a PhD in biochemistry.

Early in his training as an Ohio State University Hospital rotating intern and junior resident (1943–1946), no doubt in part because of his background in biochemistry, he developed an early interest in surgical nutrition and peptic ulcer disease. This era was several decades before the characterization and precise measurements of gastrointestinal peptide

hormones, the advent of effective antacid blockers and radiologic techniques such as computed tomography (CT) scans. Rather crude measurements of gastric acid secretion, such as an overnight gastric aspiration, often with the house officer at the bedside to maintain patency of the nasogastric tube, was the primary metric measured. His surgical residency training was interrupted by two years of military service and he was stationed from 1946 to 1948 at Fort Ord California where he was chief of the surgical section.

Ellison returned to Ohio State University Hospital to complete a final and then a super chief resident year in surgery (1950–1951) under Dr. **Robert Zollinger**, Dr. Ellison was one of the first surgical faculty hired by Dr. Zollinger, who had recently returned from overseas WWII duty in Europe to be the new department chairman. The Ohio State surgical training program was organized along the Halstedian model, along the lines developed by Dr. **Harvey Cushing** and Dr. Elliot Cutler, with whom Dr. Zollinger had worked first as a resident and then a junior faculty member at the Brigham Hospital before World War II. Dr. Cushing had been a Halsted resident before going to the Brigham Hospital in Boston and the Halsted training program influences on training surgeons passed through Drs. Cushing/Cutler to Zollinger and then to Ellison.

During his tenure at Ohio State University Hospital from 1951–1958, Ellison advanced in rank to full-time professor. He and Dr. Zollinger both had busy clinical practices and collaborated together on numerous research projects. Nutrition in the surgical patient and finding the best operation for peptic ulcer diseases were areas of interest. Dr. Ellison was one of the early authorities in nutrition, blood substitutes, as well as fluid and electrolyte balance. He was an early pioneer in bringing the flame photometer to practical use in the care of surgical patients.

As a very junior surgical faculty member, Dr. Ellison's frustrating clinical experiences with a patient who had recurrent jejunal ulcers, massive gastric acid hypersecretion and failed ulcer operations were observed in the same year (1954)

S. D. Wilson (✉)
Division of Surgical Oncology, Department of Surgery,
Froedtert Hospital/Medical College of Milwaukee,
Milwaukee, WI, USA
e-mail: swilson@mcw.edu

J. L. Pasieka, J. A. Lee (eds.), *Surgical Endocrinopathies,* DOI 10.1007/978-3-319-13662-2_49,
© Springer International Publishing Switzerland 2015

in one of Dr. Zollinger's patients. These experiences prompted Dr. Ellison to start a study of "jejunal ulcer patients."

The clinical saga, of jejunal ulcers, in only two patients and the remarkable series of events concerning their care occurring in 1954 led to the discovery of the "Zollinger –Ellison syndrome." Their hypothesis of an "ulcerogenic humoral factor of pancreatic islet origin" was reported at the 1955 Annual meeting of the American Surgical Association [1]. Not unlike the Princes of Serendip, Zollinger and Ellison had discovered by accident and sagacity something they were not in quest of; they were trying to find a better operation for jejunal ulcers [2]. Their report and hypothesis captured the imagination of and excited surgeons, clinicians, and physiologists worldwide. Details of this remarkable story describing the discovery of the Zollinger–Ellison's syndrome has been well documented and is a must read for all endocrine surgeons [3].

Dr. Ellison excelled early in his academic career, and his relationship with Dr. Zollinger was close. Their birthdays happened to occur on the same day, September the 4th. Dr. Zollinger had said "Eddie was the answer to the dream of every professor of surgery, a young associate who strived every day to please and indeed, to exceed the teacher... he gave clear evidence that he was a man of great talent and a capacity for work and for leadership" [4]. He received the Man of the Year award from the Ohio State Medical School faculty in 1957.

Dr. Ellison was recognized early as a rising star in academic surgery. He was only 39 years when Marquette University School of Medicine in Milwaukee, Wisconsin (now the Medical College of Wisconsin), initiated a recruitment process to bring him to Milwaukee. He accepted and became the first full-time professor and chairman, Department of Surgery in 1958.

Ellison was a true visionary. A major attraction of the job in Milwaukee was the promise of the imminent development of a university teaching hospital in association with the medical school. Kurtis Froedtert, a wealthy businessman, who produced grains and malt for Milwaukee's famous beers, had created the trust to build the hospital. However, the Milwaukee academic environment in the early 1960s for the new department chair was to prove most challenging. Marquette University School of medicine had limited resources and there was no medical service plan to generate revenue for the school. The surgery department had no full-time faculty. Research facilities were limited. There were eight Milwaukee hospitals with American College of Surgeons (ACS)-approved independent graduate training programs in general surgery. Several programs were only for 3 years.

Dr. Ellison, a tireless worker with enormous enthusiasm and a great charisma, had within several years recruited

full-time division chairs for neurosurgery, ophthalmology, otolaryngology, cardiothoracic surgery, transplant, orthopedics, and urology. Early funding of an NIH program project grant (1960) for gastrointestinal research was obtained by Dr. Ellison and then additional funding for a modern state-of-the-art 14,000 sq. ft. research facility. Allen Bradley Medical Science Laboratory, built in 1961 and administered by the Department of Surgery, provided the ideal environment for research.

Ellison was a great communicator for the practicing surgeons in the community and the "Town and Gown" relationships were uncommonly good. These relationships were necessary to help staff the nearly 1000-bed Milwaukee County General Hospital, which served as the primary teaching hospital for the residents and medical students, as well as a base for the growing list of new full-time surgical faculty

Nationally, a major change in the education and training of surgeons was happening. Residency standards, oversight, and accreditation were new for surgery residency program directors. Many of the free standing, nonuniversity programs in small hospitals in the Milwaukee community during the Ellison period (1958–1969) would soon not be able to meet the standards for accreditation. Dr. Ellison was able to convey his vision for a great surgical training program to the medical school and the Milwaukee community hospitals. After only a few years in Milwaukee, he was able to integrate the surgical residencies at the Milwaukee County General Hospital, the VA hospital, Milwaukee Children's Hospital and three private hospitals into one large integrated surgical postgraduate training program under a single program director with funding from participating institutions. The Marquette University Affiliated Hospital program for surgery would become a model for other academic programs in large US metropolitan centers.

The new Allen Bradley Medical Science Laboratory (ABMSL) provided an inviting environment for surgical research. Surgical faculty, full time and clinical, quickly started projects. Residents were encouraged to do research, some continuing long-term projects even during their clinical rotations as the laboratory was across the street from the hospital. The research products from this laboratory were soon presented at numerous national meetings and the research published in peer-reviewed journals.

Dr. Ellison was a skilled photographer and an artist. He was proud of the awards he received for his sketches and artwork. The importance of medical illustration and color movies was apparent to the new chairman. He recruited a medical illustrator, Robert Albertin, whom he had worked with at Ohio State. The new department of medical illustration located in the Milwaukee County General Hospital became part of the surgery department. The projected slides, initially lantern slides, and the art work seen at national meetings were unique and often recognized as being from the "Ellison program".

Dr. Ellison was a serious but gentle man. His bedside rounds with house officers, demonstrating the abdominal exam and interacting with the patient, were always instructive. He taught by precept, showing concern for the patient and family. His teaching style was very different from his mentor, Dr. Zollinger. He did not chastise the residents or medical students nor did he raise his voice. He would on occasion assemble in the middle of the night a whole group of "experts" at the bedside of a very sick patient to sort out particularly perplexing problems. He recognized the importance of other specialists in providing the best care and was particularly respectful of the radiologist and anesthesiologist.

As Ellison's surgery program grew and gained recognition, a prominent academic surgeon noted that the new young faculty and residents surrounding Ellison formed a kind of surgical Camelot in Milwaukee during the early 1960s. These were heady times as Ellison conveyed his vision of a great surgical program to the practicing Milwaukee surgical community, and nationally to his academic surgical colleagues [5]. In 1963, Ellison's accomplishments were recognized by his election to the presidency of the Society of University Surgeons. Dr. Ellison was proud to show off his residents, young faculty, and the new ABMSL to several national surgical societies, who held their annual meeting in Milwaukee. Ellison's new surgical subspecialty chairmen also made their mark with their new residency programs and research. These new programs further enhanced the medical school reputation.

However, everything in Camelot was not rosy. The promised Froedtert Hospital construction was delayed further, initially because of some probate and legal issues surrounding the trust. Ellison was frustrated and impatient and pushed hard for the grand vision of a great medical center. As early as 1961, he had presented to the Milwaukee County Board a plan that would place the medical school's basic science and administration buildings, the VA Hospital and Froedtert Hospital in a vast, largely unoccupied, Milwaukee county campus along with the Milwaukee County General Hospital. It is of interest that 2 years later he presented to the medical school board of directors a timetable for construction of the Froedtert University Hospital. The minutes of that meeting noted "that his enthusiasm was met with cautious conservatism" [6].

A new dean was appointed for the Marquette University Medical School in September of 1965. Such events sometimes herald turbulent times for surgical chairmen. Several months later Ellison was fired as chairman. The major reason given for this action was that Ellison's efforts to make the teaching hospital a reality were not always in concert with the medical school. The dean's actions caused great turmoil and protest from faculty and the surgical community. Ellison was reinstated as chairman after just 3 weeks. The conditions of his reinstatement were not made public but he abruptly discontinued his campaign to build Froedtert Hospital and kept a low profile on the medical center development [5].

In February 1966, the society of University Surgeons met in Milwaukee with Ellison back in charge. Dr. Ellison was at his best and the "local" scientific program with research by the faculty and residents was exceptional. The entire program of local papers presented by Dr. Ellison's faculty and residents was published as a special issue in the *American Journal of Surgery*. Academic surgeons in the USA now better recognized the development of this new Department of Surgery and residency program in Milwaukee.

During the next several years, Ellison continued to nurture his surgery program but the inability to have private referred patients at the county hospital and the continued delays in the progress of the medical center dream and a University Hospital caused him more frustration and depression. No construction was in sight, the medical school dean once again expressed a lack of confidence in the Department of Surgery, in large part because some of the full-time faculty operated on their private patients in community hospitals.

Ellison resigned in 1969 and he was given a sabbatical leave for one year. He had accepted a position as professor and department head at a southern hospital. Dr. Ellison took his own life April 27, 1970, shortly before he was to take the new position. He was only 51 years old. Edwin Ellison's mentor at Ohio State, Dr. Robert Zollinger, had said that "Ellison was truly ahead of his time." Ellison's vision for the medical center in Milwaukee was to eventually come true.

Within the next decade that followed after the Ellison era, an organization named the Milwaukee Regional Medical center was in place. Froedtert Hospital, the basic science and administration buildings of the medical school, as well as Children's Hospital were all located on the campus with the Milwaukee County General Hospital. The medical school became a freestanding private institution, now named the Medical College of Wisconsin. In the 50 years since the Camelot era of Ellison's rather short tenure, the Milwaukee Regional Medical Center has grown exponentially and now ranks ahead of nearly two thirds of its peers nationally and it is still growing. Edwin Ellison's dream of a great medical center did come true. The Zollinger-Ellison syndrome is certainly and important part of the Ellison legacy but his early vision and struggles to develop an academic surgery program and a great medical center in Milwaukee are perhaps the most important contributions to the Edwin H. Ellison legacy.

References

1. Zollinger RM, Ellison EH. Primary peptic ulcerations of the jejunum associated with islet cell tumors of the pancreas. Ann Surg. 1955 Oct;142(4):709–23.
2. Wilson SD. Connell's fundusectomy, Zollinger's "Dream" ulcer operation, and two princes of serendip: the discovery of the Zollinger–Ellison syndrome. In: Zieger MA, Shen WT, Fegler EA, editors. 'The Supreme Triumph of the Surgeons Art', a narrative history of endocrine surgery. California: University of California Medical Humanities Press; 2013. p. 116–29.
3. Zollinger RM, Coleman DW. The influences of pancreatic tumors on the stomach. Springfield: Charles C. Thomas; 1974.
4. Zollinger R. Eulogy for E. H. Ellison; 1970 May 2.
5. Condon RE. A short history of the Department of Surgery, Medical College of Wisconsin, Department of Surgery Archives; 1998.
6. Engbring NH. An anchor for the future: a history of the Medical College of Wisconsin, 1893–1990. Milwaukee: Medical College of Wisconsin; 1991. 500 p.

VIPoma

Anthony J. Chambers

Introduction

VIPomas are rare neuroendocrine tumors usually occurring in the pancreas associated with the increased systemic release of vasoactive intestinal polypeptide (VIP) causing symptoms of high-volume watery diarrhea. Their management is complex involving surgery, medical therapies, interventional radiology, and nuclear medicine modalities.

Historical Features

The first report of a patient with VIPoma was likely by Priest and Alexander in 1957 [1]. They reported the case of a 56-year-old male who died from complications of refractory diarrhea, hypokalemia, and hyponatremia in association with a pancreatic neuroendocrine tumor that had recurred after resection. **Verner** and **Morrison** described this constellation of clinical features in more detail in 1958, and the syndrome produced by high levels of VIP released from these tumors subsequently bears their names [2]. They reported two male patients who died with similar clinical features of chronic high-volume watery diarrhea, hypokalemia, and hyponatremia, leading to their death from complications of dehydration and electrolyte disturbance. At autopsy, both were found to have pancreatic neuroendocrine tumors, and the authors postulated that a hormonally active substance produced by these tumors was responsible for the diarrhea and electrolyte disturbance. The hormone responsible was not identified until 1970 when Said and coworkers isolated a hormonally active peptide from porcine small intestinal cells and found that it increased splanchnic blood flow, naming it VIP [3]. An association between elevated levels of VIP and the Verner–Morrison syndrome was first shown by Bloom and coworkers in 1973 [4]. They found elevated levels of circulating VIP in patients with pancreatic neuroendocrine tumors and symptoms of the Verner–Morrison syndrome, and also showed staining for VIP within these tumors on immunohistochemistry. A direct association between VIP and the clinical symptoms of this syndrome was also shown by Kane and coworkers in 1983. They were able to induce a profuse watery diarrhea and electrolyte disturbance in human volunteers after infusion of porcine VIP [5].

Incidence and Risk Factors

VIPomas are a rare form of an already uncommon family of tumors, accounting for 1% of all pancreatic neuroendocrine tumors [6]. It is estimated that they occur with an incidence of less than one case per million population per year [7, 8]. These tumors can occur at any age including childhood, with a mean age of between 40 and 50 years [9]. They occur with equal frequency in both males and females. They may be associated with other pancreatic neuroendocrine tumors, primary hyperparathyroidism and pituitary adenomas as part of the multiple endocrine neoplasia type 1 (MEN1) syndrome, occurring in 1–2% of patients with this inherited genetic mutation [10, 11]. Eleven percent of patients with VIPoma managed at the Mayo Clinic had MEN1 [12].

Pathophysiology

VIP is a peptide hormone comprising 28 amino acids and normally functions as a neurotransmitter confined within neurones of the central nervous system, gastrointestinal tract, lung, and genitourinary tract. The plasma half-life of VIP in the systemic circulation is extremely short (less than 60 s), and for this reason plasma levels of this hormone are normally very low (less than 50–100 pg/ml) and do not elevate after eating [9]. VIP acts via binding to specific receptors to increase the secretion, smooth muscle contractility, and blood flow within the gastrointestinal tract, particularly the small intestine and pancreas.

A. J. Chambers (✉)
Department of Surgical Oncology, St. Vincent's Hospital
and University of New South Wales, Suite 709 St Vincent's Clinic,
438 Victoria St, 2010 Darlinghurst, NSW, Australia
e-mail: anthonyjchambers@gmail.com

J. L. Pasieka, J. A. Lee (eds.), *Surgical Endocrinopathies,* DOI 10.1007/978-3-319-13662-2_50,
© Springer International Publishing Switzerland 2015

The high circulating levels of VIP secreted by VIPomas produce symptoms of watery diarrhea, typically more than 6–8 l/day [9]. The diarrhea does not have features of malabsorption such as steatorrhea, and persists despite fasting. The loss of electrolytes in the stool, particularly potassium and bicarbonate, leads to hypokalemia and achlorhydria. For this reason, the syndrome has been previously referred to as WDHA (watery diarrhea, hypokalemia, and achlorhydria) syndrome and pancreatic cholera. Other symptoms include weight loss (occurring in 72% of cases), generalized muscle weakness, abdominal pain (50%), hyperglycemia (40%), and cutaneous flushing (28%) [12, 13].

Although VIP is the predominant hormonally active peptide produced by VIPomas, high levels of other hormones have also been documented in as many as 66% patients with these tumors, including glucagon, pancreatic polypeptide, serotonin, calcitonin, somatostatin, insulin, gastrin, and growth-hormone-releasing hormone [12, 14].

Diagnosis and Imaging Studies

VIPomas are associated with very high circulating levels of VIP, with serum concentrations typically greater than 500 pg/ml (normal range less than 50–100) being diagnostic for these tumors [8, 15]. As for other neuroendocrine tumors, serum levels of chromogranin-A may also be elevated [16].

VIPomas occur most commonly in the pancreas, accounting for 90% of cases. Within the pancreas, the tail of the gland is the most common location (50–75%), followed by the body (8–22%) and the head (11–30%) [9, 12]. Rare sites of primary VIPomas include the duodenum, colon, bronchial tree, and liver. The adrenal glands and retroperitoneal paraganglia can also rarely be the site of these tumors particularly in children [8].

VIPomas typically form discrete masses within the pancreas. By the time of diagnosis, they have usually reached a size of more than 2 cm, with a mean size of 5 cm in one large series [9]. Local invasion into surrounding organs may be seen with larger tumors. Metastases are present in 60–80% of cases at the time of diagnosis, most commonly to regional lymph nodes and to the liver (seen in up to 78% of cases) [9, 12].

The location of the primary tumor is usually readily apparent on cross-sectional imaging using computed tomography or magnetic resonance [17]. As both primary VIPomas and their metastases are hypervascular, contrast enhancement aids in their imaging. Magnetic resonance has been recommended as superior to computed tomography scanning for the detection and staging of VIPomas [17].

VIPomas express receptors for somatostatin in 80–90% of cases, and in this way nuclear medicine scanning using radiolabeled somatostatin analogs such as octreotide can detect 91% of primary tumors and 75% of metastatic lesions [9, 18]. More recently, positron emission tomography using the 68-gallium-labeled somatostatin analogs DOTATATE and DOTATOC have been used to enhance the sensitivity of these studies [18]. Small primary tumors of the pancreas may be best located by endoscopic ultrasound, a technique that also allows for fine-needle aspiration biopsy of lesions. This technique has been particularly recommended in patients with MEN1 syndrome who may have multiple small neuroendocrine tumors of the pancreas [17].

Management

The management of VIPomas is complex and multidisciplinary, involving surgical, medical, interventional radiology, and nuclear medicine modalities. Due to the rarity of these tumors, our understanding of their management is incomplete and evolving, based largely on expert opinion, anecdotal reports, and small case series. The complexity of the management of these rare tumors means that their treatment should be confined to specialist centers that can offer the full range of treatment options.

The initial management of patients newly diagnosed with VIPoma involves correction of the fluid and electrolyte deficiencies caused by the chronic high-volume diarrhea in order to stabilize the patient [9]. In addition to intravenous fluid therapy and potassium replacement, medical therapy with antidiarrheals such as loperamide and opiates may help to control the fluid losses.

The mainstay of symptom control and palliation in patients with VIPoma is with somatostatin analog therapy [8]. These act via binding to somatostatin receptors expressed on 80–90% of VIPomas to inhibit the secretion of VIP. Short-acting agents such as octreotide can be used initially prior to initiating therapy with long-acting formulations such as octreotide LAR or lanreotide. A sustained improvement in symptoms of diarrhea can be achieved in more than 80% of cases with this therapy [19]. VIP levels can be monitored to assess the biochemical response to treatment and may normalize. Unfortunately, tachyphylaxis to these agents occurs within 12–24 months in most cases, requiring increasing dosage and eventually leading to worsening symptoms [8]. Therapy with somatostatin analogs may also have an antitumor effect, leading to prolonged periods of disease stabilization or less commonly a reduction in the size of primary lesions or metastases (seen in 20%) [19]. All patients with VIPomas should have their symptoms controlled by somatostatin analog therapy prior to undergoing surgery.

Surgery for VIPomas involves resection of the primary tumor and may be combined with cytoreductive surgery to remove metastatic disease in regional lymph nodes or the liver where this is practicable. Smith and coworkers in a series of 18 patients with VIPomas managed at the Mayo Clinic reported that surgery with a curative intent was possible in only 28% of cases, and that only 44% of patients were suitable for any attempt at surgical resection [12]. As the primary tumor is usually located within the body or tail of the pancreas, distal or subtotal pancreatectomies are the most commonly employed procedures. In patients with MEN1 where multiple small pancreatic neuroendocrine tumors may be present, subtotal pancreatectomy is the preferred procedure [12]. Hepatic metastases may be candidates for surgical resection or ablative techniques such as radiofrequency ablation [20]. Where multiple hepatic metastases are present that are not suitable for surgical intervention, hepatic artery chemoembolization or infusion with yttrium-90-radiolabeled microspheres have both been associated with symptom control, normalization of VIP levels, and a reduction in the size of metastases [13, 21]. Liver transplantation has also been reported in a patient with multiple hepatic metastases from VIPoma and was associated with a prolonged survival of 9 years [22].

In patients whose tumors and metastases express somatostatin receptors as seen by positivity on radiolabeled octreotide scanning, radionuclide therapy using the 177-lutetium-labeled somatostatin analog DOTATATE may also be used [23]. Conventional systemic therapy with cytotoxic chemotherapy agents such as streptozotocin, 5-fluorouracil, cyclophosphamide, doxorubicin, and temozolomide have been used to treat patients with metastatic VIPoma. Although response rates of 30–40% have been reported, the results of systemic chemotherapy for patients with metastatic VIPoma are generally considered to be poor [15]. More recently, newer therapies targeting the vascular endothelial growth factor receptor (bevacizumab) and tyrosine kinase signaling pathways (sunitinib, sorafenib) have been used to treat metastatic VIPoma [24, 25]. Inhibitors of mammalian target of rapamycin such as everolimus and temsirolimus have shown promise in the treatment of metastatic pancreatic neuroendocrine tumors and may also have a future role [15].

Prognosis

The prognosis of patients with VIPoma is dependent on disease stage. The presence of metastatic disease and disease not amenable to surgical resection with curative intent are associated with a worse prognosis. As 80% of cases have metastatic disease present at the time of diagnosis, the median survival of patients with VIPoma is 3–4 years [6, 12]. This is not different from the prognosis of other pancreatic neuroendocrine tumors when matched for disease stage [6]. Death typically occurs either from complications of fluid and electrolyte disturbances refractory to medical therapies or from the complications of metastatic disease progression.

Conclusion

VIPomas are exceedingly rare neuroendocrine tumors primarily occurring in the pancreas that produce symptoms of diarrhea due to their excessive secretion of VIP. The management of these tumors is complex, involving multiple treatment modalities including surgery, medical therapies, systemic targeted therapies, and radionuclide treatments. Due to the rarity of these tumors, our understanding of them and their optimal treatment is evolving.

Key Summary Points

- VIPomas are rare neuroendocrine tumors most commonly occurring in the pancreas.
- VIPomas secrete high levels of VIP, producing chronic and profuse watery diarrhea leading to electrolyte disturbances (Verner–Morrison syndrome).
- As most VIPomas have metastasized prior to diagnosis, surgical resection has a limited role in management.
- Control of symptoms of metastatic VIPoma is best achieved using somatostatin analog therapy.
- The management of metastatic VIPoma is multidisciplinary, utilizing cytoreductive surgery, medical therapies, interventional radiology, and radionuclide treatment modalities.

References

1. Priest WM, Alexander MK. Islet-cell tumour of the pancreas with peptic ulceration, diarrhoea and hypokalaemia. Lancet. 1957;270:1145–7.
2. Verner JV, Morrison AB. Islet cell tumor and a syndrome of refractory watery diarrhea and hypokalemia. Am J Med. 1958;25:374–80.
3. Said SI, Mutt V. Polypeptide with broad biological activity: isolation from small intestine. Science. 1970;169:1217–8.
4. Bloom SR, Polak JM, Pearse AG. Vasoactive intestinal peptide and watery-diarrhoea syndrome. Lancet. 1973;2:14–16.
5. Kane MG, O'Dorisio TM, Krejs GJ. Production of secretory diarrhea by intravenous infusion of vasoactive intestinal polypeptide. N Engl J Med. 1983;309:1482–5.
6. Yao JC, Eisner MP, Leary C, Dagohoy C, et al. Population-based study of islet cell carcinoma. Ann Surg Oncol. 2007;14:3492–500.
7. Friesen SR. Update on the diagnosis and treatment of rare neuroendocrine tumors. Surg Clin North Am. 1987;67:379–93.
8. Ito T, Igarashi H, Jensen RT. Pancreatic neuroendocrine tumors: clinical features, diagnosis and medical treatment: advances. Best Pract Res Clin Gastroenterol. 2012;26:737–53.
9. Ghaferi AA, Chojnacki KA, Long WD, Cameron JL, Yeo CJ. Pancreatic VIPomas: subject review and one institutional experience. J Gastrointest Surg. 2008;12:382–93.

10. Lévy-Bohbot N, Merle C, Goudet P, Delemer B, et al. Prevalence, characteristics and prognosis of MEN 1-associated glucagonomas, VIPomas, and somatostatinomas: study from the GTE (Groupe des Tumeurs Endocrines) registry. Gastroenterol Clin Biol. 2004;28:1075–81.

11. Heymann MF, Moreau A, Chetritt J, Murat A, Leborgne J, Le Neel JC, et al. Pathologic study with immunohistochemistry of 61 pancreatic endocrine tumors in 16 patients suffering from multiple endocrine neoplasia type I (MEN I): review of the literature. Ann Pathol. 1996;16:167–73.

12. Smith SL, Branton SA, Avino AJ, Martin JK, et al. Vasoactive intestinal polypeptide secreting islet cell tumors: a 15-year experience and review of the literature. Surgery. 1998;124:1050–5.

13. Case CC, Wirfel K, Vassilopoulou-Sellin R. Vasoactive intestinal polypeptide-secreting tumor (VIPoma) with liver metastases. Med Oncol. 2002;19:181–7.

14. Perry RR, Vinik AI. Clinical review 72: diagnosis and management of functioning islet cell tumors. J Clin Endocrinol Metab. 1995;80:2273–8.

15. Abood GJ, Go A, Malhotra D, Shoup M. The surgical management of neuroendocrine tumors of the pancreas. Surg Clin North Am. 2009;89:249–66.

16. Kanakis G, Kaltas G. Biochemical markers for gastroenteropancreatic neuroendocrine tumours (GEP-NETs). Best Pract Res Clin Gastroenterol. 2012;26:791–802.

17. Sundin A. Radiological and nuclear medicine imaging of gastroenteropancreatic neuroendocrine tumours. Best Pract Res Clin Gastroenterol. 2012;26:803–18.

18. Nikou GC, Toubanakis C, Nikolaou P, Giannatou E, Safioleas M, Mallas E, Polyzos A. (2005). VIPomas: an update in diagnosis and management in a series of 11 patients. Hepatogastroenterology. 2005;52:1259–65.

19. Maton PN, Gardner JD, Jensen RT. Use of long-acting somatostatin analog SMS 201–995 in patients with pancreatic islet cell tumors. Dig Dis Sci. 1989;34:28S–39S.

20. Moug SJ, Leen E, Horgan PG, Imrie CW. Radiofrequency ablation has a valuable therapeutic role in metastatic VIPoma. Pancreatology. 2006;6:155–9.

21. King J, Quinn R, Glenn DM, Janssen J, Tong D, Liaw W, Morris DL. Radioembolization with selective internal radiation microspheres for neuroendocrine liver metastases. Cancer. 2008;113:921–9.

22. Johnston PC, Ardill JE, Johnston BT, McCance DR. Vasoactive intestinal polypeptide secreting pancreatic tumour with hepatic metastases: long-term survival after orthotopic liver transplantation. Ir J Med Sci. 2010;179:439–41.

23. Kwekkeboom DJ, de Herder WW, Krenning EP. Somatostatin receptor-targeted radionuclide therapy in patients with gastroenteropancreatic neuroendocrine tumors. Endocrinol Metab Clin North Am. 2011;40:173–85

24. Duran I, Salazar R, Casanovas O, et al. New drug development in digestive neuroendocrine tumors. Ann Oncol. 2007;18:1307–13.

25. Kulke M, Lenz HJ, Meropol NJ, et al. Activity of sunitinib in patients with advanced neuroendocrine tumors. J Clin Oncol. 2008;26:3403–10.

John V. Verner Jr. and Ashton B. Morrison

1927–; 1922–2008

Michael J. Demeure

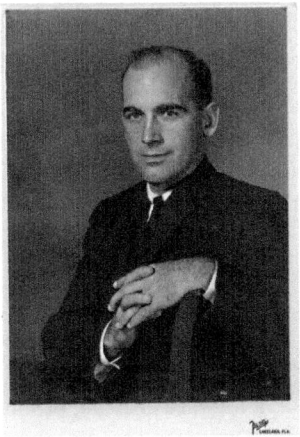

John V. Verner Jr., MD. (Courtesy John and Sally Verner)

that serendipitous happening
—John Verner MD

As relayed by Dr. John Verner [1], the groundwork for the discovery of the syndrome that was to later bear his name and that of Dr. Ashton "Archie" Morrison was the result of an intern research project that was required of the Internal Medicine residency house staff at Duke University. He credits the leadership of Dr. Eugene Stead Jr., the chair of the Department of Medicine, who encouraged clinical research and that his charges think creatively about clinical problems. Dr. Verner developed an interest in hypokalemia and asked the laboratory to alert him to any inpatients with low potassium levels. Three years a chief resident, he saw each patient admitted to the medical ward, and it was in this context that he evaluated the first of the two patients in the seminal report of the watery diarrhea, hypokalemia,

and achlorhydria (WDHA) syndrome associated with islet cell neoplasms. This man had undergone a routine herniorraphy, yet he passed away from profuse cholera-like diarrhea with profound hypokalemia and uremia. This peculiar case was later presented at the Clinical Pathological Conference (CPC). It struck Dr. Verner that the provisional clinical diagnosis of "probable chronic laxative abuse" was preposterous. The finding on autopsy of a small acorn-sized benign non-beta islet cell tumor was described as an incidental finding of no known clinical significance. Dr. Verner experienced a "eureka" epiphany and was sure in his mind that this tumor had been the cause of this patient's demise.

As chance would have it, sitting beside Dr. Verner, at the CPC that day, was Dr. Morrison, the Markley Scholar and a pathologist at Duke. Dr. Morrison's primary research interest was in kidney function, particularly in the way the kidneys handled protein and potassium [2]. He was also intrigued by this case. A second similar case was presented shortly thereafter giving birth to the idea that this was a distinct and previously unrecognized clinical syndrome. Dr. Verner reviewed the chart of a 19-year-old man who had been recently discharged from Duke Medical Center from his 19th admission for profuse diarrhea and hypokalemia. Dr. Verner discovered that the patient had missed an appointment with his psychiatrist because he had been admitted to another hospital where he subsequently died. The autopsy findings of this patient also included a small benign islet cell tumor.

Dr. Verner then embarked on a detailed search of the existing literature and was excited to find that this clinical pathologic syndrome had not been previously described. He and Dr. Morrison presented their manuscript to Dr. Stead who recognized its obvious significance and importance. He recommended that their article be submitted to the American Journal of Medicine where it was promptly published in 1958 [3]. Dr. Stead also directed Dr. Verner to submit and subsequently present their findings at a meeting of the American Federation for Clinical Research in Atlantic City on May 4, 1958. An additional report followed in 1974 in which Drs. Verner and Morrison amassed and detailed an ad-

M. J. Demeure (✉)
Integrated Cancer Genomics,
Translational Genomics Research Institute,
9475 E. Ironwood Square, Suite 102, Phoenix, AZ 85258, USA
e-mail: mdemeure@tgen.org

J. L. Pasieka, J. A. Lee (eds.), *Surgical Endocrinopathies*, DOI 10.1007/978-3-319-13662-2_51,
© Springer International Publishing Switzerland 2015

ditional 55 cases on nonbeta islet cell-induced watery diarrhea and hypokalemia [4].

Dr. John Victor Verner Jr. was born on April 26, 1927, in Greenville North Carolina. From 1944 to 1947, during World War II, Verner served as a second lieutenant in the infantry. He went on to pursue his education at Duke University where he matriculated in 1947 and then earned his BA degree in premedical studies in 1950. He attended the Duke University School of Medicine graduating with his MD degree in 1954. He stayed on, doing an internship year in internal medicine from 1954 to 1955. Verner then went to the University of Michigan in Ann Arbor from 1955 to 1956 to serve as a junior resident in internal medicine before returning to Duke as a senior resident from 1956 to 1957 and then as an instructor and chief resident in internal medicine until 1958 (Fig. 1).

Verner then signed on to work with Dr. Frank L. Engel who was a professor of medicine and the director of the division of endocrinology. John worked in Dr. Engel's laboratory as an Associate American College of Physicians Research Fellow from 1958 to 1959. He received a stipend of US$ 4500. He made an excellent impression on Dr. Engel who observed that Verner showed, "considerable skill in design and conduct of his experiments." In the clinic, Engel commented that he was "quick, bright and very enthusiastic, and carries out his work with care and precision." They published several papers together on vitamin D intoxication [5], recurrent hyperparathyroidism [6], and glucose uptake in adipose cells [7]. John applied for and received a fellowship award from the American Diabetes Association but declined the honor because he was appointed to the full-time faculty at Duke University in the Department of Medicine. Engel assigned Verner the considerable task of reorganizing their diabetes clinic and teaching program. From mutual correspondence in the years that followed, it is evident that Verner viewed Engel as his mentor and they maintained a close, cordial relationship.

Verner had a distinguished career in medicine beyond his important discovery of the syndrome that bears his name. He was awarded the Distinguished Faculty Award by Duke University. In 1962, Verner left Duke and moved to the Watson Clinic in Lakeland, Florida. He was a member of many important medical and scientific societies. He held regional and national offices including the chairman of the Department of Medicine at the Lakeland General Hospital from 1969 to 1971. Verner was the president of the Florida Society of Internal Medicine from 1972 to 1973. He was a trustee on the board of the American Society of Internal Medicine from 1974 to 1976 and a governor for the American Board of Internal Medicine from 1975 to 1981. He also served his local community as a director of the local Greater Lakeland Chamber of Commerce, a board member of the First United Methodist Church of Lakeland, and as president of the local chapter of

the Salvation Army. In 1987, John Verner Jr. retired from the practice of medicine and continued to live in Lakeland Florida with his wife Sally. They have four children.

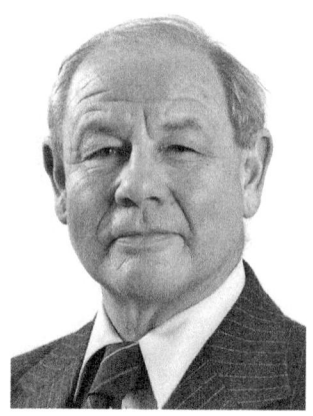

Ashton B. Morrison, MD, PhD. (From EVMS 2009 Spring Magazine, used with permission from Eastern Virginia Medical School, Norfolk, Virginia)

Dr. Ashton Morrison, who was known as Archie to his friends and close colleagues, was born in Lurgan, County Armagh, in Northern Ireland on October 13, 1922. The troubles that existed in that era shaped his life. Dr. Morrison was born into the Protestant upper class and was the only child of two teachers. As such, he was afforded many comforts and luxuries growing up, including private school, elocution lessons, and holiday trips. He began his education at the Carrick Fergus Model School, a forward thinking primary school by the sea in a lovely little town with a medieval castle. From there, he went on to grammar school at the Royal Belfast Academical Institution, also known as Isnt. The young Morrison was bright and studious.

Although his father was a teacher, and he came from a long line of teachers, Archie decided to become a physician leading to some disappointment in the family. Morrison went to medical school at Queen's University in Belfast, earning an MB degree where he was awarded the coveted "Symington Medal" which to him was one of his proudest achievements. During World War II, he did not join the military to fight in the war effort, but rather went to the USA on a Rockefeller scholarship. Initially, Morrison wanted to study medicine at Johns Hopkins University, but he was not accepted. He was, however, accepted to Duke University Medical School. In 1946, he graduated with an MD degree. He returned to earn a PhD in Biochemistry in 1950. He was trained at the Royal Victoria Hospital and at Addesbrookes Hospital in Cambridge, England. During his time as a graduate student, he worked in the Anatomy laboratory in the medical school as an instructor. While in this temporary role, he discovered a mistake in the iconic "Gray's Anatomy" text regarding the course of a nerve in the head and neck and was rewarded with a footnote for his correction.

It was at Queen's University that Morrison met Claire Morris, who was Catholic. She was born in Glenarm,

Northern Ireland, to Charles and Maggie (McEvoy) Morris [8]. Her background was half Presbyterian and half native Irish and likely Norman, but she was raised a Catholic in the Glens of Antrim. There, she was a golf champion and an outstanding student. From St Louis convent in Ballymena, she went on to Queen's University in Belfast where she got not only her MB but also did a thesis in the epidemiology of tuberculosis in mill workers and was awarded an MD with commendation. Her only "flaw" was her religion. Sir Henry Biggart, a local luminary, told Morrison that if he married Claire, his promising career in Northern Ireland would be over. Undaunted, he married her on August 28, 1950. The troubles they encountered took their toll and Morrison found that he could not thrive in his own country with his Catholic bride. A fellow Inst graduate, Robert McCance, took him in at his laboratory in Cambridge, England, and it was there that Morrison continued his work studying enzymes.

Duke beckoned again, and while Dr. Morrison accepted the offer to go stateside, his wife Claire refused initially to go to the USA. Instead, she chose to retreat to Belfast and even purchased a house there. That was her anchor to her homeland, and it was only with personal angst that she ultimately conceded to move in 1956, a year after her husband had already left for the USA. At Duke, she embarked on a distinguished career of her own as a pulmonologist. According to the Morrison family's lore, Claire Morrison became the first female fellow of Eugene Stead. Dr. Stead was the godfather of all medicine at Duke and a truly great man, who guided his charges with insight, intelligence, and kindness. Mrs. Morrison claimed that as a foreigner, perhaps she was too ignorant, to know to be afraid of Dr. Stead. She had the greatest fond admiration for him.

During his time at Duke, Morrison had an appointment in the Pathology Department, and his clinical contribution was working on the autopsy service. It was there that he and Verner found something amiss in the pancreas, and connected the islet cell tumors with the watery diarrhea and profound hypokalemia they had observed and described in what would become known as Verner Morrison syndrome. In 1958, he joined the faculty at the University of Pennsylvania as an assistant professor of pathology. He moved to the University of Rochester School of Medicine in 1961, where he became an associate professor. In 1965, he became professor and chairman of Pathology at Rutgers University. Then in 1980, he became the third dean at the Eastern Virginia Medical School until 1983 when he returned to Rutgers University as dean of the Robert Wood Johnson Medical School. During his time at Rutgers University, Dr. Morrison continued to maintain a home in Norfork, VA, where his wife Claire lived full time.

Those who knew and worked with Dr. Archie Morrison described him as upbeat, friendly, and mild-mannered. One of Morrison's students who later became a colleague, Dr. Desmond Hayes said of him, "He was one of the few faculty members that one could enjoy a pint of Guinness with on the weekends" and that, "he was an excellent clinical instructor and demanding of us." Another colleague, Dr. Robert Faulkner, who had been the chair of the Department of Pathology at Eastern Virginia Medical School recalled that, "he used to come to my office and he loved to talk, not only about the medical school, but about medicine in general." Archie Morrison was a truly humble man. He had a gentle manner and was a friend to all those who worked in the hospital from the janitor to the vice president. His humble nature is perhaps best exemplified by the fact that throughout his entire life, Dr. Morrison was adamant that the syndrome he and Dr. Verner described not be known by their eponyms but rather as the WDHA syndrome or pancreatic cholera. He felt that the syndrome for which he was most famous was a fortunate observation, and while it was for this discovery that Archie Morrison is most well known, the bulk of his lifelong research efforts was devoted to the study of renal failure using a 5/6th nephrectomized rat model he had developed [9]. He received from Duke University, the Distinguished Alumnus Award.

Morrison retired in 1989. Claire Morrison died on June 20, 2008, at the age of 88, and Archie passed away shortly afterwards on September 6, 2008, at the age of 85. They had a daughter, Dr. Mary M. Saltz who is a radiologist, and two grandchildren. Dr. Saltz described that on the occasion of the first birthday of his namesake and grandson Ashton, Dr. Morrison gave him a copy of his textbook *The Pancreas* with an inscribed message to his grandson wishing him "a useful and productive life."

Acknowledgment The author would like to express his gratitude to Dr. John and Sally Verner and to Dr. Mary Saltz for their time, assistance, and interesting recollections.

References

1. Verner JV. This week's citation classic. Curr Contents 1986;4:14.
2. Third Dean Remembered (obituary in Eastern Virginia Medical School Spring 2009 Magazine, p. 5).
3. Verner JV, Morrison AB. Islet cell tumor and a syndrome of refractory watery diarrhea and hypokalemia. Am J Med. 1958;25:374–80.
4. Verner JV, Morrison AB. Endocrine pancreatic islet disease with diarrhea: report of a case due to diffuse hyperplasia of nonbeta islet tissue and a review of 54 additional cases. Arch Intern Med. 1974;133:492–500.
5. Verner JV Jr, Engel FL, McPherson HT. Vitamin D intoxication: report of two cases treated with cortisone. Ann Intern Med. 1958;48:765–73.
6. Greenfield JC, Verner JV Jr, Engel FL. Hyperparathyroidism recurring ten years after removal of parathyroid adenoma. J Am Med Assoc. 1959;171:164–7.
7. Verner JV Jr, Engel FL. The blocking effects of ACTH and the catechol amines on glucose uptake by adipose tissue. Am J Med. 1959;27:329.
8. Obituary Dr. Claire Morrison, New York Times June 30, 2008.
9. Morrison AB. Experimentally induced chronic renal insufficiency in the rat. Lab Invest. 1962;11:321.

Glucagonoma

Peter J. Mazzaglia

History

Glucagonoma and the glucagonoma syndrome were elucidated over several decades, due to the condition's rarity. The syndrome's first description in 1942 was published in the *Archives of Dermatology* by Drs. Becker, Kahn, and Rothman, dermatologists in Chicago. They described a patient with a malignant pancreatic islet cell tumor, with a migrating erythematous rash, glossitis, stomatitis, diabetes, anemia, weight loss, depression, and venous thrombosis [1]. The next publication of a similar case did not appear until 1960, by Gössner and Korting [2]. In this report, a tumor extract was described to have a hyperglycemic effect. Several more publications appeared in the 1960s, including Dr. McGavran's classic description published in the *New England Journal of Medicine* [3].

Meanwhile, the Russian physician V. C. Zhadanov had described an identical syndrome in a patient with a malignant islet cell tumor 10 years earlier [4]. It seems as though most of these authors were unaware of the prior publications, and at that time, the rash had not been given its current name, so the respective authors were labeling it as something else. Therefore, these individual case reports were not recognized as being related until the 1970s [5].

In 1971, Dr. Darrell Wilkinson presented a patient with a psoriaform rash and a pancreatic tumor with hepatic metastases before the Dermatological Section of The Royal Society of Medicine of London [6]. Several of the physicians present recognized the combination of symptoms and physical findings as strikingly similar to ones present in patients they had treated. Based on discussions held during this meeting, one of these patients underwent a laparotomy and was found to have a limited pancreatic tumor. Post resection, the rash is reported to have improved within hours, and disappeared within a week. The patient's diabetes and anemia soon resolved, and weight gain ensued. Pathology demonstrated a pancreatic islet cell tumor, which contained glucagon. Measurement of plasma glucagon was 20 times normal preoperatively, and normalized post-op [5].

Word of these cases was spread through the British Dermatological Association, and a total of nine similar patients were identified. This series of nine was published in 1974, establishing the defining characteristics of the glucagonoma syndrome [7].

Glucagonomas are pancreatic neuroendocrine tumors that arise from pancreatic islet alpha cells. They are most well known for the paraneoplastic glucagonoma syndrome that they produce. The first descriptions of the syndrome appear in the dermatologic literature, since the development of a classic rash eventually occurs in nearly all patients. This rash, coined necrolytic migratory erythema (NME) by Dr. Wilkinson in 1973, is in fact the most likely reason for suspecting the underlying pathology. While the disease is exceedingly rare, with an incidence of only 1 in 20 million, it is very well described, in part because of its uniqueness. In addition to NME, the common features include hyperglycemia, anemia, thromboembolic disease, weight loss, depression, and stomatitis. Typically, patients present in the fifth or sixth decade, and there is an equal gender distribution.

Historically, most patients with glucagonoma presented with diabetes and dermatologic manifestations. However, because of its rarity, the pathognomonic rash associated with glucagonoma, NME, frequently goes unrecognized. Thus, these patients are often followed in dermatology clinics for lengthy periods of time prior to having a definitive diagnosis made. However, a substantial minority of patients will not have developed the rash prior to being diagnosed. In fact in the largest single institution review, including 21 patients at the Mayo Clinic, NME was a presenting complaint in only 67% [8]. For the other 33%, 7 out of the 21, presenting symptoms included weight loss, abdominal pain, diarrhea, and **Zollinger–Ellison** syndrome. Another series of

P. J. Mazzaglia (✉)
Rhode Island Hospital, Warren Alpert School of Medicine,
Brown University, 2 Dudley St., Providence, RI 02905, USA
e-mail: peterjmazzaglia@gmail.com

J. L. Pasieka, J. A. Lee (eds.), *Surgical Endocrinopathies,* DOI 10.1007/978-3-319-13662-2_52,
© Springer International Publishing Switzerland 2015

18 cases reported in the British literature by Frankton and Bloom, similarly identified NME at presentation in 72 % [9]. A second less frequent method of presentation is the finding of an incidental pancreatic lesion, or evidence of metastatic disease, identified on cross-sectional imaging obtained for other purposes.

Necrolytic Migratory Erythema

The rash is characterized not only by its appearance and tendency to migrate but also by its distribution. The name given, necrolytic migratory erythema, is based on both clinical and histologic characteristics of the rash. Dr. Wilkinson's published series contained nine patients with what was considered glucagonoma syndrome [10] (Fig. 1).

It typically originates in the perineum and lower abdomen, but may also present in the perioral area or lower extremities, especially the feet. Involvement of the thorax and upper extremities is rare. It also commonly causes angular cheilitis and glossitis, with "vermilion discoloration" of the tongue [5].

At the time of its initial appearance, the rash appears as a slightly raised, erythematous patch, which spreads within several days. Initially, it resembles an area of scalded skin, with overlying dead epithelium. Often the rash is mistaken for psoriasis, pemphigus, or eczema. Because it causes significant skin fragility, the epidermis is easily rubbed off, leaving raw, weeping surfaces. Especially prone to this, are areas of high friction, such as the perineum and feet. Other affected areas may develop superficial blisters and crusting. It is frequently painful and pruritic.

Typically, as the edge of the lesion spreads, the central areas heal with hyperpigmentation. The migrating edge of the rash tends to have a very well-demarcated appearance that is slightly raised. The process of spreading with central healing takes on a cyclical pattern lasting 7–14 days. There do not appear to be any exacerbating factors [11].

In some instances, the rash follows a more indolent pattern, with a smoldering central necrosis that becomes secondarily infected, usually with *Candida* or *Staphylococcus aureus* [12]. Perineal involvement in women causes urethral inflammation leading to urinary tract infection. In intertriginous areas, the rash becomes more lichenified and psoriaform due to the repetitive friction [13].

The histologic changes of necrolytic migratory erythema are pathognomonic. The findings are confined to the epidermis, where there is necrosis and necrolysis in the most superficial half of the epidermis. Vessicles or bullae form as the dead layer separates from the deeper viable layer. Neither evidence of an immune basis for the rash nor evidence of an ischemic origin has been established. The light microscopic

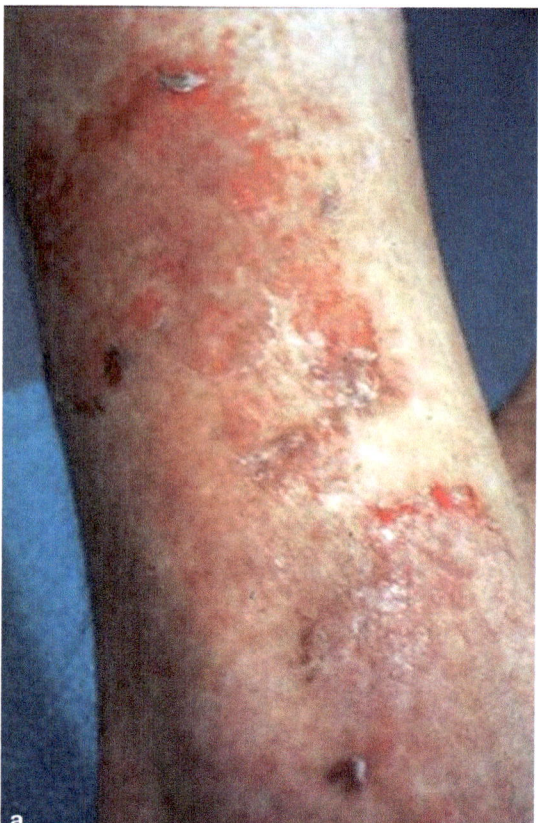
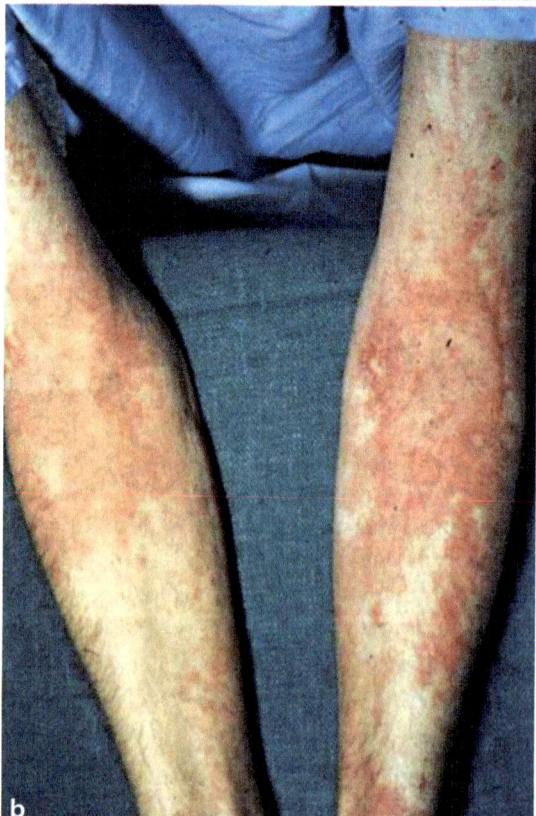

Fig. 1 **a** and **b** Necrolytic migratory erythema. (Photos courtesy of Dr. Janice Pasieka and Dr. Steve Urbanski)

patterns described by Kheir et al. include (1) superficial epidermal vacuolization and necrosis, (2) subcorneal pustule formation, (3) vascular dilatation of the papillary dermis, and (4) psoriaform hyperplasia with confluent parakeratosis [11, 14]. The findings may mimic those of acrodermatitis enteropathica, pellagra, kwashiorkor, fatty acid deficiency, and hypoalbuminemia. On electron microscopy, there is cytoplasmic vacuolization with degeneration of nuclear structures. There is widening of intercellular spaces, and the cells are smaller and have pyknotic nuclei [11].

Several theories as to the cause of the rash include activation of lysosomes in the middle layer of the epidermis, or as a result of abnormal keratinization. In order to successfully make the diagnosis, a biopsy must be taken from the edge of a fresh lesion so as to avoid the secondary changes seen in the areas of infection [15, 16].

Oral ulcers, angular cheilitis, and tongue involvement have been reported with variable frequency. In one of the first series by Mallinson, they were present in almost 90% of patients, but more recent studies suggest their prevalence in 30% [7, 8, 9]. Uncommon dermatologic findings include nail dystrophy, onycholysis, and paronychial swelling, as well as blepharitis and alopecia [12, 13].

Diabetes

The majority of patients will have impaired glucose tolerance, which may occur before the rash develops, by months or years. It is often mild, and able to be controlled through diet or oral agents. Diabetic ketoacidosis is not a feature. The typical peripheral and systemic manifestations of diabetes have not been documented in glucagonoma patients. These patients have a degree of hyperinsulinemia, which is thought to counteract the hyperglucagonemia, and they may have a normal glucose tolerance test until very late in the disease [17].

Anemia

Virtually all patients will have a normochromic normocytic anemia. Its severity correlates with the extent of disease, worsening with tumor progression, and the development of hepatic metastases. The degree of anemia also fluctuates with the activity of the rash, often approaching normal levels when the rash is quiescent. The exact cause of the anemia is unclear, and it does not seem to be related to iron deficiency. Bone marrow exams in these patients have not revealed abnormal erythropoiesis. Some have suggested a direct bone marrow suppressive effect of glucagon [8].

Venous Thrombosis

Thromboembolic events have been reported in up to 30% of cases [7, 18], and are a presenting symptom in 11–14% [8, 9].

Weight Loss

Weight loss is a common finding in most patients with glucagonoma, much more so in those with hepatic metastatic disease, as would be expected. It has been reported in 56–91% of patients [8, 19–22]. It is thought that the catabolic effects of glucagon are responsible for this finding. As with the anemia, weight seems to improve when the rash recedes.

Depression

Psychiatric symptoms occur in roughly 20% of patients. They include depression, dementia, psychosis, decreased cognitive function, agitation, nervousness, insomnia, ataxia, and muscle weakness [11]. Optic atrophy may occur, leading to decreased visual acuity [23, 24].

Uncommon Symptoms

Other symptoms that have been documented in these patients, but are not typical, include intermittent diarrhea. There are no commonly detected electrolyte abnormalities, and urinary 5-hydroxyindoleacetic acid (5-HIAA) levels are normal. Anorexia can be seen as well as abdominal pain. As with other pancreatic neuroendocrine tumors, the islet cells are capable of secreting more than one hormone. Those that have been documented with glucagonomas include insulin, gastrin, 5-HIAA, pancreatic polypeptide, chromogranin, vasoactive intestinal peptide, calcitonin, adrenocorticotropic hormone, and somatostatin [8, 9].

While most glucagonomas are sporadic, there have been rare reports of them occurring as part of the multiple endocrine neoplasia type I (MEN-I) syndrome. [8, 9, 25] These patients generally present at a younger age, and often do not suffer from the classic manifestations of the glucagonoma syndrome, possibly due to earlier detection [11].

There is a subset of patients with glucagonoma who do not develop NME. They present only with severe diabetes and a pancreatic neuroendocrine tumor. Interestingly, these patients also do not develop the other manifestations of the disease.

Diagnosis

The average time from initial presentation until diagnosis is roughly 2 years. Once the diagnosis is suspected, testing should begin with a plasma glucagon level. Circulating glucagon is comprised of several different sized molecules, all sharing the same amino terminus. The larger molecules are felt to represent pro-hormones that are later cleaved. While normal glucagon levels range from 10 to 120 mmol/mL, levels in glucagonoma patients have been reported to range from 500 to 6000 mmol/mL. While certain physiologic conditions such as burns, trauma, and diabetic ketoacidosis can elevate plasma glucagon, they do not approach the levels seen in patients with glucagonoma. Box 1 lists many of the conditions in which hyperglucagonemia can be seen, and thus these need to be ruled out as possible causes. If the level exceeds 1000 pg/mL without an obvious secondary cause, the diagnosis of glucagonoma is highly likely.

Box 1. Causes of hyperglucagonemia [11]
Other islet cell tumors
Cirrhosis
Pancreatic disease
Chronic renal failure
Myocardial infarction
Fasting
Diabetic ketoacidosis
Familial hyperglucagonemia
Celiac disease
Sepsis
Trauma
Cushing's syndrome
Danazol therapy

There is a significant variability over time. Plasma insulin levels are often elevated, as is fasting blood glucose. An oral glucose tolerance test should be performed, and is expected to be abnormal.

Of historical note, several agents have been shown to stimulate an abnormal rise in plasma glucagon levels. These include oral glucose, intravenous tolbutamide, and intravenous arginine; however, these maneuvers are not part of current clinical practice.

There is a consistent finding of reduced plasma amino acids, which is unique to this disease. It was first reported by Mallinson in 1974 [7]. The reduction is felt to be a direct consequence of the catabolic effect of hyperglucagonemia [26]. The hormone binds to receptors on hepatocytes and adipocytes, and regulates carbohydrate, protein, and fat metabolism. Normally it stimulates gluconeogenesis and glycogenolysis, which ordinarily aids in the maintenance of blood glucose levels during fasting, exercise, and stress [26]. At pathologic levels, glucagon promotes amino acid mobilization from tissues to serve as substrate for gluconeogenesis. Subsequent protein degradation leads to the low amino acid levels seen in patients with glucagonoma syndrome, and this in turn may lead to cellular necrosis in the epidermis. This is one theory on how hyperglucagonemia directly leads to NME [7].

Tumor location and characteristics: Glucagonomas are tumors of pancreatic neuroendocrine origin, specifically alpha-2 islet cells. Primary tumor sizes ranging from 2 to 25 cm have been reported [8]. They are derived from the embryonic dorsal lobe of the pancreas [5]. The majority are located in the neck, body, tail, and superior part of the head of the pancreas.

Once an elevated glucagon level is documented, radiologic studies, beginning with a pancreatic protocol computed tomography (CT) scan are indicated. Today's thin cut CT scans are highly sensitive, and will also provide images of the liver. Due to its improved sensitivity and noninvasive nature, CT scan has replaced celiac angiography, which was once a common localization technique.

Octreotide scanning has been extensively studied, and was early on the most utilized method of localization. That role has been supplanted by CT, however there is still a place for radioisotope scanning, when searching for suspected disease in CT negative patients, or when the question of miliary type hepatic metastases exists.

On histological analysis, cells are of varying sizes. Cells are pleomorphic, and may be arranged in a glandular trabecular pattern similar to normal islets, or more of a disorganized array with areas resembling rosettes and follicles. There are few mitoses, and the cytoplasm is acidophilic and finely granular [27]. Electron microscopy reveals the numerous dense round secretory granules. Immunofluorescence is confirmatory that an islet cell tumor indeed is glucagon containing. They stain positively for both glucagon and pancreatic polypeptide. Of the islet cell tumors, only glucagonomas are found to contain substantial levels of glucagon, but these levels may not be significantly higher than those found in normal pancreatic tissue. Most are well vascularized.

Thus, definitive pathologic diagnosis depends on the histologic finding of an islet cell tumor which contains secretory granules that stain positively for glucagon. Determination of malignancy, as is the case with most pancreatic neuroendocrine tumors (PNETS), depends on the finding of local tumor invasion or the development of metastases. Upwards of 70% of glucagonomas display malignant behavior [8, 9, 28]. Those that are classified as benign simply may not have had the time to develop metastases.

Treatment

As with other pancreatic neuroendocrine tumors, small lesions confined to the pancreas can often be enucleated, or removed with a partial pancreatectomy. Since a large percentage of these tumors are malignant, once a diagnosis is made, the goal should be to resect the primary lesion, in a timely fashion. While surgical dogma has traditionally deemed metastatic tumors unresectable, newer studies suggest benefit for many PNET patients, who are candidates for resection of the primary tumor, and resection or debulking of hepatic metastases [29].

When complete tumor excision is achieved, patients with NME experience dramatic and gratifying resolution of their rash, which occurs within days. Improvement is also seen in the patient's anemia, depression, weight, and glucose tolerance. Even when a patient cannot be rendered disease free due to metastatic disease, resection of the primary and debulking of metastases can be very beneficial in terms of improving the associated paraneoplastic conditions [30–32].

For patients with hepatic metastases that cannot be completely resected, a combination of surgery and ablation may be employed. Most studies group all patients with pancreatic neuroendocrine tumor liver metastases together. In one study of 63 patients with neuroendocrine liver metastases who underwent laparoscopic radiofrequency ablation, symptom relief was reported in 90% with a median 3.9-year survival. Intrahepatic recurrences are high [33].

Alternate modalities of treating unresectable liver metastases include hepatic artery embolization with chemotherapeutic agents [34], Yttrium-90 resin-based spheres (Sirspheres), or glass-based radioembolization (Theraspheres) [35]. Most studies are retrospective in nature. In a study of 148 patients from 10 institutions, disease response was stable in 23% and partial in 61%, with progression in only 5%. Median survival was 70 months [36].

Direct treatment of the rash has been mostly unsuccessful. Attempts to treat areas of superinfection with topical antibiotics are generally of little benefit. Systemic corticosteroids have also shown little improvement.

For many patients with unresectable disease, or persistent systemic disease, systemic chemotherapy has traditionally been used, but with limited efficacy. Agents include dacarbazine, 5-fluorouracil (5-FU), and streptozotocin. The latter has shown a 50% response rate in a review of 52 patients [37]. A combination of 5-FU and streptozotocin has given a 60–70% response rate [38]. However, more typical response rates are in the 10–20% range.

Reports of performing pancreatectomy and liver transplantation exist, and have demonstrated long-term disease-free survival [38, 39].

The treatment of paraneoplastic symptoms preoperatively or in patients with unresectable disease is highly effective using somatostatin analogs such as octreotide or lanreotide. These medications act to lower serum glucagon levels [40]. They are especially effective in controlling NME, where improvement can be seen in 48–72 h, and near resolution within 2 weeks. By lowering serum glucagon levels, the catabolic effects are decreased, and patients are also seen to gain weight.

Other targeted agents showing potential promise for the treatment of metastatic pancreatic neuroendocrine tumors include everolimus (RAD001), which is an inhibitor of the mammalian target of rapamycin. In a placebo-controlled trial of 410 patients, progression-free survival was 11 months in the everolimus-treated patients versus 4.6 months in the placebo group [41]. The multi-receptor tyrosine kinase inhibitor sunitinib has also been approved by the FDA for use in patients with advanced pancreatic neuroendocrine tumors, after a randomized placebo-controlled trial showed similar results to the everolimus study [42].

Lifelong surveillance is necessary, as patients are prone to late recurrences, and routine measurement of glucagon levels is thereby recommended.

Summary

Glucagonoma is one of the rarest types of pancreatic islet cell neoplasms. It is often malignant, commonly presenting with hepatic metastases. Its most well-known feature, and the one that should raise concern for the diagnosis, is necrolytic migratory erythema. Associated findings include diabetes mellitus, stomatitis, anemia, weight loss, and depression. Patients receive significant symptomatic benefit upon tumor resection, and even in cases when complete tumor resection is not possible, or there are hepatic metastases, surgery may be indicated for palliation.

Key Summary Points

- Incidence of glucagonoma is only 1 in 20 million.
- Most patients present with the pathognomonic rash, necrolytic migratory erythema, and diabetes.
- Recognition is often delayed because of its rarity, and consequent failure to distinguish the rash from more common dermatologic conditions.
- Treatment for limited disease is surgical with rapid symptom resolution.
- Metastatic disease can be effectively palliated with somatostatin analogues, and studies are demonstrating benefit for targeted biologic agents.

References

1. Becker SW, Kahn, D, Rothman, S. Cutaneous manifestations of internal malignant tumours. Arch Dermatol Syph. 1942;49:1069.
2. Goessner W, Korting GW. Metastasizing islet cell carcinoma of the A cell type in a case of pemphigus foliaceus with diabetes renalis. Dtsch Med Wochenschr. 1960;85:434–7.
3. McGavran MH, Unger RH, Recant L, Polk HC, Kilo C, Levin ME. A glucagon-secreting alpha-cell carcinoma of the pancreas. N Engl J Med. 1966;274(25):1408–13.
4. Zhdanov VS. Diabetes in tumor of islands of Langerhans. Arkh Patol. 1956;18(3):92–3.
5. Friesen SR, editor. Surgical endocrinology: clinical syndromes. Philadelphia: J. B. Lippincott Company; 1978:120–144.
6. Wilkinson GT, Prydie J, Scarnell J. Possible "orf" (contagious pustular dermatitis, contagious ecthyma of sheep) infection in the dog. Vet Rec. 1970;87(25):766–7.
7. Mallinson CN, Bloom SR, Warin AP, Salmon PR, Cox B. A glucagonoma syndrome. Lancet. 1974;2(7871):1–5.
8. Wermers RA, Fatourechi V, Wynne AG, Kvols LK, Lloyd RV. The glucagonoma syndrome. Clinical and pathologic features in 21 patients. Medicine. 1996;75(2):53–63.
9. Frankton S, Bloom SR. Gastrointestinal endocrine tumours. Glucagonomas. Baillieres Clin Gastroenterol. 1996;10(4):697–705.
10. Wilkinson DS. Necrolytic migratory erythema with carcinoma of the pancreas. Trans St Johns Hosp Dermatol Soc. 1973;59(2):244–50.
11. Chastain MA. The glucagonoma syndrome: a review of its features and discussion of new perspectives. Am J Med Sci. 2001;321(5):306–20.
12. Prinz RA, Dorsch TR, Lawrence AM. Clinical aspects of glucagon-producing islet cell tumors. Am J Gastroenterol. 1981;76(2):125–31.
13. Shupack JL, Berczeller PH, Stevens DM. The glucagonoma syndrome. J Dermatol Surg Oncol. 1978;4(3):242–7.
14. Kheir SM, Omura EF, Grizzle WE, Herrera GA, Lee I. Histologic variation in the skin lesions of the glucagonoma syndrome. Am J Surg Pathol. 1986;10(7):445–53.
15. Wilkinson DS. Necrolytic migratory erythema with pancreatic carcinoma. Proc R Soc Med. 1971;64:1196.
16. Necrolytic migratory erythema with carcinoma of the pancrease. Trans St Johns Hosp Dermatol Soc. 1973;59:244.
17. Sweet RD. A dermatosis specifically associated with a tumour of pancreatic alpha cells. Br J Dermatol. 1974;90(3):301–8.
18. Pedersen NB, Jonsson L, Holst JJ. Necrolytic migratory erythema and glucagon cell tumour of the pancreas: the glucagonoma syndrome. Report of two cases. Acta Derm Venereol. 1976;56(5):391–5.
19. Boden G. Insulinoma and glucagonoma. Semin Oncol. 1987;14(3):253–62.
20. Mozell E, Stenzel P, Woltering EA, Rosch J, O'Dorisio TM. Functional endocrine tumors of the pancreas: clinical presentation, diagnosis, and treatment. Curr Probl Surg. 1990;27(6):301–86.
21. Stacpoole PW. The glucagonoma syndrome: clinical features, diagnosis, and treatment. Endocr Rev. 1981;2(3):347–61.
22. Kaplan EL, Michelassi F. Endocrine tumors of the pancreas and their clinical syndromes. Surg Annu. 1986;18:181–223.
23. Khandekar JD, Sriratana P. Response of glucagonoma syndrome to lomustine. Cancer Treat Rep. 1986;70(3):433–4.
24. Lambrecht ER, van der Loos TL, van der Eerden AH. Retrobulbar neuritis as the first sign of the glucagonoma syndrome. Int Ophthalmol. 1987;11(1):13–5.
25. Croughs RJ, Hulsmans HA, Israel DE, Hackeng WH, Schopman W. Glucagonoma as part of the polyglandular adenoma syndrome. Am J Med. 1972;52(5):690–8.
26. Lefebvre PJ. Glucagon and its family revisited. Diabetes Care. 1995;18(5):715–30.
27. Parker CM, Hanke CW, Madura JA, Liss EC. Glucagonoma syndrome: case report and literature review. J Dermatol Surg Oncol. 1984;10(11):884–9.
28. Schwartz RA. Glucagonoma and pseudoglucagonoma syndromes. Int J Dermatol. 1997;36(2):81–9.
29. Mayo SC, de Jong MC, Pulitano C, Clary BM, Reddy SK, Gamblin TC, et al. Surgical management of hepatic neuroendocrine tumor metastasis: results from an international multi-institutional analysis. Ann Surg Oncol. 2010;17(12):3129–36.
30. Smith AP, Doolas A, Staren ED. Rapid resolution of necrolytic migratory erythema after glucagonoma resection. J Surg Oncol. 1996;61(4):306–9.
31. Edney JA, Hofmann S, Thompson JS, Kessinger A. Glucagonoma syndrome is an underdiagnosed clinical entity. Am J Surg. 1990;160(6):625–8; discussion 8–9.
32. Holmes A, Kilpatrick C, Proietto J, Green MD. Reversal of a neurologic paraneoplastic syndrome with octreotide (Sandostatin) in a patient with glucagonoma. Am J Med. 1991;91(4):434–6.
33. Mazzaglia PJ, Berber E, Milas M, Siperstein AE. Laparoscopic radiofrequency ablation of neuroendocrine liver metastases: a 10-year experience evaluating predictors of survival. Surgery. 2007;142(1):10–9.
34. Gupta S, Johnson MM, Murthy R, Ahrar K, Wallace MJ, Madoff DC, et al. Hepatic arterial embolization and chemoembolization for the treatment of patients with metastatic neuroendocrine tumors: variables affecting response rates and survival. Cancer. 2005;104(8):1590–602.
35. Saxena A, Chua TC, Bester L, Kokandi A, Morris DL. Factors predicting response and survival after Yttrium-90 radioembolization of unresectable neuroendocrine tumor liver metastases: a critical appraisal of 48 cases. Ann Surg. 2010;251(5):910–6.
36. Kennedy AS, Dezarn WA, McNeillie P, Coldwell D, Nutting C, Carter D, et al. Radioembolization for unresectable neuroendocrine hepatic metastases using resin 90Y-microspheres: early results in 148 patients. Am J Clin Oncol. 2008;31(3):271–9.
37. Broder LE, Carter SK. Pancreatic islet cell carcinoma. I. Clinical features of 52 patients. Ann Intern Med. 1973;79(1):101–7.
38. Wynick D, Hammond PJ, Bloom SR. The glucagonoma syndrome. Clin Dermatol. 1993;11(1):93–7.
39. Arnold JC, O'Grady JG, Bird GL, Calne RY, Williams R. Liver transplantation for primary and secondary hepatic apudomas. Br J Surg. 1989;76(3):248–9.
40. Jockenhovel F, Lederbogen S, Olbricht T, Schmidt-Gayk H, Krenning EP, Lamberts SW, et al. The long-acting somatostatin analogue octreotide alleviates symptoms by reducing posttranslational conversion of prepro-glucagon to glucagon in a patient with malignant glucagonoma, but does not prevent tumor growth. Clin Investig. 1994;72(2):127–33.
41. Yao JC, Shah MH, Ito T, Bohas CL, Wolin EM, Van Cutsem E, et al. Everolimus for advanced pancreatic neuroendocrine tumors. N Engl J Med. 2011;364(6):514–23.
42. Raymond E, Dahan L, Raoul JL, Bang YJ, Borbath I, Lombard-Bohas C, et al. Sunitinib malate for the treatment of pancreatic neuroendocrine tumors. N Engl J Med. 2011;364(6):501–13.

Small Bowel Neuroendocrine Tumors

Josefina C. Farra and Steven E. Rodgers

List of Abbreviations

CT Scan	Computed tomography scan
MRI	Magnetic resonance imaging
PET Scan	Positron emission tomography
NETs	Neuroendocrine tumors
WHO	World Health Organization
NCDB	National Cancer Database
SEER	Surveillance Epidemiology and End Results
5-HIAA	5-hydroxyindoleacetic acid
NCCN	National Comprehensive Cancer Network
AJCC	American Joint Committee on Cancer
TAE	Transarterial embolization
TACE	Transarterial chemoembolization
ENETS	European Neuroendocrine Tumor Society
LITT	Laser-induced thermotherapy
PRRT	Peptide-receptor radiotherapy

Introduction

Neuroendocrine tumors (NETs) originate in the endocrine cells that populate the submucosa of the gastrointestinal (GI) tract [1]. The tumors were originally described by Langhans in 1867 and Lubarsch in 1888 [2]. **Siegfried Oberndorfer** introduced the term "carcinoid" in 1907 to distinguish these tumors as less aggressive tumors of the small bowel than most carcinomas [3]. Later, Gosset and Masson demonstrated that the cells of these tumors contain silver-salt reducing granules, leading to the concept that carcinoid tumors contain argentaffin cells, which are derived from the Kulchitsky cells or enterochromaffin (EC) cells of the small intestine [3].

NETs of the small bowel can be divided into functional NETs, in which excess hormone secretion causes a clinical syndrome, and nonfunctional NETs, which are hormonally silent [1]. These are histologically and biochemically diverse tumors that usually correspond to the site of origin and hormone secreting ability of the tumor [4]. In 1963, Williams and Sander classified carcinoid tumors based on their embryonic division in the GI tract. They distinguished the tumors based on foregut (bronchial, gastric, duodenal), midgut (jejunal, ileal, cecal), and hindgut (distal colic and rectal); and described the differences in their characteristics [1, 3]. In 2000, The World Health Organization (WHO) classified these tumors into NETs and neuroendocrine carcinomas instead of carcinoids.

Epidemiology

Small bowel NETs are the most common neoplasm of the small intestine, surpassing adenocarcinoma of the small bowel. Data from the National Cancer Data Base (NCDB) and the Surveillance Epidemiology and End Results (SEER) national cancer registry indicate that over the past three decades 37.4 % of all patients with small bowel malignances had carcinoid tumors, whereas 36.9 % had adenocarcinomas. The incidence of small bowel NETs has increased fourfold in the past four decades [5]. The reported annual age-adjusted incidence of small bowel NETs increased from 1.09/100,000 in 1973 to 5.25/100,000 in 2004 [6]. The increase in incidence is thought to be in part due to improvement in classification systems, as well as increases in endoscopic procedures, improvements in imaging, and improved recognition of neuroendocrine histology [1, 6].

NETs are distributed throughout the body; however, the majority of NETs are found within the GI tract (54.5 %). An analysis of all patients diagnosed with carcinoid tumors between 1973 and 1997 was performed from the SEER national

S. E. Rodgers (✉)
Department of Surgery, University of Miami Miller School of Medicine, Clinical Research Building (C232),
1120 NW 14th Street, 4th Floor, Miami, FL 33136, USA
e-mail: srodgers@med.miami.edu

J. C. Farra
Department of Surgery, Jackson Memorial Hospital,
University of Miami Miller School of Medicine, Miami, FL, USA

J. L. Pasieka, J. A. Lee (eds.), *Surgical Endocrinopathies*, DOI 10.1007/978-3-319-13662-2_53,
© Springer International Publishing Switzerland 2015

cancer registry. Among NETs found in the GI tract, 44.7% of them were found in the small intestine, followed by the rectum (19.6%), appendix (16.7%), colon (10.6%), and stomach (7.2%). Within the small intestine, NETs were found in the ileum more than 50% of the time; they were found less frequently in the jejunum and duodenum. Interestingly, while the incidence of small bowel NETs has increased, that of NETs of the appendix has decreased from 31.8% of all carcinoids in 1973 to 12% in 1997 [4]. Another analysis of 13,715 carcinoid tumors registered in cancer registries in the USA between 1950 and 1999 found similar incidences. The majority of NETs were located in the GI tract (67%). The breakdown of those found within the GI tract demonstrated that the majority arose in the small intestine (42%), followed by the rectum (27%), colon (20%), stomach (20%), and appendix (18%) [7].

The median age at presentation for small bowel NETs is 66, and 52% of patients are male. Numerous studies have reported metastatic disease at the time of diagnosis in around 30% of patients. However, in a surgical series of 603 patients with small bowel NETs from a single high-volume center, Norlén et al. reported that 88% of patients had mesenteric lymph node metastases and 61% had liver metastases at the time of diagnosis. This may be due to selection bias or a more aggressive approach in the diagnosis of disease [4, 6, 8]. Midgut NETs have a higher proclivity to metastasize to regional lymph nodes and the liver. However, they are associated with a long life expectancy, as they proceed at an indolent pace compared to metastatic NETs originating from the foregut or hindgut [1, 5]. The most common sites of metastatic disease are liver, followed by the mesentery and peritoneum. Other sites include the skeleton, lungs, central nervous system, mediastinal lymph nodes, ovaries, breast, and skin [5].

Clinical Presentation

Patients with small bowel NETs may present with symptoms due to the local effects of the primary tumor, due to metastatic disease, or due to hormonal secretion causing carcinoid syndrome. Initially, small bowel NETs are typically asymptomatic or present with vague abdominal symptoms because they grow slowly in the intestinal wall. The most common presenting symptom is abdominal pain, which is often crampy and episodic [1]. The pain then progresses to abdominal distention, nausea and vomiting, diarrhea, and weight loss. Ultimately, patients may present with small bowel obstruction, ischemia, or bleeding [5]. This is often due to the mechanical effects of the intraluminal tumor or due to mesenteric lymph node involvement, which can produce a secondary desmoplastic response leading to bowel kinking and mesenteric ischemia (Fig. 1) [1]. In 30–45% of

patients, the diagnosis of small bowel NET is made at the time of exploration for a small bowel obstruction [5].

Carcinoid Syndrome

The term carcinoid syndrome was first described in 1954 by Thorson et al., who were the first to draw a correlation between certain unusual clinical symptoms in patients with metastatic small bowel NETs. These symptoms include flushing, diarrhea, bronchospasm, and right-sided valvular heart disease [9]. Metastatic NETs of the midgut most commonly produce the classical carcinoid syndrome [1]. These manifestations are associated with the release of various substances from the tumor, including serotonin, 5-hydroxytryptophan (HTP), histamine, dopamine, vasoactive intestinal peptide, and prostaglandins [5]. The liver detoxifies the substances that are released by primary small bowel NETs and mesenteric metastases as these pass through the portal circulation into the liver. Serotonin is metabolized in the liver to 5-hydroxyindoleacetic acid (5-HIAA), a urinary metabolite. Carcinoid syndrome occurs in patients with liver metastasis in which the tumors can secrete vasoactive substances directly into the systemic circulation and bypass the portal circulation [10].

Flushing is the most common symptom of carcinoid syndrome and occurs in 73% of patients. It presents as a diffuse erythematous flushing of the face, neck, and upper torso, which may be precipitated by exercise, stress, alcohol, or certain foods. Typically, patients experience symptoms episodically for 2–10 min. It is attributed to the release of prostaglandins, tachykinins, and serotonin from the tumors

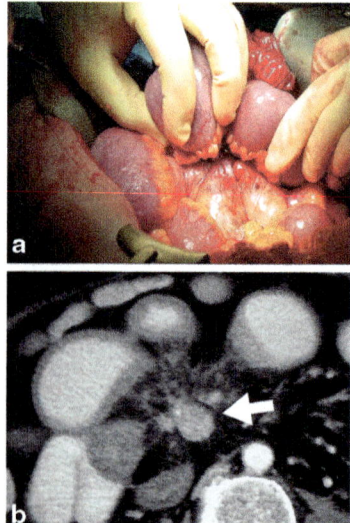

Fig. 1 (**a**) Intraoperative photo of small bowel obstruction due to kinking caused by neuroendocrine tumor. (**b**) CT scan image demonstrating the same neuroendocrine tumor (indicated by *arrow*)

[11, 12]. Diarrhea is the next most commonly observed symptom, with approximately 65% of patients affected. Serotonin, prostaglandins, histamines, and tachykinins are involved in the pathogenesis of the diarrhea by stimulating peristalsis and therefore resulting in increased colonic transit times. They may also affect intestinal fluid and electrolyte secretion via 5-HT2A receptors [13, 14]. Approximately 10% of patients develop carcinoid heart disease over time due to long-standing elevations in circulating serotonin levels. Patients may develop tricuspid regurgitation and pulmonic stenosis due to deposition of fibrotic tissue on the valves [15]. The right heart is affected preferentially over the left side due to the direct exposure to vasoactive substances secreted by liver metastases, whereas the pulmonary circulation inactivates the hormones prior to exposure of the left side of the heart [16]. Patients with carcinoid heart disease may require heart surgery or valve replacement [5]. Bronchoconstriction occurs in 8% of cases of carcinoid syndrome and is manifested as wheezing [14].

Diagnosis

Biochemical Studies

Small bowel NETs produce both functional hormones and nonfunctional proteins that are released from their secretory vesicles. These may be used as biochemical markers to aid in the diagnosis and management of patients with small bowel NETs.

Urinary 5-HIAA, a metabolite of serotonin, is useful for the diagnosis and monitoring of patients with small bowel NETs. The measurement of 5-HIAA in a 24-h urine sample collected under strict dietary restrictions has a sensitivity of 73% for localized disease and 100% for metastatic disease. It has a specificity of 100% for the presence of midgut carcinoid but is less useful for foregut and hindgut NETs, as these rarely produce serotonin [5, 14]. Although normal ranges vary by laboratory, the normal range for 24-h urine 5-HIAA is between 2 and 15 mg/day. Certain drugs such as selective serotonin reuptake inhibitors, foods rich in tryptophan, and malabsorption syndromes such as celiac disease may increase 24-h urine 5-HIAA levels and produce a false positive result. Patients with carcinoid syndrome may have levels greater than 100 mg/day [1, 17].

When urinary 5-HIAA values are equivocal, whole blood serotonin levels may be helpful in making the diagnosis. The range of normal values for whole blood fasting serotonin levels varies between 71 and 310 ng/ml and can be extremely elevated in patients with carcinoid syndrome, with values as high as 790–4500 ng/ml [18]. The sensitivity and specificity of blood serotonin assays have not been well established,

and false-positive results may occur due to the release of platelet serotonin [1].

Chromogranins are glycoproteins that are stored within secretory vesicles and released with peptides and amines from neuroendocrine tissues. Well-differentiated NETs release elevated levels of chromogranin [1]. Chromogranin A is the most sensitive among the subtypes (chromogranin A, B, and C), and it is a sensitive but not specific marker for NETs. The sensitivity and specificity of chromogranin A depend on the set cutoff value; a level greater than 32 U/L has a sensitivity of 75% and specificity of 84%. There is a correlation between chromogranin A levels and tumor burden, and a level greater than 5000 g/L is an independent predictor of poor overall survival [19]. False-positive chromogranin A levels may result from atrophic gastritis, renal dysfunction, inflammatory bowel disease, and the use of proton pump inhibitors [20, 21]. Chromogranin A is used as a tumor marker in patients with an established diagnosis of NET, rather than as a screening test due to its low specificity. Levels can be followed to monitor disease progression, response to therapy, and surveillance for recurrence [22].

Various other secretory proteins have been proposed and studied as possible useful tumor markers for small bowel NETs. These include neuron specific enolase (NSE), substance P, neurokinin A, and pancreastatin. Although some studies have found that changes in these tumor markers correlate with treatment response, tumor progression, or recurrence, chromogranin A still remains a more sensitive marker [23, 24]. The latest 2014 update of the National Comprehensive Cancer Network (NCCN) guidelines for NETs still does not recommend routine measurement of any tumor marker [25].

Imaging

Primary small bowel NETs are often small in size and therefore difficult to identify in imaging studies. Lesions are more often identified by imaging studies once there is metastatic involvement of the mesentery or the liver [5]. The primary imaging modalities used to evaluate small bowel NETs are computed tomography (CT) scan, magnetic resonance imaging (MRI), and somatostatin receptor scintigraphy (SRS). Also, several novel imaging techniques are emerging using various positron emission tomography (PET) radiotracers [1].

Small bowel NETs may produce mesenteric masses by either direct tumor involvement or metastasis to lymph nodes. These mesenteric masses are best evaluated by contrast-enhanced CT scan, which can demonstrate the dense desmoplastic fibrosis, often tethering the surrounding small bowel. Additionally, contrast enhancement aids in the evaluation

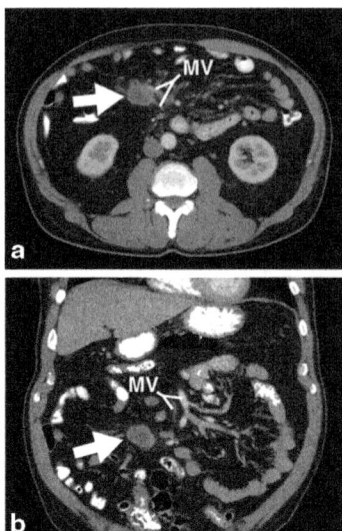

Fig. 2 Axial (**a**) and coronal (**b**) CT scan images demonstrating a neuroendocrine tumor in the mesentery (indicated by *arrow*) and its relationship to the mesenteric vessels (*MV*)

of resectability by visualizing the major mesenteric vessels and their relation to the tumor (Fig. 2) [1, 5]. CT enterography also may be employed to identify primary small bowel tumors that are not visualized on standard CT scans [26]. Triple-phase CT scans are preferred when evaluating liver metastases, as NET metastatic lesions are hypervascular and therefore exhibit a pattern of enhancement during the early arterial phase and rapid washout during the portal venous phase [27].

MRI can delineate and detect liver metastases and is more sensitive than other imaging modalities. In a series of patients with metastatic small bowel NET to liver, MRI was able to detect more hepatic metastases than CT or SRS. Additionally, MRI has the ability to detect subcentimeter hepatic lesions, which is of benefit when planning cytoreductive hepatic surgery [28].

Small bowel NETs often express somatostatin receptors, which bind to the somatostatin analogue octreotide. SRS (e.g., Octreoscan) uses indium-111-labeled octreotide to identify areas of uptake in the body. This imaging modality visualizes the entire body, enabling the detection of active lesions throughout the body. The sensitivity of SRS has been reported to be greater than 90 % [1, 5]. This imaging modality also provides useful information on the somatostatin receptor status of the tumor to determine if the patient is eligible for treatment with somatostatin analogues [29]. Improvements in CT and MRI technology have led to a decline in the use of SRS in the workup of NETs. In one series, CT and MRI were superior to SRS at detecting pathologic lesions and found that SRS was inferior at detecting metastatic lesions less than 1.5 cm with a reported sensitivity of only 35 % [28].

Recently, functional PET imaging modalities have emerged as novel methods to visualize NETs. Their advantages include improved spatial resolution over CT and SRS, and improved sensitivity for detection of small lesions. The radiotracers used are not yet widely available but include 18F-dihydroxyphenylalanine (18F-DOPA), 11C-5-hydroxytrytophan (11C-5-HTP), and 68 Ga-DOTATOC. Due to the limited availability of these radiopharmaceuticals, they are generally used only when other imaging techniques are unsuccessful. Fluorodeoxyglucose (FDG)-PET scans are typically not used in the imaging workup of NETs because FDG only accumulates in high-grade NETs [29, 30]. FDG positivity is associated with early tumor progression and a higher risk of death. Recent studies have proposed the use of FDG-PET as a method to identify tumors with a higher malignant potential [31, 32].

Pathology and Staging

The clinical behavior of small bowel NETs is closely associated with the histological grade and differentiation of the tumors. Histological grade is determined by the proliferative activity of the tumor, which is measured by the mitotic rate and the Ki-67 index. Differentiation of the tumor describes how closely the tumor cells resemble normal endocrine cells, where well-differentiated tumors closely resemble normal endocrine tissues and poorly differentiated do not. The classification of NETs has evolved over the years, and in 2007 the European Neuroendocrine Tumor Society (ENETS) proposed a formal tumor, node, metastasis (TNM) staging for tumors of the lower jejunum and ileum, as well as incorporated a histologic grade into the new classification system. In 2010, the American Joint Committee on Cancer (AJCC) adopted this classification system. The TNM classification distinguishes between tumors that remain within the submucosa and are smaller than 1 cm (T1), tumors that invade muscularis propia or are larger than 1 cm (T2), tumors that invade through the muscularis propia into the subserosa or nonperitonealized tissue (T3), and tumors that invade peritoneum or other organs (T4; Table 1) [33, 34]. The World Health Organization's pathological classification describes well-differentiated tumors as low grade (<2 mitoses per 10 high-power field [HPF] and ≤2 % Ki67 index) or intermediate grade (2–10 mitoses per 10 HPF or 3–20 % Ki67 index). Poorly differentiated tumors are high grade (>20 mitoses per 10 HPF or >20 % Ki67 index) (Table 2) [35].

A recent study by Strosberg et al. examined the prognostic validity of the AJCC staging classification by looking at 691 patients with jejunal–ileal NETs and examining overall survival based on stage. The 5-year survival rate was 100 % for stage I and II tumors, 91 % for stage III tumors, and 72 % for stage IV tumors. There was a difference in survival in the

Table 1 TNM staging classification of small bowel NETs. (From [33]. Reprinted with permission from Springer)

T1	Tumor invades lamina propia or submucosa and is 1 cm or less		
T2	Tumor invades muscularis propia or is greater than 1 cm		
T3	Tumor invades through the muscularis propia, into the subserosa, or into non-peritonealized tissue		
T4	Tumor invades the peritoneum or any other organs or structures		
N0	No regional lymph node metastasis		
N1	Regional lymph node metastasis		
M0	No distant metastasis		
M1	Distant metastasis		
Stage	*T*	*N*	*M*
I	T1	N0	M0
IIA	T2	N0	M0
IIB	T3	N0	M0
IIIA	T4	N0	M0
IIIB	Any T	N1	M0
IV	Any T	Any N	M1

T tumor, *N* node, *M* metastasis

Table 2 Pathological classification of neuroendocrine tumors. (Data from [35])

Differentiation	Grade	Criteria
Well differentiated	Low (typical)	<2 mitoses/10HPF and <2% Ki67 index
	Intermediate (atypical)	2–20 mitoses/10HPF or 3–20% Ki67 index
Poorly differentiated	High	>20 mitoses/10HPF or >20% Ki67 index

stage IIIB patients based on resectability of the tumor, with a 95% 5-year survival for resectable tumors compared to a 78% 5-year survival for unresectable tumors [36].

Management

Surgery

Management of small bowel NETs requires a multidisciplinary approach to achieve the best long-term survival rates. Aggressive management with surgery, embolization of metastases, radiotherapy, metabolic therapy, and chemotherapy can achieve long-term survival even in patients with advanced disease. Nevertheless, surgical resection with removal of the primary tumor with regional lymph nodes and resection of metastatic lesions when possible is the only hope for cure and is only possible in about 20% of cases [37]. Surgery for resection of the primary tumor may be necessary even in patients with unresectable metastases to treat or prevent local complications such as intestinal obstruction, ischemia, or bleeding, as well as to provide symptomatic control of carcinoid syndrome [38]. Although some controversy exits regarding whether resection of the primary tumor in these cases is associated with improved survival, most experts agree on resection for prevention of local complications from small bowel NETs in patients who are likely to survive long enough to experience symptoms [39].

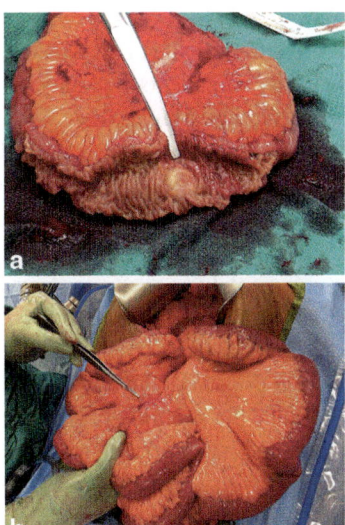

Fig. 3 Intraoperative photos demonstrating **a** primary intraluminal neuroendocrine tumor of the small bowel and **b** lymph node metastasis in the small bowel mesentery

The most common location for small bowel NETs is the ileum, followed by jejunum. Surgical resection is determined by the precise location of the tumor. Tumors in the distal ileum near the ileocecal valve are treated with right hemicolectomy. Small bowel NETs located more proximal in the small bowel are managed by partial small bowel resection (Fig. 3). Although multifocality is rare, the entire bowel should be inspected for additional synchronous lesions and lymphatic metastases. Regional mesenteric lymph nodes should be resected in conjunction with the small bowel in order to examine for lymph node metastases, a practice that has been associated with improved survival [39, 40]. Lymph node metastases at the root of the mesentery may involve the superior mesenteric vessels, and these cases should be referred to high-volume centers with surgical expertise. A laparoscopic approach may be used in certain cases to resect primary small bowel NETs and is associated with shorter hospital stays and decreased morbidity [37]. Radioguided exploration has recently been explored as a novel tool to assist in the cytoreductive surgery for metastatic small bowel NETs [41].

Duodenal NETs are less commonly encountered, and options for surgical resection depend on their size and exact location. Endoscopic resection can be used for lesions less than 1 cm in size that are superficial. Tumors between 1 and 2 cm can be treated by transduodenal excision. Larger tumors and those in close proximity to the ampulla may require pancreaticoduodenectomy (Whipple procedure) [39].

Surgery for Liver Metastasis

The liver is the predominant site of metastasis in small bowel NETs, and a majority of patients will have liver metastases at the time of presentation. Management of liver metastases may be accomplished by surgical resection, ablation, transarterial embolization (TAE) or chemoembolization (TACE), molecular targeted radiotherapy, and liver transplantation [5, 8].

Surgical resection of liver metastases remains the gold standard for patients in which it is an option. The 5-year survival for patients who undergo liver resection of metastatic small bowel NETs is 60–80%. The ENETS consensus guidelines determined that the minimum requirements for liver resection with curative intent are: (1) resectable well-differentiated liver disease with acceptable morbidity (~30%) and less than 5% mortality, (2) absence of right heart insufficiency, and (3) absence of extra-abdominal metastasis or diffuse peritoneal carcinomatosis. Several factors are involved in the decision on the type of surgical resection for liver metastases. These include the number, size, and location of the liver lesions; the patient's general condition; and estimation of adequate functional residual liver parenchyma postoperatively [42]. In experienced hands, 65–70% of whole liver volume may be resected in patients with acceptable liver function. One- or two-step procedures may be required based on the complexity of the resection, as well as in cases of bilobar liver metastases. Additionally, a combination of liver resection and ablative procedures may be employed in patients

in order to maintain adequate liver function postoperatively. Patients with carcinoid syndrome should be managed preoperatively with somatostatin analogues to prevent carcinoid crisis perioperatively [5].

Palliative debulking has a role in the management of patients in which curative resection is not possible and whose hormonal symptoms do not respond to medical therapy. However, the removal of greater than 70% of tumor volume by resection or ablative techniques is required in order to be effective, and sufficient hepatic reserve and function must be maintained [43].

Ablative Techniques

The most frequently employed ablative technique for NET liver metastases is radiofrequency ablation (RFA). It can be used either as sole therapy for liver metastasis or in combination with resection. RFA is very effective at relieving the symptoms of NET metastasis and in achieving local control of metastatic lesions. It has the advantage that it can often be performed percutaneously under image guidance and, therefore, is beneficial for patients who are poor surgical candidates [5]. It is not recommended for tumors larger than 5 cm or those near vital structures, large vessels, and central bile ducts. Although ablation may be performed multiple times within the same metastases, as tumor size increases to >3 cm, it is increasingly difficult to fully ablate the tumor. Once a tumor reaches >5 cm in size, it is considered unsuitable for RFA [42]. While surgical resection remains the most effective management of liver metastases, the combination of RFA with surgery offers the opportunity for complete tumor removal in patients who would otherwise be unresectable [44, 45].

Selective TAE or TACE can be used to treat patients with unresectable liver metastases. Objective tumor responses and symptom control are seen in over 50% of patients. There is no evidence to suggest that survival is prolonged with TACE or that it is superior to RFA [42]. The overall 5-year survival rate after TACE ranges between 50 and 86% in the literature. The cytotoxic agents used are most often doxorubicin or streptozotocin. TACE should only be performed in experienced centers, as it can be associated with significant morbidity. The procedure is contraindicated in patients with portal vein thrombosis or hepatic insufficiency [46].

Laser-induced thermotherapy (LITT) is another method of controlling liver metastases. The range of effect can be more precisely controlled than other modalities, but the heat produced by the laser limits its use for tumors adjacent to vital structures. Most centers favor the use of RFA over that of LITT due to availability and effectiveness of treatment [47].

Medical Therapy for Systemic Disease

Somatostatin analogues are effective at treating the symptoms of metastatic small bowel NETs, as they inhibit the release of neuroendocrine hormones, including serotonin. Up to 80% of patients experience symptomatic improvement [1]. In a clinical trial evaluating subcutaneous octreotide for the treatment of carcinoid syndrome, 88% of patients reported improvement of flushing and diarrhea, and 72% of patients had a decrease in urine 5-HIAA levels [48]. Side effects of somatostatin analogues include abdominal discomfort, flatulence, malabsorption, steatorrhea, and gallstone formation. Therapy is usually initiated with short-acting analogues and transitioned to long-acting depot formulations of octreotide, which can be administered once a month. The efficacy of therapy is monitored by observing symptom improvement and following levels of urinary 5-HIAA, plasma serotonin, and plasma substance P [49].

Patients with carcinoid syndrome may experience carcinoid crisis when undergoing invasive procedures or with any significant stress to the body. They may experience circulatory collapse, which is caused by the release of serotonin and other vasoactive substances into the circulation. These patients should receive prophylactic dosing of octreotide subcutaneously or intravenously before undergoing any invasive procedure to prevent the development of carcinoid crisis. Patients who develop symptoms of carcinoid crisis should be treated with bolus doses of intravenous octreotide until symptoms are controlled [50].

Somatostatin analogues have been found to have antiproliferative effects, and evidence has emerged suggesting they are capable of inhibiting tumor growth. In one study, they were effective at stabilizing tumor growth in approximately 50% of patients who had prior evidence of tumor progression [51]. The antiproliferative effects are mediated through direct interaction on somatostatin receptors, as well as through direct inhibition of insulin-like growth factor and vascular endothelial growth factor [52]. A placebo-controlled, randomized, prospective study published in 2009 found a statistically significant improvement in median time to progression between the placebo group (6 months) and the group that received long-acting octreotide (14.5 months) [53].

Interferon-alpha is another treatment available for the management of metastatic NETs. Interferons function by various mechanisms, including stimulation of T cells, inhibition of angiogenesis, and induction of cell cycle arrest. Additionally, they have been found to induce expression of somatostatin in NETs [54]. Interferon-alpha successfully controls symptoms and produces a decrease in biochemical markers in 50% of patients, but tumor responses are only seen in about 10% of patients. The treatment effect is not as rapid and the side effects are more pronounced than that of somatostatin analogues [55]. Therefore, interferon-alpha is a second-line treatment that is recommended only for functional tumors with a low proliferation rate.

Targeting somatostatin receptors with radiolabeled somatostatin analogues is the basis of peptide-receptor radiotherapy (PRRT), a promising new treatment option. Approximately 80% of well-differentiated NETs express high levels of somatostatin receptors, which is a requirement in order to receive PRRT [56]. The first radiolabeled somatostatin analogue used for PRRT was indium-111 pentetreotide, which demonstrated symptomatic improvement but poor tumor remission. 90-Y-DOTATOC, a high-energy beta particle emitter, was the next radiolabeled somatostatin analogue to emerge. It has a reported objective treatment response of 9–33% in the literature, and a median duration of response of 30 months. It produces a high level of symptom control, and 70% of patients achieved stability of disease [57]. 177-Lu-octreotate is a compound that emits beta and gamma particles with an increased affinity for somatostatin receptor 2. PRRT with 177-Lu-octreotate has demonstrated an objective response in 29% of patients; it has achieved stability of disease in 35% of patients and a median duration of response of 40 months. Treatment with 177-Lu-octreotate seems to confer a survival benefit of several years. It is an encouraging treatment for metastatic small bowel NETs [58].

Chemotherapy for NETs is indicated in patients with unresectable progressive liver metastasis and includes treatment with combinations of streptozotocin, doxorubicin, and 5-fluorouracil. The benefits for cytotoxic chemotherapy for metastatic small bowel NETs are limited, as objective response rates are seen in only about 35% of patients [42].

Summary

Small bowel NETs are the most common neoplasm of the small intestine, and their incidence has increased in the past four decades. Greater than 80% of patients with small bowel NETs may present with metastasis at the time of diagnosis. Biochemical and imaging studies are important in the diagnostic workup and surveillance of small bowel NETs. Surgical resection of the primary tumor with regional lymph nodes and resection of metastatic lesions when possible is the only hope for cure and only possible in about 20% of cases. In patients with unresectable metastases, ablative techniques exist which can achieve tumor control. Patients with systemic disease may be treated with somatostatin analogues, as well as new emerging modalities such as peptide-receptor radiotherapy. Advancements in the treatment of metastatic lesions with ablative techniques and targeted medical therapy have improved survival.

Key Summary Points

- Small bowel NETs are the most common neoplasm of the small intestine, and their incidence has increased in the past four decades.
- Biochemical and imaging studies are important in the diagnostic workup and surveillance of small bowel NETs.
- Surgical resection of the primary tumor with regional lymph nodes and resection of metastatic lesions when possible is the only hope for cure and only possible in about 20 % of cases.
- In patients with unresectable metastasis, ablative techniques exist which can achieve tumor control.
- Patients with systemic disease may be treated with somatostatin analogues, as well as new emerging modalities such as peptide-receptor radiotherapy.
- Advancements in the treatment of metastatic lesions with ablative techniques and targeted medical therapy have improved survival from small bowel NETs.

References

1. Strosberg J. Neuroendocrine tumours of the small intestine. Best Pract Res Clin Gastroenterol. 2012;26(6):755–73.
2. Lundqvist M, Wilander E. Subepithelial neuroendocrine cells and carcinoid tumours of the human small intestine and appendix. A comparative immunohistochemical study with regard to serotonin, neuron-specific enolase and S-100 protein reactivity. J Pathol. 1986;148(2):141–7.
3. Williams ED, Sandler M. The classification of carcinoid tum ours. Lancet. 1963;1(7275):238–9.
4. Maggard MA, O'Connell JB, Ko CY. Updated population-based review of carcinoid tumors. Ann Surg. 2004;240(1):117–22.
5. Cameron JL, Cameron AM. Small Bowel Carcinoid/ Neuroendocrine Tumors Current Surgical Therapy Elsevier Saunders 2011.
6. Yao JC, Hassan M, Phan A, Dagohoy C, Leary C, Mares JE, et al. One hundred years after "carcinoid": epidemiology of and prognostic factors for neuroendocrine tumors in 35,825 cases in the United States. J Clin Oncol. 2008;26(18):3063–72.
7. Modlin IM, Lye KD, Kidd M. A 5-decade analysis of 13,715 carcinoid tumors. Cancer. 2003;97(4):934–59.
8. Norlén O, Stålberg P, Öberg K, Eriksson J, Hedberg J, Hessman O, et al. Long-term results of surgery for small intestinal neuroendocrine tumors at a tertiary referral center. World J Surg. 2012;36(6):1419–31.
9. Thorson A, Biorck G, Bjorkman G, Waldenstrom J. Malignant carcinoid of the small intestine with metastases to the liver, valvular disease of the right side of the heart (pulmonary stenosis and tricuspid regurgitation without septal defects), peripheral vasomotor symptoms, bronchoconstriction, and an unusual type of cyanosis; a clinical and pathologic syndrome. Am Heart J. 1954;47(5):795–817.
10. Vinik AI, Silva MP, Woltering EA, Go VL, Warner R, Caplin M. Biochemical testing for neuroendocrine tumors. Pancreas. 2009;38(8):876–89.
11. Cunningham JL, Janson ET, Agarwal S, Grimelius L, Stridsberg M. Tachykinins in endocrine tumors and the carcinoid syndrome. Eur J Endocrinol. 2008;159(3):275–82.
12. Matuchansky C, Launay JM. Serotonin, catecholamines, and spontaneous midgut carcinoid flush: plasma studies from flushing and nonflushing sites. Gastroenterology. 1995;108(3):743–51.
13. von der Ohe MR, Camilleri M, Kvols LK. A 5HT3 antagonist corrects the postprandial colonic hypertonic response in carcinoid diarrhea. Gastroenterology. 1994;106(5):1184–9.
14. Kvols LK. Metastatic carcinoid tumors and the malignant carcinoid syndrome. Ann N Y Acad Sci. 1994;733:464–70.
15. Lundin L, Norheim I, Landelius J, Oberg K, Theodorsson-Norheim E. Carcinoid heart disease: relationship of circulating vasoactive substances to ultrasound-detectable cardiac abnormalities. Circulation. 1988;77(2):264–9.
16. Robiolio PA, Rigolin VH, Wilson JS, Harrison JK, Sanders LL, Bashore TM, et al. Carcinoid heart disease. Correlation of high serotonin levels with valvular abnormalities detected by cardiac catheterization and echocardiography. Circulation. 1995;92(4):790–5.
17. Zuetenhorst JM, Bonfrer JM, Korse CM, Bakker R, van Tinteren H, Taal BG. Carcinoid heart disease: the role of urinary 5-hydroxyindoleacetic acid excretion and plasma levels of atrial natriuretic peptide, transforming growth factor-beta and fibroblast growth factor. Cancer. 2003;97(7):1609–15.
18. Burke AP, Thomas RM, Elsayed AM, Sobin LH. Carcinoids of the jejunum and ileum: an immunohistochemical and clinicopathologic study of 167 cases. Cancer. 1997;79(6):1086–93.
19. Campana D, Nori F, Piscitelli L, Morselli-Labate AM, Pezzilli R, Corinaldesi R, et al. Chromogranin A: is it a useful marker of neuroendocrine tumors? J Clin Oncol. 2007;25(15):1967–73.
20. Conlon JM. Granin-derived peptides as diagnostic and prognostic markers for endocrine tumors. Regul Pept. 2010;165(1):5–11.
21. Sanduleanu S, De Bruine A, Stridsberg M, Jonkers D, Biemond I, Hameeteman W, et al. Serum chromogranin A as a screening test for gastric enterochromaffin-like cell hyperplasia during acid-suppressive therapy. Eur J Clin Invest. 2001;31(9):802–11.
22. Yao JC, Pavel M, Phan AT, Kulke MH, Hoosen S, St Peter J, et al. Chromogranin A and neuron-specific enolase as prognostic markers in patients with advanced pNET treated with everolimus. J Clin Endocrinol Metab. 2011;96(12):3741–9.
23. Bajetta E, Ferrari L, Martinetti A, Celio L, Procopio G, Artale S, et al. Chromogranin A, neuron specific enolase, carcinoembryonic antigen, and hydroxyindole acetic acid evaluation in patients with neuroendocrine tumors. Cancer. 1999;86(5):858–65.
24. Ito T, Igarashi H, Jensen RT. Serum pancreastatin: the long sought universal, sensitive, specific tumor marker for neuroendocrine tumors? Pancreas. 2012;41(4):505–7.
25. NCCN Guidelines: Neuroendocrine Tumors National Comprehensive Cancer Network, 2014.
26. Hakim FA, Alexander JA, Huprich JE, Grover M, Enders FT. CT-enterography may identify small bowel tumors not detected by capsule endoscopy: eight years experience at Mayo Clinic Rochester. Dig Dis Sci. 2011;56(10):2914–9.
27. Paulson EK, McDermott VG, Keogan MT, DeLong DM, Frederick MG, Nelson RC. Carcinoid metastases to the liver: role of triple-phase helical CT. Radiology. 1998;206(1):143–50.
28. Dromain C, de Baere T, Lumbroso J, Caillet H, Laplanche A, Boige V, et al. Detection of liver metastases from endocrine tumors: a prospective comparison of somatostatin receptor scintigraphy, computed tomography, and magnetic resonance imaging. J Clin Oncol. 2005;23(1):70–8.
29. Sundin A. Radiological and nuclear medicine imaging of gastroenteropancreatic neuroendocrine tumours. Best Pract Res Clin Gastroenterol. 2012;26(6):803–18.
30. Haug AR, Cindea-Drimus R, Auernhammer CJ, Reincke M, Wangler B, Uebleis C, et al. The role of 68 Ga-DOTATATE PET/CT in suspected neuroendocrine tumors. J Nucl Med. 2012;53(11):1686–92.

31. Garin E, Le Jeune F, Devillers A, Cuggia M, de Lajarte-Thirouard AS, Bouriel C, et al. Predictive value of 18F-FDG PET and somatostatin receptor scintigraphy in patients with metastatic endocrine tumors. J Nucl Med. 2009;50(6):858–64.

32. Binderup T, Knigge U, Loft A, Federspiel B, Kjaer A. 18F-fluorodeoxyglucose positron emission tomography predicts survival of patients with neuroendocrine tumors. Clin Cancer Res. 2010;16(3):978–85.

33. Rindi G, Kloppel G, Couvelard A, Komminoth P, Korner M, Lopes JM, et al. TNM staging of midgut and hindgut (neuro) endocrine tumors: a consensus proposal including a grading system. Virchows Arch. 2007;451(4):757–62.

34. Edge SB, Compton CC. The American Joint Committee on Cancer: the 7th edition of the AJCC cancer staging manual and the future of TNM. Ann Surg Oncol. 2010;17(6):1471–4.

35. Klimstra DS, Modlin IR, Coppola D, Lloyd RV, Suster S. The pathologic classification of neuroendocrine tumors: a review of nomenclature, grading, and staging systems. Pancreas. 2010;39(6):707–12.

36. Strosberg JR, Weber JM, Feldman M, Coppola D, Meredith K, Kvols LK. Prognostic validity of the American Joint Committee on Cancer staging classification for midgut neuroendocrine tumors. J Clin Oncol. 2013;31(4):420–5.

37. Figueiredo MN, Maggiori L, Gaujoux S, Couvelard A, Guedj N, Ruszniewski P, et al. Surgery for small-bowel neuroendocrine tumors: is there any benefit of the laparoscopic approach? Surg Endosc. 2014;28(5):1720–6.

38. Soreide O, Berstad T, Bakka A, Schrumpf E, Hanssen LE, Engh V, et al. Surgical treatment as a principle in patients with advanced abdominal carcinoid tumors. Surgery. 1992;111(1):48–54.

39. Kulke MH, Benson AB, 3rd, Bergsland E, Berlin JD, Blaszkowsky LS, Choti MA, et al. Neuroendocrine tumors. J Natl Compr Canc Netw. 2012;10(6):724–64.

40. Landry CS, Lin HY, Phan A, Charnsangavej C, Abdalla EK, Aloia T, et al. Resection of at-risk mesenteric lymph nodes is associated with improved survival in patients with small bowel neuroendocrine tumors. World J Surg. 2013;37(7):1695–700.

41. Wang YZ, Diebold A, Woltering E, King H, Boudreaux JP, Anthony LB, et al. Radioguided exploration facilitates surgical cytoreduction of neuroendocrine tumors. J Gastrointest Surg. 2012;16(3):635–40.

42. Steinmüller T, Kianmanesh R, Falconi M, Scarpa A, Taal B, Kwekkeboom DJ, et al. Consensus guidelines for the management of patients with liver metastases from digestive (neuro)endocrine tumors: foregut, midgut, hindgut, and unknown primary. Neuroendocrinology. 2008;87(1):47–62.

43. Chambers AJ, Pasieka JL, Dixon E, Rorstad O. The palliative benefit of aggressive surgical intervention for both hepatic and mesenteric metastases from neuroendocrine tumors. Surgery. 2008;144(4):645–51; discussion 51–3.

44. Pawlik TM, Izzo F, Cohen DS, Morris JS, Curley SA. Combined resection and radiofrequency ablation for advanced hepatic malignancies: results in 172 patients. Ann Surg Oncol. 2003;10(9):1059–69.

45. Mayo SC, de Jong MC, Pulitano C, Clary BM, Reddy SK, Gamblin TC, et al. Surgical management of hepatic neuroendocrine tumor metastasis: results from an international multi-institutional analysis. Ann Surg Oncol. 2010;17(12):3129–36.

46. Roche A, Girish BV, de Baere T, Baudin E, Boige V, Elias D, et al. Trans-catheter arterial chemoembolization as first-line treatment for hepatic metastases from endocrine tumors. Eur Radiol. 2003;13(1):136–40.

47. Vogl TJ, Straub R, Eichler K, Sollner O, Mack MG. Colorectal carcinoma metastases in liver: laser-induced interstitial thermotherapy–local tumor control rate and survival data. Radiology. 2004;230(2):450–8.

48. Kvols LK, Moertel CG, O'Connell MJ, Schutt AJ, Rubin J, Hahn RG. Treatment of the malignant carcinoid syndrome. Evaluation of a long-acting somatostatin analogue. N Engl J Med. 1986;315(11):663–6.

49. di Bartolomeo M, Bajetta E, Buzzoni R, Mariani L, Carnaghi C, Somma L, et al. Clinical efficacy of octreotide in the treatment of metastatic neuroendocrine tumors. A study by the Italian Trials in Medical Oncology Group. Cancer. 1996;77(2):402–8.

50. Kvols LK, Martin JK, Marsh HM, Moertel CG. Rapid reversal of carcinoid crisis with a somatostatin analogue. N Engl J Med. 1985;313(19):1229–30.

51. Strosberg J, Kvols L. Antiproliferative effect of somatostatin analogs in gastroenteropancreatic neuroendocrine tumors. World J Gastroenterol. 2010;16(24):2963–70.

52. Serri O, Brazeau P, Kachra Z, Posner B. Octreotide inhibits insulin-like growth factor-I hepatic gene expression in the hypophysectomized rat: evidence for a direct and indirect mechanism of action. Endocrinology. 1992;130(4):1816–21.

53. Rinke A, Muller HH, Schade-Brittinger C, Klose KJ, Barth P, Wied M, et al. Placebo-controlled, double-blind, prospective, randomized study on the effect of octreotide LAR in the control of tumor growth in patients with metastatic neuroendocrine midgut tumors: a report from the PROMID Study Group. J Clin Oncol. 2009;27(28):4656–63.

54. Detjen KM, Welzel M, Farwig K, Brembeck FH, Kaiser A, Riecken EO, et al. Molecular mechanism of interferon alfa-mediated growth inhibition in human neuroendocrine tumor cells. Gastroenterology. 2000;118(4):735–48.

55. Oberg K, Funa K, Alm G. Effects of leukocyte interferon on clinical symptoms and hormone levels in patients with midgut carcinoid tumors and carcinoid syndrome. N Engl J Med. 1983;309(3):129–33.

56. Kwekkeboom DJ, Mueller-Brand J, Paganelli G, Anthony LB, Pauwels S, Kvols LK, et al. Overview of results of peptide receptor radionuclide therapy with 3 radiolabeled somatostatin analogs. J Nucl Med. 2005;46(1):62S–6S.

57. Bushnell DL, Jr., O'Dorisio TM, O'Dorisio MS, Menda Y, Hicks RJ, Van Cutsem E, et al. 90Y-edotreotide for metastatic carcinoid refractory to octreotide. J Clin Oncol. 2010;28(10):1652–9.

58. van Essen M, Krenning EP, Kam BL, de Jong M, Valkema R, Kwekkeboom DJ. Peptide-receptor radionuclide therapy for endocrine tumors. Nat Rev Endocrinol. 2009;5(7):382–93.

Carcinoid Syndrome

Vladimir Neychev and Electron Kebebew

Introduction

The family of neuroendocrine tumors consists of a spectrum of neoplasms that can arise from the diffuse endocrine system throughout the body. The carcinoid tumor, a member of this fascinating family of tumors, is characterized by its ability to uptake (or synthesize), store, and release a variety of biogenic amines, polypeptides, and prostaglandins (Table 1). Although carcinoid tumors have been reported in essentially all tissues, the overwhelming majority of these neoplasms originate in the gastrointestinal tract [1–3]. Most carcinoid tumors have a relatively slow-growing, indolent natural history but sometimes they can behave in a highly malignant fashion, exhibiting metastatic behavior, most often to the liver and lungs [4].

The early symptoms of carcinoid tumor are nonspecific and may include abdominal pain, diarrhea, intermittent intestinal obstruction, and gastrointestinal bleeding. These often vague and generalized signs and symptoms produce a delay in diagnosis in many patients. Although symptoms may be caused by mechanical effects of the tumors, symptoms of carcinoid tumors are also caused by the effects of amine and neuropeptide substances secreted into the gastrointestinal tract or the systemic circulation [1]. The effects of these chemicals, collectively referred to as the carcinoid syndrome, are diverse and include cutaneous flushing, diarrhea, carcinoid heart disease, bronchoconstriction, hypotension, hypertension, and pellagra (Fig. 1) [1].

The classic carcinoid syndrome does not develop until a tumor has metastasized to the liver and or lung, and the hormonal products released by the tumor reach the central venous circulation in substantial concentrations [5]. Some patients with functioning gastric or bronchial carcinoids have clinical and biochemical variations from the classic syndrome [6].

Epidemiology

The incidence of classical carcinoid syndrome, which is characterized by flushing, diarrhea, abdominal cramping, and, less often, wheezing, heart-valve dysfunction, and pellagra, varies depending on the study population. While studies that include patients with localized and incidental tumors report the frequency of carcinoid syndrome to be about 10–18%, the prevalence may be as high as 50% among patients with advanced and metastatic disease [7–11]. The syndrome results from synergistic interactions between biochemical substances secreted by the tumor, and it is often observed in patients with metastatic disease or when the primary tumor site allows the secreted amines to escape enteral hepatic circulation The presence of carcinoid syndrome is associated with poor survival [10].

Biochemistry of Carcinoid Syndrome

In 1954, Pernow and Waldenstrom demonstrated the presence of serotonin in the blood and urine of two patients with carcinoid tumor during an attack of flushing [12]. Originally, the whole spectrum of symptoms was related to the production and secretion of serotonin by the tumor and its metastases [5, 12]; however, since that time, a number of hormonal substances contributing to the signs and symptoms of carcinoid syndrome have been described, and the syndrome itself has been more fully characterized [8].

Carcinoid tumors produce and secrete a great variety of bioactive compounds, including serotonin, histamine, bradykinin, tachykinin, motilin, substance P, kallikrein, prostaglandins, catecholamines, and in some cases adrenocorticotropic hormone [1, 10, 13]. Although the contribution

E. Kebebew (✉) · V. Neychev
Endocrine Oncology Branch, National Institutes of Health-National Cancer Institute, 10 Center Drive, Bethesda, MD 20892-1201, USA
e-mail: Electron.Kebebew@nih.gov

J. L. Pasieka, J. A. Lee (eds.), *Surgical Endocrinopathies,* DOI 10.1007/978-3-319-13662-2_54,
© Springer International Publishing Switzerland 2015

Table 1 Bioactive substances secreted by carcinoid tumors

Hormones	Precursor/activator	Products
Amines	Tryptophan	Serotonin
		5-Hydroxytryptophan
		5-HIAA
	Histidine	Histamine
Peptides	Kallikrein	Bradykinin
		Kallidin
	Tachykinins	Substance P
		Neurokinin A
		Neurokinin B
		Neuropeptide K
		Hemokinin-1
	–	Motilin
		ACTH
		Chromogranin A
Prostaglandins	PGE synthase	Prostaglandins E
	PGF synthase	Prostaglandins F

5-HIAA 5-hydroxyindoleacetic acid, *PGE synthase* prostaglandin E synthase, *PGF synthase* prostaglandin F synthase, *ACTH* adrenocorticotropic hormone

of each of these mediators is not yet completely understood, some of them including serotonin, histamine, tachykinins, and kallikrein are thought to play a major role in the development of the clinical picture of carcinoid syndrome.

Tryptophan and Serotonin

Tryptophan is an essential amino acid, and, therefore, must be obtained from the diet. In healthy people, as much as 99 % of dietary tryptophan is metabolized by the oxidative pathway into nicotinic acid, and 1 % or less is converted into 5-hydroxytryptophane [7, 10, 14]. In carcinoid tumors, however, a disequilibrium of tryptophan metabolism has been hypothesized whereby as much as 60–70 % of the body's tryptophan may be shunted to 5-hydroxylation and production of 5-hydroxytryptophane instead of nicotinic acid (Fig. 2) [7, 15]. This is the most constant biochemical feature of carcinoid tumors.

The typical midgut carcinoid tumors also contain aromatic amino acid decarboxylase (AADC), which catalyzes the conversion of 5-hydroxytryptophane to 5-hydroxytryptamine (serotonin) (Fig. 2). Hindgut and foregut tumors such as gastric carcinoids, however, are frequently deficient in this enzyme and release 5-hydroxytryptophane instead of serotonin. Following its release into the portal circulation, almost all circulating serotonin is rapidly metabolized by the liver enzymes monoamine oxidase and aldehyde dehydrogenase and converted into the respective inactive metabolites 5-hydroxyindoleacetaldehyde and 5-hydroxyindoleacetic acid (5-HIAA). 5-HIAA is excreted into the urine as urinary

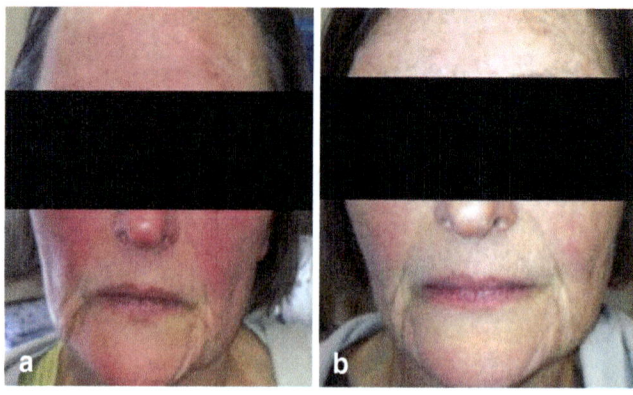

Fig. 1 A 62-year-old woman with carcinoid syndrome-related flushing, elevated urinary 5-HIAA, and an unknown primary. The image shows flushing in the patient before octreotide therapy (**a**) and after octreotide therapy (**b**)

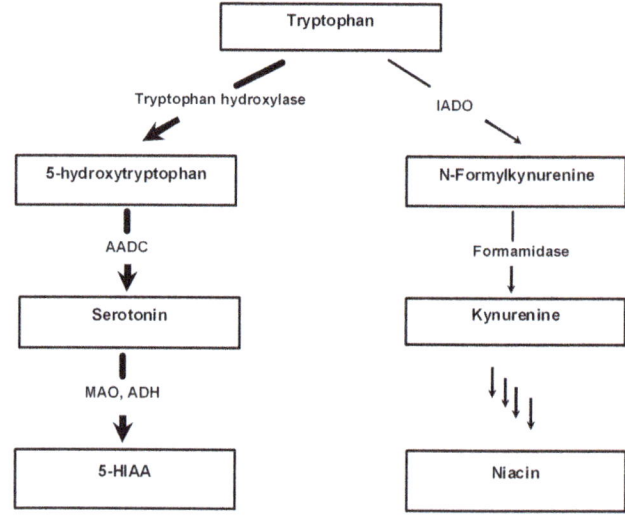

Fig. 2 Tryptophan metabolism in carcinoid tumors. *Thick lines* depict predominant tryptophan metabolic pathway in carcinoid tumors. *AADC* aromatic amino acid decarboxylase, *MAO* monoamine oxidase, *ADH* aldehyde dehydrogenase, *5-HIAA* 5-hydroxyindoleacetic acid, *IADO* Indoleamine-2,3-dioxygenase

5-HIAA, which can be used as a biomarker of the tumor activity. Although in smaller amounts, removal of serotonin from the bloodstream can also be mediated by its active uptake in the platelets.

5-Hydroxyindoleacetic Acid

5-HIAA is the end product of serotonin metabolism (Fig. 2). The measurement of 24-h urinary excretion in patients suspected to have carcinoid syndrome is a useful initial diagnostic test with a sensitivity and specificity of over 90 % [16, 17]. However, certain drugs and tryptophan/serotonin-rich foods

Table 2 Common symptoms in patients with the carcinoid syndrome: frequency and association with secreted compounds

Symptoms	Putative substances	Frequency (%)	References
Flushing	Histamine, tachykinins, kallikrein, bradykinin	>90	[5, 39, 40]
Diarrhea	Serotonin, substance P, motilin, prostaglandins	70–85	[32–34, 46–48, 50, 51]
Cardiac valvular disease	Serotonin, 5-HIAA, neurokinin A, substance P	~40–60	[52, 56, 58–60]
Telangiectasias	Serotonin, bradykinin, prostaglandins	25	[5, 7, 37]
Bronchospasm	Serotonin, bradykinin	15–19	[1, 8, 5, 10, 37]
Pellagra (dermatitis, diarrhea, dementia)	Niacin deficiency due to excess tryptophan metabolism	5–7	[5, 10, 11, 37]

5-HIAA 5-hydroxyindoleacetic acid

can lead to false positive results, and these foods should be avoided for at least 24 h prior to urine collection [18]. While the test is generally most useful in patients with midgut carcinoid tumors, its sensitivity could be lower in patients with carcinoid tumors without carcinoid syndrome [16]. The normal rate of 5-HIAA excretion ranges from 2 to 8 mg/day (10–42 µmol/day). Patients with carcinoid syndrome may have variable 5-HIAA urinary levels ranging from mildly elevated (30 mg/day) to more than 2000 mg/day [17].

Tachykinins

The peptides of the tachykinin family are one of the largest families of neuropeptides many of which are present in normal enterochromaffin cells of the gastrointestinal tract and in many neuroendocrine tumors including carcinoid tumors [11, 19–23]. Among the members of the tachykinin family are substance P, neurokinin A and B, neuropeptide K, and hemokinin-1 [24, 25]. Tachykinins have been shown to possess a number of biological activities, including smooth-muscle contraction, vasodilatation, pain transmission, activation of the immune system, and stimulation of endocrine gland secretion [20, 26].

Histamine

Although primary gastric carcinoids are frequently deficient in the enzyme AADC and lack the ability to produce serotonin, they overexpress the enzyme histidine decarboxylase, which converts the essential amino acid histidine into histamine [27]. Histamine has been suggested to be the primary causative agent for the atypical flushing and pruritus associated with these tumors [28]. This hypothesis was supported by the observation that administration of histidine markedly increased the frequency, severity, and duration of flushing [29]. In addition, this flushing can be ameliorated by combined H1 and H2 antagonists [30]. Healthy people excrete normally <20 µg of histamine per 24 h, while patents with gastric carcinoid syndrome may excrete >200 µg per 24 h [30].

Kallikrein and Prostaglandins

Series of investigations have implicated the kallikrein–kinin system in the pathogenesis of carcinoid syndrome [28, 29, 31]. Kallikrein is a protease that cleaves kininogens to form kinins (bradykinin and kallidin) plasma proteins that are further converted into vasoactive peptides. It has been shown that some carcinoid tumors contain kallikrein, and the hepatic venous blood draining carcinoid liver metastases contains bradykinin [28, 29]. Bradykinin is one of the most potent vasodilators known and may be responsible for flushing in some carcinoid patients [29]. Kinins also stimulate intestinal motility and increase vascular permeability [28].

It has been suggested that prostaglandins E and F stimulate intestinal motility and fluid secretion in the normal gastrointestinal tract [32–34]. Elevated serum prostaglandin concentrations have been found in patients with the carcinoid syndrome, suggesting that these compounds may also play a role in some aspects of the carcinoid syndrome. However, there is no direct evidence to support this hypothesis and their role in the constellation of symptoms that are present in carcinoid syndrome is uncertain [35].

Clinical Presentation of Classical Carcinoid Syndrome

Carcinoid syndrome is generally characterized by flushing, diarrhea, and, less commonly, wheezing, heart-valve dysfunction, and pellagra (Table 2) [1, 10, 23, 36]. The frequency of carcinoid syndrome correlates with the extent of the metastatic carcinoid disease, and it can be as low as 10 % in localized cases, but can occur in 40–50 % of patients with more advanced disease [7–11, 37]. The presence of carcinoid syndrome is associated with poor survival [10].

Not all patients with carcinoid tumors develop the carcinoid syndrome. Symptoms develop when the secretory products released from the tumors gain direct access to the systemic circulation, bypassing metabolism in the liver. The conditions in which such a bypass may develop include the presence of liver and lung metastases draining directly into

Table 3 Association of carcinoid syndrome with carcinoid tumor localization and secreted compounds

Site of tumor	Localization	Secreted substances	Carcinoid syndrome
Foregut	Bronchus	5-Hydroxytryptophan, histamine, peptide hormones, ACTH (bronchial, thymus)	Atypical, rarely Cushing's syndrome
	Thymus		
	Stomach		
	Duodenum		
	Pancreas		
Midgut	Jejunum	Serotonin, peptide hormones, prostaglandins	Classical
	Ileum		
	Appendix		
	Ascending colon		
Hindgut	Transverse colon	Variable peptide hormones	Rare
	Descending colon		
	Sigmoid colon		
	Rectum		

ACTH adrenocorticotropic hormone

the caval circulation, retroperitoneal disease with drainage into paravertebral veins, or primary sites of disease outside the gastrointestinal tract [37, 38]. In up to 90 % of patients, the development of the carcinoid syndrome is associated with metastatic tumors originating in the midgut [37]. In contrast, bronchial carcinoid tumors are associated with the carcinoid syndrome in approximately 10 % of cases, and nearly all hindgut tumors are hormonally silent. As many as 40 different substances have been identified in various carcinoid tumors (Table 3) [18]. Some of these tumor products are responsible for the carcinoid syndrome, but the relative contributions of each and specificity of any for particular components of the syndrome are yet unknown.

Skin Flushing

Most studies cite flushing in the skin as the most common and first discernible symptom of carcinoid syndrome that occurs in over 90 % of patients [5, 39, 40]. Four types of flushing patterns may occur including the diffuse erythematous, violaceous, prolonged, and bright red patchy type. These patterns can last from 2 to 10 min, affecting the face, neck, and upper chest, or up to 2–3 days, affecting the whole body with lacrimation, edema of the salivary glands, and hypotension [8, 10]. The diffuse erythematous flush is short-lived, lasts 2–10 min, affects the face, neck, and upper chest, and is usually associated with midgut carcinoids [8, 11]. The violaceous flush type is similar to the diffuse erythematous flush, except that attacks may be longer and patients may develop a permanent cyanotic flush with facial telangiectasias, watery eyes, and injected conjunctiva. This type of flushing is usually associated with foregut carcinoids. Prolonged flushes last up to 2–3 days, may involve the whole body, and may also be associated with profuse lacrimation, swelling of the salivary glands, hypotension, and facial edema. This type of flushing is a hallmark of bronchial carcinoids. The bright red, patchy

flushing typically seen with gastric carcinoids is the result of increased histamine production. As a consequence of prolonged vasodilatation, some patients may develop venous telangiectasia characterized by purplish vascular lesions, similar to those seen in acne and rosacea. These lesions most often occur on the nose, upper lip, and malar areas may appear late in the course of the carcinoid syndrome.

Based on the fact that serotonin is the major recognized chemical secreted by the majority of carcinoid tumors, it is commonly, but incorrectly, thought that serotonin is the cause of the flushing. It has been shown that the magnitude of the facial flushing does not correlate with the levels of serotonin present [41]. In addition, it was found that the injection of serotonin does not cause flushing, and serotonin antagonists, which ameliorate the diarrhea, do not alleviate the flushing [5, 30, 41].

A correlation between tachykinins levels and flushing has been described [19, 21, 42, 43]; however, direct proof that tachykinins can cause flushing has not yet been provided [10]. It has been shown that intraluminal tachykinin concentrations are higher in patients with carcinoid syndrome than in healthy control subjects [44]. An association between flushing and secretion of kallikrein (the enzyme producing bradykinin, one of the most powerful vasodilators known) has been reported by some investigators [7, 45] but questioned by others [31, 41].

Diarrhea

Diarrhea may occur at least as frequently, and according to some studies, more often than flushing [46–48]. Secretory diarrhea may occur in more than 80 % of patients and is one of the most debilitating components of the carcinoid syndrome [37, 46]. Stools may vary from few to more than 30 per day, are typically watery and non-bloody, and can be explosive and accompanied by abdominal cramping [39].

The abdominal cramps may be a consequence of mesenteric fibrosis or intestinal blockage by the primary tumor. The diarrhea is usually unrelated to flushing episodes. Transit time through the intestine may be extremely short [47]. The pathophysiology of diarrhea in patients with the carcinoid syndrome is not completely understood. Earlier studies have shown a role of fluid and electrolyte secretion with accelerated small bowel and colonic transit in patients with carcinoid diarrhea and no previous intestinal resections [48, 49]. Elevated levels of serotonin in plasma or of its urinary metabolite, 5HIAA, and increased plasma substance P and motilin have been documented in patients with the syndrome [47, 48, 50, 51].

Cardiac Valvular Disease

The association between malignant carcinoid tumors and right-sided cardiac lesions is well known, but the pathogenetic link between tumor bioactivity and cardiac disease remains incompletely understood [1, 18, 37, 52, 53]. The first clinical signs of carcinoid heart disease including fatigue and dyspnea on exertion are nonspecific and often subtle early in the course of the disease, and may be well tolerated for many months [54, 55]. However, right-sided heart failure with worsening dyspnea, edema, and ascites may develop with progressive disease in up to two thirds of patients with carcinoid syndrome and may be the initial presentation in up to 20 % of patients [37, 54–56].

Carcinoid heart disease is characterized by pathognomonic plaque-like deposits of fibrous tissue [57]. Plaques may develop on the endocardium of the right ventricle and atrium, the valve leaflets, and the subvalvular apparatus, including chordae and papillary muscle [56]. The preponderance of right-sided lesions suggests that causal factors may be released into the hepatic veins from the liver metastases. A growing body of evidence points toward an important role and involvement of serotonin, 5-HIAA, and plasma neurokinin A and substance P [52, 56, 58–60]. In many patients with carcinoid heart disease, the predominant terminal symptoms and death may be attributed directly to cardiac disease [54, 55, 61].

Wheezing and Bronchospasm

Bronchospasm is usually associated with flushing. Both serotonin and bradykinin have been implicated as causes of bronchospasm [1, 8, 10, 11]. It is critical to note that this bronchospasm must *not* be treated like an asthmatic bronchospasm with epinephrine because epinephrine will provoke a vasomotor attack leading to death. Steroids should be the treatment of choice instead [39].

Less Common Manifestations

Although the earliest clinical manifestations of carcinoid syndrome are usually skin flushing and diarrhea, other less common symptoms may herald this syndrome.

Rarely, the diversion of dietary tryptophan for synthesis of large amounts of serotonin instead of niacin can result in the development of pellagra [62]. This condition is manifested by rough scaly skin, glossitis, angular stomatitis, and mental confusion [39]. Diarrhea and malabsorption can exacerbate this process and lead to general muscle wasting.

The development of fibrosis in carcinoid syndrome is usually associated with fibrotic lesions of the right side of the heart involving the tricuspid and pulmonic valves; however, gross fibrosis of the peritoneum, mesentery, and bladder wall have also been associated with the carcinoid syndrome [63, 64].

Variant Carcinoid Syndrome

Gastric and bronchial carcinoids have specific biochemical characteristics that may lead to the development of variant carcinoid syndrome.

Gastric Variant

Gastric carcinoid tumors have two important biochemical features, which may explain at least in part the pathophysiological basis of variant gastric carcinoid syndrome. First, gastric carcinoids are usually unable to convert the dietary tryptophan into serotonin, because they are frequently deficient in the enzyme AADC. Serotonin has been increasingly implicated in the pathophysiology of diarrhea [47, 48, 50] and carcinoid heart disease [52, 56, 58, 60, 64]. As a consequence, the diarrhea and cardiac lesions, which are common features of classic midgut carcinoid syndrome, are unusual in gastric variant of the syndrome [6, 65]. Second, gastric carcinoids can produce large amounts of histamine [66], which has been shown to play primary role in the atypical flushing and pruritus associated with these tumors [28]. In patients with the gastric carcinoid variant, the flushes may be patchy, sharply demarcated, serpiginous, and cherry red; they are also intensely pruritic.

Bronchial Carcinoid Variant Syndrome

Bronchial carcinoids produce less serotonin than do midgut carcinoids, accounting for a lower rate of carcinoid syndrome (Table 3) [67]. Although carcinoid syndrome is encountered only rarely among patients with localized bronchial carcinoids (majority of typical carcinoids), it can be present in over 80 % of patients with liver metastases [68]. The symptoms of bronchial carcinoid syndrome may be atypical, with episodes of severe and prolonged flushing, lasting hours to days. Other related manifestations including disorientation, anxiety, tremor, lacrimation, salivation, hypotension, tachycardia, diarrhea, asthma, and edema [69]. Approximately, 1–2 % of bronchial carcinoids (both typical and atypical) are associated with Cushing's syndrome due to ectopic production of adrenocorticotropic hormone [70–72].

Carcinoid Crisis

Some patients with carcinoid tumors may develop carcinoid crisis, a life-threatening form of carcinoid syndrome, characterized by profound flushing, diarrhea, arrhythmias, extreme changes in blood pressure, bronchospasm, and altered mental status [73]. This medical emergency may occur spontaneously, during anesthesia, surgery, or chemotherapy [37, 74]. It has been hypothesized that these precipitating events may stimulate release of an overwhelming amount of bioactive compounds by the tumor, leading to a multisystem functional collapse refractory to fluid resuscitation and administration of vasopressors [37]. A great deal of precaution is needed prior to surgery, embolization, or chemotherapy, because carcinoid crisis may be precipitated by anesthesia with intraoperative complications occurring in 2 % to greater than 50 % of patients [8, 75, 76]. Octreotide should be available for intraoperative use or given preemptively, especially in patients with extensive tumor load [77]. During carcinoid crisis, an initial bolus dose of 50 mg intravenously with further increments as required can be successful in reversing the condition [37]. In addition, histamine receptor blockers may be useful in reducing histamine release [74]. Close hemodynamic monitoring may be required for patients with carcinoid heart disease, who are at risk of developing arrhythmias and extreme changes in blood pressure. Regional anesthesia and specific pharmacologic agents such as morphine, suxamethonium, beta-blockers, tubocurarine, halothane, and atracurium should be avoided [8, 37].

Key Summary Points

- Symptoms of classic carcinoid syndrome develop when bioactive products released from the carcinoid tumors gain direct access to the systemic circulation, bypassing metabolism in the liver.
- Carcinoid syndrome is generally characterized by episodic flushing and diarrhea; however, the manifestation of carcinoid syndrome may vary among individual patients and symptoms such as wheezing, heart-valve dysfunction, and pellagra may be present less frequently.
- In the majority of cases, carcinoid syndrome is associated with metastatic tumors originating in the midgut; however, some patients may have gastric or bronchial carcinoids that present with atypical carcinoid syndrome symptoms.
- The frequency of carcinoid syndrome is associated with heavy tumor burden. It can be as low as 10 % in localized cases, but can occur in 40–50 % of patients with more advanced disease.
- Carcinoid tumors produce and secrete a variety of bioactive compounds, including serotonin, histamine, bradykinin, tachykinin, motilin, substance P, kallikrein, prostaglandins, catecholamines, and in some cases adrenocorticotropic hormone; however, the contribution of each of these mediators to carcinoid syndrome is not completely understood.
- The most prominent biochemical characteristic of carcinoid tumors is the shunting of tryptophan metabolism toward the production of serotonin instead of nicotinic acid. 5-HIAA is the end product of serotonin metabolism.
- The measurement of 24-h urinary excretion of 5-HIAA is the initial diagnostic test in patients suspected to have classic carcinoid syndrome, but it may not be useful in patients with carcinoid syndrome due to foregut or bronchial carcinoid tumors.
- Some patients with carcinoid tumors may develop carcinoid crisis, a life-threatening form of carcinoid syndrome, characterized by profound flushing, diarrhea, arrhythmias, and extreme changes in blood pressure, bronchospasm, and altered mental status. This medical emergency may occur spontaneously or during surgery, biopsy, and anesthesia. Less commonly, carcinoid crisis may develop after chemotherapy, hepatic arterial embolization, or radionuclide therapy.
- Administration of prophylactic subcutaneous or intravenous octreotide in patients undergoing surgery or hepatic artery embolization for metastatic carcinoid is recommended and may reduce the incidence of carcinoid crisis.

References

1. Dierdorf SF. Carcinoid tumor and carcinoid syndrome. Curr Opin Anaesthesiol. 2003;16(3):343–7.
2. Moertel CG. Treatment of the carcinoid tumor and the malignant carcinoid syndrome. J Clin Oncol. 1983;1(11):727–0.
3. Modlin IM, Lye KD, Kidd M. A 5-decade analysis of 13,715 carcinoid tumors. Cancer. 2003;97(4):934–59.
4. Modlin IM, Shapiro MD, Kidd M. Siegfried Oberndorfer: origins and perspectives of carcinoid tumors. Hum Pathol. 2004;35(12):1440–51.
5. Creutzfeldt W. Carcinoid tumors: development of our knowledge. World J Surg. 1996;20(2):126–31.

6. Borch K, Ahren B, Ahlman H, Falkmer S, Granerus G, Grimelius L. Gastric carcinoids: biologic behavior and prognosis after differentiated treatment in relation to type. Ann Surg. 2005;242(1):64–73.

7. Caplin ME, Buscombe JR, Hilson AJ, Jones AL, Watkinson AF, Burroughs AK. Carcinoid tumor. Lancet. 1998;352(9130):799–805.

8. Memon MA, Nelson H. Gastrointestinal carcinoid tumors: current management strategies. Dis Colon Rectum. 1997;40(9):1101–18.

9. Soga J. Carcinoids and their variant endocrinomas. An analysis of 11842 reported cases. J Exp Clin Cancer Res. 2003;22(4):517–30.

10. Schnirer II, Yao JC, Ajani JA. Carcinoid—a comprehensive review. Acta Oncol. 2003;42(7):672–92.

11. Vinik AI, McLeod MK, Fig LM, Shapiro B, Lloyd RV, Cho K. Clinical features, diagnosis, and localization of carcinoid tumors and their management. Gastroenterol Clin North Am. 1989;18(4):865–96.

12. Pernow B, Waldenstrom J. Paroxysmal flushing and other symptoms caused by 5-hydroxytryptamine and histamine in patients with malignant tumors. Lancet. 1954;267(6845):951.

13. Pasieka JL, McKinnon JG, Kinnear S, Yelle CA, Numerow L, Paterson A, et al. Carcinoid syndrome symposium on treatment modalities for gastrointestinal carcinoid tumors: symposium summary. Can J Surg. 2001;44(1):25–32.

14. Bender DA. Biochemistry of tryptophan in health and disease. Mol Aspects Med. 1983;6(2):101–97.

15. Kvols LK. Metastatic carcinoid tumors and the malignant carcinoid syndrome. Ann N Y Acad Sci. 1994;733:464–70.

16. O'Toole D, Grossman A, Gross D, Delle Fave G, Barkmanova J, O'Connor J, et al. ENETS consensus guidelines for the standards of care in neuroendocrine tumors: biochemical markers. Neuroendocrinology. 2009;90(2):194–202.

17. Sjoblom SM. Clinical presentation and prognosis of gastrointestinal carcinoid tumors. Scand J Gastroenterol. 1988;23(7):779–87.

18. Modlin IM, Kidd M, Latich I, Zikusoka MN, Shapiro MD. Current status of gastrointestinal carcinoids. Gastroenterology. 2005;128(6):1717–51.

19. Cunningham JL, Janson ET, Agarwal S, Grimelius L, Stridsberg M. Tachykinins in endocrine tumors and the carcinoid syndrome. Eur J Endocrinol. 2008;159(3):275–82.

20. Bishop AE, Hamid QA, Adams C, Bretherton-Watt D, Jones PM, Denny P, et al. Expression of tachykinins by ileal and lung carcinoid tumors assessed by combined in situ hybridization, immunocytochemistry, and radioimmunoassay. Cancer. 1989;63(6):1129–37.

21. Norheim I, Oberg K, Theodorsson-Norheim E, Lindgren PG, Lundqvist G, Magnusson A, et al. Malignant carcinoid tumors. An analysis of 103 patients with regard to tumor localization, hormone production, and survival. Ann Surg. 1987;206(2):115–25.

22. Theodorsson-Norheim E, Brodin E, Norheim I, Rosell S. Antisera raised against eledoisin and kassinin detect immunoreactive material in rat tissue extracts: tissue distribution and chromatographic characterization. Regul Pept. 1984;9(4):229–44.

23. Strodel WE, Vinik AI, Jaffe BM, Eckhauser FE, Thompson NW. Substance P in the localization of a carcinoid tumor. J Surg Oncol. 1984;27(2):106–11.

24. Page NM. New challenges in the study of the mammalian tachykinins. Peptides. 2005;26(8):1356–68.

25. Improta G, Broccardo M. Tachykinins: role in human gastrointestinal tract physiology and pathology. Curr Drug Targets. 2006;7(8):1021–9.

26. Beaujouan JC, Torrens Y, Saffroy M, Kemel ML, Glowinski J. A 25 year adventure in the field of tachykinins. Peptides. 2004;25(3):339–57.

27. Kolby L, Wangberg B, Ahlman H, Modlin IM, Granerus G, Theodorsson E, et al. Histidine decarboxylase expression and histamine metabolism in gastric oxyntic mucosa during hypergastrinemia and carcinoid tumor formation. Endocrinology. 1996;137(10):4435–42.

28. Oates JA. The carcinoid syndrome. N Engl J Med. 1986;315(11):702–4.

29. Oates JA, Pettinger WA, Doctor RB. Evidence for the release of bradykinin in carcinoid syndrome. J Clin Invest. 1966;45(2):173–8.

30. Roberts LJ, 2nd, Marney SR, Jr, Oates JA. Blockade of the flush associated with metastatic gastric carcinoid by combined histamine H1 and H2 receptor antagonists. Evidence for an important role of H2 receptors in human vasculature. N Engl J Med. 1979;300(5):236–8.

31. Grahame-Smith DG. What is the cause of the carcinoid flush? Gut. 1987;28(11):1413–6.

32. Metz SA, McRae JR, Robertson RP. Prostaglandins as mediators of paraneoplastic syndromes: review and up-date. Metabolism. 1981;30(3):299–316.

33. Jaffe BM, Condon S. Prostaglandins E and F in endocrine diarrheagenic syndromes. Ann Surg. 1976;184(4):516–24.

34. Feldman JM, Plonk JW, Cornette JC. Serum prostaglandin F-2 alpha concentration in the carcinoid syndrome. Prostaglandins. 1974;7(6):501–6.

35. Sandler M, Karim SM, Williams ED. Prostaglandins in amine-peptide-secreting tumors. Lancet. 1968;2(7577):1053–4.

36. Ramage JK, Davies AH, Ardill J, Bax N, Caplin M, Grossman A, et al. Guidelines for the management of gastroenteropancreatic neuroendocrine (including carcinoid) tumors. Gut. 2005;54(Suppl 4):iv1–16.

37. Raut CP, Kulke MH, Glickman JN, Swanson RS, Ashley SW. Carcinoid tumors. Curr Probl Surg. 2006;43(6):383–450.

38. Fink G, Krelbaum T, Yellin A, Bendayan D, Saute M, Glazer M, et al. Pulmonary carcinoid: presentation, diagnosis, and outcome in 142 cases in Israel and review of 640 cases from the literature. Chest. 2001;119(6):1647–51.

39. McCormick D. Carcinoid tumors and syndrome. Gastroenterol Nurs. 2002;25(3):105–11.

40. Abreu Velez AM, Howard MS. Diagnosis and treatment of cutaneous paraneoplastic disorders. Dermatol Ther. 2010;23(6):662–75.

41. Lucas KJ, Feldman JM. Flushing in the carcinoid syndrome and plasma kallikrein. Cancer. 1986;58(10):2290–3.

42. Ahlman H, Dahlstrom A, Gronstad K, Tisell LE, Oberg K, Zinner MJ, et al. The pentagastrin test in the diagnosis of the carcinoid syndrome. Blockade of gastrointestinal symptoms by ketanserin. Ann Surg. 1985;201(1):81–6.

43. Norheim I, Theodorsson-Norheim E, Brodin E, Oberg K, Lundqvist G, Rosell S. Antisera raised against eledoisin and kassinin detect elevated levels of immunoreactive material in plasma and tumor tissues from patients with carcinoid tumors. Regul Pept. 1984;9(4):245–57.

44. Makridis C, Theodorsson E, Akerstrom G, Oberg K, Knutson L. Increased intestinal non-substance P tachykinin concentrations in malignant midgut carcinoid disease. J Gastroenterol Hepatol. 1999;14(5):500–7.

45. Varas-Lorenzo MJ, Munoz-Agel F, Espinos-Perez JC, Bardaji-Bofill M. Gastrointestinal carcinoid tumors. Rev Esp Enferm Dig. 2010;102(9):533–7.

46. Feldman JM. Carcinoid tumors and the carcinoid syndrome. Curr Probl Surg. 1989;26(12):835–85.

47. von der Ohe MR, Camilleri M, Kvols LK, Thomforde GM. Motor dysfunction of the small bowel and colon in patients with the carcinoid syndrome and diarrhea. N Engl J Med. 1993;329(15):1073–8.

48. Valdovinos MA, Thomforde GM, Camilleri M. Effect of putative carcinoid mediators on gastric and small bowel transit in rats and the role of 5-HT receptors. Aliment Pharmacol Ther. 1993;7(1):61–6.

49. Donowitz M, Binder HJ. Jejunal fluid and electrolyte secretion in carcinoid syndrome. Am J Dig Dis. 1975;20(12):1115–22.

50. Oberg K, Norheim I, Lundqvist G, Wide L. Cytotoxic treatment in patients with malignant carcinoid tumors. Response to streptozocin–alone or in combination with 5-FU. Acta Oncol. 1987;26(6):429–32.

51. Bjorck S, Ahlman H, Dahlstrom A, Phillips SF, Kelly KA. Serotonergic regulation of canine enteric motility (measured as electrical activity) and absorption: physiologic and morphologic evidence. Acta Physiol Scand. 1988;133(2):247–56.
52. Gustafsson BI, Hauso O, Drozdov I, Kidd M, Modlin IM. Carcinoid heart disease. Int J Cardiol. 2008;129(3):318–24.
53. Himelman RB, Schiller NB. Clinical and echocardiographic comparison of patients with the carcinoid syndrome with and without carcinoid heart disease. Am J Cardiol. 1989;63(5):347–52.
54. Pellikka PA, Tajik AJ, Khandheria BK, Seward JB, Callahan JA, Pitot HC, et al. Carcinoid heart disease. Clinical and echocardiographic spectrum in 74 patients. Circulation. 1993;87(4):1188–96.
55. Lundin L, Norheim I, Landelius J, Oberg K, Theodorsson-Norheim E. Carcinoid heart disease: relationship of circulating vasoactive substances to ultrasound-detectable cardiac abnormalities. Circulation. 1988;77(2):264–9.
56. Bhattacharyya S, Davar J, Dreyfus G, Caplin ME. Carcinoid heart disease. Circulation. 2007;116(24):2860–5.
57. Anderson AS, Krauss D, Lang R. Cardiovascular complications of malignant carcinoid disease. Am Heart J. 1997;134(4):693–702.
58. Jian B, Xu J, Connolly J, Savani RC, Narula N, Liang B, et al. Serotonin mechanisms in heart valve disease I: serotonin-induced up-regulation of transforming growth factor-beta1 via G-protein signal transduction in aortic valve interstitial cells. Am J Pathol. 2002;161(6):2111–21.
59. Robiolio PA, Rigolin VH, Wilson JS, Harrison JK, Sanders LL, Bashore TM, et al. Carcinoid heart disease. Correlation of high serotonin levels with valvular abnormalities detected by cardiac catheterization and echocardiography. Circulation. 1995;92(4):790–5.
60. Simula DV, Edwards WD, Tazelaar HD, Connolly HM, Schaff HV. Surgical pathology of carcinoid heart disease: a study of 139 valves from 75 patients spanning 20 years. Mayo Clin Proc. 2002;77(2):139–47.
61. Westberg G, Wangberg B, Ahlman H, Bergh CH, Beckman-Suurkula M, Caidahl K. Prediction of prognosis by echocardiography in patients with midgut carcinoid syndrome. Br J Surg. 2001;88(6):865–72.
62. Swain CP, Tavill AS, Neale G. Studies of tryptophan and albumin metabolism in a patient with carcinoid syndrome, pellagra, and hypoproteinemia. Gastroenterology. 1976;71(3):484–9.
63. Morin LJ, Zuerner RT. Retroperitoneal fibrosis and carcinoid tumor. JAMA. 1971;216(10):1647–8.
64. Bivens CH, Marecek RL, Feldman JM. Peyronie's disease—a presenting complaint of the carcinoid syndrome. N Engl J Med. 1973;289(16):844–5.
65. Gough DB, Thompson GB, Crotty TB, Donohue JH, Kvols LK, Carney JA, et al. Diverse clinical and pathologic features of gastric carcinoid and the relevance of hypergastrinemia. World J Surg. 1994;18(4):473–9; discussion 479–80.
66. Kolby L, Wangberg B, Ahlman H, Modlin IM, Granerus G, Theodorsson E, et al. Histidine decarboxylase expression and histamine metabolism in gastric oxyntic mucosa during hypergastrinemia and carcinoid tumor formation. Endocrinology. 1996;137(10):4435–42.
67. Gustafsson BI, Kidd M, Chan A, Malfertheiner MV, Modlin IM. Bronchopulmonary neuroendocrine tumors. Cancer. 2008;113(1):5–21.
68. Fischer S, Kruger M, McRae K, Merchant N, Tsao MS, Keshavjee S. Giant bronchial carcinoid tumors: a multidisciplinary approach. Ann Thorac Surg. 2001;71(1):386–93.
69. Melmon KL, Sjoerdsma A, Mason DT. Distinctive clinical and therapeutic aspects of the syndrome associated with bronchial carcinoid tumors. Am J Med. 1965;39(4):568–81.
70. DeStephano DB, Lloyd RV, Schteingart DE. Cushing's syndrome produced by a bronchial carcinoid tumor. Hum Pathol. 1984;15(9):890–2.
71. Limper AH, Carpenter PC, Scheithauer B, Staats BA. The Cushing syndrome induced by bronchial carcinoid tumors. Ann Intern Med. 1992;117(3):209–14.
72. Shrager JB, Wright CD, Wain JC, Torchiana DF, Grillo HC, Mathisen DJ. Bronchopulmonary carcinoid tumors associated with Cushing's syndrome: a more aggressive variant of typical carcinoid. J Thorac Cardiovasc Surg. 1997;114(3):367–75.
73. Basson MD, Ahlman H, Wangberg B, Modlin IM. Biology and management of the midgut carcinoid. Am J Surg. 1993;165(2):288–97.
74. Lips CJ, Lentjes EG, Hoppener JW. The spectrum of carcinoid tumours and carcinoid syndromes. Ann Clin Biochem. 2003;40(Pt 6):612–27.
75. Woodside KJ, Townsend CM, Jr, Mark Evers B. Current management of gastrointestinal carcinoid tumors. J Gastrointest Surg. 2004;8(6):742–56.
76. Tornebrandt K, Nobin A, Ericsson M, Thomson D. Circulation, respiration and serotonin levels in carcinoid patients during neurolept anaesthesia. Anaesthesia. 1983;38(10):957–67.
77. Dery R. Theoretical and clinical considerations in anaesthesia for secreting carcinoid tumors. Can Anaesth Soc J. 1971;18(3):245–63.

Sigfried Oberndorfer

1879–1944

Per Hellman

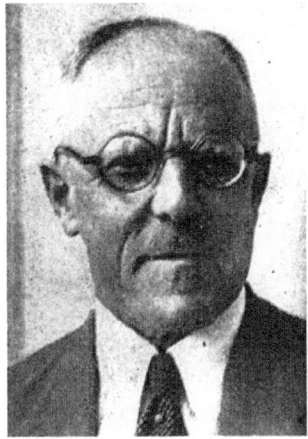

Sigfried Oberndorfer in 1936 in Istanbul

When Sigfried was 9 years old, he probably did not think that he would discover a very specific type of malignant tumor, which even today, i.e., more than 100 years after his finding, is a strange, different, and difficult-to-treat variant of the neuroendocrine tumors (NET) [1, 2].

Sigfried was born in June 1879 in Munich, Germany. His father Heinrich and mother Helene were both Jewish. Sigfried had five siblings. The health issues of his childhood were typical of the time, centered around infectious diseases and general survival. He himself survived typhoid fever at 3 years of age, but lost a sister who at the age of 25 died of ruptured appendicitis. Sigfried was probably a skilled pupil at school, interested in Greek and Latin literature. He graduated in 1895 at 16 years of age. He proceeded to medical school at the University of Munich. He presented his thesis about syphilis in 1899, and shortly after received his medical license in 1900. Already during medical school, he became interested in pathology, which he studied in Kiel with Professor Heller, and later after finishing medical school, at

the Institute of Pathology in Geneva with Professor Zahn, and in Munich with Professor Bollinger. However, he also saw living patients while working as a ship doctor on the Atlantic in 1901. To maintain a normal life and support his family, he also worked as a general practitioner for a short while. Otherwise, his main interest was pathology and he made a significant career locally, presenting research data on many topics including chronic appendicitis which also was his habilitation thesis [3]. Around this time, he met a woman named Gutta who became his wife in 1906. They later raised three children (Fig. 1).

He was the youngest Jewish physician ever appointed to the faculty in 1906. He received, at 29 years of age, *Venia Legendi* (permission to teach). His inaugural lecture was a fascinating discourse about tuberculosis in the female genital organs. Later, in 1908, he was asked to organize a new pathological institute. His successful career continued, and in 1911 he was promoted to professor of pathology and became the director of the Munich-Schwabing Hospital's Pathological Institute. Between 1911 and 1933, he continued to study medicine and pathology in his position as professor of pathological anatomy, with a break during the First World War when he volunteered and served as an army pathologist at the Western Front. The birth of his third child took Sigfried home to Munich, which probably saved him from being captured by the Allied forces, which won the Battle of Selle in 1918.

Sigfried was scientifically highly productive, releasing 333 publications encompassing an impressively wide variety of diagnoses [4–9]. He was also recognized for his educational skills, by in 1928 receiving an honorary award from the University of Munich.

Over the years, he collected a number of autopsy and pathological specimens for which a particularly strange tumor of the small intestine became his deep, personal interest. When investigating these tumors under the microscope, he noted the cancer-like appearance, and the term *karzinoid* was coined. His early studies immediately took him to Dresden

P. Hellman (✉)
Department of Surgery, University Hospital, Uppsala, Sweden
e-mail: per.hellman@surgsci.uu.se

J. L. Pasieka, J. A. Lee (eds.), *Surgical Endocrinopathies,* DOI 10.1007/978-3-319-13662-2_55,
© Springer International Publishing Switzerland 2015

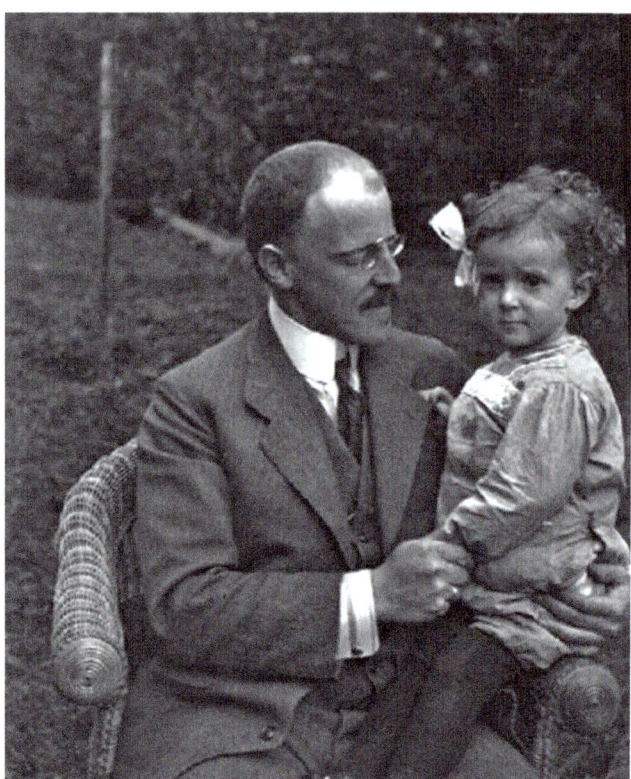

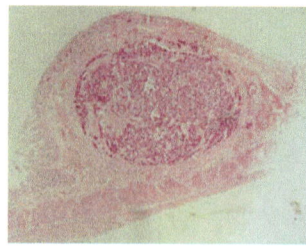

Fig. 2 Original section of Oberndorfer demonstrating a primary ileal neuroendocrine tumor. According to [17] provided by Robert Rössle (1876–1956) who was a colleague of Oberndorfer at the University of Munich. (From [17]. Reprinted with permission from Springer)

Fig. 1 Sigfried Oberndorfer and his daughter Helena in Munich 1911. (From [17]. Reprinted with permission from Springer)

in September 1907 where he presented his findings—*karzinoide*—at the annual German Pathological Society convention (Fig. 2). A paper regarding the same finding was published in the *Frankfurt Journal of Pathology* in December 1907. In it he described six small intestinal tumors which all grew very slowly without signs of metastases. He had gathered information about these tumors over many years, finding the first two from his time with Professor Zahn in Geneva in 1901, and another four from Professor Bollinger in Munich in 1904. For decades, this report was falsely cited as a report of a "benign carcinoma", partly due to Sigfried's statement that they were benign, without a tendency toward infiltration. Thus, in his initial report he happened to find cases which were amenable to surgical resection. Additionally, as a pathologist, he found them at autopsy in patients who were fairly young and who died of other causes. Sigfried worked in an era where the attention was focused around tuberculosis, infectious diseases, and death of other causes rather than cancer. However, his findings have become quite important in the modern era.

Indeed, his autopsy findings were retrospectively supported by others. For example, in 1867, Theodor Langhans (Usinger, Germany), described a 50-year-old woman who died of tuberculosis but who also had a small intestinal tumor, which was presumably a NET of the small intestine. Several

other case reports may be found which presumably describe findings of *karzinoid*, thereby supporting Sigfried. Although Sigfried was the one who coined the term *karcinoid*, others also reported the existence of these tumors before him, such as William Bayliss, Ernest Starling, and Nikolai Kulchitsky who described these endocrine cells interspersed in the bowel epithelium [10]. Somewhat later Pierre Masson described argentaffin-staining cells in small intestinal tumors and linked them to the endocrine system [11, 12]. In addition to his work on carcinoid tumors, Sigfried also recognized the difference between other lesions of the small intestine (presumably inflammatory diseases such as Crohn's disease or due to infectious agents).

Sigfried noted that small intestinal carcinoid was not very rare, and he foresaw the increased recognition of the disease, predicting the higher prevalence in the modern era. In fact, autopsy studies describing the incidence of carcinoid are sparse, with the first report after Sigfried's seminal paper was published 70 years later, in the 1970s [13].

His subsequent work revealed that *karzinoid* tumors often spread to lymph nodes and the liver. Eventually, in 1929—after 22 years of study—he presented another study of 36 *karzinoids* where he noted that these tumors did have malignant potential [14], causing him to revise his initial statement (Fig. 3). Other physicians noted this malignant potential as well with William B. Ransom (1860–1909) publishing a case of a patient who died of a small intestinal tumor with liver metastases but also features of the carcinoid syndrome in the Lancet in 1890 [15].

What Sigfried did not know at the time, but later had to realize, was the fate of being Jewish. Later in his career, world events intervened in Sigfried's life. The Nazis stated that "in the interest of German patients" Jewish physicians had to be removed from duty. It was expressed as the *Verjudung* of the Academy. Sixteen percent of German physicians were Jewish at the time (although only 0.8% of the total population was Jewish). On April 1, 1933, no Jewish physicians, lawyers, or businesses could continue to function by the order of the government. This led to the Nazis stripping Sigfried of his title. Sigfried went to Istanbul, in Turkey, where he

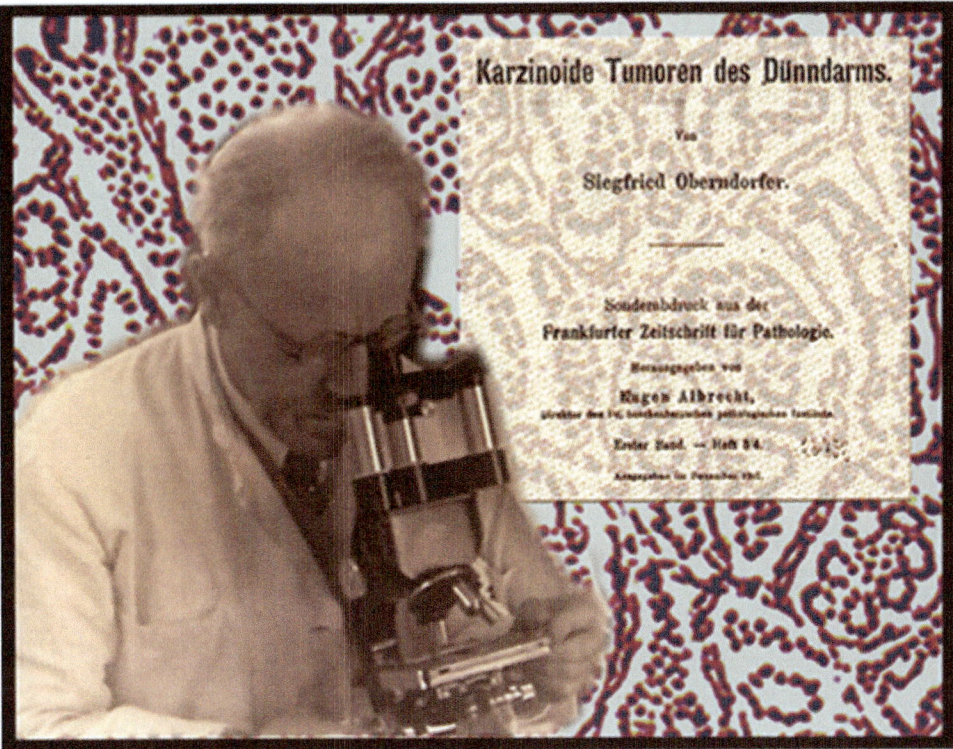

Fig. 3 Sigfried Oberndorfer at his microscope. Published after acceptance by the American Medical Association. (From [16]. Reprinted with permission from American Medical Association)

worked as chair of the Institute of Istanbul until his death in 1944. This emigration was made possible by the by Kemal Pasha ("father of Turks"; Ataturk) who took the opportunity to recruit the German academic elite by offering them asylum and working positions. Sigfried Oberndorfer was offered to post of professor in general and experimental pathology at the University of Istanbul. Although Sigfried and his wife Gutta survived, their daughter Anna and Sigfried's brother both died in German concentration camps during World War II. Sigfried continued to be successful in his profession, and received the King's Medal of King George II of Greece in 1936. His growing interest in cancer took him to cancer conferences, and in 1937 he founded the Turkish Institute for Cancer Research, and was awarded the Rudolf Virchow medal.

Sigfried died on March 1, 1944, at the age of 67 from a thoracic tumor, probably a thymoma, and is buried in Istanbul [16]. Sigfried never lived long enough to receive the recognition for his great discovery and for him to fully realize the importance of his contribution to the medical and scientific community.

Acknowledgment This contribution would not have been possible without studying the research performed by Irvin Modlin and collaborators, who by their immense and thorough investigations could bring forward interesting facts about Sigfried Oberndorfer [16, 17]. Also the work done by Joachim Katz made important contributions [18].

References

1. Akerstrom G, Hellman P. Surgery on neuroendocrine tumours. Best Pract Res Clin Endocrinol Metab. 2007;21(1):87–109.
2. Norlen O, Stalberg P, Oberg K, Eriksson J, Hedberg J, Hessman O, et al. Long-term results of surgery for small intestinal neuroendocrine tumors at a tertiary referral center. World J Surg. 2012;36(6):1419–31.
3. Oberndorfer S. Anatomie der cronischen Appendicitis Habilitatiosschrift. Mitt Grenzgeb Med Chir. 1905–1906;15:653–700.
4. Oberndorfer S. Pigment und Pigmentbildung. Zentralbl Neurol Pcychol. 1921;25:81–101.
5. Oberndorfer S. Spontangangrän des Unterarms als Unfallsfolge. Munch Med Wochenschr. 1927;74:1369–71.
6. Oberndorfer S. Meniskusverletzung durch Sprung. Monatsschr Unfallheilkd. 1927;34:255–8.
7. Oberndorfer S. Aterosklerose des Ductus Thoracicus. Verh Dtsch Ges Pathol. 1925;20:247–52.
8. Oberndorfer S. Die Anatomischen Grundlagen der Angina pectoris. Munch Med Wochenschr. 1925;72:1495–8.
9. Oberndorfer S. Zellmutationen und mutiple Geschwulstentstehungen im Lungen. Virchows Arch 1930;275:728–37.
10. Kulchitsky N. Zur Frage "ber den bau des Darmkanals. Arch Mikrosk Anat. 1897;49:7–35.
11. Gosset A, Masson P. Tumeors endocrines de l'appendice. Presse Med. 1914;25:237–40.
12. Masson P. La glande endocrin de l'intestin chez l'homme. CRAcad Sci Paris. 1914;15:59–61.
13. Berge T, Linell F. Carcinoid tumours. Frequency in a defined population during a 12-year period. Acta Pathol Microbiol Scand Sect A, Pathol. 1976;84(4):322–30.

14. Oberndorfer S. Karzinoide. Handbook of pathological anatomy. Berlin: Verlag von Julius Springer; 1929.
15. Ransom W. A case of primary carcinoma of the ileum. Lancet. 1890;2:1020–3.
16. Modlin IM, Shapiro MD, Kidd M, Eick G. Siegfried Oberndorfer and the evolution of carcinoid disease. Arch Surg. 2007;142(2):187–97.
17. Kloppel G, Dege K, Remmele W, Kapran Y, Tuzlali S, Modlin IM. Siegfried Oberndorfer: a tribute to his work and life between Munich, Kiel, Geneva, and Istanbul. Virchows Arch. 2007;451 Suppl 1:S3–7.
18. Katz JT. Leben und Werk des Pathologen Prof. Dr. Siegfried Oberndorfer, erster Chefarzt der Pathologie am Krankenhaus München-Schwabing, 2005.

von Hippel–Lindau Disease

Adriana G. Ramirez and Philip W. Smith

Introduction

von Hippel–Lindau (vHL) is an inherited autosomal dominant pleomorphic disorder characterized by the development of specific multiorgan neoplasms. The syndrome has been linked to mutations in a single tumor suppressor gene; however, the spectrum of clinical manifestations of vHL varies significantly from patient to patient. Generally, the lesions are highly vascularized tumors, may be cystic or solid, and may be benign or malignant. The organs involved most commonly are the central nervous system (CNS), eyes, kidneys, adrenal glands, pancreas, and to a lesser extent, the auditory and reproductive adnexal organs. Specifically, vHL patients are at risk of developing the lesions listed in Table 1 [1, 2].

Older estimates suggest the incidence of vHL to be 1:36,000 live births in an Anglo-Saxon population [3]. Substantial geographical variability and referral bias occur as patients live in proximity to their kindred and their care becomes increasingly concentrated at specialized centers. Thus, the true incidence is difficult to ascertain but a more recent estimate is 1:39,000–53,000 [2, 4]. The lifetime penetrance of vHL-associated disease in those with a vHL mutation is nearly 100% [5]. Complications of renal cell carcinoma (RCC, 32%) or CNS hemangioblastomas (53%) continue to be the leading causes of vHL-related mortality [1, 2].

Characterization of the natural history of the disease as well as the genetic and molecular abnormalities in vHL has resulted in substantial improvement in the management of these patients. In addition, it has led to the ability to inform genetic counseling and provide prognostic determinants based on disease subtype. The knowledge gained about the disease has become the basis for current screening and surveillance guidelines as well as impacted surgical decision making. A study of survival rates of multiple genetic neoplastic disorders comparing before and after the intensification of standardized screening demonstrates significant progress in the management of vHL. The life expectancy for vHL prior to 1990 and the establishment of a genetic registrar was 52.5 years and had the lowest expectancy of the diseases studied. A survival benefit of 16.3 years was seen in those patients diagnosed after 1990 increasing the life expectancy to 68.8 years [6]. Screening of asymptomatic vHL patients and at-risk family members identifies disease-related lesions at an earlier stage and correlates to higher cure rates for malignant lesions as well as increased options for organ-sparing interventions. Guidelines are established and are readily available to patients and providers through the vHL Family Alliance at www.vhl.org. These guidelines are summarized in Table 2 and will be revisited throughout this chapter.

The crucial importance of coordinated screening and intervention for a disease that, by definition, involves multiple organ systems makes the case that vHL patients should be referred to dedicated vHL care centers with an experienced and appropriately resourced multidisciplinary team. Specialized care centers are essential for optimum surveillance, coordinated operative and nonoperative care, and ancillary service support. The endocrine surgeon plays an important role in the management of vHL but must be placed appropriately within the context of whole-patient disease management system.

Disease Subtypes

vHL patients can be classified into clinical subtypes (Table 3) with major subtypes based on the risk of developing a pheochromocytoma. Type 1 patients may develop all other tumor types associated with vHL; however, they have a significantly reduced risk of pheochromocytoma. Type I accounts for 80–93% of the vHL population. Type 2 patients have a high lifetime risk of a pheochromocytoma and represent the

P. W. Smith (✉) · A. G. Ramirez
Department of Surgery, University of Virginia, Box 800709,
Charlottesville, VA 22908, USA
e-mail: philip@virginia.edu

A. G. Ramirez
e-mail: agr5e@virginia.edu

J. L. Pasieka, J. A. Lee (eds.), *Surgical Endocrinopathies,* DOI 10.1007/978-3-319-13662-2_56,
© Springer International Publishing Switzerland 2015

Table 1 Frequency of lesions and age of onset of vHL manifestations. (Adapted from [1, 10])

	Mean age of onset (years)	Frequency (%)
Central nervous system (CNS)		
Retinal hemangioblastomas	18	70
Craniospinal hemangioblastomas	29	60–90
Endolymphatic sac tumors	22–32	11–16
Visceral		
Pheochromocytomas	30	10–20
Pancreatic lesion	36	17–75
Pancreatic neuroendocrine tumors (PNET)	35	20
Renal cell carcinoma or cysts	34	90–95
Epididymal cystadenoma	35	42
Broad ligament cystadenoma	–	–

Table 2 Screening guidelines. (Adapted from vHL Alliance [25])

Age	Test	Comments
0	Physical examination Routine newborn hearing screening	Pediatrician assess for neurological disturbances or ophthalmic abnormalities (nystagmus, strabismus, white pupil, etc.)
1–4	Indirect ophthalmoscope (annual) Physical examination (annual)	Ophthalmologist performed eye/retinal examination Regular assessments with pediatrician that includes the above as well as blood pressure, vision, and hearing abnormalities
5–15	Same as above plus: Fractionated metanephrines or 24-h urine test (annual) Abdominal ultrasound (annual after 8 years of age) Complete audiology assessment (every 2–3 years)	If biochemical abnormalities or concerning findings on ultrasound are found, an abdominal MRI or MIBG scan is indicated If symptoms of audiovestibular disturbance are found, audiology screening frequency should be annually MRI with and without contrast of internal auditory canals in case of repeated ear infections
16+	Same as above plus: MRI of abdomen wwo contrast (every 2 years) MRI of the brain and entire neuroaxis (every 2 years)	Neuroaxis includes cervical, thoracic, and lumbar spine with thin slices through posterior fossa/temporal bone
Pregnancy	Retinal screening (periodic) Fractionated metanephrines or 24-h urine test (per trimester) MRI of brain and spine (4th month of gestation)	Hemangioblastomas are known to have accelerated growth during pregnancy Important to ensure the absence of a pheochromocytoma during pregnancy and prior to delivery

MRI magnetic resonance imaging, *MIBG* metaiodobenzylguanidine

Table 3 vHL disease subtypes

Type 1	Reduced risk of pheochromocytoma
Types 2	Increased risk of pheochromocytoma
Type 2A	Increased risk of pheochromocytoma + low risk of RCC
Type 2B	Increased risk of pheochromocytoma + high risk of RCC
Type 2C	Pheochromocytoma only

other 7–20 % of vHL patients [2]. Type 2 patients can be further subdivided into groups (A, B, or C) on the basis of the likelihood of developing RCC. Within the type 2A subgroup, there is a predominance of pheochromocytomas with a low risk of RCC versus in type 2B where there is a high risk of RCC, retinal, and cerebral disease in addition to a significant risk of developing a pheochromocytoma. The only manifestation of vHL in type 2C patients is pheochromocytoma. Despite these general classifications, due to variable penetrance in patients with the same mutation, screening and management guidelines are not currently tailored based on subtype classification.

Diagnosis, Molecular Biology, and Genetics

vHL exhibits autosomal dominant inheritance with >95 % penetrance of disease specific manifestation by age 65. The involved gene in vHL maps to the short arm of chromosome 3, specifically 3p25-p26 [7]. There also exists a prominent modifier of the vHL gene by CCND1 on 11q13.3. The vHL gene is a tumor suppressor gene and, as such, the germline mutation in one allele is not adequate to result in emergence of tumors. Per Knudson's two-hit hypothesis, a second mutation must occur with the normal vHL allele resulting in "loss of heterozygosity" that causes complete loss of the gene's normal downstream products and effects [8]. This "second hit" results in loss of tumor suppressor function and subsequent tumor development.

The vHL gene is fundamental in the response to hypoxia and serves as a cellular oxygen sensor. It is important in angiogenesis, erythropoiesis, and cell cycle regulation [9, 10]. The protein product (pVHL) is a component of an E3 ubiquitin ligase complex, which normally mediates degradation of the hypoxia-inducible factor (HIF) transcriptional complex via poly-ubiquitination in oxygen-replete cells. In contrast, its function is suppressed in hypoxic cells, which allows for activation of the HIF target genes associated with angiogenesis, growth, and mitogenic factors, extracellular matrix control, and microtubule regulation, as well enhanced glucose uptake [9–11]. In vHL, regulation of HIF is lost. The affected tissues behave as if in a chronically oxygen-depleted environment with an uncontrolled growth stimulus. The most pronounced impact is seen in highly vascularized areas such as the CNS, retina, medulla, kidneys, and pancreas [12].

Genetic testing has revealed over 100 germline mutations associated with vHL among known kindreds. Frequent mutations include R238Q and R238W, which is associated with a 62% incidence of pheochromocytoma, as well R167Q and R167W, which are associated with developing both pheochromocytoma and renal cell carcinoma. Generally, type I disease is more associated with deletions, nonsense, and frameshift mutations, whereas type II disease is associated with missense mutations. While these examples demonstrate that there is a correlation between specific mutation and disease manifestations, the same mutation in different individuals may have different clinical manifestations. Due to the overall poor correlation between genotype and phenotype, the specific mutation cannot be used to tailor screening recommendations, or treatment strategies, at this time [13, 14].

If the patient has a previously described mutation in the vHL gene, genetic testing can confirm the diagnosis with near 100% specificity [15]. In the absence of an already confirmed mutation status, the established clinical criteria may be used to establish diagnosis. In the setting of a positive family history, the patient in question must present with any one major disease-related lesion, which include a CNS hemangioblastoma, retinal hemangioblastomas, pheochromocytoma, or RCC. In the setting of no family history, the diagnosis requires two vHL-associated lesions, which can include two or more CNS hemangioblastomas or one CNS hemangioblastoma and one visceral tumor [2].

Specific Manifestations

We will individually address the organ-specific manifestations of vHL, progressing generally from cephalad to caudad. We will address greatest attention to those neoplasms that are of greatest clinical impact to the patient, as well as those of particular interest to the endocrine surgeon.

Cerebral and Spinal Hemangioblastoma

Hemangioblastomas of the CNS are capillary-rich, circumscribed, benign neoplasms. Although benign, due to their location in the neuraxis, they can cause major morbidity and mortality due to mass effect of the lesion (as seen in the patient in Fig. 1), associated cysts, or from hemorrhage. CNS hemangioblastomas are the most prevalent neoplasms in vHL, developing in 60–90% of patients [16]. These present at a younger average age than sporadic hemangioblastomas (mean of 29 years in vHL) and more often are multifocal [17]. Both sporadic and vHL-associated hemangioblastomas typically are infratentorial (Figs. 1 and 2). A prospective evaluation of 250 vHL patients with CNS hemangioblastomas demonstrated a median of eight lesions per patient, with 1% supratentorial, 6% in the brainstem, 45% in the cerebellum, and the remaining 48% caudal to that (spinal cord, cauda equina, and nerve roots). These patients developed a median of 0.3 new lesions/patient-year [16]. Although also infratentorial, a larger proportion (>80%) of sporadic CNS hemangioblastomas are cerebellar [17].

Other than presentation with a symptomatic lesion, identification of CNS hemangioblastoma occurs by imaging. The majority of lesions are clinically asymptomatic and there are no available screening laboratory studies. CT is not an adequate test for this entity and contrast-enhanced magnetic resonance imaging (MRI) is the preferred modality. Current guidelines for screening in vHL patients are for ≥1.5 T MRI scans with and without contrast to include the brain and whole spine with thin cuts through the posterior fossa. These are to start by age 16 and be performed every 2 years. This interval is then shortened in those with demonstrated lesions.

The majority of these lesions are asymptomatic and do not require intervention. However, due to the presence of multiple lesions per patient, many vHL patients will harbor at least one symptomatic lesion. At final evaluation in a prospective series, while only 6% of all detected lesions had associated symptoms requiring intervention, they were distributed across one-third of the patient population [16]. The rate of growth of vHL-associated CNS hemangioblastoma varies with the anatomic location of the tumor, with more rapid progression for those in the brainstem and cerebellum [16]. These lesions may develop cysts in some cases (12%) and the presence of a cystic component is associated with faster growth and a greater likelihood of developing symptoms [16].

It is not universally agreed when to intervene on these lesions, but most believe that they should be closely observed radiographically, and correlated with history or physical exam findings for specifically associated neurologic symptoms, and that onset of symptoms should prompt treatment of the causative lesion [16]. While there are some clinical vari-

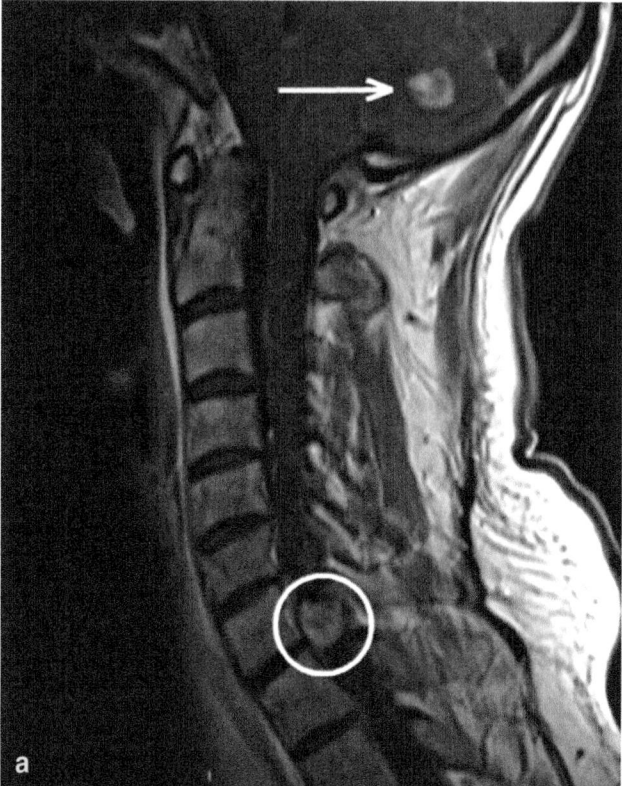
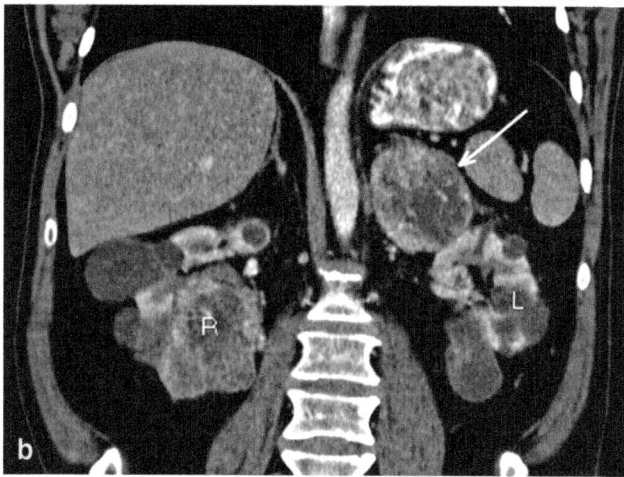

Fig. 1 Radiographic findings all from a single 47-year-old male without prior diagnosis of von Hippel–Lindau (vHL), but a suggestive family history, who presented with chief complaint of headache. Imaging demonstrates two cerebellar hemangioblastomas, one causing obstructive hydrocephalus (*arrow* in image **a**), as well as spinal hemangioblastomas (including at C7 in *circle* in image **a**). Recent-onset hypertension and clinical suspicion based on multiple hemangioblastomas prompted biochemical testing and abdominal imaging. Computerized tomography (CT) demonstrated 7 cm left adrenal lesion consistent with pheochromocytoma (*arrow* in image **b**), an unremarkable right adrenal gland and multiple bilateral renal cysts and masses consistent with RCC (see *R* and *L* in image **b**). Twenty-four-hour urine collection demonstrates norepinephrine 557 (15–80 µg/24 h), epinephrine <5 (0.5–20 p/24 h), and normetanephrines + metanephrines 5.4 (0.17–0.70 mg/24 h)

ables that are associated with lesion progression [16], these are neither sensitive nor specific. Therefore, radiographic and clinical follow up is mandatory. When treatment of CNS hemangioblastoma is deemed necessary, surgical resection is the primary modality. Due to the morbidity and difficulty in surgical access to some of these lesions, stereotactic radiosurgery has also been employed. Although this therapy was well tolerated, stereotactic radiosurgery demonstrated diminished ability to control lesions over time. Therefore it is recommended that stereotactic radiosurgery be reserved for those symptomatic lesions not amenable to surgical therapy [18]. Although the vascular nature of the lesions raised hope that antiangiogenic therapy would be effective, there does not currently exist a demonstrated effective option for medical therapy.

While the presence of multiple CNS hemangioblastomas should very strongly raise the concern for vHL, an apparently sporadic CNS hemangioblastoma may be the index presentation of a previously unknown germline vHL mutation. In one series, this occurred in 4 % of patients otherwise thought to have sporadic CNS hemangioblastomas, all of whom presented at an age less than 40 years. A further 5 % of these patients who tested negative for germline mutation subsequently developed another vHL-related lesion, which may have been the result of mosaicism [19]. Given the importance of appropriate screening for other vHL-associated lesions, this is of clear importance for those patients in whom a germline vHL mutation is detected. For this reason, it is reasonable to submit all patients with retinal or CNS hemangioblastoma for vHL testing, even if these initially are believed to be sporadic lesions.

Retinal Capillary Hemangioblastomas

Hemangioblastomas also occur in the eyes of vHL patients and can be complicated by vision loss. These are frequently the earliest manifestation of vHL, and most vHL patients do not develop new retinal hemangioblastomas late in life. However, cumulatively, 70 % of vHL patients have retinal hemangioblastomas by age 60 and they frequently are bilateral. Compared to patients with sporadic retinal hemangioblastomas, they occur at an earlier age (18 vs. 36 years) and more frequently are multifocal and bilateral (about 50 %) [16, 20].

Retinal hemangioblastomas are not initially clinically apparent and are only detected by dilated ophthalmologic exam. Due to subretinal edema, traction, and hemorrhage, these lesions can result in vision loss. Monitoring and therapy aim to prevent or minimize vision loss. Treatment of most of these lesions is laser photocoagulation. There is not universal agreement and some recommend treating asymptomatic lesions while others recommend that small asymptomatic

Fig. 2 Radiographic findings all from a single patient from a known vHL kindred. He underwent bilateral total adrenalectomy at age 10 for bilateral pheochromocytoma (*circle* and *arrow* image **a**). At that time his biochemical workup included 24- h urine with epinephrine <5 (<25); NorEpinephrine 552 (<100); NorMet+Met 3.5. He was lost to formal follow up until re-presenting at age 20 following a school entrance physical. Imaging at that time demonstrates a large pelvic paraganglioma (image **b**), cerebellar and spinal hemangioblastomas (image **c**), three head of pancreas PNETs (image **d**), and two tail of pancreas PNETs. Biochemical evaluation revealed no evidence of functional PNET, and urine normetanephrines 1.2 nMol/L (<0.9), urine metaneprhines <0.20 nMol/L

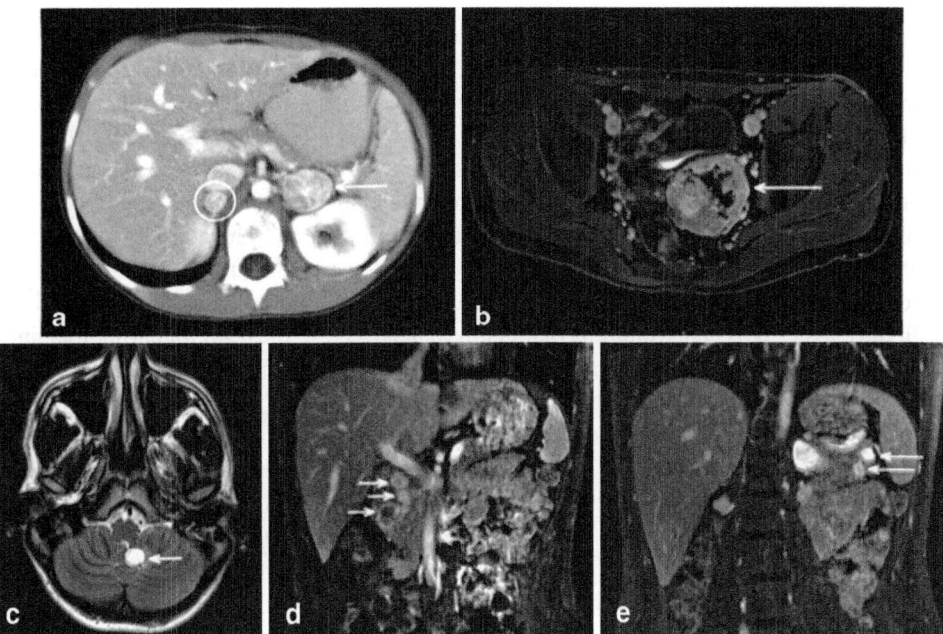

lesions may be closely monitored for growth or symptoms [16, 21]. As with CNS hemangioblastoma, investigations into antiangiogenesis therapies have demonstrated some potential role, but are not yet adequately studied.

Although not universally agreed upon, it is reasonable to offer vHL testing to patients with otherwise apparently sporadic retinal hemangioblastoma. In the presence of a known vHL germline mutation, screening for retinal hemangioblastoma is recommended annually starting at age 1 and in the hands of an ophthalmologist with expertise in these lesions.

Endolymphatic Sac Tumors of the Middle Ear

Tumors of the endolymphatic sac (ELST) are an overgrowth of the papillary epithelium of the endolymphatic system located within the middle ear. These tumors are characterized as highly vascular and locally aggressive. While rare in the general population, they are detected in 11–16% of vHL patients, 22 with an age at onset of 22–32 years [23]. vHL is the only condition associated with bilateral ELSTs [23]. Patients may present with acute-onset hearing loss, tinnitus, pain, vertigo, facial paresis, and aural fullness [22–24]. The mechanism for the audiovestibular dysfunction's sudden onset is hypothesized to be acute intralabyrinthine hemorrhage. However a more gradual decline in hearing secondary to otic capsule invasion and/or hydrops formation also is reported [22, 23]. Regardless of mechanism, hearing loss usually is permanent.

Screening for ELSTs begins at birth with the routine newborn hearing screening. Periodic assessments of hearing should be performed by the child's pediatrician. Starting at age 5, a formal audiology examination should be completed

every 2–3 years, and more frequently if symptoms arise. The vHL Alliance also recommends an MRI with contrast of the internal auditory canal with thin cuts in cases of recurrent ear infections every 2 years after age 16 which is concurrent with the exam for CNS hemangioblastoma [25]. Indications for surgery include patients with radiologic evidence of a tumor on computed tomography (CT) or MRI that either have preserved hearing, or for deaf patients with persistent neurological symptoms associated with an ELST [22]. Surgical resection does not improve hearing but has been shown to prevent further damage, and improve other associated neurological symptoms. Of vHL patients who complain of audiovestibular symptoms, 60% do not have findings on imaging and surgical intervention of these patients remains controversial [22].

Pheochromocytoma and Paraglanglioma

Pheochromocytoma has a reported incidence of 0.1–0.5% in the general population which correlates to 2–8 people per million per year. The "rule of 10s" previously supported the belief that approximately 10% of pheochromocytomas occur in the setting of heritable familial syndromes. This has proven to be an underestimate as more syndromes have been recognized and testing has become more frequent [26]. Some estimates suggest that 24–30% of sporadic pheochromocytomas occur within familial syndromes including vHL, neurofibromatosis 1, multiple endocrine neoplasias type 2, and succinate dehydrogenase mutations [27, 28]. More recently, this statistic has been contested citing referral and catchment area bias, and revised estimates are between 11.6 and 19%. Within vHL patients, the rate of pheochromocytomas is 10–20 % [14]. However, the true risk of developing a pheochromocytoma depends on the type of vHL, varies among kindreds, and ranges from 0 % to upward of 57 %.

The demographics and manifestations of pheochromocytoma in vHL differ significantly compared to patients with sporadic disease, as well as when compared to other familial pheochromocytomas. The mean age of presentation is 30 years but has been reported prior to the age of 10 [14]. Pheochromocytomas in vHL patients are less likely to present with the classic signs and symptoms (palpitations, headache, diaphoresis, hypertension, tachycardia, pallor, and nausea) than sporadic pheochromocytoma. Over one-third of pheochromocytoma in vHL are clinically asymptomatic. Most pheochromocytomas in vHL are within the adrenal gland and up to 50 % of vHL patients have bilateral intra-adrenal disease. However, extra-adrenal paragangliomas also are more prevalent compared to sporadic disease, with 12 % of vHL patients having extra-adrenal disease, and some patients having bilateral intra-adrenal as well as extra-adrenal disease (Fig. 2). Paragangliomas can arise in the glomus jugulare, carotid body, and the periaortic tissues. Pheochromocytoma in vHL is less likely to have malignant transformation than pheochromocytoma in sporadic disease, with a rate of 3.3 %.

Patients with a diagnosis of vHL or at-risk family members with a known carrier status for a germline mutation should undergo routine screening for pheochromocytoma regardless of their disease subtype. Screening for pheochromocytoma should include both biochemical and radiographic testing. Biochemical screening is recommended to begin annually no later than 5 years of age with some studies suggesting initiating screening even earlier [14]. Serum chromogranin A is a nonspecific marker with poor sensitivity and is not a standard part of screening. Plasma-free metanephrines and normetanephrines are used as the first-line screening tool in vHL as in sporadic disease with a sensitivity of 97–100 % and specificity of 85–89 %. As with testing in sporadic disease, attention must be given to the medication list and testing environment to limit the rate of false-positive results. If the results from the serum testing are equivocal, the patient should conduct a 24-h urine collection for catecholamines. When performed correctly, urine biochemical studies have a sensitivity and specificity of 98 and 98 %, respectively, for pheochromocytoma; however, they are cumbersome for the patient to collect and are prone to errors in collection.

Regardless of the method of testing, pheochromocytoma in vHL has a predictable biochemical signature, with elevations in norepinephrine and normetanephrine, without elevations in epinephrine and metanephrine levels (as demonstrated by both patients in Figs. 1 and 2). In contrast, sporadic disease and other familial syndromes such as multiple endocrine neoplasia (MEN) have concurrent elevations of epinephrine and metanephrine [29]. The reason for primary production of norepinephrine in vHL patients is the relative

lack of phenylethanolamine-N-methyltransferase (PNMT) responsible for the conversion of norepinephrine to epinephrine found exclusively within the adrenal medulla. vHL patients also express less tyrosine hydroxylase (the rate-limiting enzyme in catecholamine synthesis) than do patients with MEN2.

The age for initiating radiographic imaging for intra-abdominal manifestations of vHL is no later than 8 years of age. Family history and physical examination may suggest the need for earlier imaging as well as biochemical testing on a case-by-case basis and left to the discretion of the individual's physician. The imaging modality of choice for screening of at-risk (known mutation carriers with no previous intra-abdominal lesions and negative biochemical studies) and asymptomatic established vHL patients is abdominal ultrasonography. If biochemical abnormalities are found, the most appropriate follow-up imaging study is an abdominal MRI in an effort to minimize the cumulative ionizing radiation exposure over a lifetime of repeated imaging studies. This is in contrast with sporadic disease, which can be evaluated with a dedicated adrenal protocol CT of the abdomen and pelvis with intravenous and oral contrast if there are no allergic or renal contraindications to intravenous contrast. CT and MRI have been shown to be equally efficacious.

In cases where CT/MRI are negative but there is high clinical suspicion or abnormalities in biochemical studies, a metaiodobenzylguanidine (MIBG) scan can be performed for localization with sensitivity of 95 % [30]. Recently, using CT/positron emission tomography (PET) with 18F-Dopa to localize pheochromocytomas has been studied. Small studies have shown a nearly 100 % sensitivity for pheochromocytomas. Unfortunately, the availability and acceptance of the test have been inhibited in part due to high cost and difficulty of synthesizing the 18F-Dopa [31]. All imaging modalities will have a lower sensitivity for small-volume disease.

Some image-detected pheochromocytomas in vHL do not result in elevated biochemical levels of catecholamines and there is no consensus on intervention or observation in that scenario. While some will intervene on any detected pheochromocytoma, others advocate withholding surgical intervention until the 24-h urine catecholamine excretion is double the upper limit of normal, or to remove nonfunctional pheochromocytoma if the tumor has grown to greater than 3.5 cm in diameter, the patient is to undergo an abdominal operation for another pathology, or if the patient desires to become pregnant or becomes pregnant [32].

Traditionally, the treatment of intra-adrenal pheochromocytoma is ipsilateral adrenalectomy, which classically was performed using an open technique by either a transabdominal or a posterior approach. With the advent of laparoscopy, today's standard is a laparoscopic approach by either the lateral transabdominal or the posterior retroperitoneal approach, depending on the preference and expertise of the surgeon and center. There also are experiences with single port, robotically assisted, and single port robotic approaches to this procedure through both the transabdominal and retroperitoneal approaches. It is the opinion of these authors that there is at most marginal superiority of any one of these variations on minimally invasive adrenalectomy, beyond the significant benefit that resulted with dissemination of minimally invasive adrenalectomy techniques in general. Regarding the transabdominal versus the retroperitoneal approach, we select the approach best suited to the patient's anatomy and prior operative history.

Traditionally, adrenalectomy is performed as a complete extirpation of the gland in question. Either sequential or simultaneous total adrenalectomy renders the patient surgically an-adrenal, and thus completely dependent on exogenous steroids, with associated quality-of-life impairment and risk for Addisonian crisis. This approach mandates thorough patient counseling and education. More recently, multiple large case series have demonstrated partial adrenalectomy (i.e., cortical-sparing adrenalectomy) via open, lateral or posterior laparoscopy, and robotic-assisted approaches to be safe and efficacious [33–35]. This involves removing the target lesion from the adrenal gland and leaving behind the grossly and radiographically normal portion of the gland. The main adrenal vein may be spared or sacrificed depending on the location of the tumor. The venae comitantes running with the arterial supply are adequate to maintain drainage even if the main adrenal vein is sacrificed, and as little as 10 % of a viable single adrenal gland has been shown to maintain adequate function to handle stress without requiring exogenous steroids [36]. Cortical-sparing adrenalectomy has been validated in the pediatric population with hereditary forms of pheochromocytoma [37]. The ability to leave a viable cortical remnant allows patients the opportunity to retain adrenocortical function, without dependence on exogenous steroids, while achieving comparable biochemical responses. Rates of Addisonian crises and long-term steroid replacement are significantly lower compared to complete adrenalectomy [33, 36, 38, 39]. As expected, recurrence rates are higher and time to recurrence is shorter with partial adrenalectomy. Outcomes data suggest these rates to be within an acceptable range and successfully treated with surveillance screening and additional surgery. The National Cancer Institute published their experience on hereditary pheochromocytoma as having a 6 % recurrence rate, which has been reproduced at other high-patient volume centers [38, 40]. In patients with vHL, the recurrence rate after partial adrenalectomy has been reported to be from 10 to 20 % after at least a 5-year follow up [39, 41]. The recent acceptance of cortical-sparing adrenalectomies makes it impossible to comment on the rates of patients that subsequently develop malignant pheochromocytoma and underscores the ongoing need for lifelong surveillance after surgical resection. In instances where addi-

tional pheochromocytomas develop, the benefit of adrenalsparing surgery lies in delaying the development of adrenal insufficiency and subsequent lifetime duration of exposure to exogenous steroid. Therefore, the decision to perform cortical-sparing adrenalectomy versus total adrenalectomy must be made with consideration of the patient's willingness and ability to tolerate adrenal insufficiency versus recurrence of disease with subsequent reoperation. The ultimate success of both approaches demands ongoing patient follow up.

Surveillance recommendations for pheochromocytoma recurrence after resection have not been defined for vHL. Frequency of testing and type of imaging study is largely dependent on provider preference and experience at the institution. Below are the author's most conservative recommendations in conjunction with the vHL Alliance, based on the available published literature. After surgery, patients should undergo corticotropin-stimulation testing to assess the need for steroid replacement therapy prior to discharge if an adrenal-sparing procedure was performed and receive appropriate follow up with a medical endocrinologist. Some patients will need short-term replacement, which can be subsequently tapered over several months postoperatively. In addition, a routine postoperative MRI should be performed in addition to biochemical testing between 3 and 6 months after surgery. If no abnormalities are noted and the patient remains asymptomatic, imaging can appropriately be extended to an annual basis.

The importance of lifelong surveillance and screening for disease cannot be overemphasized. Patients who are followed up routinely have smaller and less functionally active tumors at diagnosis, which has a direct impact on their quality of life, treatment options, and prognosis [14]. Those vHL patients lost to follow up or who do not receive appropriate screening and surveillance later present at a larger tumor size and higher incidence of associated symptoms than sporadic disease of similar size [14]. This is well demonstrated in the patient in Fig. 1 who was not diagnosed until age 47 and then presented with a large adrenal pheochromocytoma, and in Fig. 2 in which the patient had been lost to follow up for 10 years before presenting with a large paraganglioma.

Pancreatic Lesions

Pancreatic lesions occur in 17–75 % of vHL patients and include cysts, microcystic adenomas with complete cystic replacement, and pancreatic neuroendocrine tumors (PNET) [42–44]. Though rare, metastatic disease to the pancreas particularly from RCC also has been documented and should be considered in the differential diagnosis. Patients and providers should be reassured that the diagnosis of vHL does not increase the risk of pancreatic adenocarcinoma. While the most prevalent pancreatic lesions in vHL patients are benign simple cysts and serous cystadenomas, we will focus on PNETs due to their greater clinical significance.

PNETs account for 1.3 % of all pancreatic tumors in the general populations, but 8–17 % of pancreatic lesions in patients with vHL [43]. The lifetime risk of developing one or more PNETs in vHL patients is 20 %, and in 6–8 % of vHL patients, it is the only manifestation of the disease [45]. PNETs in vHL present at a younger average age (35 years, see Fig. 2) compared to sporadic disease (58.5 years) [43, 46]. The specific vHL mutation has clinical implication with PNETs being more frequent in patients with missense mutations, and patients with exon 3 mutations being more likely to suffer metastasis from PNET [42, 47]. The majority of PNETs in vHL are nonfunctional and asymptomatic with a Surveillance, Epidemiology, and End Results (SEER) database review demonstrating biochemical function in 9.2 % [46]. When they are symptomatic, the most frequent complaints are changes in stool and epigastric pain related to mass effects of the tumor rather than syndromes of hormone excess. Pancreatic insufficiency and obstructive jaundice are rare presentations as are symptoms of malabsorption and diabetes [43].

Laboratory values such as chromogranin A and pancreatic polypeptide (PP) are not reliable for detection of PNET in vHL. For this reason, as well as lack of clinical symptomatology, the diagnosis is typically made by radiographic appearance or pathologic analysis. In symptomatic patients, biochemical studies, discussed in greater detail in a previous chapter, should be obtained to identify hormone excess and facilitate perioperative management. If the patient is not symptomatic on careful review of systems, serum hormone testing is not absolutely required, but frequently is performed [42]. When found on routine imaging, approximately two-third of PNETs in vHL are solitary pancreatic lesions, but also can be multiple as seen in Fig. 2. PNETs in vHL have a frequent concurrent presentation with pheochromocytomas with a rate of 33–63 % captured on the same imaging study [47].

Typical features of PNET on contrasted CT include an early enhancing, well-circumscribed, solid mass with rounded or lobulated borders. The early enhancement (or increased intensity with the arterial phase) correlates with the tumor's rich vascular supply [45]. When considering the cumulative lifelong radiation exposure, MRI is the preferred imaging modality [25]. A pancreatic lesion concerning for PNET on MRI will show increased signal intensity of T2-weighted images. The current guidelines recommend an abdominal MRI every 2 years for assessment of the kidneys, pancreas, and adrenals with annual ultrasound starting at age 16 [25]. However, clinical suspicion or family history may warrant earlier evaluation. Other imaging modalities that can be used to assess a pancreatic lesion are endoscopic ultrasound (which allows biopsy when the diagnosis is in question) and

somatostatin receptor scintigraphy. A recent evaluation by the NIH suggests that 18FDG-PET may detect metastatic disease not detected by other modalities [48].

The natural history remains unpredictable with PNET in sporadic or genetically linked cases. Nonlinear growth patterns have been documented in the literature numerous times. One study demonstrated that 20 % decrease in size, 20 % showing no interval change, and the 60 remaining percent have significant rates of tumor growth and activity within vHL patients [49]. To add an additional layer of complexity, the growth pattern or growth rate is not associated with tumor grade or malignant transformation as partial and complete spontaneous regressions of malignant PNET have also been documented. While histologic staining for hormonal markers does not correlate with the functional secretory state of the lesion, staining with anti-chromogranin A and anti-synaptophysic antibodies is used to assist in confirming the diagnosis [43].

Simple cystic lesions of the pancreas can generally be followed with observation and routine imaging regardless of size-reserving intervention for symptomatic lesions [43]. Since PNETs in vHL typically are nonfunctional, slow-growing, and the majority are benign, it is important to carefully weigh the decision to observe or to subject the patient to a major surgical intervention. However, this is balanced against the fact that aggressive surgical intervention offers the best potential for a cure and prevention of metastatic disease. This is another area in which there is no consensus, but Libutti et al. developed guidelines based on genetic analysis and tumor characteristics to distinguish which patients would benefit from early surgical intervention and which patients could safely be observed. Based on these data from the NIH series, observation is recommended if the solid pancreatic lesion is less than 3 cm in size, the mutation is not within exon 3, and tumor doubling time is greater than 500 days. Using these guidelines, they showed that 0 of their 25 patients with PNET that met surgical criteria had any signs of metastatic disease following resection over a follow-up period of 4–110 months [44]. They recommend resection if the tumor is greater than 3 cm (or greater than 2 cm in the pancreatic head) without evidence of metastatic disease, or if the patient is undergoing a laparotomy for management of another process in the same surgical field (such as left adrenalectomy for a tail of pancreas lesion). If these criteria are not met, the tumor can be followed with annual imaging [44].

The surgical approaches for PNET are based on location and include pancreaticodudenectomy (**Whipple** procedure), distal pancreatectomy, central pancreatectomy, total pancreatectomy, and enucleation. Despite the concern by some that enucleation has a prohibitive rate of pancreatic fistula, enucleation is considered by many others to be the treatment of choice when technically feasible. To attempt to limit the rate of pancreatic fistula, the target lesion must be greater than 2–3 mm from the pancreatic duct. Intraoperative ultrasound may aid in these cases to assess the relationship of the tumor to the pancreatic duct. In vHL patients, the possibility of a concurrent pheochromocytoma and renal cell cancer should be investigated with biochemical testing and careful review of preoperative imaging. If a pheochromocytoma is found, resection of the PNET should be done only after the removal of the pheochromocytoma, but this may be done under the same anesthetic depending on hemodynamic stability.

A PNET that manifests metastasis (typically to the liver) is malignant by definition, occurring in 2–17% of vHL patients that develop a neuroendocrine tumor. Malignant transformation of PNET is associated with a poor prognosis with a survival average of 1–3 years. This again underscores the importance of appropriate follow up and lifelong surveillance in vHL [44, 45]. In such cases, resection (even incomplete), ablation, hepatic artery ligation, and embolization and/or isolated hepatic chemotherapeutic perfusion should be considered as treatment options. Resection is preferred if the patient is a reasonable operative candidate, the lesions are technically resectable, and there is adequate hepatic reserve, while the non-extirpative options are used adjunctively. Intervention is rarely curative but has been associated with survival benefit. In the case of symptomatic disease, a significant percentage of patients have improvements or resolution of their symptoms.

The current surveillance recommendations in vHL patients with known lesions or post-resection include a pancreatic protocol abdominal CT or MRI. Imaging should be performed annually in patients who had a solid pancreatic lesion and every 2 years for complex or cystic lesions [25].

Renal Cell Carcinoma

Intra-tumoral vHL gene mutations are well known even in sporadic RCC occurring in 34–78% [50, 51]. Germline vHL mutations predispose to markedly high rates of RCC. vHL patients have a lifetime risk of 90–95% of developing cystic or solid renal lesions and 24–45% develop RCC [52]. RCC is responsible for 13–42% of all-cause mortality in this population [53, 54]. vHL-associated RCC is exclusively of the clear cell morphology and accounts for 1.6% of all RCC [5].

The tumors' manifestation and behavior vary significantly when comparing sporadic versus vHL-associated RCC. The average age at presentation in vHL is 34; 25 years earlier than sporadic RCC [5]. In vHL patients, RCC is more likely to be associated with renal cysts, to be bilateral (71–83%), and to be multifocal (92%) [5, 54]. Careful pathologic examination reveals as many as 1100 cystic lesions, and 600 clear cell neoplasms in a vHL kidney [51, 55]. Although RCC is the most common metastatic lesion in vHL, com-

pared to sporadic RCC, tumors are slow growing and have a lower incidence of metastasis. The 10-year disease-specific survival of vHL associated RCC was 94 versus 74% in sporadic RCC [5].

Recognizing RCC at earlier stages remains critical to preserving renal function. Initial screening can be performed using ultrasound and reliably distinguishes lesions into two categories; simple cysts and everything else. RCC commonly presents as a complex cystic lesion and is characterized per the radiographic Bosniak classification. Concerning features on imaging include thickened irregular or abnormal enhancement on the walls or septa as well as enhancing soft-tissue components adjacent to the cyst [51]. Lesions biopsies are not routinely performed. Further evaluation is necessary when other types of lesions are found and can be adequately imaged through CT or MRI, with preference for MRI to avoid cumulative ionizing radiation.

Management options for a suspected RCC lesion in a vHL patient include observation, radical nephrectomy (unilateral or bilateral) with or without renal transplantation, nephron-sparing or partial nephrectomy, enucleation, and more recently, radiofrequency ablation and cryoablation [51, 52, 56–58]. In general, management strategies have moved away from radical resection and toward nephron-sparing approaches. Current recommendations are that surgical intervention is indicated after the largest solid lesion reaches 3 cm or greater in diameter [52]. This threshold has been shown to be associated with minimal risk of metastasis, more frequent ability to perform parenchymal-sparing procedures, preservation of renal function, and minimizes the number of procedures for the patient [53]. Identified solid lesions measuring less than the 3 cm threshold can be safely monitored with CT or MRI every 6–12 months. While cystic lesions may have islands of disease, their presence is not factored into the decision to operate.

Tissue-sparing techniques such as enucleation and partial nephrectomy are the most common interventions. Enucleation has been associated with decreased rate of positive margins compared to partial nephrectomy likely secondary to the predictable, well-defined pseudocapsule surrounding the lesion [58]. At the time of surgery, the target lesion is removed in addition to all other accessible cysts. Use of an intraoperative ultrasound may be used to localize any additional resectable lesions at the time of surgery [53]. Complications tend to be temporary; however, renal atrophy and need for dialysis has been documented [52]. The patient undergoing a tissue-sparing procedure should understand that surgery is not curative as the remainder of the kidney is highly probable to develop, or already harbor, other sites of RCC. The chance of local recurrence is high (29 vs. 85% at 5 and 10 years, respectively) compared to 4–9% in sporadic cases [52, 54]. Thus, patients should be counseled on the necessity of ongoing surveillance and the likelihood of additional surgeries. However, this likelihood of local recurrence is not associated with a decrement in 10-year survival. When this information is coupled with the many downsides of dialysis dependence, it is understandable that prophylactic bilateral nephrectomies have no role in the management of the disease [54]. While the latter has the advantage of removing all involved tissue, vHL patients have a 65% 5-year survival on renal replacement after this surgery compared to 71–86% in the general population [51]. Renal transplantation has been explored, but there is limited long-term data.

Papillary Cystadenoma of the Epididymis, Broad Ligament, and Mesosalpinx

Papillary cystadenomas are rare, benign, but locally invasive epithelial tumors of mesonephric origin [59]. The presence of a papillary cystadenoma within the adnexal reproductive structures particularly the epididymis, broad ligament, and mesosalpinx is considered a vHL-associated lesion. Approximately one-third of male vHL patients have epididymal lesions. These present at a mean age of 35 (range of 16–76) and are located within the efferent ductules of the head of the epididymis. Lesions may occur unilaterally, but the apparently sporadic discovery of bilateral papillary cystadenomas should be considered highly suggestive of vHL [60]. Frequently, the lesions are asymptomatic and found during routine examination. If symptomatic, the patients most frequently describe painless, gradual scrotal swelling and occasionally note tenderness or infertility [59, 61, 62]. Ultrasound is the preferred imaging modality for characterization of papillary adenomas [60]. Demographic information on the female-associated manifestations of papillary cystadenoma is limited based on the lack of available published data on small case series [63].

Because they are benign and most are asymptomatic, resection is not usually indicated. When symptomatic, management is surgical resection and includes testicle-sparing excision versus orchiectomy. Microscopically, the epithelial cells contain glycogen or fat creating the appearance of a central clearance [61]. Due to similar histological appearance, it is important to differentiate a papillary cystadenoma from metastatic clear cell RCC [59, 63]. No surveillance guidelines have been reported.

Special Considerations

Pregnancy

A diagnosis of vHL carries unique implications for the pregnant patient. An analysis of maternal and fetal outcomes in a vHL cohort found fetal survival rate to be 96.4% and a maternal morbidity rate of 5.4–17% that was directly associated with a known vHL lesion [64, 65]. No maternal mortalities are reported in the small published case series [64–67]. As such, pregnancy should not be discouraged on the grounds of a prior vHL diagnosis. However, genetic and prenatal counseling are appropriate when a patient is contemplating pregnancy with a known diagnosis, or as a member of an established kindred. The involved parties should understand the risk the fetus has of inheriting the disease and possible fetal complications such as growth restriction and fetal demise. Parents should be made aware that antenatal diagnosis is possible. In addition, the patient would benefit from referral to a specialized care center with a multidisciplinary team experienced in vHL patients. While there are not established prenatal or screening guidelines for vHL, this is an important opportunity to perform a thorough evaluation of the mother and delineate management strategies of existing lesions or potential risks. Intense prenatal care and counseling has been shown to decrease fetal mortality and maternal morbidity [67].

Several studies have documented that pregnancy is associated with growth of vHL associated lesions with particular attention to hemangioblastomas and pheochromocytoma [65]. The accelerated growth of hemangioblastomas has been linked to hormonal changes and increases in venous pressure during pregnancy causing venous distension and subsequent release and stimulation of angiogenic factors [65, 66]. Case reports of pancreatic and renal lesions that develop or become symptomatic during pregnancy also exist but are less likely to require prepartum surgical attention and do not appear to be adversely impacted by pregnancy.

In the case of a pheochromocytoma, the lesion should be removed if at all possible prior to pregnancy. Exacerbation of pregnancy-related hypertensive disorders such as eclampsia has been documented and is among the most common and serious vHL complications encountered in this patient population. Medical management of hypertension is the same as in sporadic pheochromocytoma with focus on alpha-blockade [65, 67]. In cases of an adrenal mass, in the absence of biochemical evidence of pheochromocytoma, in a normotensive and otherwise asymptomatic gravid patient, increased surveillance of the fetus and mother is warranted but surgery is not immediately indicated.

All other vHL lesions should be carefully monitored for onset or worsening symptomatology during pregnancy. Frequent fetal monitoring with nonstress testing, Doppler studies, and routine ultrasounds are recommended [67]. Surgical intervention for many lesions may be delayed until close to expected delivery date. It is important to remember the potential for preterm labor postoperatively particularly in the third trimester of pregnancy as well as the anesthetic concerns in cases with a CNS lesion [66, 67]. If surgery is unavoidable, delivery of the baby has been safely performed via either vaginal delivery or cesarean section with concurrent or peripartum surgical management of the vHL lesion.

Synchronous Multiorgan Visceral Tumors

Synchronous lesions can and do occur at time of diagnosis or during routine surveillance (patients in Figs. 1 and 2). The incidence of concurrent lesions within the abdominal viscera is of particular interest to the endocrine surgeon and presents a unique management scenario. As previously outlined, the pancreas, adrenals, and kidneys have defined criteria for timing of surgical resection. However, it may be appropriate to address multiple lesions during the same surgical intervention despite not all lesions meeting individual surgical indications [32]. The advantages to a single-stage procedure are to decrease the number of major abdominal surgeries for the patient, decrease the difficulty of multiple stage procedures from adhesions and scarring, decrease exposure to anesthesia and avoid delay of definite surgery for potentially metastatic or deleterious lesions [32]. Decisions of which lesions to address during an individual procedure should be tailored to the patient's particular combination of lesions. Preoperative planning should include order of procedures to be performed. Removal of a pheochromocytoma should be prioritized followed by any renal and pancreatic lesions depending on size and metastatic potential [32]. Overall complication rates of combined procedures have been shown to be comparable to that of the same procedures performed separately. The simultaneous availability of experienced specialists to address all planned lesions is yet another reason to manage vHL patients at a center experienced in their care.

Key Summary Points

- vHL is an autosomal inherited disorder linked to chromosome 3. The tumor suppressor gene product mediates the response to hypoxemia by upregulating angiogenesis, erythropoiesis, and the cell cycle.
- Neoplastic manifestations of vHL include neuraxial hemangioblastoma, retinal hemangioblastoma, endolymphatic sac tumors, pheochromocytoma, extra-adrenal paraganglioma, renal cell carcinomas, pancreatic cysts, pancreatic neuroendocrine tumors, epididylmal cysts, adenomas, and broad ligament cyst adenomas.
- Standardization of screening guidelines has been shown to increase life expectancy for vHL patients and is crucial in the appropriate care of these patients. Although there are disease subtypes with different patterns of penetrance, the screening guidelines are universal for all subtypes.
- CNS hemangioblastomas and RCC are the top causes of disease-related mortality in vHL.

- Compared to sporadic pheochromocytoma, those occurring in vHL present at a younger age, and more often are bilateral and extra-adrenal.
- The biochemical signatures of vHL-associated pheochromocytomas are elevated norepinephrine and normetanephrine without elevation in epinephrine and metanephrine. CT or MRI has been shown to be equally efficacious for imaging of the adrenals.
- Cortical-sparing adrenalectomy should be considered for vHL patients with pheochromocytoma.
- PNETs develop in 20 % of vHL patients and usually are nonfunctional and asymptomatic.
- Observation of PNET is recommended if the solid pancreatic lesion is less than 3 cm in size, the mutation is not within exon 3, and tumor doubling time is greater than 500 days.
- When taking a vHL patient to the operating room for any reason, it is important to evaluate first for pheochromocytoma.
- If multiple synchronous lesions are present, it may be appropriate to address multiple lesions in a single-stage operation despite not all lesions meeting individual surgical indications.

References

1. Lonser R. Glenn G. von Hippel-Lindau disease. Lancet. 2003;361:2059–67.
2. Friedrich C. Von Hippel-Lindau syndrome. A pleomorphic condition. Cancer. 1999;86:2478–82.
3. Maher E. Von Hippel-Lindau disease: a genetic study. J Med Genet. 1991;28:443–7.
4. Neumann H. Prevalence, morphology and biology of renal cell carcinoma in von Hippel-Lindau disease compared to sporadic renal cell carcinoma. J Urol. 1998;160:1248–54.
5. Maher E. Clinical features and natural history of von Hippel-Lindau disease. Q J Med. 1990;77:1151–63.
6. Wilding A. Life expectancy in hereditary cancer predisposing diseases: an observational study. J Med Genet. 2012;49:264–9.
7. Latif F. Identification of the von Hippel-Lindau disease tumor suppressor gene. Science. 1993;260:1317–20.
8. McKusick V. Mendelian inheritance in man and its online version, OMIM. Am J Hum Genet. 2007;80(4):588–604.
9. Jaakkola P. Targeting of HIF-alpha to the von Hippel-Lindau ubiquitylation complex by O_2-regulated prolyl hydroxylation. Science. 2001;292:468–72.
10. Barry R. The von Hippel-Lindau tumour suppressor: a multi-faceted inhibitor of tumourigenesis. Trends Mol Med. 2004;10:466–72.
11. Kim W. Role of VHL gene mutation in human cancer. JCO. 2004;22:4991–5004.
12. Corless C. Immunostaining of the von Hippel-Lindau gene product in normal and neoplastic human tissues. Hum Pathol. 1997;28:459–64.
13. Webster A. An analysis of phenotypic variation in the familial cancer syndrome von Hippel–Lindau disease: evidence for modifier effects. Am J Hum Genet. 1998;63:1025–35.
14. Walther M. Clinical and genetic characterization of pheochromocytoma in von Hippel-Lindau families: comparison with sporadic

pheochromocytoma gives insight into natural history of pheochromocytoma. J Urol. 1999;162:659–64.

15. Stolle C. Improved detection of germline mutations in the von Hippel-Lindau disease tumor suppressor gene. Hum Mutat. 1998;12:417–23.

16. Lonser R. Prospective natural history study of central nervous system hemangioblastomas in von Hippel-Lindau disease. J Neurosurg. 2014;120:1055–62.

17. Neumann H. Hemangioblastomas of the central nervous system. A 10-year study with special reference to von Hippel-Lindau syndrome. J Neurosurg. 1989;70:24–30.

18. Asthagiri A. Prospective evaluation of radiosurgery for hemangioblastomas in von Hippel-Lindau disease. Neuro-Oncol. 2010;12:80–86.

19. Woodward E. VHL mutation analysis in patients with isolated central nervous system haemangioblastoma. Brain. 2007;130:836–42.

20. Singh A. Retinal capillary hemangioma: a comparison of sporadic cases and cases associated with von Hippel-Lindau disease. Ophthalmology. 2001;108:1907–11.

21. Singh A. Treatment of retinal capillary hemangioma. Ophthalmology. 2002;109:1799–806.

22. Lonser R. Tumors of the endolymphatic Sac in von Hippel–Lindau disease. N Engl J Med. 2004;350:2481–6.

23. Butman J. Mechanisms of morbid hearing loss associated with tumors of the endolymphatic sac in von Hippel-Lindau disease. JAMA. 2007;298:41–8.

24. Choo D. Endolymphatic sac tumors in von Hippel-Lindau disease. J Neurosurg. 2004;100:480–7.

25. VHL Alliance Web site. The VHL Handbook, What you need to know about VHL. A reference handbook for people with von Hippel-Lindau disease, their families, and support personnel. http://www.vhl.org/wordpress/patients-caregivers/resources/vhl-handbooks/. Updated July 17, 2014. Accessed 1 Aug 2014.

26. Elder E. Pheochromocytoma and functional paraganglioma syndrome: no longer the 10 % tumor. J Surg Oncol. 2005;89:193–201.

27. Neumann H. Germ-line mutations in nonsyndromic pheochromocytoma. N Engl J Med. 2002;346:1459–66.

28. Mazzaglia P. Hereditary pheochromocytoma and paraganglioma. J Surg Oncol. 2012;106:580–5.

29. Eisenhofer G. Pheochromocytomas in von Hippel-Lindau syndrome and multiple endocrine neoplasia type 2 display distinct biochemical and clinical phenotypes. J Clin Endocrinol Metab. 2001;86:1999–2008.

30. Neumann H. Pheochromocytomas, multiple endocrine neoplasia type 2, and von Hippel-Lindau disease. N Engl J Med. 1993;329:1531–8.

31. Nanni C. 18F-DOPA PET and PET/CT. J Nucl Med. 2007;48:1577–9.

32. Hwang, J. Surgical management of multi-organ visceral tumors in patients with von Hippel-Lindau disease: a single stage approach. J Urol. 2003;169:895–8.

33. Walther M. Laparoscopic partial adrenalectomy in patients with hereditary forms of pheochromocytoma. J Urol. 2000;164:14–7.

34. Boris R. Robot-assisted laparoscopic partial adrenalectomy: initial experience. Urology. 2011;77:775–80.

35. Julien J. Robot-assisted cortical-sparing adrenalectomy in a patient with von Hippel-Lindau disease and bilateral pheochromocytomas separated by 9 years. J Laparoendosc Adv Surg Tech. 2006;16:473–7.

36. Baghai M. Pheochromocytomas and paragangliomas in von Hippel–Lindau disease: a role for laparoscopic and cortical-sparing surgery. Arch Surg. 2002;137:682–9.

37. Rogers C. Concurrent robotic partial adrenalectomy and extra-adrenal pheochromocytoma resection in a pediatric patient with von Hippel-Lindau disease. J Endourol. 2008;22:1501–4.

38. Grubbs E. Long-term outcomes of surgical treatment for hereditary pheochromocytoma. J Am Coll Surg. 2013;216:280–9.

39. Benhammou J. Functional and oncologic outcomes of partial adrenalectomy for pheochromocytoma in patients with von Hippel-Lindau syndrome after at least 5 years of followup. J Urol. 2010;184:1855–9.

40. Diner E. Partial adrenalectomy: the National Cancer Institute experience. Urology. 2005;66:19–23.

41. Yip L. Surgical management of hereditary pheochromocytoma. J Am Coll Surg. 2004;198:525–34.

42. Blansfield J. Clinical, genetic and radiographic analysis of 108 patients with von Hippel-Lindau disease (VHL) manifested by pancreatic neuroendocrine neoplasms (PNETs). Surgery. 2007;142:814–8.

43. Hammel P. Pancreatic involvement in von Hippel-Lindau disease. The Groupe Francophone d'Etude de la Maladie de von Hippel-Lindau. Gastroenterology. 2000;119:1087–95.

44. Libutti S. Clinical and genetic analysis of patients with pancreatic neuroendocrine tumors associated with von Hippel-Lindau disease. Surgery. 2000;128:1022–7.

45. Hough D. Pancreatic lesions in von Hippel-Lindau disease: prevalence, clinical significance, and CT findings. AJR. 2013;162:1091–4.

46. Halfdanarson T. Pancreatic neuroendocrine tumors (PNETs): incidence, prognosis and recent trend toward improved survival. Ann Oncol. 2008;19:1727–3.

47. Curley S. Surgical decision-making affected by clinical and genetic screening of a novel kindred with von Hippel-Lindau disease and pancreatic islet cell tumors. Ann Surg. 1998;227:229–35.

48. Sadowski S. Prospective evaluation of the clinical utility of 18-fluorodeoxyglucose PET CT scanning in patients with von hippel-lindau-associated pancreatic lesions. J Am Coll Surg. 2014;218:997–1003.

49. Weisbrod A. Assessment of tumor growth in pancreatic neuroendocrine tumors in von hippel lindau syndrome. J Am Coll Surg. 2014;218:163–9.

50. Schraml P. VHL mutations and their correlation with tumour cell proliferation, microvessel density, and patient prognosis in clear cell renal cell carcinoma. J Pathol. 2002;196:186–93.

51. Meister M. Radiological evaluation, management, and surveillance of renal masses in Von Hippel-Lindau disease. Clin Radiol. 2009;64:589–600.

52. Herring J. Parenchymal sparing surgery in patients with hereditary renal cell carcinoma: 10-year experience. J Urol. 2001;165:777–81.

53. Duffey B. The relationship between renal tumor size and metastases in patients with von Hippel-Lindau disease. J Urol. 2004;172:63–5.

54. Steinbach F. Treatment of renal cell carcinoma in von Hippel-Lindau disease: a multicenter study. J Urol. 1995;153:1812–6.

55. Walther M. Prevalence of microscopic lesions in grossly normal renal parenchyma from patients with von Hippel-Lindau disease, sporadic renal cell carcinoma and no renal disease: clinical implications. J Urol. 1995;154:2010–5.

56. Shingleton W. Percutaneous renal cryoablation of renal tumors in patients with von Hippel-Lindau disease. J Urol. 2002;167:1268–70.

57. Klatte T. The contemporary role of ablative treatment approaches in the management of renal cell carcinoma (RCC): focus on radiofrequency ablation (RFA), high-intensity focused ultrasound (HIFU), and cryoablation. World J Urol. 2014;32:597–605.

58. Longo N. Simple enucleation versus standard partial nephrectomy for clinical T1 renal masses: perioperative outcomes based on a matched-pair comparison of 396 patients (RECORd project). Eur J Surg Oncol. 2014;40:762–8.

59. Mehta G. Progression of epididymal maldevelopment into hamartoma-like neoplasia in VHL disease. Neoplasia. 2008;10:1146.

60. Choyke P. Epididymal cystadenomas in von Hippel-Lindau disease. Urology. 1997;49:926–31.

61. Odrzywolski K. Papillary cystadenoma of the epididymis. Arch Pathol Lab Med. 2010;134:630–3.

62. Cox R. Papillary cystadenoma of the epididymis and broad ligament: morphologic and immunohistochemical overlap with

clear cell papillary renal cell carcinoma. Am J Surg Pathol. 2014;38:713–8.

63. Nogales F. An analysis of five clear cell papillary cystadenomas of mesosalpinx and broad ligament: four associated with von Hippel-Lindau disease and one aggressive sporadic type. Histopathology. 2012;60:748–57.

64. Grimbert P. Pregnancy in von Hippel-Lindau disease. Am J Obstet Gynecol. 1999;180:110–1.

65. Frantzen C. Pregnancy-related hemangioblastoma progression and complications in von Hippel-Lindau disease. Neurology. 2012;79:793–6.

66. Hayden M. Von Hippel-Lindau disease in pregnancy: a brief review. J Clin Neurosci. 2009;16:611–3.

67. Kolomeyevskaya N. Pheochromocytoma and Von Hippel-Lindau in pregnancy. Am J Perinatol. 2010;27:257–63.

Eugen von Hippel and Arvid Lindau

1867–1939; 1892–1958

Steven K. Libutti

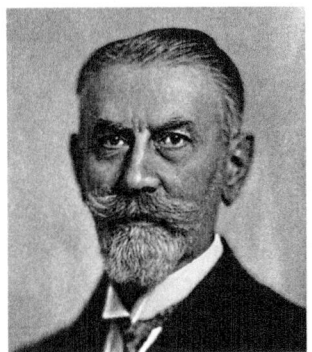

Professor Eugen von Hippel. (Courtesy of VHL Family Alliance)

Introduction

An autosomal dominant familial cancer syndrome, von Hippel–Lindau (vHL), affects numerous organs, most prominently the central nervous system (CNS; angiomas and hemangioblastomas), the ear (endolymphatic sac tumors), the pancreas (cysts, microcystic adenomas, pancreatic neuroendocrine tumors), the adrenal glands (pheochromocytomas), and the kidneys (cysts and renal cell carcinoma). For over a century, our understanding of this disease has evolved from observational and linkage analysis to a more complete genetic and molecular picture of the pathogenesis of the syndrome. Recommendations for screening (clinical, imaging, and genetic) and management have evolved and new agents are being developed and are the subject of clinical trials. With all these advances, it is important to understand how this inherited cancer syndrome was first recognized and to appreciate the physicians whose astute observations laid the foundation for our current approaches and advances.

S. K. Libutti (✉)
Surgery and Genetics, Albert Einstein College of Medicine, Broonx, USA

Department of Surgery, Montefiore Einstein Center for Cancer Care, Montefiore Medical Center, Greene Medical Arts Pavilion, 3400 Bainbridge Ave., 4th Floor, Broonx, 10467 NY, USA
e-mail: slibutti@montefiore.org

Eugen von Hippel was born in Königsberg, Germany (now Kaliningrad, Russian Federation), in 1867. Königsberg was a city on the eastern edge of Germany until it was captured by the Soviet Union at the close of World War II. Eugen was the son of Arthur von Hippel (1841–1916) a respected ophthalmologist and an early pioneer of corneal transplantation.

The younger von Hippel pursued formal education in some of the most prestigious institutions of his day. He studied in Giessen, Freiburg, Berlin, Heidelberg, and Göttingen, receiving his doctorate in medicine in 1890. Following medical school, he first pursued the study of pathology under the mentorship of Professor Arnold in Heidelberg. His primary focus at that time was on the effects of severe infections in cadavers. However, undoubtedly influenced by his father's example, Eugen began to specialize in ophthalmology in 1892 under the guidance of Professor Theodore Leber. Leber is best known for his descriptions of congenital amaurosis and hereditary optic neuropathy.

While working with Leber, von Hippel became interested with disorders in the formation of the eye, notably hydrophthalamus, corneal defects, cataracts, corectopia, and finally angiomatosis of the retina. Given his background in pathology, he was fascinated not only with his anatomic observations of these conditions but also in a broader understanding on their pathogenesis and embryonic origins. His work led to his seminal publication in 1904 [1]. The work described in detail a very rare disease of the retina that von Hippel termed "angiomatosis retinae."

Perhaps, what makes this work so impactful was not only von Hippel's description of the physical manifestations in great detail but also his observations of a linkage to a possible hereditary cause through his documentation of the presence of this rare condition in members of the same families. These keen strengths of observation, documentation, and attention to detail made Eugen von Hippel a very well-respected professor and teacher in his own right. He was known to create a very rich learning environment in his clinic and in his laboratory. He was well respected by his students and staff for encouraging discussion and debate while maintaining an inclusive interaction, which was unusual for the time.

J. L. Pasieka, J. A. Lee (eds.), *Surgical Endocrinopathies,* DOI 10.1007/978-3-319-13662-2_57,
© Springer International Publishing Switzerland 2015

He was not the typical professor of his era, as he welcomed being challenged. Dr. von Hippel was also known for being a caring and compassionate physician, often sought after to care for complicated problems.

Dr. von Hippel was devoted to his family. He was known for providing medical care to them for eye conditions as well as involving them in his work. One particular instance bears repetition as it illustrates the juxtaposition of work and family. When he was a child, Arthur von Hippel, Eugen's nephew, broke his glasses while playing ball. A small piece of glass was in his eye and he was brought to his uncle's laboratory to have it removed. While waiting in the laboratory for Dr. von Hippel to arrive, Arthur became bored and noticed a cage of monkeys in the back of the laboratory, no doubt subjects of an observational study. As young boys can often become victims of their own curiosity, the door to the cage was opened, and the monkeys quickly began to exercise their freedom by rampaging throughout the laboratory. When Dr. von Hippel arrived, he too had to exercise both literally to catch the monkeys and figuratively in restraining his displeasure. As Arthur had successfully assisted in recapturing the monkeys, he was not disciplined.

While Professor von Hippel is remembered for the syndrome that bears his name, he made other important contributions during his career. After spending 1909–1914 teaching at Halle and expanding his understanding of the signs and diagnostic approaches to retinal angiomatosis, he moved back home to become the head of the University Eye Clinic in Göttingen, a post his father had held for many years. While leading the Eye Clinic, he conducted a series of studies on tuberculosis of the eye, sympathetic ophthalmia, and chorioid membrane sarcoma. His writings focused on diseases of the optic nerve as well as the anatomy of the cornea.

Arvid Vilhelm Lindau was born in Malmö, Sweden, in 1892. His father was a regiment physician and after completing his undergraduate studies, Arvid pursued training as a military officer and physician. He completed his medical degree in Lund in 1923 and went on to receive a PhD in 1926. Lindau also studied bacteriology at the University of

Professor Arvid Lindau (1892–1958). (Courtesy of VHL Family Alliance)

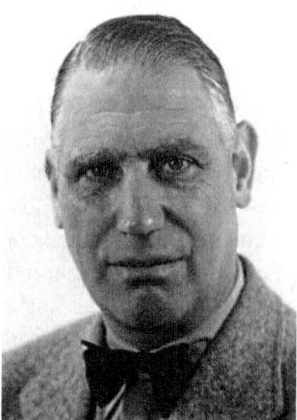

Copenhagen and at Harvard University on a Rockefeller Scholarship. He was both a pathologist at Lund and a military physician from 1924 to 1933.

Professor Lindau was a prolific researcher throughout his career on subjects in pathology, neurology, and bacteriology. His work in infectious diseases focused on bovine tuberculosis, Boeck's sarcoid, and Wasserman reaction. However, it was his work in neuropathology that would leave the most lasting impact.

Lindau was studying an association between angiomas of the retina and cerebellum. He noted their presentation appeared to occur together in families and postulated that the condition was heritable. In 1927, he published his doctoral thesis, a study of the association of cerebellar cysts with retinal angiomas [2]. This work would form the basis of much of the modern study of vHL.

Lindau's work came to the attention of Dr. **Harvey Cushing**, who had treated a patient with the condition Lindau described. Cushing visited Lindau's laboratory and invited Lindau to visit him in Baltimore. During the visit, they made rounds on Cushing's patients, one of whom thanked Cushing for saving his life. Cushing noted that it was not he who should be thanked, but rather Professor Lindau who had described the patient's condition. Lindau and Cushing remained friends and colleagues and corresponded throughout their careers.

Arvid Lindau was very active in his community. He held political office in his town and was a referee for local soccer games. He received numerous awards and honors and was the secretary of the Lund Medical Society. He was known for riding his bicycle to work and was fond of cars and motorcycles. He had a 1942 two-door Studebaker coupe and a motorcycle with a sidecar.

Lindau's most cited contribution is the observations linking the various CNS manifestations of vHL. However, throughout his career, he made substantive contributions to the fields of pathology and bacteriology publishing over 40 papers. In 1933, he became the chair of pathology, bacteriology, and general health science at Lund.

While the contributions of Eugen von Hippel and Arvid Lindau to the description of the familial syndrome that bears their names are unquestioned, it would be inaccurate not to mention the important work performed by others throughout the nineteenth and twentieth centuries that helped form the foundation of our modern understanding of vHL. Early observations by the English neurologist John Hughlings Jackson in 1872, and by the German ophthalmologist Hugo Magnus in 1874, helped to identify the eye lesions characteristically associated with the syndrome. Both Ernest Fuchs in 1882 and Treacher Collins in 1894 made contributions to the description of retinal manifestations and the apparent inherited nature of the lesions, respectively. The ophthalmologist, Wilhelm Czermak of Prague, observed an association between angiomas of the retina and cerebellar lesions in 1905.

The term "Lindau's disease," may have been first coined by Harvey Cushing in a published report of a case of a cerebellar hemangioma, where he made reference to Lindau's observations [3]. The syndrome was not termed von Hippel–Lindau until a 1936 publication by Davison, Brock, and Dyke [4]. Even then, it was not until the latter half of the twentieth century that the term gained widespread use. Finally, the understanding of the genetics of the disease was advanced by the work of Dr. Berton Zbar and Dr. Marston Linehan of the US National Cancer Institute.

References

1. von Hippel E. Uber eine sehr seltene Erkrankung der Netzhaut. Klin Beobachtungen Arch Ophthalmol. 1904;59:83–106.
2. Lindau A. Zur Frage der Angiomatosis retinae und ihrer Hirnkomplikationen. Acta Ophthalmol. 1927;4193–226.
3. Cushing H, Bailey P. Hemangiomas of the cerebellum and retina (lindau's disease); with the report of a case. Arch Ophthalmol. 1928;57:447–63.
4. Davison C, Brock S, Dyke CG. Retinal and centralfckLRnervous hemangioblastomatosis with visceral changes (von Hippel-Lindau's disease). Bull Neurol Instit NY. 1936;5:72–9.

Additional Sources

Personal correspondence Joyce Graff, VHL Family Alliance

Personal correspondence Dr. Eric von Hippel, Massachusetts Institute of Technology.

Jan Lindau, proceedings MEN/VHL Conference in Leeuwenhorst, the Netherlands, June 1997.

Overview of Eugen von Hippel, prepared by Joyce Graff, Dr. Harmut P.H. Neumann, Dr. Harry H. Wilcox and Mr. Richard Wolfe.

EyeWiki—www.eyewiki.aao.org

Multiple Endocrine Neoplasia Type 1

Kuan-Chi Wang and Mark Sywak

Introduction

Multiple endocrine neoplasia type 1 (MEN-1) is an autosomal-dominant disorder with synchronous or metachronous neoplasms of endocrine and non-endocrine organs. It predominantly manifests as a syndrome of parathyroid hyperplasia, pancreatic neuroendocrine tumors (pNETs), and/or pituitary adenoma. MEN-1 is a rare disorder with a prevalence of 2–3 cases per 100,000 [1].

The clinical presentation of MEN-1 was first noted by Jacob Erdheim in 1903 during the autopsy of an acromegalic man which showed a synchronous pituitary tumor with three enlarged fat-depleted parathyroid glands [2]. Half a century later, with advances in hormone assays, imaging, and histopathology, the syndromic manifestations were observed by Underdahl in a report of eight patients with tumors of the pituitary, parathyroid, and pancreatic glands [3]. Then in 1954, a year later, **Paul Wermer** first acknowledged these cases as a genetic disorder with "dominant hereditary transmission" through which "one autosomal-dominant gene (with high penetrance) is responsible for the whole pathologic picture" [4]. Despite naming this disease entity as multiple endocrine adenomatosis, his discovery led MEN-1 to be known as Werner syndrome. However, the nomenclature to classify the three different types of "multiple endocrine neoplasia" did not occur until 6 years later in 1968 by Steiner et al. [5]. Furthermore, recent studies examining germ-line mutations (*CDKN1B*) have led to the discovery of a distinct subset of MEN-1-like syndrome that was formally named MEN-4 in 2007 [6, 7].

Molecular Genetics of MEN-1

Molecular support for Werner's observation of this genetic syndrome arose in 1988 where linkage analysis was able to localize the MEN-1 gene to the long arm of chromosome 11 (11q13) [8]. In their study, Larsson et al. suggested that tumors in MEN-1 were probably caused by "loss of function." Systematic narrowing of the candidate gene interval and positional cloning of these intervals for the next 10 years allowed Chandrasekharappa to discover the MEN-1 gene in 1997 [9]. The MEN-1 gene is 9.8 kb long and consists of ten exons with an 1830-base-pair coding region. It is a tumor suppressor gene that encodes a unique 610-amino-acid protein named *menin*. *Menin* is unique as it is not homologous to any other proteins or peptides found, as such its putative function could not be easily elucidated. Studies have shown that *menin* is located primarily in the nucleus in nondividing cells, and there are at least two independent nuclear localization signals in the C-terminal of the protein [10, 11]. Its interactions with transcription factors such as JunD, C-Jun, Activating protein-1, and Smad3 indicate that *menin* is important in transcriptional regulation, genome stability, and cell division [12–17].

It is believed that mutations in the MEN-1 gene progress to disease via Knudson's two-hit hypothesis [18]. Specifically, this requires an inherited or somatically acquired inactivating mutation (first hit) and then another mutation at the same genetic locus (second hit). Thus, both copies of the MEN-1 gene are inactivated causing tumorigenesis. Usually, the "first hit" involves small mutations of only one or a few bases [19]. In around 75 % of cases, these mutations cause truncation of the *menin* protein causing loss of the C-terminal nuclear-localizing signal [10]. While the "second hit" is usually associated with large-scale loss of chromosomal material in somatic tissues during life, inactivation of both alleles compromises the nuclear localization of *menin* leading to its inactivation or absence and subsequently loss of function. The consequence of this is an increase in proliferation rate and transition from G0/G1 to S phase of the affected cells [20].

M. Sywak (✉) · K.-C. Wang
Endocrine Surgical Unit, University of Sydney, AMA House,
Suite 202, 69 Christie St, St. Leonards, NSW, Australia
e-mail: marksywak@nebsc.com.au

J. L. Pasieka, J. A. Lee (eds.), *Surgical Endocrinopathies*, DOI 10.1007/978-3-319-13662-2_58,
© Springer International Publishing Switzerland 2015

There are over 1000 MEN-1 gene mutations identified; approximately 45% are frame-shift deletions or insertions, 22% of these are due to nonsense mutations, 18% are missense mutations, 8% are in-frame deletions or insertions, and 7% are splice-site mutations [21–23]. It should be noted that in approximately 10% of cases, MEN-1 mutations arise de novo without any family history of the syndrome [23]. Furthermore, clinical manifestations of MEN-1 can occur without identifiable mutations in a known MEN-1 gene in 10% of cases. This can be explained by deletions or mutations in noncoding regions such as promotor and untranslated regions, whole-exon deletion or duplication, and inheritance through alternative MEN-1 locus [9, 23–25]. As such, care must be taken not to exclude patients with normal MEN-1 sequencing analysis when strong clinical features are present. Mutations in the MEN-1 gene show variable but high penetrance. By the age 20 and 40, approximately 50 and 100% of carriers with MEN-1 mutations will, respectively, have symptomatic or biochemically apparent disease [23]. In addition, MEN-1 mutations also show variable expression as studies have not been able to demonstrate a clear genotype–phenotype correlation [22]. This is in contrast to the well-described correlations which occur in MEN type 2. Consequently, it is difficult to predict the natural history of patients and families exhibiting MEN-1 disease.

Table 1 Percentage of clinical penetrance and presentation of MEN-1 patients

Pathology	Penetrance
Endocrine	
Parathyroid	>95%
Enteropancreatic	
Gastrinoma	30–40%
Insulinoma	10%
Functional	2%
Nonfunctional	20%
Pituitary	
Prolactinoma	20%
Other functional	10%
Nonfunctional	5%
Foregut neuroendocrine	
Gastric	10%
Thymic	6%
Bronchial	3%
Adrenal	
Nonfunctioning	20–30%
Pheochromocytoma	<1%
Non-Endocrine	
Facial angiofibromas	85%
Collagenomas	70%
Lipomas	10–30%
Leiomyomas	10%
Meningiomas	5%
Ependymomas	1%

Clinical Presentation and Diagnosis

MEN-1 patients today can present with clinical disease, which is typically due to primary hyperparathyroidism (HPT) or as a consequence of genetic screening. Clinical diagnosis in an index case requires at least two of the three principal endocrine organs to have evidence of tumor development. Genetic testing is confirmatory. For individuals within a known MEN-1 kindred, disease in one of the principal endocrine organs is considered diagnostic.

MEN-1 is known by its classic triad of tumorigenesis in the parathyroid (95%), enteropancreas (50–70%), and anterior pituitary glands (30–55%) [26–29]; however, tumorigenesis is not limited to these endocrine organs. Less commonly, MEN-1 patients have also been shown to have nonfunctioning foregut carcinoid (thymic, bronchial, and gastric), adrenal adenoma, facial angiofibroma, collagenoma, subcutaneous lipomas, leiomyomas, meningiomas, and ependymomas (Table 1). More than half of patients with MEN-1 present with two or more diseased organs, while 12–20% have demonstrated three affected organs [27]. The clinical manifestations of MEN-1 depend upon the site of tumorigenesis and associated hormonal hypersecretion. While any of the three principal organs can give rise to the initial presentation in an MEN-1 case, hyperparathyroidism is most often the first clinical problem [26–28, 30]. The

typical presenting problems in decreasing order of frequency include hypercalcemia, nephrolithiasis, peptic ulcer disease, hypoglycemia, headache, visual field loss, hypopituitarism, acromegaly, galactorrhea, amenorrhea, and *Cushing*'s syndrome [31]. It should be stressed that because of the variable expression of MEN-1 mutations, the combination of organs affected and the associated clinical manifestations have been shown to differ between family members, even twins [19, 27]. MEN-1 can first become apparent at a variety of ages with first presentations reported to occur from as young as 5 years up to 81 years of age [23, 32]. For females, the peak incidence occurs in the third decade of life, while for males it peaks during the fourth decade [29]. Biochemical abnormalities can be detected years before symptomatic disease becomes apparent [33, 34]. This makes careful biochemical screening an important part of the care of individuals from a known MEN-1 kindred. Diagnostic DNA analysis is not only helpful in confirming the clinical diagnosis of MEN-1 but also identifying at-risk patients for surveillance.

Patients with MEN-1 have lower life expectancy with a 50% mortality rate by the age of 50 years [35–37]. Death in MEN-1 is most commonly due to the malignant progression of pancreatic disease [35, 37]. While parathyroid and pituitary lesions can cause significant morbidity, they account for a smaller proportion of the overall mortality rate.

The main principles of managing patients with MEN-1 are to treat the hormone excess and preventing malignant progression of tumors. These are discussed below within each affected organ system.

Parathyroid Tumors

Clinical Presentation

Primary HPT is the most common clinical manifestation in individuals with MEN-1. Studies have shown that by 40 years of age, approximately 95 % of patients with MEN-1 mutations have parathyroid disease [27, 30]. HPT is also the most common initial presentation of MEN-1, accounting for 60–90 % of presenting complaints. The rate of symptomatic hypercalcemia is markedly decreased to 30 % in those patients within a known MEN-1 kindred who are known to be at risk and are undergoing regular biochemical surveillance. MEN-1 HPT accounts for only 2–4 % of all HPT cases in the community and 10 % of those with multiglandular disease [38]. MEN-1-related HPT differs from sporadic cases, and these differences have implications for the surgical management of this disease. First, the typical age of presentation is approximately 20–25 years of age, which is in marked contrast to sporadic HPT, which most commonly occurs during the fifth decade of life [27, 30]. Second, the sex distribution for MEN-1-related HPT is equal with males just as likely to have HPT as females [30, 32]. In contrast, sporadic HPT is three times more common in females. Thirdly, the pattern of parathyroid enlargement differs between MEN-1 and sporadic HPT. In sporadic HPT, approximately 90 % of cases are due to a single adenoma, while, in comparison, HPT in MEN-1 presents with multiglandular disease [39, 40]. The development of parathyroid hyperplasia in MEN-1 is asynchronous in nature with all four glands ultimately involved but at varying times. This gives rise to a pattern of asymmetrical disease with some glands showing significant growth, while others appear initially to be macroscopically normal [40, 41]. MEN-1 parathyroid disease is associated with supernumerary glands and ectopic glands in up to 15 % [42–44]. This pattern of multiglandular involvement and frequent occurrence of extra glands supports the traditional surgical approach of four-gland parathyroid exploration with cervical thymectomy. This approach has been challenged more recently with some groups advocating focused parathyroidectomy in selected cases [45]. Histopathologically, the enlarged glands show multiple monoclonal tumors, which have developed from polyclonal hyperplasia [46]. MEN-1 patients appear to demonstrate markedly increased levels of parathyroid mitogenic factor found within the serum of MEN1 patients. This mitogenic factor is similar to fibroblast growth factor and influences growth of the endothelial component of parathyroid glands [47]. Despite this mitogenic influence, it is unusual for HPT cases in MEN-1 to progress to parathyroid cancer [48–52].

Aside from the differences in age and sex distribution at presentation, the symptoms of MEN-1-associated HPT do not differ significantly from those seen in the sporadic form of the disease. In the past, up to 50 % of MEN-1 cases have presented with symptomatic renal calculi; however, with the advent of genetic testing and aggressive screening protocols, more patients are being managed with subclinical disease. The typical symptoms of HPT including bone abnormalities, musculoskeletal complaints, fatigue, and change in mental state are also seen. MEN-1 patients with HPT may complain of fatigue, polydipsia, polyuria, joint pain, bone pain, constipation, and sometimes depression.

Diagnosis

Inappropriately elevated intact serum parathyroid hormone levels in conjunction with hypercalcemia (raised ionized or total-albumin corrected serum calcium) are the principal biochemical characteristic in the diagnosis of HPT. Biochemical confirmation of HPT should always include measurement of 24-h urinary calcium to exclude benign familial hypocalciuric hypercalcemia. Determination of 1,25-dihydroxyvitamin D3 levels and serum blood urea and nitrogen and glomerular filtration rate (GFR) are important to rule out secondary causes of HPT. Screening for other elements of the MEN-1syndrome in patients considered a risk such as gastrin, insulin, Chromogranin A, pancreatic polypeptide (PP), IGF-1, VIP, glucagon, and prolactin can be obtained. Screening also includes cross-sectional imaging of the pancreas, adrenal glands, thymus, and pituitary. With the advent of minimally invasive surgery and focused parathyroid exploration for sporadic HPT, localization studies with ultrasound, sestamibi scintigraphy, or 4-D CT (four-dimensional computerized tomography) are now well established in the preoperative workup of sporadic cases. However, the role of localization studies for parathyroid tumors in MEN-1 is more controversial. This is because HPT in MEN-1 is multiglandular and traditional surgical approaches have required bilateral exploration. Parathyroid imaging for preoperative localization has not traditionally been advocated as a thorough four-gland exploration is the most widely adopted surgical approach [26, 53, 54]. However, the frequency of supernumerary glands and ectopic parathyroid locations challenges this view, and our practice more recently has been to routinely perform ultrasound and sestamibi scintigraphy prior to parathyroid surgery in MEN-1. This approach may also provide the surgeon and patient with the option of undertaking focused or minimally invasive parathyroid surgery if the imaging points to enlarged parathyroid glands confined to just one side of the neck [45]. Careful preoperative imaging is very important in planning surgery for patients with recurrent or persistent HPT, and in this setting concordant functional and anatomical imaging should be sought.

Management

The indications for parathyroid surgery generally follow the guidelines suggested for the management of asymptomatic HPT [55]. MEN-1 patients with Zollinger–Ellison syndrome should be considered for early parathyroid surgery as hypercalcemia is a potent stimulus for gastrin secretion, and normalizing parathyroid hormone levels improves control of hypergastrinemia [56, 57]. With the advent of easily available hormone assays, DNA analysis, improved imaging modalities, and surveillance of known MEN-1 kindreds, patients are increasingly presenting with mild HPT and are often asymptomatic. The question in these cases is when to initiate surgical intervention.

The ideal surgical approach to parathyroid disease in MEN-1 should strike a balance between minimizing the incidence of persistent or recurrent disease and avoiding permanent hypoparathyroidism. Surgery should be initiated in a timely fashion prior to the development of significant renal or skeletal complications. Prophylactic parathyroidectomy is generally not supported, and it is important that the surgeon understands that the outcome of permanent hypoparathyroidism may be worse than the disease itself considering there is rarely any malignant potential to parathyroid tumors in MEN-1 HPT. The timing of surgery and the specific surgical approaches are important and debatable. Some groups have suggested that delaying surgery until hypercalcemia worsens or symptoms develop allows the pathological glands to enlarge making success at the first operation greater and reduces the need for subsequent reoperations. However, proponents for early surgical intervention argue that normalization of hypercalcemia may not only decrease gastrin production but also help to avoid the skeletal and renal complications of HPT [57–62].

The main operative approaches at initial surgery are total parathyroidectomy with autotransplantation of a portion of parathyroid tissue (total parathyroidectomy; tPTX) or subtotal parathyroidectomy (sPTX; Fig. 1). In both procedures, cervical thymectomy is recommended to allow inspection of the thymus for supernumerary glands as well as potentially reducing the chance of thymic carcinoid tumors developing. In a small number of cases where preoperative imaging suggests asymmetric parathyroid disease, and parathyroid enlargement is confined to one side of the neck, we have undertaken unilateral parathyroid exploration with removal of the ipsilateral thymus via a small cervical incision [45]. This approach certainly avoids the problem of hypoparathyroidism; however, its long-term durability requires longer follow-up.

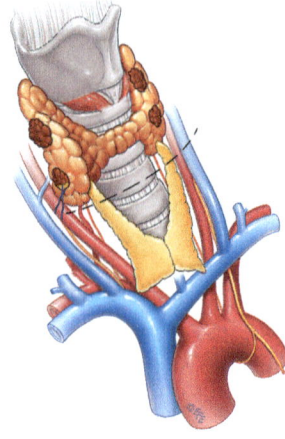

Fig. 1 Subtotal parathyroidectomy and bilateral cervical thymectomy. Incision is made over the *dotted line*. Then all four parathyroid glands are visualized with excision of all but approximately 50 mg of right inferior gland which is *marked with suture*. Bilateral cervical thymectomies are performed at the same time

The operative approach requires a delicate balance between avoiding recurrence and preventing hypoparathyroidism. The two main surgical approaches for MEN-1 HPT are tPTX or sPTX (Fig. 1). Procedures which involve a lesser approach to parathyroidectomy (<sPTX) than tPTX or sPTX are associated with higher (>50%) persistent or recurrent rates and lower disease-free intervals (7 years for<sPTX vs. 16.5 years for tPTX or sPTX) [63]. However, in selected cases, we have undertaken unilateral minimally invasive parathyroidectomy (MIP) with a resulting improvement in the complication profile and acceptable control of HPT [45]. Figure 2 illustrates a case in which unilateral parathyroidectomy has been performed with thymectomy.

The technique for total parathyroidectomy involves removing all visible parathyroid glands with autotransplantation of small fragments of parathyroid tissue from the most normal-appearing gland either into the brachioradialis muscle of the forearm or into the sternocleidomastoid muscle of the neck. Once all four parathyroids have been located, cervical thymectomy is undertaken and a portion of the most normal-appearing gland weighing approximately 50 mg is transplanted into the brachioradilais muscle of the nondominant upper limb via a longitudinal incision placed over the forearm [64]. This autotransplantation site is marked with titanium clips to facilitate excision in the event of graft hyperfusion. The remaining glands are removed and sent for histological assessment with a portion of tissue also saved for cryopreservation. The benefits of using cryopreserved tissue in hypoparathyroid patients have also been questioned by other groups who have demonstrated poor success rates after transplantation of cryopreserved tissue [65–69].

sPTX (Fig. 1), in which three and a half glands are removed with a small parathyroid remnant equal to approximately 50 mg left in situ on a vascularized pedicle, is utilized

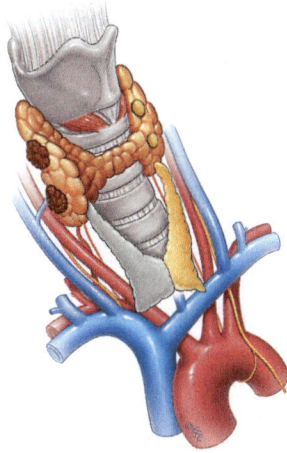

Fig. 2 Minimally invasive parathyroidectomy. In patients with localizing imaging, a focused or unilateral parathyroidectomy approach through minimal incision is recommended. In this procedure, all unilateral glands are explored and resected if found enlarged and at the same time unilateral cervical thymectomy is performed

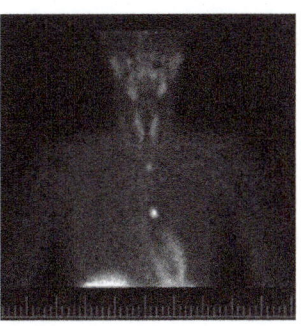

Fig. 3 4-D CT of patient with mediastinal hyperparathyroid. 4-D CT 4-dimensional computerized tomography

by many especially in the younger patients. Once the viability of the retained gland is established, the remaining glands are removed and the in situ parathyroid is marked with a nonabsorbable Prolene suture. At this point, a cervical thymectomy is performed. Cervical thymectomy has the theoretical advantage of decreasing the rate of MEN-1-associated thymic carcinoid tumors as well as increasing the disease-free survival rates [70–72]. However, it should be noted that cases of thymic carcinoid have been documented in patients with prior cervical thymectomy [73–76].

sPTX is associated with lower rates of hypoparathyroidism on the order of 1–10% compared with rates of 10–30% seen in tPTX. However, MEN-1 patients treated with sPTX have been shown to have recurrence rates within 10–12 years between 40 and 60% of patients, in comparison to sporadic HPT with rates of <5% [41, 77–84].

Persistent HPT in MEN-1 is typically due to the failure to identify and resect supernumerary or ectopic glands at the first procedure [85]. In addition, the development of hyperfunction in autotransplanted tissue or parathyroids which were retained at sPTX is a frequent cause of recurrence [85]. Index cases of MEN-1 who undergo surgery for what appears at initial presentation to be sporadic disease are at risk of recurrence as a result of the widespread use of minimally invasive techniques for parathyroidectomy and because hyperplasia may not have been appreciated at the initial procedure. As such, screening patients who present with HPT at a young age, <40 years for MEN-1, is appropriate. Imaging studies are essential for planning reoperative surgery in contrast to primary cases and having two concordant imaging modalities are ideal prior to proceeding to reoperative parathyroidectomy. Useful modalities include two or more of the following: CT, sestamibi, cervical ultrasonography,

MRI with sensitivities of 70–85, 70–85, 25–90, and 60–80%, respectively [86–90] (Fig. 3). In cases where forearm autotransplantation has been performed, graft hyperfunction can be demonstrated by drawing blood from both arms, while a tourniquet is applied to the side which carries the autotransplanted tissue. Known as the Casanova test, this approach can confirm differential PTH readings between the grafted forearm and peripheral blood and can direct the surgeon to either repeat cervical surgery or removal of the forearm graft. In difficult cases of recurrent disease, where ultrasound, sestamibi, 4-D CT, and MRI are unhelpful, we undertake selective venous sampling (SVS). This modality requires an experienced interventional radiologist and the mapping of PTH gradients from multiple sites along the internal jugular and mediastinal veins. SVS has been shown to correctly localize hyperfunctioning parathyroids in 60–85% of cases [91–94]. In cases where imaging has failed to confidently localize the site of recurrence, undirected cervical reoperation is usually best avoided, and we prefer to observe the patient for a period of 6 months before repeating our imaging algorithm.

After adequate preoperative imaging, reoperation for HPT in MEN-1 can often be undertaken as a focused procedure without the need for extensive dissection. The majority of recurrent intrathymic parathyroid tumors sit within the upper anterior mediastinum and can be successfully removed via cervical exploration. For tumors located deeper in the middle and posterior mediastinum and aorticopulmonary window, minimally invasive thoracic approaches and even formal sternotomy is necessary to establish safe surgical access.

Achieving normocalcemia after revision surgery for HPT in MEN-1 has been described in up to 70% of cases [72, 95]. Recurrences following reoperation are frequent and occur in 30–60% of patients with 10–30% of patients acquiring permanent hypoparathyroidism and 1–5% with permanent recurrent laryngeal nerve injury. In cases where surgery is not feasible or the patient is not a suitable operative candidate, ethanol ablation and angiographic embolization have been used with some success. Medical therapy with the calcimimetic agent Cinacalcet can be used to manage refractory cases where operative intervention is not appropriate.

Pancreaticoduodenal Neuroendocrine Tumors

Pancreatic and duodenal neuroendocrine tumors (PNETs) are the second most prevalent clinical manifestations of MEN-1 disease with clinical penetrance of 50–70% [27, 96]. However, autopsy studies have shown that almost 100% of MEN-1 patients, by the age of 40 years, have multiple nonfunctioning macroadenomas [97]. PNETs can present with clinical syndromes of hormone excess, most commonly from gastrinoma accounting for 30–40% of cases. However, nonfunctional tumors account for 20%. Other functioning PNETs include insulinoma (10%) and rarely glucagonoma, VIPoma, and somatostatinoma (2%; Table 1) [26].

In contrast to sporadic disease, MEN-1-related PNETs are solid, multifocal, and heterogeneous. Most are micro-adenomas (<0.5m) scattered throughout the pancreas and surround a larger macroadenoma. It has been theorized that these microadenomas may arise from pancreatic duct precursor cells because microadenomas are often surrounded by dysplastic (proliferating) exocrine ducts. Histologically, these lesions do not show normal islet-cell architecture and on immunohistochemistry can stain positively for numerous proteins such as chromogranin A, synaptophysin, neuron-specific enolase, as well as multiple hormones such as PP, glucagon, insulin, and somatostatin [98–101]. In addition, submucosal duodenal carcinoids are detected in >50% of patients with MEN-1-associated PNETs which have important implications during surgical intervention [102].

PNETs are the most frequent cause of mortality in MEN-1. At the time of clinical diagnosis, 30–50% of patients have lymph node or liver metastasis [34, 96, 103, 104]. Furthermore, studies have shown that nearly 50% of MEN-1-associated deaths before 50 years of age are due to pancreatic malignancy predominantly with liver metastasis [35–37, 104, 105]. Studies looking at the progression of PNETs have shown that they are an important factor in the long-term survival of MEN-1 patients [106, 107]. It remains controversial whether there is a correlation between tumor size and risk of metastasis. However, the French GTE (*Groupe d'etudes des tumeurs endocrines*) register did reveal that a tumor size of >3 cm correlated with a higher rate of metastasis (15–52%) [105, 108–111]. Interestingly, a recent Swedish study did not show any survival difference between MEN-1 PNET patients compared with similar sporadic cases and that survival itself can be correlated to tumor, node, metastasis (TNM) staging and Ki67 proliferation index [112]. Furthermore, it showed that nonfunctioning tumors had poorer survival. Whether this decreased survival is due to delayed presentation as they are asymptomatic, or that the disease itself is more aggressive, needs to be elucidated.

Functioning Pancreaticoduodenal Endocrine Tumors

Gastrinoma

Zollinger and **Ellison** in 1955 first described two patients with non-β islet cell pancreatic tumors with marked gastric acid production and subsequent recurrent peptic ulceration [113]. Then in 1960, Gregory was able to extract a gastric secretagogue, otherwise known as Gastrin, from these tumors [114, 115]. As such, gastrinoma is synonymous with the Zollinger–Ellison syndrome. Gastrinoma is a common presentation of MEN-1, and approximately 20–25% of patients with gastrinoma have MEN-1 disease [116]. The syndrome comprises tumors of the pancreas or duodenum that secrete gastrin and gastrin precursors, thereby mimicking gastrin secreted by G cells in the gastric antrum.

Similarly, to MEN-1 HPT disease, PNETs in these patients differ to sporadic cases, in that age of presentation is usually 10 years younger and that the disease is often multifocal [102, 117]. Gastrinomas in MEN-1 are commonly found in the duodenum (>90%) as small, multiple, and nodular, predominantly in the first and second part which is not dissimilar to sporadic cases [118]. Rarely, gastrinomas can be seen in the pancreas, and these are often large and associated with early liver metastasis.

Studies have shown that many MEN-1 patients have biochemical hypergastrinemia without clinical sequelae of Zollinger–Ellison syndrome. Approximately, 30–50% of symptomatic patients have nodal or liver metastasis [96, 103, 111, 119]. Those that have metastasized to the liver have a 50% 5-year survival rate [120]. Despite the multifocal and metastatic potential of gastrinomas in MEN-1, studies have not detected an expected worsened prognosis compared to sporadic cases; 5-year survival rates for all gastrinoma patients range between 62 and 75% [112]. However, currently there has been no correlation between genotype and disease progression as it can often differ significantly even between family members [34, 111]. Features associated with a worse prognosis are pancreatic primary, liver metastasis, ectopic Cushing's syndrome, or markedly elevated plasma gastrin concentrations [120].

Localization of gastrinoma may be challenging as these lesions are often small and multifocal. Investigations include CT, MRI, somatostatin receptor scintigraphy, gallium positron emission tomography (Ga-PET) scan and endoscopic ultrasound. CT and MRI are important in evaluating the pancreas, liver, lymph node status, and overt peritoneal disease. Figure 4 is an example of a CT scan of a patient with PNETs. Endoscopic ultrasound also has high sensitivity of up to 90%

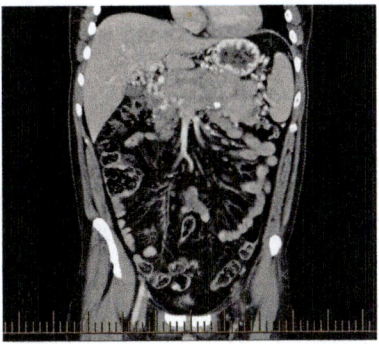

Fig. 4 CT scan in coronal view demonstrating enteropancreatic endocrine tumor. As can be seen the multifocal nature of the pancreatic lesions can be appreciated. *CT* computerized tomography

and has the added advantage of incorporating fine-needle biopsy of the suspected lesions [121–123]. Endoscopic ultrasound and intraoperative ultrasound have become the most reliable modalities for isolating pancreatic and duodenal lesions in our experience. Fluorodeoxyglucose (FDG) PET scan has a limited role in detecting most primary PNETs as they are commonly negative due to lesions being less than 5 mm. However, FDG PET is useful for evaluating metastatic disease. The recent use of Gallium 68-labeled octreotide scintigraphy (Ga-68 1,4,7,10-tetraazacyclododecane-NI,NII,NIII,NIIII-tetraacetic acid (D)-Phe1-thy3-octreotide (DOTATOC)) allows functional detection of the lesions and can often identify up to 35 % of occult tumors not seen in anatomical imaging [124]. It has a sensitivity of around 85 % and specificity of up to 100 % [124–126].

Treatment of gastrinoma involves managing the hypergastrinemia and surveillance for the development of malignancy. Medical treatment with acid inhibitors, such as proton pump inhibitors (PPIs), has markedly reduced the rate of death resulting from hypergastrinemia-induced metabolic complications. However, medical treatment does not prevent malignant transformation or metastatic disease, and this is where surgical intervention may play a role.

The aim of surgical intervention is to provide eugastrinemia as well as removing malignant or premalignant disease. There are several controversies regarding surgical management of gastrinoma in MEN-1, and these include timing and indication of surgery, type of surgery, and surgery for advanced disease. PNETs in MEN-1 are multifocal and as such curative excision of gastrinomas is unlikely. Norton, in 1999, in a prospective study showed that cure rates were 5 % at 5 years and 0 % at 10 years [118]. In comparison, sporadic cases had a cure rate of 34 % at 10 years. Furthermore, postoperative analysis demonstrated no survival benefit or decrease in rate of liver metastasis in patients who had undergone surgical excision [118, 127]. However, it should be noted in these studies, indications for surgery were lesions greater than 3 cm and/or symptoms of obstruction. Propo-

nents for delayed surgical intervention argue that even with metastatic disease, there is a 15-year survival rate of 52 % [128]. Lowney, in a recent study of MEN-1 patients, could not demonstrate a correlation between size of tumor and metastatic potential in general, only those with tumors of >2 cm had liver metastasis [105]. This raises the question whether earlier surgical intervention may actually produce survival benefit in the form of reducing liver metastasis. Studies in support of this idea involved resection of lesions >1 cm and have shown no development of liver metastasis after a median follow-up of 83 months [111]. Finally, it has been suggested that there should be a delay in operating in small PNETs because surgery itself has a mortality rate of up to 15 %. However, it should be noted there have been numerous studies with little or no mortality associated with surgical intervention [111, 129–131].

There have been many surgical approaches advocated in the literature, and the most commonly described is that of **Dr. Norman Thompson**. This surgical approach is primarily based on two unique characteristics of PNET. The first is that gastrinomas are usually located in the duodenum and within the "gastrinoma triangle" between the junction of the cystic and common bile ducts, junction of second and third parts of duodenum, and junction of the neck and body of the pancreas. Second, concomitant nonfunctioning tumors are usually found in patients with gastrinoma. Consequently, Thompson proposed that intraoperative ultrasound should be used to investigate lesions in the pancreas, and those found in the pancreatic head are enucleated. At the same time, an 80 % distal pancreatectomy with splenic preservation is per-

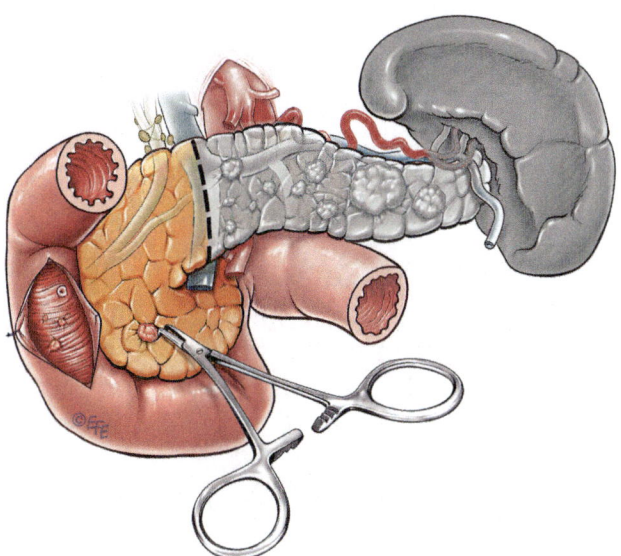

Fig. 5 Surgical management of large distal pancreatic lesions. This includes distal pancreatectomy (80 %) with enucleation of smaller lesions in pancreatic head. Patients who have a raised gastrin level will then proceed to have a duodenotomy to allow identification and enucleation of duodenal gastrinomas

formed (Fig. 5). Those with Zollinger–Ellison syndrome are further subjected to duodenotomy, whereby the entire duodenum is examined and the typical small submucosal lesions are enucleated. A regional lymphadenectomy is also undertaken. Initial results reported by Thompson using this technique in 40 patients have demonstrated that 68% of patients remain eugastrinemic and that only one person developed a solitary liver metastasis with no mortality in follow-up as long as 19 years [121, 122]. However, long-term follow-up of these patients have demonstrated a high recurrence rate of PNETs in the remaining pancreas [132]. There is a 10–20% risk of pancreatic pseudocyst and fistula which are often dealt with adequately with drainage and time. Controversy exists whether routine distal pancreatectomy should be performed. The theoretical advantage of distal pancreatectomy in patients without evidence of distal pancreatic disease has been questioned with studies like that of Norton et al. showing excellent survival rates without routinely performing distal pancreatectomy. In their study of 81 patients, 25 of these with PNET <2.5 cm had 15-year survival of 100%, 17 patients with PNET <6 cm had survival of 100%, and 31 patients with ≥2 tumors or >6 cm had survival of 89% [106, 133].

For MEN-1 cases with larger lesions in the head of the pancreas which are not amenable to conservative enucleation, pylorus preserving pancreaticoduodenectomy (PPPD) is required (Fig. 6). Rarely, patients with multiple large malignant pancreatic lesions may require total pancreatectomy; however, these cases are almost always associated with significant endocrine and exocrine insufficiency, have higher complication rates, and should be reserved for those kindreds where a strong history of metastatic disease is apparent [131, 134].

Patients with recurrent disease can often undergo reoperation with either further enucleations or pancreaticoduo-

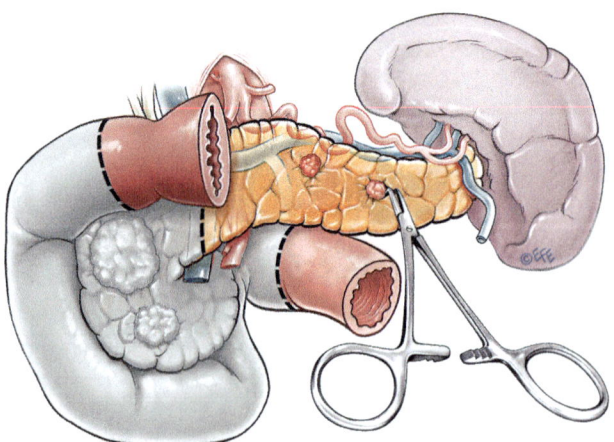

Fig. 6 Surgical management of large lesions in pancreatic head. This involves pylorus-preserving pancreaticoduodenectomy with enucleation of distal pancreatic lesion

denectomy. A study by Jaskowiak exploring reoperations in patients with recurrent disease found that the 2.5-year follow-up cure rate was lower at 23% (vs. 47% in those with only a primary operation) [135]. The authors suggested that cure rates of 23% were a clear indication that surgery should be attempted to allow patients to be "disease free." However, 15-year survival rates of 93% are seen in postoperative patients and as such reoperation may not change survival [133]. Furthermore, the role of surgical intervention in hepatic metastasis is evolving. Surgical debulking and/or radiofrequency ablation of hepatic metastasis with acceptable morbidity and low mortality is generally recommended as it may increase survival as well as help manage Zollinger–Ellison syndrome. For patients with disseminated disease, hormonal control with long-acting octreotide, PPIs, chemotherapy agents, such as streptozotocin and 5-fluorouracil or doxorubicin, have been used with some success for palliation [136].

Insulinoma

Insulinoma are β islet cell tumors that secrete insulin and are the second most common functional PNETs seen in MEN-1 patients with a prevalence of 10% (Table 1) [27, 29]. MEN-1-associated insulinoma accounts for only 4% of all patients with insulinoma. Patients are younger at presentation (less than 20 years of age) which is in contrast to those sporadic cases which typically present greater than 40 years of age. Clinically, they present with hormonal effects of hyperinsulinemia, hypoglycemia, especially after fasting or exertion. Diagnosis requires supervised 72-h fasting with inappropriately elevated insulin C-peptide and proinsulin concentrations. MEN-1 insulinoma is usually caused by a single dominant and benign tumor and is typically 2–3 cm in size but can be located anywhere in the pancreas [29, 137]. However, it is often associated with multiple other nonfunctioning lesions. Surgical excision remains the most effective treatment for insulinoma in order to prevent life-threatening hypoglycemia.

Preoperative localization studies include endoscopic ultrasound, CT, celiac axis angiography, pre- and perioperative transhepatic portal venous sampling, selective intra-arterial stimulations with hepatic venous sampling, and intraoperative direct pancreatic ultrasonography. Operative management is dependent upon the site, size, and proximity to the pancreatic duct of the dominant lesion. Cure rates are greater than 90% with median follow up of 10 years and conservative resections as expected have a higher incidence of recurrence versus subtotal resections [138–140].

VIPoma, glucagonoma, PPoma, Somatostatinoma, and GHRHoma

Pancreatic tumors which secrete vasoactive intestinal peptide (VIP), the so-called Verner–Morrison syndrome, glucagon, PP, somatostatin, and growth-hormone-releasing hormone (GHRH) occur infrequently. These are all rare and together have a prevalence of less than 2% in MEN-1 syndrome [27, 141]. In PPoma and somatostatinoma, secretion of these enzymes usually does not translate into any apparent endocrinopathy. In contrast, tumors that secrete growth-hormone-releasing hormone (GHRH) have rarely been reported in MEN-1 and when they arise can be found >50% in the lung, 30% in pancreas, and 10% in small intestine. Glucagonoma usually presents as hyperglycemia, anorexia, glossitis, anemia, diarrhea, venous thrombosis and necrolytic migratory erythema. By the time patients present, the lesions are large and have often metastasized and palliative surgery, and ablative procedures are typically necessary.

VIPomas secrete VIPs causing watery diarrhea, hypokalemia, and achlorhydria. As these lesions are usually located in the tail of the pancreas, surgical excision has been curative. Unfortunately, unlike insulinomas, these rarer PNETs are often asymptomatic until the tumor is large and metastasis to visceral organs is present. The GTE registry showed that these tumors were twice as likely to be >3 cm in size and visceral metastasis were also more frequently seen in comparison to other types of MEN-1-associated PNETs (40 and 15%, respectively). These characteristics translate to a poorer survival that is equivalent to that of nonfunctioning tumors. The 10-year disease-related survival rates for the various PNETS is as follows: glucagonomas, VIPomas, or somatostatinomas 54%; gastrinomas 81.7%; insulinomas 91.4%; and nonfunctioning PNET 62.2% (141).

Nonfunctioning Pancreaticoduodenal Endocrine Tumors

The prevalence of nonfunctioning PNETs in MEN-1 is around 20–35% and clinical presentation has been detected as early as 12 and 14 years of age [26, 27, 108]. Despite its asymptomatic nature, they have a high-malignant potential and subsequently need to be monitored and resected before malignant progression. The 10-year survival rate for patients with nonfunctioning PNETs has been found to be around 62% [108, 141]. Furthermore, the rate of survival can be correlated to tumor size and metastasis. Tumors with diameters of <1, 1–3, and >3 cm had metastasized in 4, 28, and 43% of patients, respectively. This correlated with 8-year survival rates of approximately 100, 80, and 40%, respectively [108]. Studies by Triponez and colleagues have recommended surgical excision in those that are ≥2 cm. However, in their study, 4% of patients with tumors, less than 1 cm had metastasis [108, 109]. Due to this, some have called for earlier intervention on lesions >1 cm. Whether preventing metastasis by more aggressive and earlier surgical intervention is improving survival has yet to be elucidated.

Pituitary Tumors

Anterior pituitary tumors are found in about 30% of MEN-1 patients and account for 25% of its initial presentation [26, 27]. Among all pituitary adenomas which proceed to surgical resection, 2–3% occurs in the setting of MEN-1. In the French GTE registry, out of 324 patients, 42% presented with pituitary adenomas with mean age of onset of 38 years but ranged from 12 to 83 years of age [108, 110]. The distribution of the types of pituitary adenoma is similar to sporadic cases; prolactinoma in 62%, somatotropinoma in 9%, Cushing's disease in 4%, and nonsecreting in 15% [110, 142]. MEN-1-associated pituitary adenomas were generally seen to be larger, and more commonly invasive than sporadic cases. In addition, there have been reported cases of double adenomas and multi-hormonal associations such as prolactin and adrenocorticotropic hormone (ACTH) or prolactin/growth hormone (GH) and follicle stimulating hormone/luteinizing hormone (FSH/LH) which are all atypical [143]. Clinical manifestations and treatment are similar to those with sporadic pituitary tumors. Surgery, medical therapy with dopamine agonists, and radiotherapy have all been used. The preferred treatment depends on the tumor size and invasion, visual impairment, the presence of hormonal hypersecretion, and response to medical treatment.

Other MEN-1-Associated Tumors

Carcinoid Tumors

Carcinoid tumors in MEN-1 patients are found predominately in the foregut (gastric, thymic, and bronchial). Carcinoids occur in about 15% of MEN-1 patients [26, 27, 29]. MEN-1 carcinoid tumors also have strong gender-specific distribution; thymic carcinoids are found predominantly in males and bronchial carcinoids in females [24, 71, 144, 145]. Furthermore, unlike other MEN-1 associated tumors, the average age of onset is much later in the 40s [146]. This reflects the lack of hormonal oversecretion and compression-induced symptoms. These tumors have malignant potential and represent the second most common case of tumor-related deaths. Thymic carcinoids are more often malignant than bronchial carcinoids (70 vs. 20%, respectively).

Thymic carcinoids are usually found at an advanced stage as a large invasive mass as can be seen in Fig. 7. Patients with MEN-1 thymic carcinoid have a poor prognosis with reported median survival of 28 months and 5-year survival rate of less than 30%. As such, it has been suggested that routine transcervical thymectomy should be performed as part of procedures for parathyroid disease [70–72]. However, resection does not prevent development of thymic carcinoids as there have been many reported cases of post-

Fig. 7 CT scan of a patient with thymic carcinoid. *CT* computerized tomography

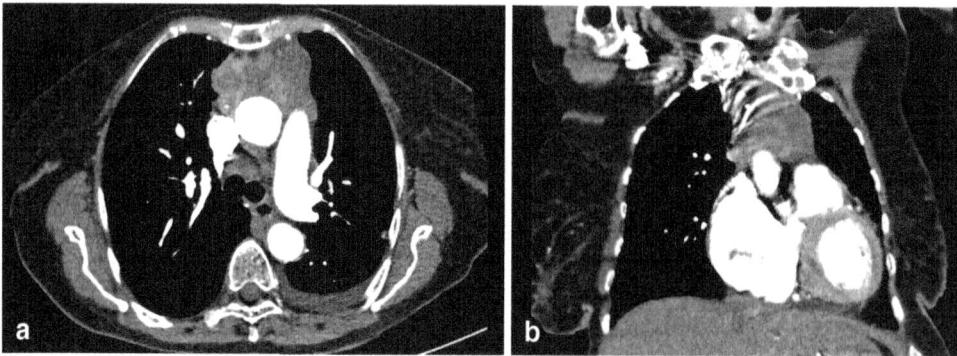

cervical thymectomized patients with thymic carcinoids [73–76]. It seems rational therefore to carefully monitor for progression of thymic disease. Bronchial carcinoids on the other hand are more indolent. Gastric carcinoids are tumors of enterochromaffin-like cells, and they occur in 10% of MEN-1 patients. They can be found either as an incidental finding on endoscopy or cause hormonal sequelae by its excessive secretion of serotonin and histamine. Also known as type II gastric neuroendocrine tumours, they have a 5-year disease free survival rate of 78%. Lesions smaller than 2 cm are recommended for endoscopic removal; however, larger ones require surgical excision.

Cutaneous Tumors

MEN-1-associated cutaneous tumors include angiofibroma, collagenoma, lipoma, leiomyoma, meningiomas, and ependymoma in decreasing order of frequency [147–149]. Angiofibroma are found in 85% of MEN-1 patients and half of these have > 5 papules on the face that do not regress and can extend beyond the vermilion border of the lips. Collagenomas are seen in 70% of MEN-1 patients and present as whitish, macular lesions seen on the trunk. Thirty percent of MEN-1 patients have lipomas which are usually dermal and small. Leiomyoma of the esophagus, lung, rectum or uterus are reported in 10% of MEN-1, and those of the esophagus and uterus are pathognomonic of MEN-1 syndrome. Rarer tumors such as cranial meningioma and spinal cerebellar ependymoma are usually benign and small and require no intervention [150–154].

Adrenal Tumors

Nonfunctioning adrenal cortical tumors have a prevalence of 20% in MEN-1 patients [27, 155]. They are usually bilateral, hyperplastic, and located in the cortex of the adrenal gland. While Pheochromocytoma are very rare with only a few reported cases; these are usually unilateral and nonfunctional. Adrenocortical carcinomas have been identified rarely (< 1%) in some kindreds, and this is increased to 13%

for larger adrenal lesions [155–158]. Surgical indications include size of > 4 cm, significant growth, or atypical imaging characteristics [53].

Surveillance

Surveillance for MEN-1 disease requires prevention of malignant transformation and screening. This includes primary prevention to identify individuals with MEN-1 mutation, recognizing asymptomatic disease in known carriers, managing those with nonfunctional disease before the progression to malignancy.

Genetic testing is indicated to identify patients that have a high potential to develop MEN-1 disease, specifically as carriers of mutated MEN-1 allele. Patients who should be screened include all first-degree relatives and even second-degree relatives if testing of the first-degree link is not available [26]. It should be noted that in around 15%, no germ-line mutation is demonstrated. However, in individuals where MEN-1 mutations are not seen, further haplotype analysis around the MEN-1 locus may be helpful in elucidating a genetic cause. Furthermore, as MEN-1 disease is autosomal dominant in nature, genetic screening can also help eliminate a lifetime of unnecessary biochemical and imaging surveillance in noncarriers. These genetic tests can be done at any age and are usually carried out promptly to allow proper secondary screening of individuals.

Secondary screening occurs as early as 5 years of age to detect pituitary tumors or insulinomas with annual prolactin, insulin-like growth factor 1, fasting glucose, and insulin levels (Table 2). Then by age 8, biochemical screening should include ionized calcium and parathyroid hormone levels. Enteropancreatic tumors are screened at 20 years of age with gastrin, Chromogranin A, glucagon, and proinsulin levels. Since nonfunctional or biochemically silent disease is common in MEN-1, screening for these with cross-sectional imaging of the chest and abdomen are recommended every 3 years regardless of biochemical results. With the advent of genetic screening, improved biochemical markers, and imaging modalities, more presymptomatic patients are being identified.

Table 2 Surveillance program for patients at high risk. (Data from Brandi et al. [26])

Pathology		Age of onset	Tests	
			Bloods (annually)	Imaging (3 yearly)
Parathyroid hyperplasia		8	iCa, PTH	None
Enteropancreatic tumour	Gastrinoma	20	Gastrin, gastric acid[a] output, secretin stimulation test[a]	None
	Insulinoma	5	Fasting glucose, insulin	
	Pancreatic Polypeptide	20	Chromogranin-A, pancreatic polypeptide	
	Other (nonfunctioning PETs)	20	Glucagons, somatostatin, proinsulin, VIP	MRI, CT, Octreotide scan[b]
Anterior pituitary	Prolactinoma	5	Prolactin	MRI
	Growth hormone	5	IGF-1	
Foregut carcinoid		20	None	CT/MRI

iCa serum-ionized calcium, *PTH* parathyroid hormone, *IGF* insulin-like growth factor, *CT* computed tomography, *MRI* magnetic resonance imaging; Indium In 111 pentetate (IN-DTPA), *VIP* vasoactive intestinal peptide, *PETs* positron emission tomographies

[a] Only tested if gastrin is high

[b] Octreotide scan: [111Indium-DTPA-D-Phe1]-Octreotide Scintigraphy

Conclusion

MEN-1 is an autosomal-dominant disorder in which patients are primarily at risk of parathyroid hyperplasia, pituitary adenoma, and enteropancreatic tumors. It is a disease that has a high morbidity and mortality rate as its manifestations often recur and can be malignant. Consequently, management of patients with MEN-1 is a lifelong process with careful and diligent screening of patients and their relatives and subsequent treatment of its clinical manifestations. Treatment of MEN-1 often requires surgical excision of the affected organ and as such a delicate balance must be achieved between preventing malignancy and avoiding the complications of treatment.

Key Summary Points

- MEN-1 is an autosomal-dominant disorder with mutations of the MEN-1 gene causing clinical triad of tumorigenesis in the parathyroids, enteropancreas, and pituitary. Patients are diagnosed clinically if two out of the three organs are involved or if known MEN-1 kindred, only one out of three is diagnostic. Genetic testing confirms diagnosis but is not exclusive.
- Primary hyperparathyroids in MEN-1 is different to sporadic cases, in that it appears in younger patients, has a female predominance, and is histologically an asymmetrical multigland disease.
- Management classically includes either total parathyroidectomy with autotransplantation or sPTX, both with cervical thymectomy. Recently, it has been suggested that a staged unilateral minimally invasive approach may also be appropriate.

- MEN-1-related PNETs are usually multifocal solid microadenomas surrounding a larger macroadenoma. They are the most frequent cause of mortality in MEN1 and 30–50 % have lymph node of liver metastasis at clinical presentation. The most common types are gastrinoma, Insulinoma, and nonfunctioning PNETs.
- Gastrinoma has clinical penetrance of 30–40 % and usually presents 10 years younger than sporadic cases. They are commonly multiple, small, and nodular lesions in the first and second part of duodenum and rarely the pancreas.
- Treatment of gastrinoma includes symptomatic control with PPIs and surgical resection. Surgical management include 80 % distal pancreatectomy and enucleation of lesions found in pancreatic head and duodenum. Those with large pancreatic head lesion should have PPPD instead. Reoccurrence rates are high and cure rates of 0 % at 10 years are found postoperatively.
- Insulinomas are the second most common MEN-1 PNETs (10 %). Patients usually are less than 20 years of age on presentation and insulinomas usually occur due to single 2–3 cm lesion in the pancreas. Operative management is indicated to prevent life-threatening hypoglycemia and cure rates of > 90 % at 10 years have been shown.
- Nonfunctioning PNETs are demonstrated in 20–35 % of MEN-1 and although patients are asymptomatic, their high malignant potential denotes a stringent surveillance and early surgical intervention.
- Pituitary tumors are seen in 30 % of MEN-1 patients and the types of pituitary adenoma and their management are similar to sporadic cases.
- Foregut carcinoids have a clinical penetrance of 15 % and have a strong gender-specific distribution (thymic for males and bronchial for females). They are the second most common tumor-related deaths in MEN-1 patients and as such survival rates are poor (5 years of less than

30%). Consequently, routine surgical excision during parathyroidectomies has been recommended.

- Genetic testing should be carried out in all first-degree relatives and secondary screening to identify disease manifestations should occur as early as 5 years of age.

References

1. Wilkinson S, Young M, Shepherd JJ. The prevalence of MEN-1 in Tasmania. Aust N Z J Surg. 1996;66(3):141–3.
2. Erdheim J. Zur normalen und pathologischen Histologie der Glandula thyreoidea, parathyroidea und Hypophysis. Beit Z Path Anat Z Alllg Path. 1903;33:78.
3. Underdahl LO, Woolner LB, Black BM. Multiple endocrine adenomas; report of 8 cases in which the parathyroids, pituitary and pancreatic islets were involved. J Clin Endocrinol Metab. 1953;13(1):20–47.
4. Wermer P. Genetic aspects of adenomatosis of endocrine glands. Am J Med. 1954;16(3):363–71.
5. Steiner AL, Goodman AD, Powers SR. Study of a kindred with pheochromocytoma, medullary thyroid carcinoma, hyperparathyroidism and Cushing's disease: multiple endocrine neoplasia, type 2. Medicine 1968;47(5):371–409.
6. Pellegata NS, Quintanilla-Martinez L, Siggelkow H, Samson E, Bink K, Hofler H, et al. Germ-line mutations in p27Kip1 cause a multiple endocrine neoplasia syndrome in rats and humans. Proc Nat Acad Sci U S A. 2006;103(42):15558–63.
7. Georgitsi M, Raitila A, Karhu A, van der Luijt RB, Aalfs CM, Sane T, et al. Germline CDKN1B/p27Kip1 mutation in multiple endocrine neoplasia. J Clin Endocrinol Metab. 2007;92(8):3321–5.
8. Larsson C, Skogseid B, Oberg K, Nakamura Y, Nordenskjold M. Multiple endocrine neoplasia type 1 gene maps to chromosome 11 and is lost in insulinoma. Nature 1988;332(6159):85–7.
9. Chandrasekharappa SC, Guru SC, Manickam P, Olufemi SE, Collins FS, Emmert-Buck MR, et al. Positional cloning of the gene for multiple endocrine neoplasia-type 1. Science 1997;276(5311):404–7.
10. Guru SC, Goldsmith PK, Burns AL, Marx SJ, Spiegel AM, Collins FS, et al. Menin, the product of the MEN1 gene, is a nuclear protein. Proc Natl Acad Sci U S A. 1998;95(4):1630–4.
11. La P, Silva AC, Hou Z, Wang H, Schnepp RW, Yan N, et al. Direct binding of DNA by tumor suppressor menin. J Biol Chem. 2004;279(47):49045–54.
12. Agarwal SK, Guru SC, Heppner C, Erdos MR, Collins RM, Park SY, et al. Menin interacts with the AP1 transcription factor JunD and represses JunD-activated transcription. Cell 1999;96(1):143–52.
13. Agarwal SK, Kennedy PA, Scacheri PC, Novotny EA, Hickman AB, Cerrato A, et al. Menin molecular interactions: insights into normal functions and tumorigenesis. Horm Metab Res. 2005;37(6):369–74.
14. Gobl AE, Berg M, Lopez-Egido JR, Oberg K, Skogseid B, Westin G. Menin represses JunD-activated transcription by a histone deacetylase-dependent mechanism. Biochim Biophys Acta. 1999;1447(1):51–6.
15. Gallo A, Cuozzo C, Esposito I, Maggiolini M, Bonofiglio D, Vivacqua A, et al. Menin uncouples Elk-1, JunD and c-Jun phosphorylation from MAP kinase activation. Oncogene 2002;21(42):6434–45.
16. Yumita W, Ikeo Y, Yamauchi K, Sakurai A, Hashizume K. Suppression of insulin-induced AP-1 transactivation by menin accompanies inhibition of c-Fos induction. Int J Cancer. 2003;103(6):738–44.
17. Kaji H, Canaff L, Lebrun JJ, Goltzman D, Hendy GN. Inactivation of menin, a Smad3-interacting protein, blocks transforming growth factor type beta signaling. Proc Natl Acad Sci U S A. 2001;98(7):3837–42.
18. Knudson AG Jr. Mutation and cancer: statistical study of retinoblastoma. Proc Natl Acad Sci U S A. 1971;68(4):820–3.
19. Agarwal SK, Debelenko LV, Kester MB, Guru SC, Manickam P, Olufemi SE, et al. Analysis of recurrent germline mutations in the MEN1 gene encountered in apparently unrelated families. Hum Mutat. 1998;12(2):75–82.
20. Schnepp RW, Mao H, Sykes SM, Zong WX, Silva A, La P, et al. Menin induces apoptosis in murine embryonic fibroblasts. J Biol Chem. 2004;279(11):10685–91.
21. Pannett AA, Thakker RV. Multiple endocrine neoplasia type 1. Endocr-Relat Cancer. 1999;6(4):449–73.
22. Lemos MC, Thakker RV. Multiple endocrine neoplasia type 1 (MEN1): analysis of 1336 mutations reported in the first decade following identification of the gene. Hum Mutat. 2008;29(1):22–32.
23. Bassett JH, Forbes SA, Pannett AA, Lloyd SE, Christie PT, Wooding C, et al. Characterization of mutations in patients with multiple endocrine neoplasia type 1. Am J Hum Genet. 1998;62(2):232–44.
24. Abe T, Yoshimoto K, Taniyama M, Hanakawa K, Izumiyama H, Itakura M, et al. An unusual kindred of the multiple endocrine neoplasia type 1 (MEN1) in Japanese. J Clin Endocr Metab. 2000;85(3):1327–30.
25. Cavaco BM, Domingues R, Bacelar MC, Cardoso H, Barros L, Gomes L, et al. Mutational analysis of Portuguese families with multiple endocrine neoplasia type 1 reveals large germline deletions. Clin Endocrinol. 2002;56(4):465–73.
26. Brandi ML, Gagel RF, Angeli A, Bilezikian JP, Beck-Peccoz P, Bordi C, et al. Guidelines for diagnosis and therapy of MEN type 1 and type 2. J Clin Endocrinol Metab. 2001;86(12):5658–71.
27. Trump D, Farren B, Wooding C, Pang JT, Besser GM, Buchanan KD, et al. Clinical studies of multiple endocrine neoplasia type 1 (MEN1). QJM 1996;89(9):653–69.
28. Benson L, Ljunghall S, Akerstrom G, Oberg K. Hyperparathyroidism presenting as the first lesion in multiple endocrine neoplasia type 1. Am J Med. 1987;82(4):731–7.
29. Marx S, Spiegel AM, Skarulis MC, Doppman JL, Collins FS, Liotta LA. Multiple endocrine neoplasia type 1: clinical and genetic topics. Ann Intern Med. 1998;129(6):484–94.
30. Marx SJ, Vinik AI, Santen RJ, Floyd JC, Jr., Mills JL, Green J, 3rd. Multiple endocrine neoplasia type I: assessment of laboratory tests to screen for the gene in a large kindred. Medicine 1986;65(4):226–41.
31. Doherty GM. Multiple endocrine neoplasia type 1. J Surg Oncol. 2005;89(3):143–50.
32. Machens A, Schaaf L, Karges W, Frank-Raue K, Bartsch DK, Rothmund M, et al. Age-related penetrance of endocrine tumours in multiple endocrine neoplasia type 1 (MEN1): a multicentre study of 258 gene carriers. Clin Endocrinol. 2007;67(4):613–22.
33. Lairmore TC, Piersall LD, DeBenedetti MK, Dilley WG, Mutch MG, Whelan AJ, et al. Clinical genetic testing and early surgical intervention in patients with multiple endocrine neoplasia type 1 (MEN 1). Ann Surg. 2004;239(5):637–45; discussion 45–7.
34. Skogseid B, Eriksson B, Lundqvist G, Lorelius LE, Rastad J, Wide L, et al. Multiple endocrine neoplasia type 1: a 10-year prospective screening study in four kindreds. J Clin Endocrinol Metab. 1991;73(2):281–7.
35. Doherty GM, Olson JA, Frisella MM, Lairmore TC, Wells SA, Jr., Norton JA. Lethality of multiple endocrine neoplasia type I. World J Surg. 1998;22(6):581–6 (discussion 6–7).
36. Wilkinson S, Teh BT, Davey KR, McArdle JP, Young M, Shepherd JJ. Cause of death in multiple endocrine neoplasia type 1. Arch Surg. 1993;128(6):683–90.
37. Dean PG, van Heerden JA, Farley DR, Thompson GB, Grant CS, Harmsen WS, et al. Are patients with multiple endocrine neoplasia

type I prone to premature death? World J Surg. 2000;24(11):1437–41.

38. Uchino S, Noguchi S, Sato M, Yamashita H, Yamashita H, Watanabe S, et al. Screening of the Men1 gene and discovery of germline and somatic mutations in apparently sporadic parathyroid tumors. Cancer Res. 2000;60(19):5553–7.

39. Cope O. The study of hyperparathyroidism at the Massachusetts General Hospital. New Engl J Med. 1966;274(21):1174–82.

40. Marx SJ, Menczel J, Campbell G, Aurbach GD, Spiegel AM, Norton JA. Heterogeneous size of the parathyroid glands in familial multiple endocrine neoplasia type 1. Clin Endocrinol. 1991;35(6):521–6.

41. Rizzoli R, Green J 3rd, Marx SJ. Primary hyperparathyroidism in familial multiple endocrine neoplasia type I. Long-term follow-up of serum calcium levels after parathyroidectomy. Am J Med. 1985;78(3):467–74.

42. d'Alessandro AF, Montenegro FL, Brandao LG, Lourenco DM, Jr., Toledo Sde A, Cordeiro AC. Supernumerary parathyroid glands in hyperparathyroidism associated with multiple endocrine neoplasia type 1. Rev Assoc Med Bras (1992). 2012;58(3):323–7.

43. Akerstrom G, Malmaeus J, Bergstrom R. Surgical anatomy of human parathyroid glands. Surgery 1984;95(1):14–21.

44. Stalberg P, Carling T. Familial parathyroid tumors: diagnosis and management. World J Surg. 2009;33(11):2234–43.

45. Versnick M, Popadich A, Sidhu S, Sywak M, Robinson B, Delbridge L. Minimally invasive parathyroidectomy provides a conservative surgical option for multiple endocrine neoplasia type 1-primary hyperparathyroidism. Surgery 2013;154(1):101–5.

46. Friedman E, Sakaguchi K, Bale AE, Falchetti A, Streeten E, Zimering MB, et al. Clonality of parathyroid tumors in familial multiple endocrine neoplasia type 1. New Engl J Med. 1989;321(4):213–8.

47. Brandi ML, Aurbach GD, Fitzpatrick LA, Quarto R, Spiegel AM, Bliziotes MM, et al. Parathyroid mitogenic activity in plasma from patients with familial multiple endocrine neoplasia type 1. New Engl J Med. 1986;314(20):1287–93.

48. Agha A, Carpenter R, Bhattacharya S, Edmonson SJ, Carlsen E, Monson JP. Parathyroid carcinoma in multiple endocrine neoplasia type 1 (MEN1) syndrome: two case reports of an unrecognised entity. J Endocrinol Invest. 2007;30(2):145–9.

49. Frank-Raue K, Leidig-Bruckner G, Lorenz A, Rondot S, Haag C, Schulze E, et al. [Hereditary variants of primary hyperparathyroidism—MEN1, MEN2, HPT-JT, FHH, FIHPT]. Dtsch Med Wochenschr (1946). 2011;136(38):1889–94.

50. Shih RY, Fackler S, Maturo S, True MW, Brennan J, Wells D. Parathyroid carcinoma in multiple endocrine neoplasia type 1 with a classic germline mutation. Endocr Pract. 2009;15(6):567–72.

51. Dionisi S, Minisola S, Pepe J, De Geronimo S, Paglia F, Memeo L, et al. Concurrent parathyroid adenomas and carcinoma in the setting of multiple endocrine neoplasia type 1: presentation as hypercalcemic crisis. Mayo Clin Proc. 2002;77(8):866–9.

52. del Pozo C, Garcia-Pascual L, Balsells M, Barahona MJ, Veloso E, Gonzalez C, et al. Parathyroid carcinoma in multiple endocrine neoplasia type 1. Case report and review of the literature. Hormones (Athens, Greece). 2011;10(4):326–31.

53. Thakker RV, Newey PJ, Walls GV, Bilezikian J, Dralle H, Ebeling PR, et al. Clinical practice guidelines for multiple endocrine neoplasia type 1 (MEN1). J Clin Endocrinol Metab. 2012;97(9):2990–3011.

54. Nilubol N, Weinstein L, Simonds WF, Jensen RT, Phan GQ, Hughes MS, et al. Preoperative localizing studies for initial parathyroidectomy in MEN1 syndrome: is there any benefit? World J Surg. 2012;36(6):1368–74.

55. Bilezikian JP, Khan AA, Potts JT, Jr. Guidelines for the management of asymptomatic primary hyperparathyroidism: summary statement from the third international workshop. J Clin Endocrinol Metab. 2009;94(2):335–9.

56. Jensen RT. Management of the Zollinger-Ellison syndrome in patients with multiple endocrine neoplasia type 1. J Intern Med. 1998;243(6):477–88.

57. Norton JA, Venzon DJ, Berna MJ, Alexander HR, Fraker DL, Libutti SK, et al. Prospective study of surgery for primary hyperparathyroidism (HPT) in multiple endocrine neoplasia-type 1 and Zollinger-Ellison syndrome: long-term outcome of a more virulent form of HPT. Ann Surg. 2008;247(3):501–10.

58. Burgess JR, David R, Greenaway TM, Parameswaran V, Shepherd JJ. Osteoporosis in multiple endocrine neoplasia type 1: severity, clinical significance, relationship to primary hyperparathyroidism, and response to parathyroidectomy. Arch Surg. 1999;134(10):1119–23.

59. Coutinho FL, Lourenco DM, Jr., Toledo RA, Montenegro FL, Correia-Deur JE, Toledo SP. Bone mineral density analysis in patients with primary hyperparathyroidism associated with multiple endocrine neoplasia type 1 after total parathyroidectomy. Clin Endocrinol. 2010;72(4):462–8.

60. Lourenco DM, Jr., Coutinho FL, Toledo RA, Goncalves TD, Montenegro FL, Toledo SP. Biochemical, bone and renal patterns in hyperparathyroidism associated with multiple endocrine neoplasia type 1. Clinics (Sao Paulo, Brazil). 2012;67(Suppl 1):99–108.

61. Lourenco DM, Jr., Toledo RA, Mackowiak, II, Coutinho FL, Cavalcanti MG, Correia-Deur JE, et al. Multiple endocrine neoplasia type 1 in Brazil: MEN1 founding mutation, clinical features, and bone mineral density profile. Eur J Endocrinol. 2008;159(3):259–74.

62. Kann PH, Bartsch D, Langer P, Waldmann J, Hadji P, Pfutzner A, et al. Peripheral bone mineral density in correlation to disease-related predisposing conditions in patients with multiple endocrine neoplasia type 1. J Endocrinol Invest. 2012;35(6):573–9.

63. Elaraj DM, Skarulis MC, Libutti SK, Norton JA, Bartlett DL, Pingpank JF, et al. Results of initial operation for hyperparathyroidism in patients with multiple endocrine neoplasia type 1. Surgery 2003;134(6):858–64; discussion 64–5.

64. Feldman AL, Sharaf RN, Skarulis MC, Bartlett DL, Libutti SK, Weinstein LS, et al. Results of heterotopic parathyroid autotransplantation: a 13-year experience. Surgery 1999;126(6):1042–8.

65. Shepet K, Alhefdhi A, Usedom R, Sippel R, Chen H. Parathyroid cryopreservation after parathyroidectomy: a worthwhile practice? Ann Surg Oncol. 2013;20(7):2256–60.

66. Borot S, Lapierre V, Carnaille B, Goudet P, Penfornis A. Results of cryopreserved parathyroid autografts: a retrospective multicenter study. Surgery 2010;147(4):529–35.

67. Caccitolo JA, Farley DR, van Heerden JA, Grant CS, Thompson GB, Steriott S. The current role of parathyroid cryopreservation and autotransplantation in parathyroid surgery: an institutional experience. Surgery 1997;122(6):1062–7.

68. Wells SA, Jr., Burdick JF, Hattler BG, Christiansen C, Pettigrew HM, Abe M, et al. The allografted parathyroid gland: evaluation of function in the immunosuppressed host. Ann Surg. 1974;180(6):805–13.

69. Wells SA, Jr., Christiansen C. The transplanted parathyroid gland: evaluation of cryopreservation and other environmental factors which affect its function. Surgery 1974;75(1):49–55.

70. Ferolla P, Falchetti A, Filosso P, Tomassetti P, Tamburrano G, Avenia N, et al. Thymic neuroendocrine carcinoma (carcinoid) in multiple endocrine neoplasia type 1 syndrome: the Italian series. J Clin Endocrinol Metab. 2005;90(5):2603–9.

71. Teh BT, Zedenius J, Kytola S, Skogseid B, Trotter J, Choplin H, et al. Thymic carcinoids in multiple endocrine neoplasia type 1. Ann Surg. 1998;228(1):99–105.

72. Hellman P, Skogseid B, Oberg K, Juhlin C, Akerstrom G, Rastad J. Primary and reoperative parathyroid operations in hyperparathyroidism of multiple endocrine neoplasia type 1. Surgery 1998;124(6):993–9.

73. Goudet P, Murat A, Cardot-Bauters C, Emy P, Baudin E, du Boullay Choplin H, et al. Thymic neuroendocrine tumors in multiple endocrine neoplasia type 1: a comparative study on 21 cases among a series of 761 MEN1 from the GTE (Groupe des Tumeurs Endocrines). World J Surg. 2009;33(6):1197–207.

74. Recuero Diaz JL, Embun Flor R, Menal Munoz P, Hernandez Ferrandez J, Arraras Martinez MJ, Rivas de Andres JJ. Thymic carcinoid associated with multiple endocrine neoplasia syndrome type I. Arch Bronconeumol. 2013;49(3):122–5.

75. Gibril F, Chen YJ, Schrump DS, Vortmeyer A, Zhuang Z, Lubensky IA, et al. Prospective study of thymic carcinoids in patients with multiple endocrine neoplasia type 1. J Clin Endocrinol Metabol. 2003;88(3):1066–81.

76. Burgess JR, Giles N, Shepherd JJ. Malignant thymic carcinoid is not prevented by transcervical thymectomy in multiple endocrine neoplasia type 1. Clin Endocrinol. 2001;55(5):689–93.

77. Hellman P, Skogseid B, Juhlin C, Akerstrom G, Rastad J. Findings and long-term results of parathyroid surgery in multiple endocrine neoplasia type 1. World J Surg. 1992;16(4):718–22 (discussion 22–3).

78. Prinz RA, Gamvros OI, Sellu D, Lynn JA. Subtotal parathyroidectomy for primary chief cell hyperplasia of the multiple endocrine neoplasia type I syndrome. Ann Surg. 1981;193(1):26–9.

79. van Heerden JA, Kent RB, 3rd, Sizemore GW, Grant CS, ReMine WH. Primary hyperparathyroidism in patients with multiple endocrine neoplasia syndromes. Surgical experience. Arch Surg. 1983;118(5):533–6.

80. Lambert LA, Shapiro SE, Lee JE, Perrier ND, Truong M, Wallace MJ, et al. Surgical treatment of hyperparathyroidism in patients with multiple endocrine neoplasia type 1. Arch Surg. 2005;140(4):374–82.

81. Waldmann J, Lopez CL, Langer P, Rothmund M, Bartsch DK. Surgery for multiple endocrine neoplasia type 1-associated primary hyperparathyroidism. Br J Surg. 2010;97(10):1528–34.

82. Schreinemakers JM, Pieterman CR, Scholten A, Vriens MR, Valk GD, Rinkes IH. The optimal surgical treatment for primary hyperparathyroidism in MEN1 patients: a systematic review. World J Surg. 2011;35(9):1993–2005.

83. Tonelli F, Marcucci T, Giudici F, Falchetti A, Brandi ML. Surgical approach in hereditary hyperparathyroidism. Endocr J. 2009;56(7):827–41.

84. Rudberg C, Akerstrom G, Palmer M, Ljunghall S, Adami HO, Johansson H, et al. Late results of operation for primary hyperparathyroidism in 441 patients. Surgery 1986;99(6):643–51.

85. Salmeron MD, Gonzalez JM, Sancho Insenser J, Goday A, Perez NM, Zambudio AR, et al. Causes and treatment of recurrent hyperparathyroidism after subtotal parathyroidectomy in the presence of multiple endocrine neoplasia 1. World J Surg. 2010;34(6):1325–31.

86. Shepherd JJ, Burgess JR, Greenaway TM, Ware R. Preoperative sestamibi scanning and surgical findings at bilateral, unilateral, or minimal reoperation for recurrent hyperparathyroidism after subtotal parathyroidectomy in patients with multiple endocrine neoplasia type 1. Arch Surg. 2000;135(7):844–8.

87. Levin KE, Gooding GA, Okerlund M, Higgins CB, Norman D, Newton TH, et al. Localizing studies in patients with persistent or recurrent hyperparathyroidism. Surgery 1987;102(6):917–25.

88. Kelly HR, Hamberg LM, Hunter GJ. 4D-CT for preoperative localization of abnormal parathyroid glands in patients with hyperparathyroidism: accuracy and ability to stratify patients by unilateral versus bilateral disease in surgery-naive and re-exploration patients. AJNR Am J Neuroradiol. 2014;35(1):176–81.

89. Carty SE, Norton JA. Management of patients with persistent or recurrent primary hyperparathyroidism. World J Surg. 1991;15(6):716–23.

90. Cheung K, Wang TS, Farrokhyar F, Roman SA, Sosa JA. A meta-analysis of preoperative localization techniques for patients with primary hyperparathyroidism. Ann Surg Oncol. 2012;19(2):577–83.

91. Witteveen JE, Kievit J, van Erkel AR, Morreau H, Romijn JA, Hamdy NA. The role of selective venous sampling in the management of persistent hyperparathyroidism revisited. Eur J Endocrinol. 2010;163(6):945–52.

92. Ogilvie CM, Brown PL, Matson M, Dacie J, Reznek RH, Britton K, et al. Selective parathyroid venous sampling in patients with complicated hyperparathyroidism. Eur J Endocrinol. 2006;155(6):813–21.

93. Reidel MA, Schilling T, Graf S, Hinz U, Nawroth P, Buchler MW, et al. Localization of hyperfunctioning parathyroid glands by selective venous sampling in reoperation for primary or secondary hyperparathyroidism. Surgery 2006;140(6):907–13 (discussion 13).

94. Chaffanjon PC, Voirin D, Vasdev A, Chabre O, Kenyon NM, Brichon PY. Selective venous sampling in recurrent and persistent hyperparathyroidism: indication, technique, and results. World J Surg. 2004;28(10):958–61.

95. Kivlen MH, Bartlett DL, Libutti SK, Skarulis MC, Marx SJ, Simonds WF, et al. Reoperation for hyperparathyroidism in multiple endocrine neoplasia type 1. Surgery 2001;130(6):991–8.

96. Shepherd JJ. The natural history of multiple endocrine neoplasia type 1. Highly uncommon or highly unrecognized? Arch Surg. 1991;126(8):935–52.

97. Majewski JT, Wilson SD. The MEA-I syndrome: an all or none phenomenon? Surgery 1979;86(3):475–84.

98. Kloppel G, Willemer S, Stamm B, Hacki WH, Heitz PU. Pancreatic lesions and hormonal profile of pancreatic tumors in multiple endocrine neoplasia type I. An immunocytochemical study of nine patients. Cancer. 1986;57(9):1824–32.

99. Le Bodic MF, Heymann MF, Lecomte M, Berger N, Berger F, Louvel A, et al. Immunohistochemical study of 100 pancreatic tumors in 28 patients with multiple endocrine neoplasia, type I. Am J Surg Pathol. 1996;20(11):1378–84.

100. Anlauf M, Schlenger R, Perren A, Bauersfeld J, Koch CA, Dralle H, et al. Microadenomatosis of the endocrine pancreas in patients with and without the multiple endocrine neoplasia type 1 syndrome. Am J Surg Pathol. 2006;30(5):560–74.

101. Thompson NW, Lloyd RV, Nishiyama RH, Vinik AI, Strodel WE, Allo MD, et al. MEN I pancreas: a histological and immunohistochemical study. World J Surg. 1984;8(4):561–74.

102. Pipeleers-Marichal M, Somers G, Willems G, Foulis A, Imrie C, Bishop AE, et al. Gastrinomas in the duodenums of patients with multiple endocrine neoplasia type 1 and the Zollinger-Ellison syndrome. New Engl J Med. 1990;322(11):723–7.

103. Lips CJ, Koppeschaar HP, Berends MJ, Jansen-Schillhorn van Veen JM, Struyvenberg A, Van Vroonhoven TJ. The importance of screening for the MEN 1 syndrome: diagnostic results and clinical management. Henry Ford Hosp Med J. 1992;40(3–4):171–2.

104. Skogseid B, Oberg K, Eriksson B, Juhlin C, Granberg D, Akerstrom G, et al. Surgery for asymptomatic pancreatic lesion in multiple endocrine neoplasia type I. World J Surg. 1996;20(7):872–6 (discussion 7).

105. Lowney JK, Frisella MM, Lairmore TC, Doherty GM. Pancreatic islet cell tumor metastasis in multiple endocrine neoplasia type 1: correlation with primary tumor size. Surgery 1998;124(6):1043–8 (discussion 8–9).

106. Norton JA, Jensen RT. Resolved and unresolved controversies in the surgical management of patients with Zollinger-Ellison syndrome. Ann Surg. 2004;240(5):757–73.

107. Tomassetti P, Campana D, Piscitelli L, Casadei R, Santini D, Nori F, et al. Endocrine pancreatic tumors: factors correlated with survival. Ann Oncol. 2005;16(11):1806–10.

108. Triponez F, Dosseh D, Goudet P, Cougard P, Bauters C, Murat A, et al. Epidemiology data on 108 MEN 1 patients from the GTE with isolated nonfunctioning tumors of the pancreas. Ann Surg. 2006;243(2):265–72.

109. Triponez F, Goudet P, Dosseh D, Cougard P, Bauters C, Murat A, et al. Is surgery beneficial for MEN1 patients with small (<or =2 cm), nonfunctioning pancreaticoduodenal endocrine

110. tumor? An analysis of 65 patients from the GTE. World J Surg. 2006;30(5):654–62 (discussion 63–4).

110. Goudet P, Murat A, Binquet C, Cardot-Bauters C, Costa A, Ruszniewski P, et al. Risk factors and causes of death in MEN1 disease. A GTE (Groupe d'Etude des Tumeurs Endocrines) cohort study among 758 patients. World J Surg. 2010;34(2):249–55.

111. Lopez CL, Waldmann J, Fendrich V, Langer P, Kann PH, Bartsch DK. Long-term results of surgery for pancreatic neuroendocrine neoplasms in patients with MEN1. Langenbeck's Arch Surg. 2011;396(8):1187–96.

112. Ekeblad S, Skogseid B, Dunder K, Oberg K, Eriksson B. Prognostic factors and survival in 324 patients with pancreatic endocrine tumor treated at a single institution. Clin Cancer Res. 2008;14(23):7798–803.

113. Zollinger RM, Ellison EH. Primary peptic ulcerations of the jejunum associated with islet cell tumors of the pancreas. Ann Surg. 1955;142(4):709–23 (discussion 24–8).

114. Gregory RA, Grossman MI, Tracy HJ, Bentley PH. Nature of the gastric secretagogue in Zollinger-Ellison tumours. Lancet 1967;2(7515):543–4.

115. Gregory RA, Tracy HJ, French JM, Sircus W. Extraction of a gastrin-like substance from a pancreatic tumour in a case of Zollinger-Ellison syndrome. Lancet 1960;1(7133):1045–8.

116. Farley DR, van Heerden JA, Grant CS, Miller LJ, Ilstrup DM. The Zollinger-Ellison syndrome. A collective surgical experience. Ann Surg. 1992;215(6):561–9 (discussion 9–70).

117. Roy PK, Venzon DJ, Shojamanesh H, Abou-Saif A, Peghini P, Doppman JL, et al. Zollinger-Ellison syndrome. Clinical presentation in 261 patients. Medicine. 2000;79(6):379–411.

118. Norton JA, Fraker DL, Alexander HR, Venzon DJ, Doppman JL, Serrano J, et al. Surgery to cure the Zollinger-Ellison syndrome. New Engl J Med. 1999;341(9):635–44.

119. Akerstrom G, Stalberg P, Hellman P. Surgical management of pancreatico-duodenal tumors in multiple endocrine neoplasia syndrome type 1. Clinics (Sao Paulo, Brazil). 2012;67 Suppl 1:173–8.

120. Yu F, Venzon DJ, Serrano J, Goebel SU, Doppman JL, Gibril F, et al. Prospective study of the clinical course, prognostic factors, causes of death, and survival in patients with long-standing Zollinger-Ellison syndrome. J Clin Oncol. 1999;17(2):615–30.

121. Thompson NW. Management of pancreatic endocrine tumors in patients with multiple endocrine neoplasia type 1. Surg Oncol Clin North Am. 1998;7(4):881–91.

122. Thompson NW. Current concepts in the surgical management of multiple endocrine neoplasia type 1 pancreatic-duodenal disease. Results in the treatment of 40 patients with Zollinger-Ellison syndrome, hypoglycaemia or both. J Intern Med. 1998;243(6):495–500.

123. Wamsteker EJ, Gauger PG, Thompson NW, Scheiman JM. EUS detection of pancreatic endocrine tumors in asymptomatic patients with type 1 multiple endocrine neoplasia. Gastrointest Endosc. 2003;58(4):531–5.

124. Naswa N, Sharma P, Soundararajan R, Karunanithi S, Nazar AH, Kumar R, et al. Diagnostic performance of somatostatin receptor PET/CT using 68 Ga-DOTANOC in gastrinoma patients with negative or equivocal CT findings. Abdom Imaging. 2013;38(3):552–60.

125. Gomez M, Ferrando R, Vilar J, Hitateguy R, Lopez B, Moreira E, et al. [99mTc-OCTREOTIDE in patients with neuroendocrine tumors from the GI tract]. Acta Gastroenterol Latinoam. 2010;40(4):332–8.

126. Bhate K, Mok WY, Tran K, Khan S, Al-Nahhas A. Functional assessment in the multimodality imaging of pancreatic neuro-endocrine tumours. Minerva Endocrinol. 2010;35(1):17–25.

127. Li ML, Norton JA. Gastrinoma. Curr Treat Options Oncol. 2001;2(4):337–46.

128. Norton JA, Fraker DL, Alexander HR, Gibril F, Liewehr DJ, Venzon DJ, et al. Surgery increases survival in patients with gastrinoma. Ann Surg. 2006;244(3):410–9.

129. Doherty GM. Multiple endocrine neoplasia type 1: duodenopancreatic tumors. Surg Oncol. 2003;12(2):135–43.

130. Doherty GM, Thompson NW. Multiple endocrine neoplasia type 1: duodenopancreatic tumours. J Intern Med. 2003;253(6):590–8.

131. Bartsch DK, Fendrich V, Langer P, Celik I, Kann PH, Rothmund M. Outcome of duodenopancreatic resections in patients with multiple endocrine neoplasia type 1. Ann Surg. 2005;242(6):757–64 (discussion 64–6).

132. Hausman MS, Jr., Thompson NW, Gauger PG, Doherty GM. The surgical management of MEN-1 pancreatoduodenal neuroendocrine disease. Surgery 2004;136(6):1205–11.

133. Norton JA, Alexander HR, Fraker DL, Venzon DJ, Gibril F, Jensen RT. Comparison of surgical results in patients with advanced and limited disease with multiple endocrine neoplasia type 1 and Zollinger-Ellison syndrome. Ann Surg. 2001;234(4):495–505 (discussion -6).

134. Tonelli F, Fratini G, Falchetti A, Nesi G, Brandi ML. Surgery for gastroenteropancreatic tumours in multiple endocrine neoplasia type 1: review and personal experience. J Intern Med. 2005;257(1):38–49.

135. Jaskowiak NT, Fraker DL, Alexander HR, Norton JA, Doppman JL, Jensen RT. Is reoperation for gastrinoma excision indicated in Zollinger-Ellison syndrome? Surgery 1996;120(6):1055–62 (discussion 62–3).

136. Ito T, Igarashi H, Uehara H, Jensen RT. Pharmacotherapy of Zollinger-Ellison syndrome. Expert Opin Pharmacother. 2013;14(3):307–21.

137. Demeure MJ, Klonoff DC, Karam JH, Duh QY, Clark OH. Insulinomas associated with multiple endocrine neoplasia type I: the need for a different surgical approach. Surgery 1991;110(6):998–1004 (discussion -5).

138. Mehrabi A, Fischer L, Hafezi M, Dirlewanger A, Grenacher L, Diener MK, et al. A systematic review of localization, surgical treatment options, and outcome of insulinoma. Pancreas 2014;43(5):675–86.

139. Giudici F, Nesi G, Brandi ML, Tonelli F. Surgical management of insulinomas in multiple endocrine neoplasia type 1. Pancreas 2012;41(4):547–53.

140. Crippa S, Zerbi A, Boninsegna L, Capitanio V, Partelli S, Balzano G, et al. Surgical management of insulinomas: short- and long-term outcomes after enucleations and pancreatic resections. Arch Surg. 2012;147(3):261–6.

141. Levy-Bohbot N, Merle C, Goudet P, Delemer B, Calender A, Jolly D, et al. Prevalence, characteristics and prognosis of MEN 1-associated glucagonomas, VIPomas, and somatostatinomas: study from the GTE (Groupe des Tumeurs Endocrines) registry. Gastroenterol Clin Biol. 2004;28(11):1075–81.

142. Verges B, Boureille F, Goudet P, Murat A, Beckers A, Sassolas G, et al. Pituitary disease in MEN type 1 (MEN1): data from the France-Belgium MEN1 multicenter study. J Clin Endocrinol Metab. 2002;87(2):457–65.

143. Trouillas J, Labat-Moleur F, Sturm N, Kujas M, Heymann MF, Figarella-Branger D, et al. Pituitary tumors and hyperplasia in multiple endocrine neoplasia type 1 syndrome (MEN1): a case-control study in a series of 77 patients versus 2509 non-MEN1 patients. Am J Surg Pathol. 2008;32(4):534–43.

144. Sachithanandan N, Harle RA, Burgess JR. Bronchopulmonary carcinoid in multiple endocrine neoplasia type 1. Cancer 2005;103(3):509–15.

145. Harpole DH, Jr., Feldman JM, Buchanan S, Young WG, Wolfe WG. Bronchial carcinoid tumors: a retrospective analysis of 126 patients. Ann Thorac Surg. 1992;54(1):50–4 (discussion 4–5).

146. Teh BT. Thymic carcinoids in multiple endocrine neoplasia type 1. J Intern Med. 1998;243(6):501–4.

147. Vidal A, Iglesias MJ, Fernandez B, Fonseca E, Cordido F. Cutaneous lesions associated to multiple endocrine neoplasia syndrome type 1. J Eur Acad Dermatol Venereol. 2008;22(7):835–8.

148. Asgharian B, Turner ML, Gibril F, Entsuah LK, Serrano J, Jensen RT. Cutaneous tumors in patients with multiple endocrine neoplasm type 1 (MEN1) and gastrinomas: prospective study of frequency and development of criteria with high sensitivity and specificity for MEN1. J Clin Endocrinol Metab. 2004;89(11):5328–36.

149. Darling TN, Skarulis MC, Steinberg SM, Marx SJ, Spiegel AM, Turner M. Multiple facial angiofibromas and collagenomas in patients with multiple endocrine neoplasia type 1. Arch Dermatol. 1997;133(7):853–7.

150. Skogseid B, Rastad J, Gobl A, Larsson C, Backlin K, Juhlin C, et al. Adrenal lesion in multiple endocrine neoplasia type 1. Surgery 1995;118(6):1077–82.

151. Asgharian B, Chen YJ, Patronas NJ, Peghini PL, Reynolds JC, Vortmeyer A, et al. Meningiomas may be a component tumor of multiple endocrine neoplasia type 1. Clin Cancer Res. 2004;10(3):869–80.

152. Funayama T, Sakane M, Yoshizawa T, Takeuchi Y, Ochiai N. Tanycytic ependymoma of the filum terminale associated with multiple endocrine neoplasia type 1: first reported case. Spine J. 2013;13(8):e49–54.

153. Al-Salameh A, Francois P, Giraud S, Calender A, Bergemer-Fouquet AM, de Calan L, et al. Intracranial ependymoma associated with multiple endocrine neoplasia type 1. J Endocrinol Invest. 2010;33(5):353–6.

154. Kato H, Uchimura I, Morohoshi M, Fujisawa K, Kobayashi Y, Numano F, et al. Multiple endocrine neoplasia type 1 associated with spinal ependymoma. Intern Med. 1996;35(4):285–9.

155. Gatta-Cherifi B, Chabre O, Murat A, Niccoli P, Cardot-Bauters C, Rohmer V, et al. Adrenal involvement in MEN1. Analysis of 715 cases from the Groupe d'etude des Tumeurs Endocrines database. Eur J Endocrinol. 2012;166(2):269–79.

156. Kharb S, Pandit A, Gundgurthi A, Garg MK, Brar KS, Kannan N, et al. Hidden diagnosis of multiple endocrine neoplasia-1 unraveled during workup of virilization caused by adrenocortical carcinoma. Indian J Endocrinol Metab. 2013;17(3):514–8.

157. Griniatsos JE, Dimitriou N, Zilos A, Sakellariou S, Evangelou K, Kamakari S, et al. Bilateral adrenocortical carcinoma in a patient with multiple endocrine neoplasia type 1 (MEN1) and a novel mutation in the MEN1 gene. World J Surg Oncol. 2011;9:6.

158. Haase M, Anlauf M, Schott M, Schinner S, Kaminsky E, Scherbaum WA, et al. A new mutation in the menin gene causes the multiple endocrine neoplasia type 1 syndrome with adrenocortical carcinoma. Endocrine 2011;39(2):153–9.

Paul Wermer

1898–1975

Miguel F. Herrera and Elpidio Manuel Barajas-Fregoso

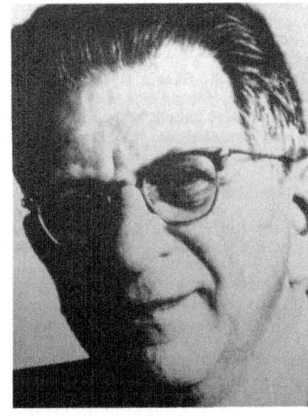

Paul Wermer. (From [14]. Reprinted with permission from ABC-CLIO Inc)

Paul Wermer, son of Leopold Wermer and Sophie nee Goldsterm, was born on February 3, 1898, in Vienna, Austria, and died on November 18, 1975, in Europe. He married Eva Raundnitz in 1925 and had a son, Hans Wermer. His native language was Hungarian.

Dr. Wermer studied at the faculty of medicine from the summer of 1918 throughout the winter semester of 1921 [1]. During his final semester, he studied at the University of Heidelberg, passed his final exams with honors, and obtained his medical degree from the medical school of the University of Vienna in 1922 [2]. For further education, Dr. Wermer moved to Ann Arbor, Michigan, obtaining the degree of Endocrine Physiologist from Michigan University in 1933. He then moved to New York in 1942 to do research in the Department of Medicine of Columbia University. He was part of the College of Physicians and Surgeons from 1947 to 1963 [3].

Paul Wermer participated in research projects in many hospitals (Fig. 1), including the Vanderbilt Clinic, the Delafield Hospital, the Bellevue Hospital, and the Presbyterian Hospital. With the aim of providing an appropriate forum for educational and disseminating the results of his biological research, Dr. Paul Wermer joined the Federation of American Societies for Experimental Biology in 1954 [3]. He retired from professional life on June 30, 1963 [2].

A constellation of multiple endocrine tumors was first reported by Jakob Erdheim in 1903. He described the autopsy of a patient with acromegaly, a pituitary tumor, thyroid goiter, three enlarged parathyroid glands, and pancreatic necrosis [4]. There were several reports of patients with multiple endocrine tumors to follow, but a true syndrome was not identified until 1953. Underhal and others from the Mayo Clinic reported eight patients with multiple endocrine adenomas that included parathyroid tumors in all, acromegaly in two, and severe peptic ulcer disease due to Zollinger–Ellison syndrome (ZES) in 3 [5].

Dr. Wermer wrote several papers in the field of endocrine disease. Perhaps his most relevant contribution was his description of the "Genetic Aspects of Adenomatosis of the Endocrine Glands," which was published in the *American Journal of Medicine* in 1954. In this publication, he described what is known today as the multiple endocrine neoplasia type 1 (MEN-1), a syndrome that includes pituitary, pancreatic, and parathyroid tumors and that was subsequently named after him (Wermer syndrome). In his paper, he described a family in which the MEN-1 syndrome occurred in several family members spanning two generations. In his conclusions, he highlighted the hereditary pattern of the syndrome as autosomal dominant suggesting that one single autosomal gene would be responsible for the disease. This hypothesis was later confirmed with the discovery of the menin gene at 11q13 [6, 7].

Zollinger and **Ellison** [8] in one of their initial reports underlined the high prevalence of ZES in the MEN-1 syndrome. This important finding was in accordance with Wermer's finding that 19 of 20 patients from his reported

M. F. Herrera (✉) · E. M. Barajas-Fregoso
Endocrine Surgery, Department of Surgery, Instituto Nacional de Ciencias Medicas y Nutricion "Salvador Zubiran", Tlalpan D.F., Mexico D.F., Mexico
e-mail: miguelfherrera@gmail.com

J. L. Pasieka, J. A. Lee (eds.), *Surgical Endocrinopathies,* DOI 10.1007/978-3-319-13662-2_59,
© Springer International Publishing Switzerland 2015

```
VC:Volunteer Med.Feb.'41
   Asst.Phys.'43'44                              1a

PH:Asst.Phys.1/1/47,'47-'57                      1a
   Asst.Att.Phys.'58 '59'60'61'62-6/30/63//      1b


DELAFIELD:Asst.Vis.Phys.1/1/50-12/31/56//        1a
```

a

```
Wermer, Paul
        M.D. 1922 U.Wien, Austria
PHARM:Volunteer Research 5/5/42
MED:(Belle)Asst.'46'47                          1a
        Instr.'48-'54
        Assoc.'55-'58'59
        Asst.Clin.Prof.'60'61'62
                -retired 6/30/63//              1b
DECEASED: 11/18/75                              1b
BELLE:1st Med.Div.Clin.Asst.Vis.Phys.
        '44-'47                                 1a
        Asst.Vis.Phys.'48-12/31/50
        Assoc.Vis.Phys.1/1/51,
        1/1/52-1/1/59,1/1/60
        1/1/61,1/1/62,1/1/63
```
b   `-retired 6/30/63//    -OVER-`

Fig. 1 Paul Wermer's employee card at Columbia University

family had ZES and led to a subsequent publication titled "Endocrine Adenomatosis and Peptic Ulcer in a Large Kindred. Inherited Multiple Tumors and Mosaic Pleiotropism in Man" [8]. One additional contribution by Wermer was the identification of multiple lipomas and gastrointestinal carcinoid tumors as part of the MEN-1 syndrome (Fig. 2) [5–12].

Interestingly, according to the 1940 US census, the last residence of Dr. Wermer was in New York City, Manhattan Borough Assembly District 7, corner of Amsterdam Av and W 85th (Fig. 3) [13]; however, the Social Security Death Index indicates that his last residence was at the US consulate in Bern, Switzerland.

References

1. Archiv der Universität Wien. Librarian for science and biology and physics. Vienna University Library. Universitätsring 1A-1010 Wien. http://bibliothek.univie.ac.at/archiv/vienna_university_archive. html. Accessed 2 May 2014.
2. Archives & Special Collections Augustus C. Long Health Sciences Library, Columbia University Medical Center. 701 West 168th Street, New York, NY 10032. http://vesta.cumc.columbia.edu/ library/archives/index.html. Accessed 23 May 2014.
3. US National Archives. National Register of Scientific and Technical Personnel Files. Record group 307. 2013. www.moncavo.com. Accessed 26 May 2014.
4. Erdheim J. Zur normalen und pathologischen histologie der glandula thyreoidea, parathyreoidea und hypophysis. Beitr Anat Pathol. 1903;33:158.
5. Lairmore T. Multiple endocrine neoplasia. In: Norton J, Barie P, Randal R, et al., editors. Essential practice of surgery. Basic science and clinical evidence. 2nd edn. New York: Springer; 2008. pp. 417–420.

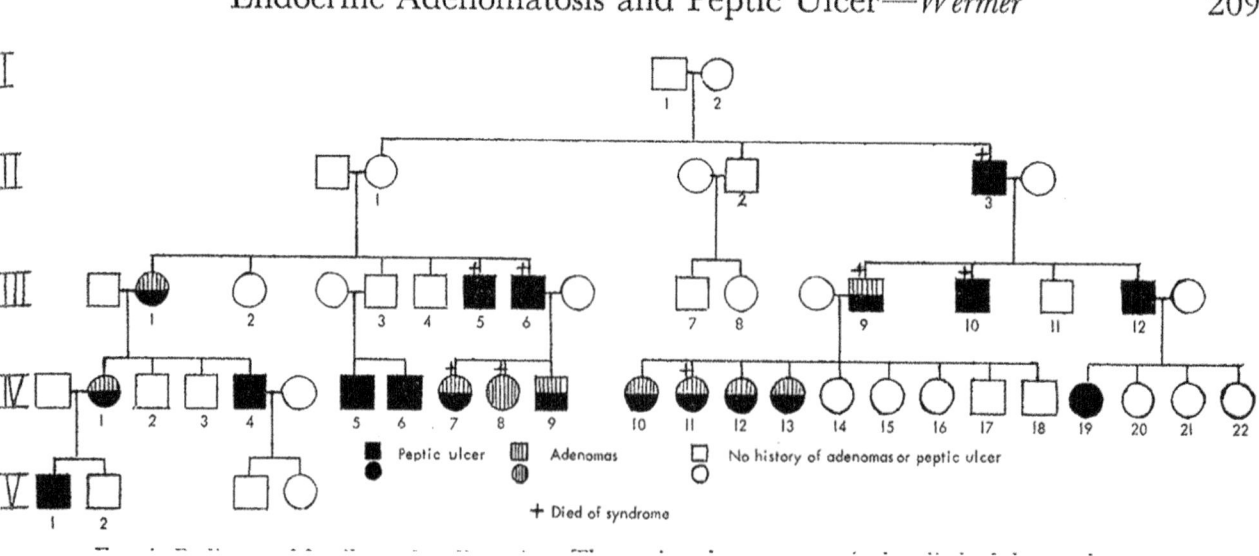

Endocrine Adenomatosis and Peptic Ulcer—*Wermer*   209

Fig. 2 Wermer's original illustration of familiar pedigree with inheritance pattern in endocrine adenomatosis and peptic ulcer

Fig. 3 US Census from 1940, New York City

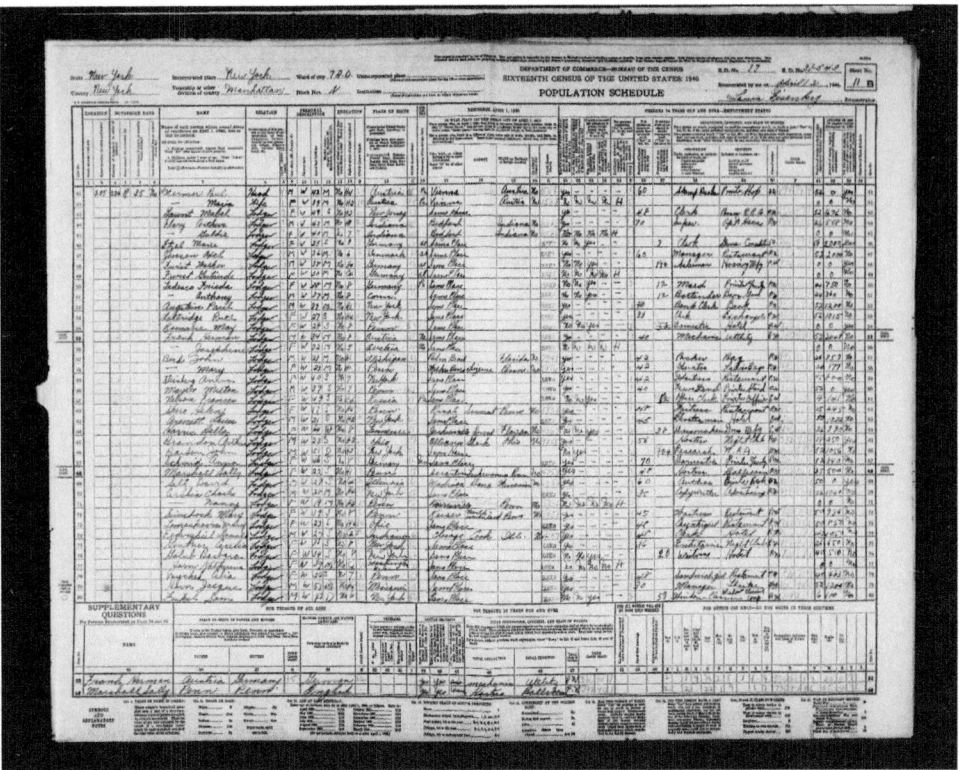

6. Wermer P. Genetic aspects of adenomatosis of endocrine glands. Am J Med. 1954 ;16(3):363–71.

7. Thompson G, Young W. Multiple endocrine neoplasia type 1. In: Clark O, Duh Q, Kebebew E, editors. Textbook of endocrine surgery. 2nd ed. Philadelphia: Elsevier Saunders; 2005. pp. 673–690.

8. Wermer P. Endocrine adenomatosis and peptic ulcer in a large kindred. Inherited multiple tumors and mosaic pleiotropism in man. Am J Med. 1963;35:205–12.

9. Zubrod CG, Wermer P, Pieper W, Hilbish TF. Acromegaly, jejunal ulcers and hypersecretion of gastric juice: clinical-pathological conference at the National Institutes of Health. Ann Intern Med. 1958;49(6):1389–409.

10. Wermer P. Duality of pancreatogenous peptic ulcer. N Engl J Med. 1968;278(7):397–8.

11. Wermer P. The diagnosis of polyadenomatosis of endocrine glands. Radiol Clin North Am. 1967;5(2):349–54.

12. Wermer P. Familiar polyendocrine adenomatous hyperplasia syndrome. Actual Endocinol. 1973;13:5–13.

13. United States census, 1940. https://familysearch.org/pal:/MM9.3.1/ TH-1942-27839-20734-3?cc=2000219. Accessed 26 May 2014.

14. Wellbourn RB. The history of endocrine surgery. Westport: Praeger; 1990.

Norman W. Thompson

1932–

Gerard M. Doherty

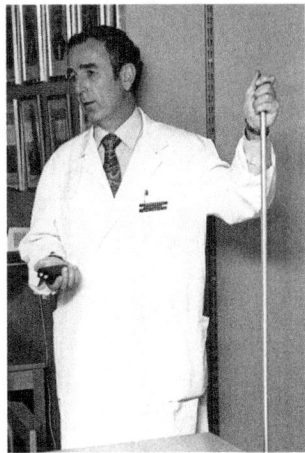

Dr. Norman W. Thompson in one of his frequent teaching moments

Dr. Norman W. Thompson (NWT) is one of the most beloved figures in endocrine surgery. His examples of patient care, mentorship, devotion to his craft, and affable nature have influenced hundreds of surgeons and affected the lives of thousands of patients. He advanced the field through his scientific research and his organizational ability. He is among a small group that can be considered the founders of the specialty of endocrine surgery.

Academic Career

NWT graduated from Hope College (located in Holland, Michigan) in 1953; he has remained a loyal supporter since. He was a member of the board of trustees from 1973 to 1988, and was awarded a Distinguished Alumni Award in 2004. He and Marcia (Hope College, Class of 1956) have endowed a science laboratory and a scholarship at Hope College (Fig. 1). Following college, he went on to the School of Medicine at the University of Michigan, receiving his medi-

cal degree in 1957. Dr. Thompson was recruited to stay at the University first in 1957 as a trainee and then in 1962 as a faculty member. He spent his entire career in Ann Arbor, despite opportunities to take leadership positions elsewhere. He retired from active practice in 2002, becoming professor emeritus. An endowed professorship was established in his honor[1].

When NWT joined the faculty in 1962, endocrine surgery did not exist as a subspecialty of general surgery. Most hormones could not be easily measured in patients, and the imaging to identify tumors was rudimentary by current standards. His initial practice was broad, and his publica-

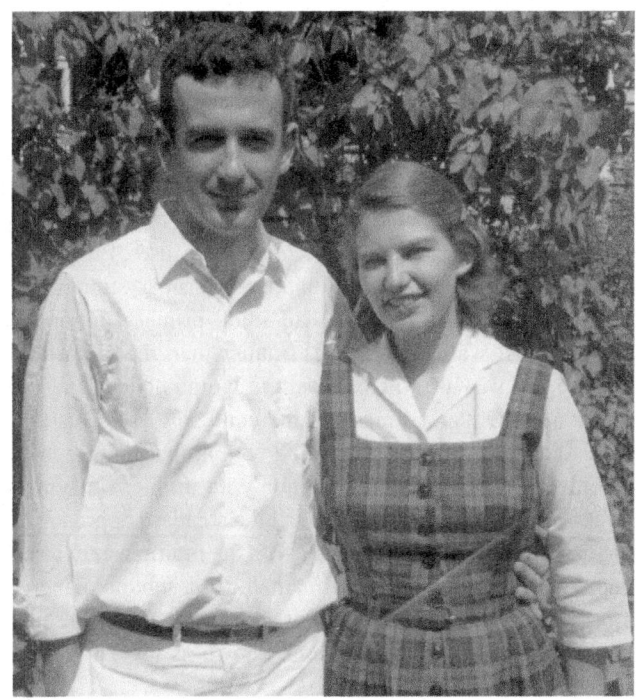

Fig. 1 Norman and Marcia during NWT's internship at the University of Michigan (ca. 1957)

G. M. Doherty (✉)
Department of Surgery, Boston University, 88 East Newton St C-500, Boston, MA 02118, USA
e-mail: dohertyg@bu.edu

[1] The author was the inaugural Norman W. Thompson professor of surgery at the University of Michigan from 2002 to 2012.

J. L. Pasieka, J. A. Lee (eds.), *Surgical Endocrinopathies,* DOI 10.1007/978-3-319-13662-2_60,
© Springer International Publishing Switzerland 2015

tions from his first decade of practice reflect his interests in general surgery, trauma, and vascular diseases. However, he was influenced by contact with faculty colleagues who were making important observations in patients with endocrine tumors, including Drs. Beierwaltes and Sisson (nuclear medicine/thyroidology), Nishiyama (pathology), Schteingart (endocrinology/adrenal), and Vinik (endocrinology/pancreas). These collaborations placed him at the center of a large group that made routine the precise measurement and interpretation of hormone levels, and developed the imaging tests needed to identify the tumors. As his experience and fascination with these tumors grew, his endocrine surgery practice squeezed out his other clinical and academic interests. He became devoted to the nascent field.

Clinical and Scientific Contributions

NWT made many of the initial observations that underpin the field of endocrine surgery as we now know it. He had a very broad endocrine surgery practice, a keen set of observational skills, and an uncanny memory for patient situations. He practiced the full spectrum of endocrine surgery, including thyroid, parathyroid, pancreas, and adrenal tumors, as well as tumors of the diffuse neuroendocrine system. His position in Ann Arbor, where the first metaiodobenzylguanidine (MIBG) scans were performed, gave him a vast experience with pheochromocytoma, one of the areas to which he made many contributions [1]. He went on to describe novel presentation of pheochromocytomas, methods for perioperative preparation, and operative techniques.

Similarly, he took his personal observations of a very rare disease (gastrinoma causing *Zollinger–Ellison* syndrome) and was among the first to determine the cause of the large proportion of patients with no apparent primary tumor. He identified that many patients had small primary tumors in the duodenal wall, often much smaller than the metastatic disease that was also often present in lymph nodes [2]. This observation explained many of the confusing concepts that investigators in this area struggled with at the time, such as whether gastrinoma could commonly be primary in lymph nodes. In related work, he developed a standard approach to the pancreatic tumors associated with the multiple endocrine neoplasia type 1 syndrome. This included a subtotal pancreatectomy and removal of the duodenal disease that he had described; this procedure became known as the Thompson operation [3].

Throughout his endocrine surgery career, NWT demonstrated his skill as a careful and thoughtful surgeon most frequently by his management of thyroid and parathyroid disease. From his early contributions cataloguing the complications of thyroidectomy, to later collaborations on the genetics of familial syndromes and molecular changes in

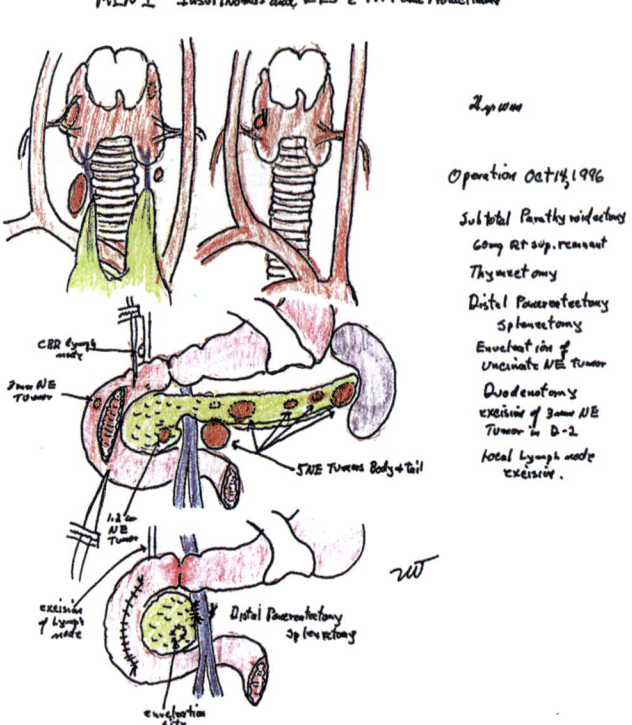

Fig. 2 A colored pencil drawing by NWT of one of his MEN-1 operations. (Courtesy of Norman W. Thompson)

thyroid cancer, NWT always stayed current and found ways to contribute [4, 5]. His intraoperative discussions are legendary, as he was able to think aloud through complex situations, teaching as he went along. At the completion of his operations, he often made a colored pencil drawing of what he had found and done (Fig. 2).

Mentorship

One of the key contributions that NWT made to the field was through his mentorship of surgeons in Ann Arbor and around the world. He was a beloved teacher of surgery at the University of Michigan and helped to train over 265 chief residents in surgery. He had an endocrine surgery fellowship in Ann Arbor that was one of the first, and the very few, to devote dedicated training time to the field. The fellowship was tailored to meet the needs and opportunity of the trainee; it could range from 3 to 12 months, and was often funded by the trainee's home institution. Many current leaders in endocrine surgery spent time in Ann Arbor with NWT in this way, including Janice Pasieka, Peter Angelos, Gary Talpos, John Kukora, and Jay Harness. NWT also spread his mentorship around the world. He has been a prolific speaker, serving as a visiting professor at 135 institutions, and delivering over 300 other invited lectures. He has received numerous honorific titles and awards. His approachability and clarity of explanation has endeared him to surgeons and to patients.

IAES and AAES

NWT was one of the founding members of both the International Association of Endocrine Surgeons (IAES), and the American Association of Endocrine Surgeons (AAES). Both of these groups can trace their lineage to the San Francisco Congress of the International Society of Surgery in September 1979 [6]. At that meeting, a group of international surgeons interested in endocrine surgery gathered, and determined that the time was right for a group dedicated to their interests. From that, the IAES was born, under the watchful eye of NWT as the inaugural council-coordinator, and subsequently the IAES president. During that same meeting in San Francisco, a smaller group of American surgeons had lunch, and decided that a similar group focused on North American-based surgeons could make important contributions to the field. The first meeting was held in Ann Arbor in May of 1980, and included a two-day scientific program, with local arrangements by NWT, who was also elected the first AAES president. As the AAES has grown, much of the credit goes to NWT, as he faithfully attended the sessions, learned the names and interests of junior surgeons from all over, and was always prepared with an opinion or comment for the papers. He helped to create the welcoming, collegial atmosphere that predominates at both the AAES and the IAES meetings. The major donors to the AAES Foundation are grouped as the Norman Thompson Fellows in his honor, to reflect the many contributions that he made to the group.

Family

NWT has remained in Ann Arbor for more than 50 years, with his wife Marcia (née Veldman), a fellow student at Hope College (Fig. 3). They have four children, all of whom attended Hope College: Robert (Hope 1979), Karen (Hope 1983), Susan (Hope 1987), and Jennifer (Hope 1989). Travel with his family, often also including visits to members of his endocrine surgery "family," was a frequent indulgence, but has been curtailed by recent health issues. The Thompsons' generosity has helped to support Hope College, the University of Michigan, and the AAES, among many other worthy causes.

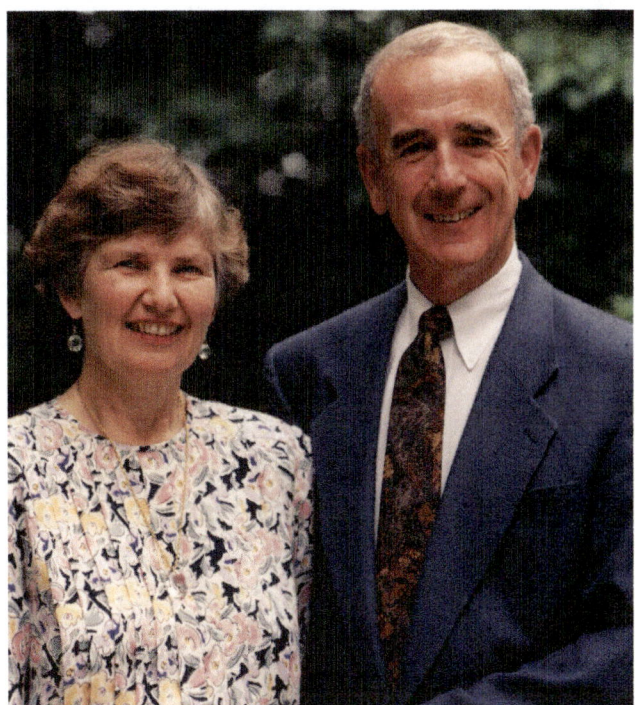

Fig. 3 Norman and Marcia in 2002

The legacy that NWT has created has influenced the lives of many; his patients, and the patients of all to whom he has given so much of himself. He has helped to create a vibrant field of endocrine surgery. He recognized it before it existed, he nurtured it in its infancy, and he shaped the future leaders of the field by both his direct contributions and his personal example. We each owe him our admiration and gratitude.

References

1. Sisson JC, et al. Scintigraphic localization of pheochromocytoma. N Engl J Med. 1981;305(1):12–7.
2. Thompson NW, Vinik AI, Eckhauser FE. Microgastrinomas of the duodenum. A cause of failed operations for the Zollinger–Ellison syndrome. Ann Surg. 1989;209(4):396–404.
3. Thompson NW, et al. The surgical treatment of gastrinoma in MEN I syndrome patients. Surgery. 1989;106(6):1081–5; discussion 1085–6.
4. Thompson NW, Harness JK. Complications of total thyroidectomy for carcinoma. Surg Gynecol Obstet. 1970;131(5):861–8.
5. Li C, et al. Does BRAF V600E mutation predict aggressive features in papillary thyroid cancer? Results from four endocrine surgery centers. J Clin Endocrinol Metab. 2013;98(9):3702–12.
6. Thompson NW. The founding of the American Association of Endocrine Surgeons: the time was right. Surgery. 2011;150(6):1303–7.

Multiple Endocrine Neoplasia 2 Syndromes

Latha V. Pasupuleti and Jennifer H. Kuo

Historical Overview

Multiple endocrine adenopathies were first documented as early as 1903. Over the next 50 years, multiple case reports involving varying associations of pituitary, parathyroid, and pancreatic islet tumors came to light, and in 1953 the term "multiple endocrine adenomas" (MEA) was born. In 1960, the Mayo Clinic documented a patient with bilateral pheochromocytomas and thyroid cancer with amyloid stroma, later to be defined as medullary thyroid cancer (MTC). In 1961, **John Sipple** was the first to report a 33-year-old man with bilateral pheochromocytomas, a follicular thyroid cancer, and an enlarged parathyroid on autopsy [1, 2]. Over the next decade, additional cases and familial clusters of MTC, pheochromocytomas, and hyperparathyroidism were identified and the term multiple endocrine neoplasia 2 (MEN 2) was coined since this pattern of endocrinopathies was distinct from multiple endocrine neoplasia 1 (MEN 1). Around the same time, a number of patients in the USA were noted to have MTC and pheochromocytomas, along with a number of distinct physical characteristics, among them mucosal neuromas and a marfanoid body habitus. Simultaneously, family clusters with the same constellation of endocrine tumors and physical features were found in Europe. In 1975, surgeons at the Mayo Clinic proposed that MEN 2 syndrome be reclassified as two distinct phenotypic patterns: MEN 2A and MEN 2B.

MEN 2 has been reported in approximately 500–1000 families worldwide, and the prevalence has been estimated at approximately 1:30,000–35,000 [3, 4]. These syndromes are relatively rare, but have high morbidity and mortality due primarily to the aggressive nature of MTC.

This chapter reviews the phenotypic manifestations of the MEN 2 syndrome subtypes, changes in the diagnoses and clinical management of the involved endocrine tumors (MTC, pheochromocytoma, hyperparathyroidism), genotypic and phenotypic correlations of the most common rearranged during transfection (RET) proto-oncogene mutations, and current screening and treatment recommendations.

Phenotypic Manifestations of MEN 2

The phenotypic manifestations of MEN 2 present as a number of unique patterns of endocrine disease. MEN 2 syndromes are divided into three subtypes: MEN 2A, MEN 2B, and familial MTC (FMTC). MEN 2A is the most common, accounting for more than 80–90 % of all MEN 2 cases, while MEN 2B accounts for just 5 % of all cases. Familial MTC makes up the remaining cases of hereditary MTC [5]. Table 1 summarizes and compares the typical unifying and distinguishing clinical manifestations of the three MEN 2 subtypes, including the proportion of patients who exhibit a certain feature.

MEN 2A

MEN 2A is also known as Sipple syndrome named after John Sipple, a pulmonary physician who first reported this endocrinopathy [1, 2]. This syndrome includes MTC, pheochromocytoma, and primary hyperparathyroidism. MTC is the most common clinical presentation of MEN 2A, with nearly 100 % of patients affected. The average age of presentation of a patient with sporadic MTC is in the sixth decade. In contrast, the average age of presentation for a patient with MEN 2A syndrome is 20–40 years, with some more aggressive forms presenting by age 5 [6].

Less commonly, patients present with symptoms due to pheochromocytomas. Pheochromocytomas are present in approximately 50 % of patients with MEN 2A and cause various symptoms including palpitations, headaches, hypertension, and flushing. Hyperparathyroidism occurs in 15–30 %

J. H. Kuo (✉) · L. V. Pasupuleti
Surgery Department, New York Presbyterian Hospital,
Columbia University Medical Center, 161 Fort Washington Ave,
8th Floor, New York, NY 10032, USA
e-mail: jhk2029@cumc.columbia.edu

J. L. Pasieka, J. A. Lee (eds.), *Surgical Endocrinopathies,* DOI 10.1007/978-3-319-13662-2_61,
© Springer International Publishing Switzerland 2015

Table 1 Phenotypic manifestations of the MEN 2 subtypes

Typical manifestations	MEN 2 subtypes		
	MEN 2A (%)	MEN 2B (%)	FMTC (%)
Medullary thyroid cancer	100	100	95–100
Pheochromocytoma	50	50	–
Primary hyperparathyroidism	15–30	–	–
Gangliotomosis of GI tract	–	100	–
Mucosal neuromas	–	100	–
Marfanoid habitus	–	75	–

MEN multiple endocrine neoplasia, *FMTC* familial medullary thyroid carcinoma, *GI* gastrointestinal

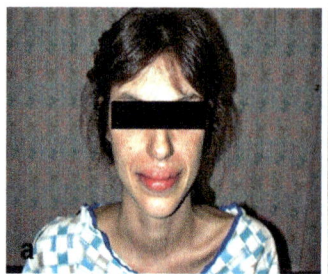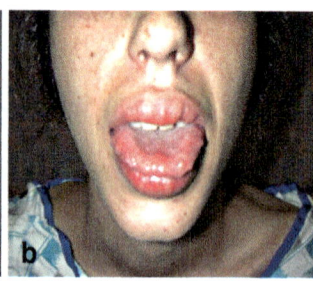

Fig. 1 Some distinct physical characteristics of MEN 2B patients. **a** MEN 2B patient with typical thin, marfanoid habitus, prognathic jaws, and prominent lips. **b** Mucosal neuromas are often found on the lips and tongue. (Courtesy of Quan-Yang Duh, UCSF, Department of Surgery)

of MEN 2A patients, with the peak incidence in the third or fourth decade. Multiglandular hyperplasia is the most common histologic finding, although single gland adenomas are present in some patients [4, 5, 7]. In addition, rare variants of MEN 2A exist, which include the above-listed endocrine tumors, along with either cutaneous lichen amyloidosis or Hirschsprung's disease [8, 9].

MEN 2B

Like MEN 2A, MEN 2B patients have MTC and pheochromocytomas, but they do not present with parathyroid disease. Instead, MEN 2B patients exhibit various unique physical features, most commonly mucosal neuromas and a marfan-like physical constitution.

MTC in MEN 2B also manifests in nearly 100 % of patients. MTC develops earlier and more aggressively than in MEN 2A. Metastatic disease has been reported before age 1, and death may occur in the second or third decade of life [4, 5]. Pheochromocytomas occur in more than half of MEN 2B patients with similar presentations as in MEN 2A. There are no well-documented examples of parathyroid disease in MEN 2B patients.

The mucosal neuromas and marfanoid body habitus are the most distinctive features of MEN 2B and are recognizable in childhood. Patients can have prominent lips and prognathic jaws (Fig. 1). The corneal nerves can also be quite enlarged. The marfanoid habitus combined with facial features is unique, and often unrelated affected individuals look strikingly similar. Neuromas are present on the tip of the tongue, buccal mucosa, under the eyelids, and throughout the gastrointestinal (GI) tract. The most common presentation in children relates to GI symptomatology, including intermittent colic, pseudo-obstruction, and diarrhea. Some children present with failure to thrive secondary to these persistent GI symptoms [5, 10]. Almost 75 % of patients will have skeletal abnormalities that give them a marfanoid body habitus [11]. Mucosal neuromas or GI gangliomas are present in nearly 100 % of MEN 2B patients [12]. Confirmation

of these various clinical features can be made by biopsy of the mucosal neuromas, rectal biopsy, or slit-lamp examination for medullated corneal nerves [6].

FMTC

Once thought to be a distinct entity, first described by **John Farndon**, FMTC is now considered a common subvariant of MEN 2A, in which MTC is the only manifestation. The clinical diagnosis of FMTC is established by the presence of MTC in greater than four family members over multiple generations without any evidence of pheochromocytoma or hyperparathyroidism. The clinical course of MTC in FMTC patients is more benign than in MEN2A and MEN2B, with a late onset or no clinical manifestation of disease. Thus, the overall prognosis is relatively good and better than the other MEN 2 subtypes [8, 9].

Since the penetrance of pheochromocytoma is 50 % in MEN 2A, it is possible that MEN 2A could masquerade as FMTC in small kindreds. It is important to consider this, because failure to recognize this scenario could lead to serious morbidity and mortality from an undiagnosed pheochromocytoma in an affected family member [4, 5].

Medullary Thyroid Cancer

Up to 75 % of all MTCs are thought to be sporadic; the rest are hereditary in the form of MEN 2 syndromes [5]. MTC is present in nearly all patients with MEN 2A and MEN 2B and is often the first presenting disease of the syndrome. The calcitonin-producing cells (C-cells) of the thyroid, which are derived from the neural crest, are considered to be the precursor cells from which MTC arises. This tumor usually develops in childhood, beginning as hyperplasia of the C-cells [5]. The C-cells secrete calcitonin and carcinoembryonic antigen (CEA), which serve as tumor markers for the disease. While sporadic MTC can present as a solitary nodule, hereditary MTC tends to be multicentric. The disease spreads regionally from central to lateral neck lymph nodes and then to the liver, lung, bone, and brain [8].

Initially, biochemical testing with basal and stimulated levels of calcitonin was used as the primary screening method for diagnosis of hereditary MTC. Secretion of calcitonin can be stimulated 3–20-fold with intravenous (IV) pentagastrin, calcium, or both [7]. The effectiveness of pentagastrin-stimulated calcitonin screening increases progressively with age, though, unfortunately, lacks sensitivity where it is needed most—in young children. Thus, its use as screening for MEN 2 syndrome in children before the age of 5 has its limitations [4, 6]. More recently, advances in genetic analysis of the RET oncogene mutations has led to direct DNA analysis becoming the primary screening method for MTC. Calcitonin screening is still used by some to determine the timing of prophylactic thyroidectomy for patients with certain RET mutations [8]. After surgical resection, plasma calcitonin and CEA levels are used to monitor disease progression. Normalization of these tumor markers has a favorable prognosis, whereas progressive increases in calcitonin or CEA indicate persistent or recurrent disease [8, 9, 13]. Calcitonin and CEA tend to rise together, but in some cases of recurrent disease, calcitonin will no longer be elevated, while CEA levels are. This is considered a sign of tumor dedifferentiation [4, 8].

Due to the poor prognosis of advanced stage MTC, early prophylactic surgery is recommended before the disease is clinically evident or becomes regionally advanced. For patients with MEN 2A and FMTC under the age of 5 with no clinically evident lymph nodes, prophylactic total thyroidectomy alone is the recommended operation. For both node-negative MEN 2A and FMTC patients older than 8 years and all MEN 2B patients, prophylactic total thyroidectomy with central neck (level VI) dissection is indicated. In newly diagnosed adult MEN 2 patients with MTC, total thyroidectomy should be performed with node dissection based on extent of disease. In patients with no evidence of local invasion or local cervical metastases, total thyroidectomy and prophylactic central neck lymph node dissection is advocated. In patients with limited locally advanced disease, lateral neck dissection is also supported [4]. Recommendations for timing of surgical resection based on genotype are discussed later in the chapter.

Pheochromocytoma

Pheochromocytomas are present in about 50 % of both MEN 2A and MEN 2B patients. The characteristics of the tumors and clinical manifestations are similar in the two subvariants. Pheochromocytomas arise in the adrenal medulla from neural crest-derived chromaffin cells which primarily secrete the catecholamines epinephrine and norepinephrine. Tumors tend to be benign with metastasis being uncommon. Tumors are commonly bilateral. If they do not present simultaneously, more than 50 % of patients who have had unilateral adrenalectomy later develop a pheochromocytoma in the contralateral gland within a decade. A distinguishing feature from hereditary paraganglioma syndromes is that the pheochromocytomas in MEN 2 are almost always found within the adrenal gland, not as extra-adrenal tumors [4, 5, 7]. Clinical presentation is similar to sporadic forms with patients having symptoms from catecholamine excess such as headaches, palpitations, hypertension, tachycardia, and flushing.

Screening for pheochromocytoma involves measuring plasma or 24-h urinary levels of metanephrines and normetanephrines. If the biochemical diagnosis is confirmed, the patient should get imaging to localize the tumor with either computed tomography (CT) or magnetic resonance imaging (MRI) [4]. Further localization and staging for metastatic disease is performed with radiolabeled metaiodobenzylguanidine (MIBG) scintigraphy and positron emission tomography (PET) with different radiotracers such as fluorine-18-dopamine ($[^{18}F]DA$), fluorine-18-dihydroxyphenylalanine ($[^{18}F]DOPA$) or fluorine-18-fluorodeoxyglucose ($[^{18}F]$ FDG). MIBG scans have historically been the most widespread functional imaging technique used for localization of pheochromocytomas and paragangliomas with high sensitivity and specificity [14, 15]. However, recent studies have shown that MIBG has lower sensitivity for certain conditions such as familial pheochromocytoma and paraganglioma syndromes and malignant disease. Increasing evidence suggests that fluorine dopamine (FDA)-PET, fluorodeoxyglucose (FDG)-PET, and dihydroxyphenylalanine (DOPA)-PET are superior localization studies for pheochromocytoma and are helpful in the above scenarios when MIBG fails to demonstrate disease, though suspicion for disease is high (Fig. 2). MIBG is still the most widely used functional imaging technique and has the added advantage of selecting for patients with metastatic disease who are suitable for MIBG nuclear therapy [14, 15].

Because of the possible coexistence of pheochromocytoma, it is essential to screen for these tumors before thyroidectomy for MTC. There is significant morbidity and mortality from an undiagnosed pheochromocytoma. Before the association of pheochromocytomas and MTC in MEN 2 was recognized, many patients died from a hypertensive crisis during or after thyroidectomy secondary to unrecognized disease [1]. In fact, before advances in screening, pheochromocytoma, not MTC, was the leading cause of death in MEN 2A patients. If a patient has both a pheochromocytoma and MTC, adrenalectomy should be performed first to avoid an intraoperative adrenal crisis during thyroidectomy [4].

After appropriate preoperative preparation of the patient with alpha blockade, adrenalectomy should be performed. Patients who have unilateral pheochromocytoma on a localizing study should have a unilateral laparoscopic adrenalectomy. However, patients with bilateral adrenal tumors should have bilateral laparoscopic adrenalectomy. If tech-

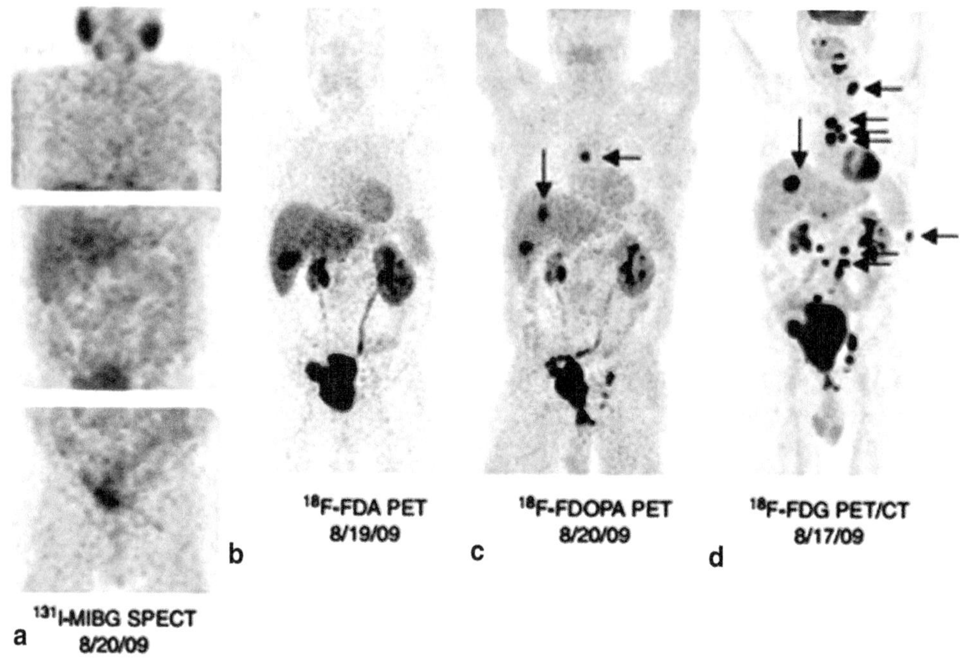

Fig. 2 Comparison of detection of metastatic pheochromocytoma by various nuclear imaging techniques. Nuclear imaging studies of a 55-year-old male with metastatic pheochromocytoma who tested negative for succinate dehydrogenase B, C, and D mutations. His primary tumor was located in the bladder and was initially resected in 2005. In 2009, he presented with metastatic disease. His 131 I-MIBG SPECT was negative (**a**), but his other nuclear imaging studies show metastatic disease: [^{18}F]-FDA PET (**b**), [^{18}F]-FDOPA PET (**c**), and especially [^{18}F]-FDG PET/CT (**d**). (From [16]. Reprinted with permission from Bioscientifica, Ltd)

nically feasible, a cortical-sparing adrenalectomy may be considered to avoid long-term steroid dependence and to reduce the risk of an Addisonian crisis, given that the risk of recurrence is relatively low [17–19]. Laparoscopic adrenalectomy can be performed via either the transabdominal or retroperitoneal approach. For a number of reasons, the retroperitoneal approach is increasingly being preferred. Both approaches have similar clinical outcomes and low rates of perioperative complications [20, 21]. The retroperitoneal approach has additional benefits of not contributing to intrabdominal adhesion formation and eliminating the need for repositioning when performing bilateral adrenalectomy [20, 21].

Primary Hyperparathyroidism

Primary hyperparathyroidism occurs in 15–30 % of patients with MEN 2A, with the peak incidence in the third or fourth decade. It is most often clinically occult with more than 85 % of patients being asymptomatic. Rarely is primary hyperparathyroidism the first manifestation of the syndrome. When present, hypercalcemia is usually mild [8]. Multiglandular hyperplasia is the most common histologic finding, though adenomas are present in some patients.

Diagnosis is established by the presence of hypercalcemia, hypophosphatemia, hypercalciuria, and high serum parathyroid hormone (intact parathyroid hormone, iPTH) [4, 5, 7]. Serum ionized or albumin-corrected calcium and parathyroid hormone levels are used to screen for asymptomatic hyperparathyroidism [4].

Surgical resection is the recommended treatment for primary hyperparathyroidism in MEN 2A. Since four-gland hyperplasia is the more common presentation, treatment is with three-and-a-half-gland excision, or four-gland excision with autotransplantation in the forearm. Autotransplantation in the arm is preferred due to increased morbidity and risk of permanent hypoparathyroidism associated with reoperative neck surgery in these patients [4, 5]. When only a single abnormal gland is found, a more focused approach utilizing intraoperative parathyroid hormone (PTH) can be done. If hyperparathyroidism is diagnosed at the same time as MTC, parathyroidectomy is performed with thyroidectomy, reducing risks and challenges of reoperative neck surgery later in life.

Genotypic Manifestations of MEN 2

In 1987, it was discovered that MEN 2 syndromes are caused by germ-line mutations in the RET proto-oncogene [9]. When RET was initially identified as the susceptibility gene for MEN 2, it was the first time that a proto-oncogene was implicated in the etiology of an inherited cancer syndrome. This discovery has led to major advances in the understanding, screening, and clinical management of MEN 2 syndromes [6].

In June 1994, the International RET Mutation Consortium first convened and pooled together the worldwide RET mutation data for joint genotype–phenotype analysis. Eighteen centers from across North America, Europe, Australia, and Asia submitted data from 477 MEN 2 families. More than 98 % of the MEN 2A families, 95 % of the MEN 2B families, and 85 % of the FMTC families had germ-line RET mutations, thus confirming a clear relationship between the RET gene and MEN 2 syndromes [13].

The RET proto-oncogene, located on chromosome 10q11.2, encodes a receptor tyrosine kinase expressed in tissues and tumors derived from the neural crest, including C-cells of the thyroid and chromaffin cells in the adrenal medulla [9]. The most common mutated codons are 609, 611, 618, 620, 630, 634, 768, 790, 791, 804, 883, 891, and 918. These codons are encoded by exons 10–16 [13]. Mutations in cysteine residues in the RET extracellular domain are primarily associated with MEN 2A, and sometimes FMTC, and involve codons 609, 611, 618, 620, 630, and 634 [22]. Approximately, 80–90 % of patients with MEN 2A have a mutation in codon 634, which causes a more aggressive form of MTC. RET intracellular kinase domain mutations are mainly associated with FMTC and MEN 2B. Mutations in the intracellular codons 768, 790, 791, 804, and 891 correlate to FMTC, and occur less commonly in patients with MEN 2A. Specific mutations of codon 918 or 883 are exclusive to MEN 2B and account for the vast majority of cases [8, 9, 22] (Fig. 3).

MEN 2 syndromes are inherited in an autosomal dominant fashion. Before DNA-based testing, MEN 2 was diagnosed either when an individual presented with the signs and symptoms of the syndrome or through annual biochemical screening of all unaffected first-degree relatives of known MEN 2 patients for MTC, pheochromocytoma, and primary hyperparathyroidism. The knowledge of transmission of mutated RET proto-oncogenes has allowed molecular diagnosis and presymptomatic DNA-based testing to become possible. RET testing is the clinical standard of care for MEN 2 in the USA and worldwide.

DNA-based testing has distinct advantages, such as not having age-dependent sensitivity, being useful as a diagnostic test to confirm a clinical diagnosis of MEN 2, and, most importantly, being used as a predictive test for asymptomatic clinically at-risk individuals [4, 6]. Predictive testing for RET mutations in MEN 2 kindreds is performed using polymerase chain reaction-based protocols. Barring administrative errors, DNA-based predictive testing is nearly 100 % accurate [6].

Genotypic Phenotype Correlations and Screening

In addition to correlations between RET codon mutations and disease subtype, clear associations have been found between specific RET genotypes and the aggressiveness and age of onset of MTC and presence of other endocrine neoplasms such as pheochromocytoma or primary hyperparathyroidism [9]. For example, patients with codon 634 mutations are at significantly higher risk for development of primary hyperparathyroidism and pheochromocytoma [8, 9, 22]. All cases of MEN 2A/Hirschsprung's disease are associated with mutations on exon 10 (codons 609, 611, 618, 620) [9]. Over 95 % of MEN 2B cases are associated with the same methionine to threonine change at codon 918 (M918 T) in the RET extracellular kinase domain [22]. A second point mutation at codon 883, A883 F, has been identified in several MEN 2B patients without a M918 T mutation. MTC in patients with A883 F mutation is less aggressive than those MEN 2B patients with the M918 T mutation [8, 9, 22].

These genotypic–phenotypic correlations between genes, age of onset of MTC, and associated endocrine tumors have been used to determine age of prophylactic thyroidectomy for MTC and screening guidelines for pheochromocytoma and hyperparathyroidism. One of the most widely used guidelines for management of MEN 2 syndromes was developed by the American Thyroid Association (ATA) and divides risk levels from A to D, with A being the least aggressive and D the most aggressive and conferring the highest risk of mortality. Patients with level A risk, which mainly consists of FMTC patients, have the lowest risk of early aggressive MTC; level B risk correlates to MEN 2A and FMTC patients who have intermediate risk; level C risk patients are those MEN 2A patients with codon 634 mutations that have higher risk of early aggressive MTC; and level D risk patients are MEN 2B patients with the highest risk of development of early, fast-growing MTC [4, 9].

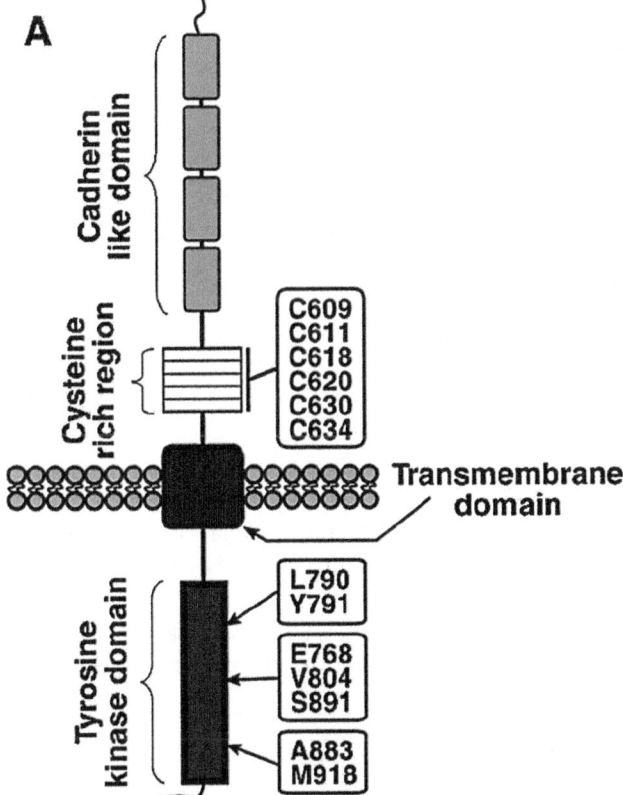

Fig. 3 Schematic diagram depicting RET tyrosine kinase receptor domains and the location of recurrent oncogenic mutations. The RET protein has a large extracellular domain containing a cysteine-rich region and a series of cadherin homology domains, a transmembrane domain, and an intracellular tyrosine kinase domain. The positions of the most common mutations found in patients with multiple endocrine neoplasia type 2 are depicted. (From [22]. Reprinted with permission from CLINICS)

Table 2 Timing for prophylactic thyroidectomy by American Thyroid Association (ATA) risk levels

ATA risk level	MEN 2 subtype	Associated codons	Treatment time line[a]
A	FMTC	768, 790, 791, 804, 891	Age 5–10[b]
B	MEN 2A, FMTC	609, 611, 618, 620, 630	Age 5
C	MEN 2A	634	Before age 5
D	MEN 2B	918, 883	Before age 1

FMTC familial medullary thyroid carcinoma, *MEN* multiple endocrine neoplasia

[a] ATA-recommended time line for performing prophylactic thyroidectomy

[b] Surgery for risk level A cases can be delayed when patient exhibits normal calcitonin, neck ultrasound

Based on these guidelines, MEN 2 patients with the lowest risk, ATA risk level A, should have prophylactic thyroidectomy between ages 5 and 10. With diligent screening for MTC using calcitonin and neck ultrasounds, this surgery can be delayed beyond this age window. On the other hand, patients with the highest risk, MEN 2B patients with ATA D risk level, should undergo prophylactic thyroidectomy before age 1 and often in the first months of life before there is clinical evidence of disease [4, 9]. The four ATA risk levels, associated MEN 2 subtypes and codons, and recommended treatment time line for prophylactic total thyroidectomy are summarized in Table 2.

In addition to risk stratification for prophylactic surgery, the ATA guidelines confer screening recommendations for the associated endocrine tumors. FMTC risk level A patients should undergo periodic screening for pheochromocytoma and hyperparathyroidism at age 20. MEN 2A and FMTC patients in risk level B should start at age 20 with annual screening for pheochromocytoma and periodic screening for hyperparathyroidism. For more aggressive forms of MEN 2A and for MEN 2B, the age to begin screening drops to childhood. MEN 2A with codon 634 mutations fall into ATA risk level C and require annual screening for pheochromocytoma and hyperparathyroidism starting at age 8. ATA risk level D patients with MEN 2B require annual screening for pheochromocytoma starting at 8 years of age [4, 9]. The ATA risk levels, associated MEN 2 subtypes and codons, and recommended treatment screening time line for pheochromocytoma and primary hyperparathyroidism are summarized in Table 3.

These recommendations are for management of at-risk individuals with MEN 2 syndrome who test positive for the RET proto-oncogene and specific codon mutations. The current practice for a patient without known family history of a MEN 2 syndrome that is diagnosed with MTC is to undergo genetic screening for RET mutations to determine if they have sporadic or hereditary MTC. If positive for a RET mutation, they should undergo biochemical screening for pheochromocytoma and primary hyperparathyroidism, particularly the former to determine if adrenalectomy should be performed before thyroidectomy [4].

Summary

Much has changed in our understanding of MEN 2 since the index case of Sipple's syndrome in 1961. Today, when we discuss MEN 2 syndromes, we refer to three distinct disease patterns known as MEN 2A, MEN 2B, and FMTC. The discovery that these disorders are transmitted via specific mutations in the RET proto-oncogene has changed both our understanding of MEN 2 syndromes' variable disease penetrance and our clinical approach to diagnosis, screening, and management of at-risk individuals. The endocrine surgery community has used these unique genotypic–phenotypic correlations to create management guidelines that have led us to aggressively screen and treat at-risk individuals at a preclinical disease state, before the morbidity and mortality from MTC can adversely affect these patients. Increased understanding of the RET proto-oncogene codon mutations will allow us to continue to gain more insight into these endocrine syndromes and further decrease the morbidity these diseases can cause to affected individuals and their families.

Key Summary Points

- Over the past half century, the definition of MEN 2 has changed from one syndrome unique from MEN 1 to three distinct MEN 2 subtypes: MEN 2A, MEN 2B, and FMTC.
- Increased understanding of the RET proto-oncogene's common codon mutations and their direct correlation to

Table 3 MEN 2 screening recommendations by ATA risk levels

ATA risk level	MEN 2 subtype	Associated codons	Screening for pheochromocytoma	Screening for primary hyperparthyroidism
A	FMTC	768, 790, 791, 804, 891	Start age 20, periodically	Start age 20, periodically
B	MEN 2A, FMTC	609, 611, 618, 620, 630	Start age 20, annually	Start age 20, periodically
C	MEN 2A	634	Start age 8, annually	Start age 8, annually
D	MEN 2B	918, 883	Start age 8, annually	n/a

MEN multiple endocrine neoplasia, *FMTC* familial medullary thyroid carcinoma, *ATA* American Thyroid Association specific MEN 2 phenotypes has changed the clinical management and screening of this disease.

References

1. Welbourn, Richard B. The history of endocrine surgery. Praeger: New York; 1990. p. 270–275.
2. Sipple, John H. The association of pheochromocytoma with carcinoma of the thyroid gland. Am J Med. 1961;31(1):163–6.
3. Marini F, Falchetti A, Del Monte F, et al. Multiple endocrine neoplasia type 2. Orphanet J Rare Dis. 2006;1:45.
4. Kloos RT, Eng C, Evans DB, Francis GL, Gagel RF, Gharib H, Moley JF, Pacini F, Ringel MD, Schlumberger M, Wells SA Jr. Medullary thyroid cancer: management guidelines of the American Thyroid Association. Thyroid. 2009;19(6):565–612.
5. Moore FD, Scoinski MA, Joste NE. Endocrine tumors and malignancies. In: Skarin A, editor. Atlas of diagnostic oncology. 3rd ed. Philadelphia: Elsevier Science; 2003.
6. Eng, Charis. RET proto-oncogene in the development of human cancer. J Clin Oncol. 1999;17:380–93.
7. Gagel RF, Shefelbine S, Hayashi H, Cote G. Multiple endocrine neoplasia type 2. In: Runge MS, Patterson C, editors. Principles of molecular medicine. Ch. 40. NJ: Humana; 2006. p 393–9.
8. Wells SA Jr, Pacini F, Robinson BG, Santoro M. Multiple endocrine neoplasia type 2 and familial medullary thyroid carcinoma: an update. J Clin Endocrinol Metab. 2013;98(8):3149–64.
9. Raue F, Frank-Raue K. Genotype-phenotype correlation in multiple endocrine neoplasia type 2. Clinics. 2012;67(1):69–75.
10. Rimoin DL, Schimke, RN. Genetic disorders of the endocrine glands. St. Louis: CV Mosby; 1971. pp. 136–8.
11. Morrison PJ, Nevin NC. Multiple endocrine neoplasia type 2B (mucosal neuroma syndrome, Wagenmann-Froboese syndrome). J Med Genetics. 1996;33(9):779–82.
12. Mulligan LM1, Marsh DJ, Robinson BG, Schuffenecker I, Zedenius J, Lips CJ, Gagel RF, Takai SI, Noll WW, Fink M, et al. Genotype-phenotype correlation in multiple endocrine neoplasia type 2: report of the International RET Mutation Consortium. J Intern Med. 1995;238(4):343–6.
13. Salehian B, Samoa R. RET gene abnormalities and thyroid disease: who should be screened and when. J Clin Res Pediatr Endocrinol. 2013;5(Suppl 1):70–8.
14. Rufini V, Treglia G, Castaldi P, Perotti G, Giordano A. Comparison of metaiodobenzylguanidine scintigraphy with positron emission tomography in the diagnostic work-up of pheochromocytoma and paraganglioma: a systematic review. Q J Nucl Med Mol Imaging. 2013;57(2):122–33.
15. Rufini V, Treglia G, Castaldi P, Perotti G, Calcagni ML, Corsello SM, Galli G, Fanti S, Giordano A. Comparison of 123I-MIBG SPECT-CT and 18 F-DOPA PET-CT in the evaluation of patients with known or suspected recurrent paraganglioma. Nucl Med Commun. 2011;32(7):575–82.
16. Fonte JS1, Robles JF, Chen CC, Reynolds J, Whatley M, Ling A, Mercado-Asis LB, Adams KT, Martucci V, Fojo T, Pacak K. False-negative ^{123}I-MIBG SPECT is most commonly found in SDHB-related pheochromocytoma or paraganglioma with high frequency to develop metastatic disease. Endocr Relat Cancer. 2012;19(1):83–93.
17. Gertner ME, Kebebew E. Multiple endocrine neoplasia type 2. Curr Treat Options Oncol. 2004;5(4):315–25.
18. Asari R, Scheuba C, Kaczirek K, Niederle B. Estimated risk of pheochromocytoma recurrence after adrenal-sparing surgery in patients with multiple endocrine neoplasia type 2A. Arch Surg. 2006;141(12):1199–205; discussion 1205.
19. Yip L, Lee JE, Shapiro SE, Waguespack SG, Sherman SI, Hoff AO, Gagel RF, Arens JF, Evans DB. Surgical management of hereditary pheochromocytoma. J Am Coll Surg. 2004;198(4):525–34; discussion 534–5.
20. Nagesser SK, Kievit J, Hermans J, Krans HM, van de Velde CJ. The surgical approach to the adrenal gland: a comparison of the retroperitoneal and the transabdominal routes in 326 operations on 284 patients. Jpn J Clin Oncol. 2000;30(2):68–74.
21. Nigri G, Rosman AS, Petrucciani N, Fancellu A, Pisano M, Zorcolo L, Ramacciato G, Melis M. Meta-analysis of trials comparing laparoscopic transperitoneal and retroperitoneal adrenalectomy. Surgery. 2013;153(1):111–9.
22. Wagner SM, Zhu S, Nicolescu AC, Mulligan LM. Molecular mechanisms of RET receptor-mediated oncogenesis in multiple endocrine neoplasia 2. Clinics. 2012;67(1):77–84.

John H. Sipple

1930–

Sonia L. Sugg

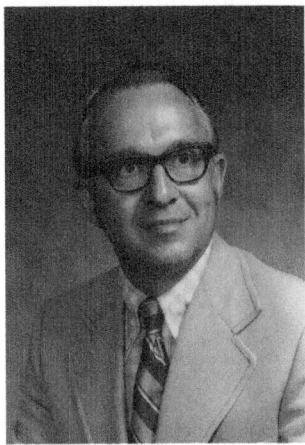

John H. Sipple, MD in 1976, president of Couse Irving Memorial medical staff

Introduction

Multiple endocrine neoplasia type 2A (Sipple syndrome) was first described by John H. Sipple in 1961 [1]. It may be surprising to some that he was not an endocrinologist, pathologist, or surgeon, but a pulmonologist. He encountered the index patient as a third-year medical resident, established an association between thyroid cancer and pheochromocytoma through meticulous research into the literature, and published a case report identifying a syndrome named after him.

Editors' Note: Much of the source material for this excellent chapter came from direct interviews that Dr. Sugg held with Dr. Sipple himself.

S. L. Sugg (✉)
Department of Surgery, Division of Surgical Oncology and Endocrine Surgery, University of Iowa Carver College of Medicine, Iowa City, IA, USA
e-mail: sonia-sugg@uiowa.edu

Childhood

John Harrison Sipple was born on July 1, 1930, in Cleveland, OH, and grew up in Lakewood, a suburb of Cleveland. His grandparents immigrated to the USA from Germany. His father John was a banker and lawyer, and his mother Marie was a homemaker. He had an older brother Richard. Sipple attended Lakewood High School, graduating as class valedictorian. In high school, he sustained a football injury and was treated with a full-body cast for 6 weeks. This experience as a patient sparked his interest in medicine as a career. He applied and was accepted to Northwestern, Colgate, and Cornell Universities. He chose to attend Cornell because he was offered a full scholarship for 4 years.

Education, Training, and Professional Career

At Cornell University, Sipple was a zoology major, and participated in football, lacrosse, and the men's Glee club. At the time, it was possible at Cornell to combine the last year of college and the first year of medical school, thereby obtaining both Bachelor's and M.D. degrees in 7 years. This allowed Sipple to have his first year of medical school supported by his undergraduate scholarship, and he therefore decided to continue his studies at Cornell University Medical College.

During medical school, Sipple was especially interested in internal medicine. The required diagnostic acumen was particularly appealing. He cites Dr. David P. Barr (1897–1977), professor and chairman of the Department of Medicine at The New York Hospital–Cornell Medical Center as a role model. He vividly recalled being impressed by an interesting patient brought in for demonstration to the class by Dr. Barr. This patient had thyrotoxicosis with classical findings of Graves' disease. He matched into a rotating internship at the State University of New York Medical Center (SUNY) in Syracuse in 1955. He was very pleased with his internship and the Department of Medicine at Syracuse and so opted to

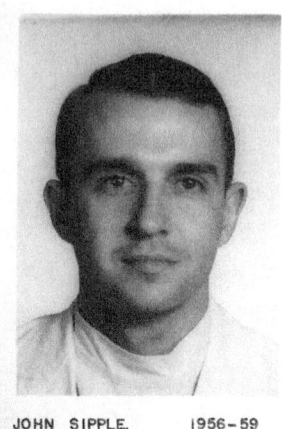

JOHN SIPPLE.   1956-59

Fig. 1 John H. Sipple, M.D. in 1956, SUNY Syracuse

take his residency in internal medicine in Syracuse, completing it in 1959 (Fig. 1). Sipple recalls, "The residency was excellent. It stressed learning, responsibility, teaching, and research in the teaching hospital, community hospitals, and a veterans' hospital. We were on call every other night early on and maybe one of five by the third year. The main emphasis was on being competent as a diagnostician and consultant in internal medicine but also developing skills (clinical and research) in a subspecialty was encouraged." His experiences during residency profoundly influenced his professional life: (1) though he was interested in all the subspecialties, he was presented with opportunities to work in the pulmonary laboratory in his spare time and he worked well with the pulmonologists; (2) he met the two men who would become his future partners; and (3) it was during his third year in residency that he encountered and decided to describe the patient in a manuscript entitled "The Association of Pheochromocytoma with Carcinoma of the Thyroid Gland" [1].

Having deferred his military obligation during medical school and residency, Sipple served in the US Air Force from 1959 to 1961 as chief of medicine at the 2845th USAF Hospital at Griffiss AFB in Rome, New York. This was between the Korean and Vietnam wars. At the conclusion of his military service, he accepted a 2-year National Institutes of Health (NIH)-sponsored pulmonary fellowship at Johns Hopkins Hospital, under Dr. Richard L. Riley (1911–2001), the prominent pulmonary physiologist and leader in pulmonary medicine. He was highly productive as a resident and fellow, publishing six papers on respiratory physiology and pulmonary topics. One year into the fellowship, he was offered a position as a pulmonary specialist by the two cardiologists that he had met as a resident in Syracuse, and whom he greatly respected. Faced with this choice, Sipple felt that he would derive greater satisfaction from practicing clinical medicine rather than continuing to perform research. He therefore joined the physician group Internist Associates of

Central New York and began practicing internal medicine in 1962. In addition to establishing a thriving practice, he became a prominent member of the medical community in Syracuse. He developed an interest in the electronic medical record in the 1980s and designed his own system for the office. He held a number of important administrative and committee positions at Crouse Irving Memorial Hospital as well as at the University Hospital. He was active in the medical school. He was attending physician for one of the medical teams and made teaching and work rounds with the team 3 months each year. In addition, he made intensive care unit (ICU) pulmonary rounds with house staff, students, and respiratory therapists throughout the year. He also taught physical diagnosis to medical students yearly. He rose up the ladder of appointments and became a full clinical professor of medicine in 1977 at SUNY Syracuse. He was active in the Upstate New York Region of the American College of Physicians, serving as governor from 1989 to 1993. He became president of his practice group Internist Associates of Central New York from 1995 until his retirement in 2000 at age 70.

Family

Sipple married in 1955, the year he graduated from medical school. He met his wife Joy in Ohio, having attended the same high school though he graduated several years before her. She attended Kent State University, and majored in liberal arts (Fig. 2). She is an artist and avid gardener. Sipple states, "We have a great marriage. We work together to have a warm home environment and she took much of the responsibility for our home and children." They had six children, four boys and two girls and 18 grandchildren. One son, Michael Sipple, followed in his father's footsteps and became a practicing gastroenterologist in Syracuse, New York.

Description of Sipple Syndrome

In 1959, during his last year in residency, Sipple was consulted on a patient who was hypertensive after neurosurgery for an arteriovenous malformation (AVM) of the brain. The patient was a 33-year-old man, from a community near Syracuse, and had a wife and several young children. He presented to the Syracuse Veterans Administration Hospital after an onset of a severe headache, nausea, and vomiting, followed by left-sided weakness and lethargy. A lumbar puncture revealed bloody spinal fluid and elevated pressure. A large AVM was seen on a right carotid angiogram. A craniotomy was done to evacuate the hematoma. Postoperatively he developed fever, restlessness, and fluctuating blood pressure, as high as 240/120. Seventeen days later, he underwent a second craniotomy to relieve elevated intracranial pressure,

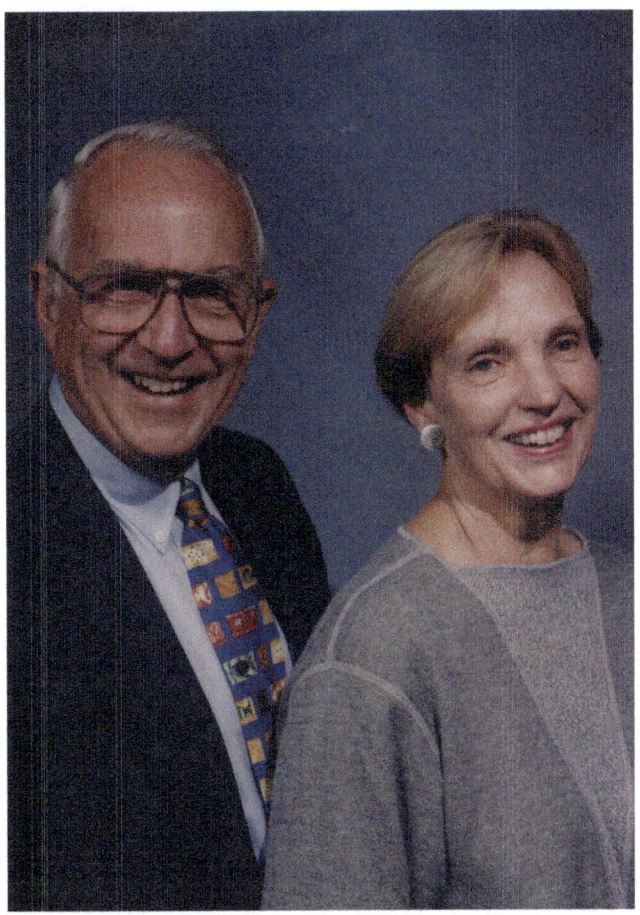

Fig. 2 John H. Sipple M.D. in 1988, at his 50th high school reunion, with his wife Joy

another hematoma was evacuated, but the patient died 3 h later. A family history could not be obtained at the time of his hospitalization. Subsequently, a detailed family pedigree was obtained [2].

Sipple became intensely interested in this case after observing the striking findings at the patient's autopsy. He states, "As I stood at the autopsy table, I knew I was looking at something special although I did not understand it. I doubted very much that it was a chance occurrence." [2] The patient was found to have large adrenal tumors bilaterally, a 2-cm "pale tan mass" in the mid-portion of each thyroid lobe, and nodular enlargement of the single parathyroid gland measuring 0.9 by 0.6 cm was identified. The adrenal glands weighed 58 and 68 g and were diagnosed as pheochromocytoma by histology. Furthermore, Myron Brin, a biochemist at Syracuse, was able to measure elevated tissue epinephrine and norepinephrine levels from the adrenal tumors. The thyroid tumors were noted to be poorly differentiated and invasive, and diagnosed as follicular adenocarcinoma of the thyroid on the pathology report. Medullary carcinoma of the thyroid gland (MTC) was just described in 1959 by Hazard, Hawk, and **Crile** [3] from the Cleveland Clinic, and therefore the patient's thyroid cancer was not recognized as such at the

time. Subsequent pathologic analysis by Schimke confirmed the tumor from this patient to be medullary carcinoma [4] and **Carney** showed that it stained positive for calcitonin [5]. There were no serum calcium or phosphorus levels ordered. Since Sipple could not find any existing literature showing association of thyroid, adrenal, and parathyroid tumors, he decided that this case deserved investigation and description.

Sipple began his research into this case during residency, finishing and publishing the paper in 1961 during his Air Force service. His methodology consisted of looking up all the published cases of pheochromocytoma, specifically looking for additional cases with concomitant thyroid carcinomas. After reviewing 20 years of Index Medicus, he found 537 cases of pheochromocytoma and of those, five (in addition to his case) were associated with thyroid carcinomas. Sipple noted that the occurrence of thyroid cancer in this series of patients with pheochromocytomas was at least 14 times the expected incidence, whereas the incidence of other cancers was not increased. He hypothesized that the thyroid cancer may have been caused by fluctuating levels of epinephrine. Among the cases he reported, the earliest dated back to 1932. Four of the six cases had bilateral pheochromocytomas confirmed at autopsy, the average age of presentation in this series was 34.5 years (range 17–63), the average age at death was 39.2 years (range 24–63). He wrote up his observations and research as the only author, and the three-page case report was accepted for publication without revisions to the *American Journal of Medicine* (AKA the Green Journal) in 1961 [1]. Sipple noted that he received many reprint requests for this article, indicating that there was a high level of interest from the medical community. In 1962, Cushman from Rochester, New York, reported a family in which the father had pheochromocytoma, MCT, and parathyroid adenoma, the son had pheochromocytoma and MCT, and the granddaughter had MCT, and it became apparent this syndrome was genetically inherited in an autosomal dominant fashion [6]. Other cases were reported [7], and the combination of pheochromocytoma and thyroid cancer became known as Sipple syndrome [5]. After the MEN2A mutation was identified in 1993 [8], the proband's family was studied [9], and 7 of 15 members who underwent genetic testing were found to have the C634R mutation of RET. It was proposed that the proband's mother had the disease, since she died at age 39 of unknown causes and was thought to have hypertension. Further research by Carney into the cases described by Sipple found that one patient had a sister who died at age 28 with a "rare disorder of the sympathetic system" and a thyroidectomy. No other patient had parathyroid disease described. Carney also identified that another of the patients included by Sipple likely had MEN 2B, having ganglioneuromatosis of the gut and enlarged lips [5]. In 1968, the term "multiple endocrine neoplasia" (MEN) was introduced by Steiner et al. to describe diseases with multiple endocrine tumors, and Sipple syndrome was designated as MEN 2. In 1974, Sizemore et al. further classified Sipple syndrome as MEN 2A, recognizing its distinction from MEN 2B [5]. Dr. Sipple kept up with work on this disease for many years, corresponding with Barry D. Nelkin, Ph.D. of Johns Hopkins, and Carl D. Malchoff, M.D. of the University of Connecticut over various projects. At the First International Workshop on MEN 2 in Ontario, Dr. Sipple gave a historical perspective [2] on his discovery of the syndrome and stated that "this workshop on MEN-2 illustrates that observations in one case can lead to the contributions of many workers in the field."

It is interesting to note that subsequent reports have demonstrated Sipple syndrome to be present in patients described earlier in the literature, though not recognized as a syndrome. Neumann et al. [10] reported that the first case of pheochromocytoma described in the literature in 1886 by Frankel had MEN 2A. The authors hypothesized that since the patient was young (18 years old) and had bilateral disease, she had an inherited condition. The relatives of the patient were traced through historical research, and the germ-line RET mutation TGC>TGG (Cys634Trp) was found in four descendants. Sisson et al. [11] reported that investigation of the subsequent medical and family history of a proband who was initially reported in 1939 for a hyperfunctioning parathyroid adenoma revealed MEN 2A. The patient was reported by Barker and Brines [12] as an 18-year-old with osteitis fibrosa cystica who had a parathyroid tumor excised. Further investigation revealed that she underwent a thyroidectomy for probable MTC at age 29 and subsequently died of "progressive cancer" at age 70. Her children developed MTC, pheochromocytomas, and parathyroid hyperplasia. Genetic testing of her descendants revealed the RET 634 TGC>CGC mutation.

This biography of Sipple shows that a young physician's keen sense of observation and curiosity combined with persistence in researching the literature resulted in identifying a previously unrecognized syndrome. It also illustrates the rapid medical progress over a single physician's four-decade career; from the description of an interesting case, to definition of the syndrome and its pathology, to the identification of calcitonin as a tumor marker for MTC, to identification of the genetic mutations in MEN 2A. With the ability to diagnose affected patients before cancer develops and with the use of prophylactic surgery, the lives of MEN 2A patients are improved and extended as a result of this progress.

Quotations

Sipple's inquisitiveness paid off.
(J. Aidan Carney, pathologist of Carney's syndrome)

Eponyms are flattering, sometimes embarrassing, and certainly not descriptive.... The paper I wrote in 1959 was my only venture into endocrinology.... So much outstanding work has been done by so many investigators in this field, and my contribution was so minimal, that remembering the name MEN-2 is more meaningful to a medical student than remembering an eponym. (John H. Sipple)

Reflections

How do you feel about having a syndrome named after you?

I got a lot of mileage out of a little case report. I don't think any of my grandchildren would consider me famous for a case report. I don't build it up. At the medical school, they were sure to teach about Sipple syndrome, and point me out as an example of "local man makes good".

How would you like to be remembered?

As somebody who was interested in seeing what they could do with their life, plugged along, had some breaks, and had a lot of fun.

References

1. Sipple JH. The association of pheochromocytoma with carcinoma of the thyroid gland. Am J Med. 1961;31:163–6.
2. Sipple JH. Multiple endocrine neoplasia type 2 syndromes: historical perspectives. Henry Ford Hospital Med J. 1984;32(4):219–21.
3. Hazard JB, Hawk WA, Crile G Jr. Medullary (solid) carcinoma of the thyroid; a clinicopathologic entity. J Clin Endocrinol Metab. 1959;19(1):152–61.
4. Schimke RN, et al. Syndrome of bilateral pheochromocytoma, medullary thyroid carcinoma and multiple neuromas. A possible regulatory defect in the differentiation of chromaffin tissue. New Engl J Med. 1968;279(1):1–7.
5. Carney JA. Familial multiple endocrine neoplasia: the first 100 years. Am J Surg Pathol. 2005;29(2):254–74.
6. Cushman P, Jr. Familial endocrine tumors; report of two unrelated kindred affected with pheochromocytomas, one also with multiple thyroid carcinomas. Am J Med. 1962;32:352–60.
7. Manning PCJ, et al. Pheochromocytoma, hyperparathyroidism and thyroid carcinoma occurring coincidentally. Report of a case. New Engl J Med. 1963;168:68–72.
8. Mulligan LM, et al. Germ-line mutations of the RET proto-oncogene in multiple endocrine neoplasia type 2A. Nature. 1993;363(6428):458–60.
9. Hughes JM, et al. The Sipple syndrome: from clinical description to genetic analysis in the index family. Endocrinologist. 1996;6(6):427–30.
10. Neumann HP, et al. Evidence of MEN-2 in the original description of classic pheochromocytoma. New Engl J Med. 2007;357(13):1311–5.
11. Sisson JC, et al. First description of parathyroid disease in multiple endocrine neoplasia 2A syndrome. Endocr Pathol. 2008;19(4):289–93.
12. Barker VL, Brines OA. Hyperfunctioning adenoma of an ectopic parathyroid gland. Arch Surg. 1939;39:205–13.

Index

Printed by Printforce, the Netherlands